Recent Developments in Skeletal Muscle Physiology

Recent Developments in Skeletal Muscle Physiology

Editor: Jean Turner

AMERICAN
MEDICAL PUBLISHERS
www.americanmedicalpublishers.com

AMERICAN
MEDICAL PUBLISHERS
www.americanmedicalpublishers.com

Cataloging-in-Publication Data

Recent developments in skeletal muscle physiology / edited by Jean Turner.
p. cm.
Includes bibliographical references and index.
ISBN 979-8-88740-422-6
1. Musculoskeletal system--Physiology. 2. Muscles--Physiology. 3. Musculoskeletal system--Anatomy.
4. Muscles--Anatomy. I. Turner, Jean.
QP301 .R43 2023
612.044--dc23

American Medical Publishers,
41 Flatbush Avenue,
1st Floor, New York,
NY 11217, USA

ISBN 979-8-88740-422-6 (Hardback)

Contents

Preface ... VII

Chapter 1 **The effects of obesity on skeletal muscle regeneration** ... 1
Dmitry Akhmedov and Rebecca Berdeaux

Chapter 2 **New roles for old enzymes: Killer caspases as the engine of cell behavior changes** ... 13
Patrick F. Connolly, Richard Jäger and Howard O. Fearnhead

Chapter 3 **Novel excitation-contraction coupling related genes reveal aspects of muscle weakness beyond atrophy—New hopes for treatment of musculoskeletal diseases** ... 23
Heather Manring, Eduardo Abreu, Leticia Brotto, Noah Weisleder and Marco Brotto

Chapter 4 **Nuclear positioning in muscle development and disease** ... 35
Eric S. Folker and Mary K. Baylies

Chapter 5 **Skeletal muscle as a regulator of the longevity protein, Klotho** ... 45
Keith G. Avin, Paul M. Coen, Wan Huang, Donna B. Stolz, Gwendolyn A. Sowa, John J. Dubé, Bret H. Goodpaster, Robert M. O'Doherty and Fabrisia Ambrosio

Chapter 6 **Skeletal muscle heat shock protein 70: Diverse functions and therapeutic potential for wasting disorders** ... 54
Sarah M. Senf

Chapter 7 **Emerging gene editing strategies for Duchenne muscular dystrophy targeting stem cells** ... 59
Carmen Bertoni

Chapter 8 **Structural alterations of skeletal muscle in COPD** ... 76
Sunita Mathur, Dina Brooks and Celso R. F. Carvalho

Chapter 9 **Advancements in stem cells treatment of skeletal muscle wasting** ... 84
Mirella Meregalli, Andrea Farini, Clementina Sitzia and Yvan Torrente

Chapter 10 **Skeletal muscle wasting with disuse atrophy is multi-dimensional: The response and interaction of myonuclei, satellite cells and signaling pathways** ... 96
Naomi E. Brooks and Kathryn H. Myburgh

Chapter 11 **Diabetic myopathy: Impact of diabetes mellitus on skeletal muscle progenitor cells** ... 110
Donna M. D'Souza, Dhuha Al- Sajee and Thomas J. Hawke

Chapter 12 **Isolation, characterization and molecular regulation of muscle stem cells** ... 117
So-ichiro Fukada, Yuran Ma, Takuji Ohtani, Yoko Watanabe, Satoshi Murakami and Masahiko Yamaguchi

Chapter 13 **Muscle hypertrophy is associated with increases in proteasome activity that is independent of MuRF1 and MAFbx expression** 133
Leslie M. Baehr, Matthew Tunzi and Sue C. Bodine

Chapter 14 **More than a bystander: The contributions of intrinsic skeletal muscle defects in motor neuron diseases** 141
Justin G. Boyer, Andrew Ferrier and Rashmi Kothary

Chapter 15 **Docosahexaenoyl ethanolamide improves glucose uptake and alters endocannabinoid system gene expression in proliferating and differentiating C2C12 myoblasts** 154
Jeffrey Kim, Morgan E. Carlson and Bruce A. Watkins

Chapter 16 **Roles of nonmyogenic mesenchymal progenitors in pathogenesis and regeneration of skeletal muscle** 168
Akiyoshi Uezumi, Madoka Ikemoto-Uezumi and Kunihiro Tsuchida

Chapter 17 **Molecular and cell-based therapies for muscle degenerations: A road under construction** 179
Emanuele Berardi, Daniela Annibali, Marco Cassano, Stefania Crippa and Maurilio Sampaolesi

Chapter 18 **CD13 promotes mesenchymal stem cell-mediated regeneration of ischemic muscle** 192
M. Mamunur Rahman, Jaganathan Subramani, Mallika Ghosh, Jiyeon K. Denninger, Kotaro Takeda, Guo-Hua Fong, Morgan E. Carlson and Linda H. Shapiro

Chapter 19 **Sphingosine 1-phosphate axis: A new leader actor in skeletal muscle biology** 204
Chiara Donati, Francesca Cencetti and Paola Bruni

Chapter 20 **A metabolic link to skeletal muscle wasting and regeneration** 214
René Koopman, C. Hai Ly and James G. Ryall

Permissions

List of Contributors

Index

Preface

This book aims to highlight the current researches and provides a platform to further the scope of innovations in this area. This book is a product of the combined efforts of many researchers and scientists, after going through thorough studies and analysis from different parts of the world. The objective of this book is to provide the readers with the latest information of the field.

Skeletal muscles are organs of the vertebrate muscular system that are commonly connected to bones of the skeleton by tendons. They are present throughout the body and respond to stimuli by contracting. They are also found in the eye socket, tongue, upper esophagus and diaphragm. Skeletal muscles have a variety of functions, such as maintaining the position and posture of the body, nutrient storage, generating movement, joint stabilization, and regulating body temperature. These muscles comprise muscle and nerve fibers, connective tissue and blood vessels, which allow humans to move and carry out daily tasks. Additionally, they are also critical for breathing mechanics. The dysfunction in skeletal muscles can cause a variety of medical diseases ranging from dysphagia to tremors, myopathies, weakness, tendon ruptures, ataxia, etc. This book explores the recent studies on skeletal muscle physiology. It will serve as a reference to a broad spectrum of readers.

I would like to express my sincere thanks to the authors for their dedicated efforts in the completion of this book. I acknowledge the efforts of the publisher for providing constant support. Lastly, I would like to thank my family for their support in all academic endeavors.

Editor

1

The effects of obesity on skeletal muscle regeneration

_Dmitry Akhmedov and Rebecca Berdeaux_*

Department of Integrative Biology and Pharmacology and Graduate School of Biomedical Sciences, University of Texas Health Science Center at Houston, Houston, TX, USA

***Correspondence:**
Rebecca Berdeaux, Department of Integrative Biology and Pharmacology and Graduate School of Biomedical Sciences, University of Texas Health Science Center at Houston, 6431 Fannin St., MSE R366, Houston, TX 77030, USA
e-mail:
rebecca.berdeaux@uth.tmc.edu

Obesity and metabolic disorders such as type 2 diabetes mellitus are accompanied by increased lipid deposition in adipose and non-adipose tissues including liver, pancreas, heart and skeletal muscle. Recent publications report impaired regenerative capacity of skeletal muscle following injury in obese mice. Although muscle regeneration has not been thoroughly studied in obese and type 2 diabetic humans and mechanisms leading to decreased muscle regeneration in obesity remain elusive, the initial findings point to the possibility that muscle satellite cell function is compromised under conditions of lipid overload. Elevated toxic lipid metabolites and increased pro-inflammatory cytokines as well as insulin and leptin resistance that occur in obese animals may contribute to decreased regenerative capacity of skeletal muscle. In addition, obesity-associated alterations in the metabolic state of skeletal muscle fibers and satellite cells may directly impair the potential for satellite cell-mediated repair. Here we discuss recent studies that expand our understanding of how obesity negatively impacts skeletal muscle maintenance and regeneration.

Keywords: obesity, type 2 diabetes, lipids, skeletal muscle, muscle regeneration, satellite cells, leptin, lipotoxicity

Obesity and associated disorders are quickly reaching a global epidemic scale. Over 500 million people worldwide are overweight or obese (World Health Organization, 2013). Obesity is highly associated with development of metabolic syndrome, type 2 diabetes, non-alcoholic fatty liver disease (NAFLD) and cardiovascular disorders (Kahn et al., 2006; Lavie et al., 2009; Samuel and Shulman, 2012). In obese individuals, lipids excessively accumulate in adipose tissues and ectopically accumulate in non-adipose tissues including skeletal muscle (Unger et al., 2010). Lipids in skeletal muscle have been extensively studied in the context of insulin sensitivity. However, lipid overload in muscle appears to affect not only insulin signaling, but also muscle maintenance and regeneration. The underlying mechanisms are not fully understood, but recent experimental data suggest that multiple factors such as accumulation of toxic lipid metabolites and low-grade inflammation result in impaired muscle regeneration under conditions of obesity. The impact of obesity on skeletal muscle maintenance and physiology has been addressed in rodent models of obesity, including leptin-deficient $Lep^{ob/ob}$ mice (commonly termed "*ob/ob*"), leptin receptor-deficient $Lepr^{db/db}$ mice (termed "*db/db*") and obese Zucker rats (which also have a leptin receptor mutation) (Kurtz et al., 1989; Tschop and Heiman, 2001), as well as in mice and rats fed a high-fat diet. All of these animals have increased whole body lipid content and develop hyperglycemia and insulin resistance, a phenotype similar to type 2 diabetes (reviewed in Unger, 2003).

Here we will discuss the sources of lipids that directly affect skeletal muscle, review studies investigating muscle regeneration in obesity models, and discuss possible mechanisms underlying impaired regenerative capacity of skeletal muscle in obese animals (summarized in **Figure 1**).

OBESITY AND SKELETAL MUSCLE LIPID ACCUMULATION

Obesity is characterized by elevated adipose storage in subcutaneous and visceral adipose depots and non-adipose organs, a phenomenon called ectopic lipid accumulation (Van Herpen and Schrauwen-Hinderling, 2008). In addition, obese individuals have increased circulating fatty acids (Boden and Shulman, 2002; Mittendorfer et al., 2009) and high ectopic lipid deposition in skeletal muscle partially resulting from increased fatty acid uptake from the circulation (Goodpaster et al., 2000b; Sinha et al., 2002; Bonen et al., 2004; reviewed in Goodpaster and Wolf, 2004). Lipids within skeletal muscle are comprised of two pools: extramyocellular lipids (EMCL) localized in adipose cells between myofibers and intramyocellular lipids (IMCL) located within muscle cells (Sinha et al., 2002; Boesch et al., 2006). A portion of EMCL comprises adipose tissue closely associated with the muscle, referred to as intermuscular adipose tissue (IMAT) (Goodpaster et al., 2000a). Although IMAT accumulation in obese patients is positively correlated with insulin resistance and reduced muscle performance (Goodpaster et al., 2000a; Hilton et al., 2008), this adipose depot does not appear to affect muscle mass (Lee et al., 2012a), and its effects on muscle regeneration have not been addressed. IMCL are comprised of neutral lipids triacylglycerols (TAG) and cholesterol esters, mainly localized to lipid droplets (reviewed in Fujimoto et al., 2008; Thiele and Spandl, 2008) as well as lipid metabolites, such as long-chain acyl CoAs, diacylglycerols and ceramides. Elevated TAG content and increased numbers of lipid droplets have been observed in muscle biopsies from obese people (Simoneau et al., 1995; Malenfant et al., 2001). Genetically obese mice (*ob/ob* and *db/db*) and obese Zucker rats also have increased IMCL (Kuhlmann et al., 2003; Unger, 2003; Fissoune et al., 2009; Ye et al., 2011). Long-chain

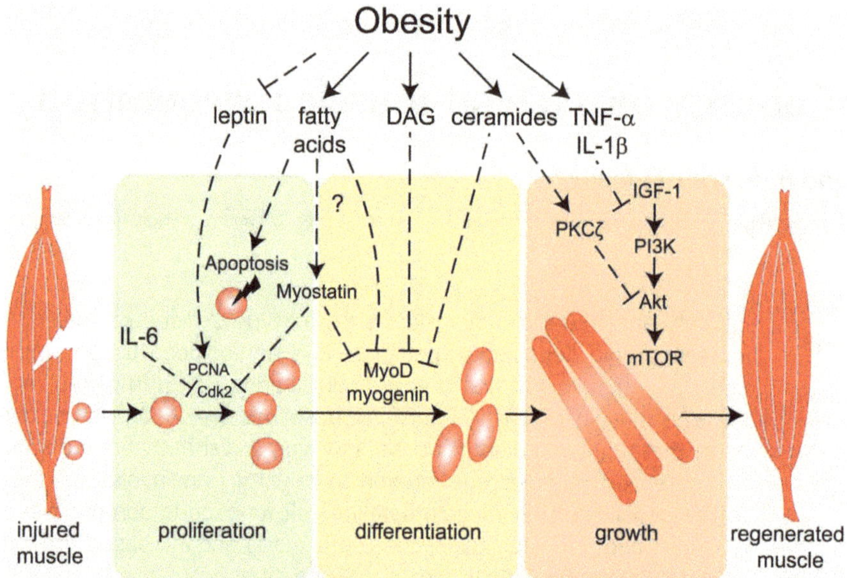

FIGURE 1 | Major mechanisms linking obesity with impaired muscle regeneration. Obesity is associated with insulin and leptin resistance, elevated circulating and intramuscular fatty acids, diacylglycerols, ceramides and pro-inflammatory cytokines. Following muscle injury, satellite cells (depicted adjacent to muscle on left) are activated, proliferate, differentiate and form myofibers that grow and replace damaged tissue. Impairment of these processes underlies inefficient muscle regeneration in obese rodents. Defective leptin signaling can contribute to decreased satellite cell proliferation and impaired muscle hypertrophy, but the molecular mechanisms are not known. Fatty acids, diacylglycerols (DAG) and ceramides induce apoptosis and decrease myoblast proliferation and differentiation, possibly via activation of myostatin and inhibition of MyoD and myogenin expression and/or activity. Ceramides and pro-inflammatory cytokines inhibit muscle growth in part by inhibiting the IGF-1/Akt /mTOR pathway.

acyl CoAs, diacylglycerols and ceramides accumulate in skeletal muscles of obese humans, *ob/ob* and *db/db* mice and obese Zucker rats (Turinsky et al., 1990; Hulver et al., 2003; Adams et al., 2004; Holland et al., 2007; Magnusson et al., 2008; Lee et al., 2013; Turner et al., 2013) and negatively affect cell signaling and metabolism; the defects are collectively referred to as lipotoxicity (Lelliott and Vidal-Puig, 2004; Kusminski et al., 2009). In skeletal muscle, lipotoxic species interfere with insulin signaling and are thought to be partly responsible for insulin resistance in obesity (reviewed in Timmers et al., 2008; Bosma et al., 2012; Coen and Goodpaster, 2012). However, it remains largely unknown what other physiologic processes are impaired by these lipid metabolites in skeletal muscle. In the following sections we will focus on recent findings on how obesity, and in some cases lipids, impair muscle progenitor cell function and muscle regeneration and regrowth.

EFFECTS OF OBESITY ON MUSCLE PROGENITOR CELLS

Insulin resistance and mitochondrial and metabolic dysfunction are perhaps the most prominent muscle abnormalities that negatively impact whole body metabolism and physical performance in states of obesity and type 2 diabetes. Skeletal muscle maintenance depends on ongoing repair, regeneration and growth, all of which decline during aging (reviewed in Jang et al., 2011). Obesity rates increase with aging, which is also accompanied by reduced regenerative capacity and muscle strength. Thus, as average life span increases, it is of growing clinical importance to understand whether obesity impacts muscle maintenance and regeneration and to identify mechanisms that may be targeted for therapeutic benefit.

Skeletal muscle regeneration after injury requires the activity of muscle stem cells and satellite cells, which remain associated with skeletal myofibers after development (reviewed in Wang and Rudnicki, 2012). Muscle regeneration is commonly experimentally induced by intramuscular injection of a myotoxic agent, such as cardiotoxin, notexin or barium chloride. Freeze-induced injury is an alternative model of muscle injury entailing application of steel cooled to the temperature of dry ice to the muscle (Warren et al., 2007). In normal animals, these injuries cause local myofiber necrosis and inflammation, followed by satellite cell activation, proliferation, differentiation, fusion and ultimately regrowth of myofibers to approximately the same size as the original within about three weeks (**Figure 1** and Charge and Rudnicki, 2004). Satellite cells are required for regenerative myogenesis (Lepper et al., 2011; Gunther et al., 2013). Currently there is a controversy regarding requirement of satellite cells for skeletal muscle hypertrophy. Load-induced hypertrophy in humans and rodents is accompanied by satellite cell activation, proliferation and fusion with existing myofibers (Rosenblatt et al., 1994; Kadi et al., 2004; Petrella et al., 2008; Bruusgaard et al., 2010). However, genetic ablation studies in mice demonstrated that satellite cells do not appear to be required for hypertrophy induced by mechanical overload (McCarthy et al., 2011; Jackson et al., 2012; Lee et al., 2012b). Although efficient hypertrophy in rodents does not strictly require satellite cell fusion to myofibers, nuclear accretion due to satellite cell fusion is thought to promote hypertrophy by supporting the growing cytoplasm. In addition, muscle regenerative capacity declines with aging, and this is thought to be due in part to reduced satellite cell function (reviewed in Jang et al., 2011). Thus, although it is still not settled to what extent this specific progenitor population is required for maintenance of adult muscle, it is clear that identification of therapeutic targets to stimulate and maintain activity of these cells has potential to improve metabolism and strength in aging and obese humans. Recent data indicate that skeletal muscle regeneration is significantly impaired in models of diabetes and obesity, possibly due to impaired muscle progenitor cell function.

LIPOTOXICITY IN MYOBLASTS

Several groups have modeled lipid overload by incubating cultured muscle cells with fatty acids or lipid metabolites. During differentiation of L6 myoblasts, exogenous ceramides markedly reduce expression of the myogenic transcription factor myogenin, likely via inhibition of phospholipase D, while inhibitors of ceramide synthesis potentiate myogenin expression and accelerate myotube formation (Mebarek et al., 2007). In addition, several studies showed that increasing ceramide pools either by palmitate loading or silencing of stearoyl-CoA desaturase 1 (SCD1), which normally desaturates fatty acids and reduces the pool of saturated fatty acids that are converted to ceramides, results in increased apoptosis in differentiated L6 and C2C12 muscle cells (Turpin et al., 2006; Rachek et al., 2007; Peterson et al., 2008b; Henique et al., 2010; Yuzefovych et al., 2010). These findings suggest that the elevated fatty acids in obesity could directly harm the muscle fibers and satellite cells.

To test the effect of intracellular free fatty acid accumulation on myoblast viability and myogenesis, Tamilarasan, et al. used C2C12 cells stably transfected with human lipoprotein lipase (LPL), which converts TAGs to free fatty acids and glycerol (Tamilarasan et al., 2012). In spite of an approximately tenfold increase in intracellular free fatty acids and TAGs, cell viability and proliferation were similar to control cells. However, LPL-expressing cells showed defective differentiation accompanied by markedly decreased expression of *MyoD*, *myogenin*, and myosin heavy chain as well as a reduced number of myotubes (Tamilarasan et al., 2012). In mice, acute triglyceride infusion resulted in increased plasma free fatty acid and diacylglycerol levels and increased caspase-3 activity in gastrocnemius muscle (Turpin et al., 2009). However, in the same study, *ob/ob* mice and mice fed high-fat diet for 12 weeks did not show increased apoptosis, autophagy or proteolysis in muscle despite elevated plasma free fatty acids, muscle diacylglycerols and ceramides (Turpin et al., 2009). In contrast with this result, another group observed increased caspase-3 activation in gastrocnemius muscle in mice after 16 weeks of high-fat diet feeding (Bonnard et al., 2008), probably secondary to elevated reactive oxygen species (ROS), oxidative stress and mitochondrial dysfunction. Because cell viability and apoptosis were not directly assessed in this study, it is difficult to conclude if caspase-3 activation was accompanied by increased apoptosis (Bonnard et al., 2008). It is possible that pro-apoptotic effects of caspase-3 in muscle from obese animals are counteracted by increased expression of pro-survival Bcl2 and transcriptional downregulation of other pro-apoptotic genes, such as *caspase8*, *caspase14*, *Fadd*, and multiple genes involved in TNF-α signaling (Turpin et al., 2009). Therefore, although fatty acids and ceramides induce apoptosis in muscle cells *in vitro*, it appears that elevated lipid metabolites do not impair muscle cell viability *in vivo*. *In vitro* studies have raised the interesting possibility that fatty acids and possibly other lipid metabolites interfere with the myogenic differentiation program, suggesting that perhaps differentiation during muscle regeneration would be impaired in obese animals.

MUSCLE REGENERATION IN OBESITY MODELS

Several recent studies have employed myotoxins and freeze injury to evaluate muscle regeneration in obese or diabetic mice. In mice fed high-fat diet for 8 months, Hu, et al. observed reduced tibialis anterior (TA) muscle mass after cardiotoxin injury, associated with smaller myofibers, larger interstitial spaces and increased collagen deposition compared with lean mice (Hu et al., 2010). Similarly, a short period of high-fat diet (3 weeks) in young mice (aged 3–6 weeks) resulted in reduced numbers of satellite cells and impaired regeneration of TA muscle after cold-induced injury (Woo et al., 2011). A similar effect on satellite cell number and regeneration was observed in young mice with prenatal malnutrition, which also results in elevated adiposity (Woo et al., 2011). Although proliferation rates were not directly assessed in this study, the data collectively suggest that high adiposity depresses proliferative capacity of satellite cells either due to intrinsic metabolic properties of the muscle or satellite cells or alterations of circulating metabolites after high-fat feeding. However, in other studies, intermediate durations (12 weeks) of high fat feeding did not markedly impair the size of regenerating fibers of extensor digitorum longus (EDL) muscle after cardiotoxin injury (Nguyen et al., 2011). Collagen deposition was not evaluated, but there do appear to be larger interstitial spaces in histological sections of regenerating muscle from the 12 week high-fat diet-fed animals (Nguyen et al., 2011) consistent with the findings of Hu et al. (2010). It is notable when comparing these studies that Hu, et al. and Woo, et al. evaluated regeneration of TA muscle while Nguyen, et al. analyzed EDL muscle. While both muscle groups are comprised of predominantly fast-twitch IIB/X fiber types, TA contains a larger proportion of oxidative type IIA fibers (Bloemberg and Quadrilatero, 2012). The choice of muscle group is an important consideration, as slow twitch muscles contain higher numbers of satellite cells per fiber (Gibson and Schultz, 1983). Thus, effects of high-fat diet feeding on different functional aspects of muscle regeneration may depend on the muscle studied and the type of analysis performed. Ultimate conclusions will depend on additional analyses of multiple parameters of muscle regeneration in high-fat diet fed animals, including careful analysis of proliferation, muscle progenitor number, as well as resolution of inflammation, fibrosis and fiber caliber during regrowth.

Effects of lipid overload on skeletal muscle regeneration have specifically been assessed in transgenic mice overexpressing LPL in skeletal muscle (Levak-Frank et al., 1995; Tamilarasan et al., 2012). Overexpression of LPL in muscle results in an approximately eightfold increase in LPL activity, increased free fatty acid uptake and three- to fourfold increases in free fatty acid and TAG concentrations in gastrocnemius muscle. By two months of age, transgenic mice develop severe myopathy, which is detected histologically as regenerating myofibers with centrally localized nuclei, in addition to perturbed sarcomere structure, excessive glycogen storage, increased protein degradation and apoptotic nuclei (Levak-Frank et al., 1995; Tamilarasan et al., 2012). Ten days after cardiotoxin injury, myofiber cross-sectional area in LPL-transgenic mice is reduced compared to wild-type mice, indicating that intracellular lipid accumulation impairs muscle regeneration (Tamilarasan et al., 2012), either directly or indirectly. The defect in regeneration might result from reduced differentiation of progenitor cells, as LPL overexpression blocks myogenic differentiation of C2C12 cells (Tamilarasan et al., 2012) as described above. This, however, has not yet been tested. The pronounced muscle degenerative phenotype in LPL-expressing mice is most likely explained by lipotoxicity caused by the several-fold increase in intracellular free fatty acid and TAG concentrations. In comparison, high-fat diet feeding usually results in a 30–50% increase in intramuscular TAG in rodents (Marotta et al., 2004; Bruce et al., 2009; Ussher et al., 2010). The ultimate extent of lipotoxicity in skeletal muscle *in vivo* will therefore likely depend on the extent of lipid infiltration.

LEPTIN SIGNALING

In genetically obese *ob/ob* and *db/db* mice, which have more severe insulin resistance than high-fat diet-fed mice, EDL myofiber regeneration after cardiotoxin injury is blunted (Nguyen et al., 2011). This finding could suggest that leptin signaling is important for skeletal muscle regeneration. In support of this model, injury-induced satellite cell proliferation is specifically impaired in leptin signaling-deficient mouse models, but not in the two high-fat diet models (Hu et al., 2010; Nguyen et al., 2011). Notably, *ob/ob* and *db/db* mice show defects of early regeneration stages: decreased proliferation and reduced MyoD expression are most evident at day 5 post-injury (Nguyen et al., 2011). In agreement with this result, basal rates of satellite cell proliferation are reduced in both mice and obese rats with leptin signaling deficiencies (Purchas et al., 1985; Peterson et al., 2008a), suggesting reduced proliferative capacity. Recombinant leptin stimulates proliferation and *MyoD* and *myogenin* expression in myoblasts from wild-type mice, but myoblasts from mice lacking all forms of the leptin receptor (referred to as POUND mice) show decreased expression of *MyoD* and *myogenin* transcripts and decreased myotube formation during differentiation *ex vivo* (Arounleut et al., 2013). Moreover, administration of recombinant leptin to *ob/ob* mice restores expression of the proliferation markers proliferating cell nuclear antigen (PCNA) and cyclin D1, which may account for the muscle growth-promoting effect of recombinant leptin in leptin-deficient animals (Sainz et al., 2009). In C2C12 myoblasts, leptin also stimulates proliferation but does not appear to promote MyoD or myogenin expression or differentiation (Pijet et al., 2013). Although leptin clearly has stimulatory effects on mouse myoblasts and muscle, it is not clear whether leptin promotes myoblast proliferation in all species. Leptin receptors are poorly abundant in porcine muscle, and recombinant leptin has no effect on proliferation of primary porcine myoblasts cultured in serum free medium or on protein accretion as these cells differentiated (Will et al., 2012). In line with this finding, lean and obese leptin receptor-deficient Zucker rats exhibit comparable BrdU incorporation, expression of myogenic regulatory factors, activation of pro-hypertrophic signaling pathways and gain of muscle mass in response to overload, demonstrating that leptin signaling *per se* is not required for satellite cell activation and muscle hypertrophy, at least in rats (Peterson et al., 2008a).

In addition to the activity of satellite cells, macrophages also contribute to regeneration of injured muscle by facilitating removal of tissue debris (Arnold et al., 2007). Leptin stimulates proliferation and activation of macrophages (Santos-Alvarez et al., 1999; Raso et al., 2002), pointing to another possible mechanism by which leptin resistance could impair muscle regeneration. Nguyen, et al. provided data supporting this hypothesis: in injured muscle of *ob/ob* and *db/db* mice, macrophage accumulation is decreased during early regeneration (Nguyen et al., 2011). In addition, these authors observed markedly decreased angiogenesis after injury in *ob/ob* and *db/db* mice (Nguyen et al., 2011). The data suggest that leptin could potentiate muscle regeneration by regulating macrophage activity and/or by stimulating vascularization. Vascularization potentiates regrowth of regenerating muscle in mice (Ochoa et al., 2007; Deasy et al., 2009). It appears that vascularization is not only important for nutrient availability but also myofiber growth. Vascular endothelial growth factor (VEGF), elevated during angiogenesis, promotes regeneration by directly stimulating myofiber growth (Arsic et al., 2004; Messina et al., 2007). As leptin resistance is often observed in obese and type 2 diabetic humans (Maffei et al., 1995; reviewed in Martin et al., 2008) it is possible that lack of leptin signaling could contribute to poor vascularity and compromised satellite cell function.

INFLAMMATION

In skeletal muscle, inflammation is activated after injury and is coordinated with myogenic differentiation to achieve efficient muscle regeneration (reviewed in Mann et al., 2011; Kharraz et al., 2013). Immediately after muscle injury, an acute inflammatory stage ensues characterized by infiltration of pro-inflammatory M1 macrophages that remove tissue debris. Later, a different population of macrophages (M2) resolves inflammation. Accumulating data show that macrophages not only mediate inflammation but also support satellite cells during skeletal muscle regeneration. In mice, deletion of chemokine receptor-2 (CCR-2) impairs macrophage infiltration after muscle injury and results in inefficient muscle regeneration (Warren et al., 2005). In co-culture experiments *in vitro*, macrophages stimulate satellite cell proliferation (Cantini et al., 1994; Massimino et al., 1997; Merly et al., 1999). When transplanted together with satellite cells into muscle of Dmd^{mdx} mice, a mouse model of human Duchenne muscular dystrophy, macrophages stimulate satellite cell survival and proliferation (Lesault et al., 2012). This potentiation effect is likely mediated, at least in part, by pro-inflammatory cytokines TNF-α and IL-6, which promote myoblast proliferation and migration *in vitro* (Li, 2003; Torrente et al., 2003; Wang et al., 2008; Toth et al., 2011). However, TNF-α and another pro-inflammatory cytokine IL-1α also prevent myogenic differentiation

(Miller et al., 1988; Layne and Farmer, 1999; Langen et al., 2001; Trendelenburg et al., 2012). During later stages of regeneration, TGF-β and IL-10 secreted by anti-inflammatory M2 macrophages promote myogenic differentiation (Arnold et al., 2007; Deng et al., 2012). Thus, the interplay between macrophages and satellite cells is precisely temporally orchestrated during skeletal muscle regeneration.

Obesity is recognized as a state of chronic inflammation with increased circulating pro-inflammatory cytokines TNF-α, IL-1β and IL-6 (reviewed in Wellen and Hotamisligil, 2005; Gregor and Hotamisligil, 2011). The effects of chronically elevated cytokines on satellite cell maintenance, activation and proliferation are not well understood, but it appears that chronic exposure to cytokines has distinct effects on myoblast proliferation and differentiation from acute exposure. For example, in a mouse model of chronic inflammation in which TNF-α is constitutively expressed in lung and becomes chronically elevated in the circulation, skeletal muscle becomes atrophic and myoblast proliferation and differentiation are reduced in response to mechanical loading (Langen et al., 2006). Similarly, chronic, local delivery of IL-6 to muscle of young rats inhibits muscle growth and stimulates expression of cyclin-dependent kinase inhibitor *p21*, suggesting decreased satellite cell proliferation, although this has not been tested (Bodell et al., 2009). It is possible that in chronic inflammation the normal coordination between macrophages and muscle satellite cells is impaired and contributes to impaired satellite cell function. It would be interesting to manipulate cytokine signaling in obesity models to determine whether the chronic inflammation that accompanies obesity in fact does impair muscle satellite cell proliferation and differentiation and ultimately muscle growth.

MYOSTATIN

Myostatin is a member of the TGF-β family of secreted proteins known to prevent muscle regeneration and growth (reviewed in Joulia-Ekaza and Cabello, 2006; Kollias and McDermott, 2008). Interestingly, myostatin expression is increased in skeletal muscle of extremely obese women (Hittel et al., 2009) and of *ob/ob* and high-fat diet-fed mice (Allen et al., 2008). In C2C12 myoblasts, recombinant or overexpressed myostatin decreases proliferation most likely by stimulating expression of the cyclin-dependent kinase inhibitor p21, resulting in inhibition of Cdk2 and impaired G1 to S phase transition (Thomas et al., 2000; Taylor et al., 2001; Joulia et al., 2003). Moreover, proliferation of satellite cells in *myostatin*-null mice is markedly increased (McCroskery et al., 2003). Myostatin also represses transcription of myogenic regulatory factors through direct activation of Smad2/3 proteins, which repress expression of *MyoD* and *myogenin*. In addition, Smad3 represses MyoD activity through direct interaction (Liu et al., 2001; Langley et al., 2002). Elevated myostatin in obese people correlates with increased phosphorylation of Smad2/3 proteins and an approximately two-fold decrease in *MyoD* and *myogenin* transcript levels (Watts et al., 2013). Thus, increased myostatin in obese animals may contribute to defects in regeneration and maintenance of muscle mass (**Figure 1**).

The source and mechanism by which myostatin becomes elevated in obese subjects remain obscure. Expression of the *myostatin* gene is stimulated in myocytes by several pathways including glucocorticoid signaling (Salehian et al., 2006) possibly via C/EBP-δ (Allen et al., 2010) or repression of miR-27a/b (Allen and Loh, 2011). *Myostatin* expression in muscle cells has also been reported to be stimulated by FoxO1 and TGF-β/Smad3 (Allen and Unterman, 2007), MyoD (Spiller et al., 2002) and a JNK/p38-mediated signaling pathway (Han et al., 2010). It is not known which, if any, of these pathways may mediate the increase in circulating myostatin in obese patients, but it is tempting to speculate that elevated glucocorticoids commonly observed in metabolic syndrome and obesity (Anagnostis et al., 2009) could stimulate *myostatin* expression by promoter regulation (Allen et al., 2010) and modulation of miR-27a/b (Allen and Loh, 2011). Alternatively, insulin resistance may result in derepression of *myostatin* via constitutive activation of FoxO1 (Allen and Unterman, 2007); this model would be consistent with the observation of elevated myostatin in insulin resistant type 2 diabetic patients and non-obese hyperinsulinemic subjects (reviewed in Allen et al., 2011). Although skeletal muscle expresses far more *myostatin* than other tissues, it is noteworthy that *myostatin* mRNA increases by at least fifty fold in adipose tissue (primarily adipocytes) and only twofold in skeletal muscle of obese mice (Allen et al., 2008). Thus, it is possible that in obesity a large amount of myostatin could be secreted from adipose as a result of hypercortisolemia. Although myostatin is well known for its role in regulation of muscle growth, it is not clear to what extent myostatin contributes to impaired muscle regeneration observed in rodent models of obesity. Genetic manipulations disrupting myostatin signaling, such as expressing a dominant negative form of the myostatin receptor in satellite cells in an obesity model, will help to answer this question.

ADIPOGENESIS

Fibro/adipogenic progenitor (FAP) cells comprise a recently identified population of progenitors that reside in the muscle and become activated after muscle damage in mice (Joe et al., 2010; Heredia et al., 2013). Unlike myogenic progenitors, FAP cells do not fuse or differentiate into myofibers. Instead, FAP cells support myogenesis likely by enhancing proliferation and differentiation of myogenic progenitors through secretion of factors such as IL-6 (Joe et al., 2010). The signals that regulate FAP cell differentiation are incompletely understood. FAP cells spontaneously differentiate into adipocytes *in vitro* and when transplanted into skeletal muscle with fatty infiltration, but not when transplanted into healthy skeletal muscle (Joe et al., 2010). Using a co-culture system, Uezumi, et al. found that muscle satellite cells inhibit adipogenic differentiation of FAP cells likely by direct physical interaction (Uezumi et al., 2010), though the signal is unknown. If the same regulation occurs *in vivo*, then a decrease in satellite cell number, activity or proximity to FAP cells could result in increased adipogenic conversion of FAP cells and IMAT accumulation. Alternatively, exciting work by Heredia, et al. demonstrated that after skeletal muscle injury, eosinophil-derived anti-inflammatory cytokines IL-4/IL-13 promote FAP proliferation and inhibit their differentiation to adipocytes (Heredia et al., 2013). It is possible that under the pro-inflammatory conditions of obesity, the ability of satellite cells or eosinophils to inhibit adipogenic differentiation of FAP cells is compromised.

As a result, FAP cells activated during injury could differentiate into adipocytes, contribute to increased IMAT, and occupy areas of the tissue once filled with skeletal myofibers. Indeed, it has been shown that muscle side population cells from dystrophic or injured tissue differentiate in culture to FAP cells and lose myogenic capacity (Penton et al., 2013). It is notable in this regard that in patients with Duchenne muscular dystrophy, the skeletal muscle eventually loses capacity for ongoing regeneration and myofibers are replaced by fatty infiltrate and collagen (Radley et al., 2007). It will be important for future studies to examine the action of FAP cells in obese animals and humans.

METABOLISM

Recently it has been recognized that satellite cells exhibit different intrinsic metabolic properties in states of quiescence, proliferation and differentiation (reviewed in Ryall, 2013). In the quiescent state, satellite cells have low energy demands, low oxygen consumption and low ATP production. In low nutrient conditions, elevated NAD^+ levels stimulate the deacetylase SIRT1, which in turn promotes myoblast proliferation and prevents myogenic differentiation, in part via MyoD deacetylation (Fulco et al., 2003). Culturing mouse myoblasts in low glucose medium similarly prevents differentiation at least in part through SIRT1 activation (Fulco et al., 2008; reviewed in Ryall, 2012). It thus can be hypothesized that in low energy states, limited nutrient supply and the associated increase in SIRT1 activity would be beneficial to maintain a pool of muscle satellite cells. On the other hand, obesity and nutrient overload would be expected to provide unfavorable conditions for maintenance of quiescent satellite cells or for proliferation after acute injury.

Cerletti, et al. tested the corollary to this hypothesis by evaluating muscle satellite cell metabolism and function in mice after short-term (12 weeks) caloric restriction. They showed that short-term caloric restriction in mice increases both the number and myogenic capacity of muscle-associated satellite cells and enhances regeneration after freeze injury (Cerletti et al., 2012). Satellite cells isolated from calorie-restricted animals had higher mitochondrial content, enhanced oxidative metabolism and reduced glycolytic capacity accompanied by elevated SIRT1 expression. Muscle stem cells harvested from calorically restricted mice also displayed improved engraftment in dystrophin-deficient Dmd^{mdx} mice that had not been previously subjected to caloric restriction (Cerletti et al., 2012). Thus, the altered cellular metabolic state of the satellite cells from a calorie-restricted animal was sufficient to confer benefits on a normal recipient. The beneficial effects of calorie restriction were not, however, limited to the satellite cells. Transplanted muscle stem cells had much higher engraftment efficiency when transplanted into healthy uninjured skeletal muscle of animals undergoing calorie restriction, possibly as a result of reduced inflammation in the muscle (Cerletti et al., 2012).

These findings strongly suggest that (1) muscle satellite cell metabolism is profoundly altered by the systemic nutritional environment and (2) the metabolic/ inflammatory state of the organism, and therefore of the mature myofibers, also affects the health or fusion capacity of satellite cells. Accumulation of SIRT1 protein in the satellite cells from calorically restricted mice could theoretically stimulate proliferation and oxidative metabolism, resulting in a larger satellite cell pool. In obesity, perturbations of intrinsic satellite cell metabolism could negatively affect the proliferation and activity of the satellite cell pool, but this exciting field is still emerging.

MUSCLE REGROWTH AFTER INJURY IN OBESE ANIMALS

A common finding among the aforementioned *in vivo* studies of skeletal muscle regeneration in obese animals is reduced recovery of muscle mass and function after injury (Hu et al., 2010; Nguyen et al., 2011; Tamilarasan et al., 2012). This may occur secondary to reduced satellite cell function or as a result of defective hypertrophic growth after initial satellite cell differentiation and fusion. In this section, we will discuss some potential mechanisms underlying defective muscle regrowth after injury in obese animals.

IGF-1/Akt SIGNALING

In normal skeletal muscle, the balance between muscle hypertrophy and atrophy is largely regulated by the IGF-1/Akt signaling pathway (reviewed in Glass, 2010), which stimulates mTOR-dependent protein synthesis and inhibits FOXO-dependent transcription of muscle-specific E3 ubiquitin ligases (Bodine et al., 2001; Sartorelli and Fulco, 2004; Bodine, 2006). The balance between muscle growth and atrophy is dysregulated in obesity. In obese mice and Zucker rats, muscle growth in response to mechanical loading is reduced due to decreased activation of Akt, p70S6 kinase and mTOR (Sitnick et al., 2009; Paturi et al., 2010). Similar mechanisms might impair muscle regrowth after injury. Indeed, in high-fat diet-fed mice, Hu, et al. found that PIP_3 levels and PI(3)-kinase activity are reduced and expression of the lipid and protein phosphatase PTEN is increased (Hu et al., 2010). These combined changes would result in decreased Akt and mTOR activity and reduced hypertrophy. *Pten* deletion in muscle is sufficient to restore Akt phosphorylation and remarkably improves muscle growth in high-fat diet-fed mice (Hu et al., 2010). These findings clearly demonstrate that dysregulated PI(3)-kinase/Akt pathway activity in muscle of obese mice not only impairs insulin signaling but also interferes with muscle growth.

On the other hand, Nguyen, et al. observed impaired muscle growth after injury in obese *ob/ob* and *db/db* and but not in high-fat diet-fed mice (Nguyen et al., 2011). Since both *ob/ob* and *db/db* mice are deficient in leptin signaling, one interpretation is that leptin signaling is necessary for normal muscle regeneration. The authors point out that leptin could promote muscle growth by activation of PI(3)-kinase and ERK1/2 pathways (Nguyen et al., 2011). Consistently, administration of recombinant leptin to mice or C2C12 myoblasts activates janus kinase 2 (JAK2), which potentiates phosphorylation of insulin receptor substrates IRS1 and IRS2, activity of PI(3)-kinase, and phosphorylation of Akt and glycogen synthase kinase 3 (GSK3) (Kellerer et al., 1997; Kim et al., 2000; Maroni et al., 2003, 2005). These studies suggest the hypothesis that leptin-dependent activation of Akt is important for regulation of muscle growth or regrowth after injury. In further support of this model, leptin treatment of *ob/ob* mice increases the mass of multiple skeletal muscle groups, including gastrocnemius, EDL and soleus, with concomitant decreased expression of muscle-specific E3 ubiquitin ligases MAFbx and MuRF1 in gastrocnemius muscle (Sainz et al., 2009).

The toxic lipid metabolites diacylglycerols and ceramides also impair IGF-1/Akt signaling. In skeletal muscle and liver, diacylglycerols activate PKCε and PKCθ, which phosphorylate multiple serine residues of insulin receptor substrate-1 (IRS-1) directly or via JNK and IKKβ ultimately leading to insulin resistance (Yu et al., 2002; Li et al., 2004; reviewed in Samuel et al., 2010; Turban and Hajduch, 2011). Interestingly, PKCθ deletion in dystrophic Dmd^{mdx} mice increases expression of myogenin and myosin heavy chain and decreases necrotic areas in the muscle (Madaro et al., 2012). Similarly, stable PKCθ knockdown in C2C12 cells increases expression of *myogenin* and myosin heavy chain and potentiates myotube formation *in vitro* (Marino et al., 2013). The other major class of toxic lipid intermediates, ceramides, inhibits Akt by two distinct mechanisms. In C2C12 myoblasts, 3T3-L1 adipocytes and PC-12 cells, ceramides activate protein phosphatase 2A, leading to Akt dephosphorylation (Salinas et al., 2000; Cazzolli et al., 2001; Chavez et al., 2003; Stratford et al., 2004). In L6 myotubes, ceramides induce PKCζ-dependent Akt phosphorylation on Thr34, which blocks Akt translocation to the plasma membrane (Hajduch et al., 2001; Powell et al., 2003, 2004; reviewed in Bikman and Summers, 2011). In addition, ceramides impair amino acid uptake in L6 myotubes by decreasing the amount of the membrane-associated amino acid transporter SNAT2, with concomitant reduction of p70S6 kinase phosphorylation and protein synthesis (Hyde et al., 2005). All of these events would be expected to inhibit myofiber growth. It is likely that a similar mechanism contributes to impaired muscle regrowth during regeneration in obese animals (**Figure 1**).

INFLAMMATION

Pro-inflammatory cytokines TNF-α, IL-1β and IL-6 inhibit IGF-1/Akt signaling and de-repress transcription of muscle ubiquitin ligases *Mafbx* and *Murf1* and potentiate skeletal muscle atrophy (reviewed in Glass and Roubenoff, 2010). Thus, in addition to the possible negative effects on myoblast proliferation and differentiation, increased circulation of TNF-α, IL-1β and IL-6 could counteract anabolic growth of skeletal muscle during regeneration in obese animals (**Figure 1**). For example, treatment of human, porcine or mouse (C2C12) myoblasts with TNF-α or IL-1β prevents IGF-1-stimulated protein synthesis (Frost et al., 1997; Broussard et al., 2003, 2004). In rats, 16 weeks of high-fat diet feeding results in decreased Akt and mTOR phosphorylation and increased apoptosis that correlates with upregulation of TNF-α receptors in the muscle (Sishi et al., 2011). Interestingly, TNF-α treatment increases ceramide synthesis in C2C12 myoblasts and L6 myotubes, and exogenous ceramides cause atrophy of L6 myotubes (Strle et al., 2004; De Larichaudy et al., 2012). In support of the idea that ceramides mediate effects of TNF-α on myotubes, ceramide synthesis inhibitors block the inhibitory effect of TNF-α on IGF-1-stimulated protein synthesis (Strle et al., 2004) and prevent TNF-α induced atrophy (De Larichaudy et al., 2012). It is therefore possible that in obese animals, elevated TNF-α impairs IGF-1 signaling and muscle regrowth via ceramides and toxic lipid intermediates, which also directly inhibit satellite cell activity.

CONCLUDING REMARKS

The influence of obesity on skeletal muscle regeneration and maintenance is an emerging area that is poorly mechanistically understood. So far, this topic has been primarily addressed in studies on obese rodents. Regenerative capacity is particularly impaired by severe obesity such as in genetically obese *ob/ob* and *db/db* mice. Identifying factors that specifically block muscle regeneration in obese animals is challenging because obesity is accompanied by several abnormalities, including but not limited to ectopic accumulation of multiple lipid species, insulin and leptin resistance, chronic inflammation and metabolic disturbances (**Figure 1**). Using genetic models and pharmacological approaches to block synthesis of specific lipid species and modulate production and signaling of cytokines will help to determine which lipid species and cytokines specifically impair regeneration in obese animals. Another challenge is determining how obesity affects different steps during regeneration such as satellite cell activation and proliferation, myoblast differentiation, fusion and myofiber growth. In this regard, intriguing new studies linking global metabolism, cellular metabolism and satellite cell capacity for engraftment may facilitate identification of new molecular mechanisms that could be targeted therapeutically. An important open question is whether and to what extent obesity impairs muscle regeneration in humans and whether impaired muscle regeneration contributes to poor wound healing in type 2 diabetic patients (reviewed in Greenhalgh, 2003), or whether poor vascular function itself impairs satellite cell function and skeletal muscle regeneration in obese and type 2 diabetic people. In obese and type 2 diabetic patients, exercise and low calorie diet aimed at reducing lipid oversupply and stimulating metabolism could be beneficial not only by improving whole body metabolism but also perhaps by promoting anabolic growth of muscle via improved satellite cell viability and function. Stimulation or preservation of satellite cells could, in turn, enable these individuals to become stronger and more active and to possibly prevent further IMAT accumulation. In addition to abnormalities discussed here, obese and type 2 diabetic individuals suffer from complications, such as peripheral neuropathy, which we do not address directly in this review (reviewed in Vincent et al., 2011; Ylitalo et al., 2011). As innervation is required for skeletal muscle maintenance and regeneration in rodents (d'Albis et al., 1988; Rodrigues Ade and Schmalbruch, 1995; Billington, 1997), it is possible that peripheral neuropathy contributes to impaired skeletal muscle regeneration in obese and type 2 diabetic humans and could prevent putative salutary effects of strategies to promote satellite cell function. Ultimate conclusions about the effects of obesity on muscle regeneration await the results of the next generation of experiments that explore signaling mechanisms and more fully characterize muscle regeneration in obese rodents and humans.

ACKNOWLEDGMENTS

This publication was supported by the National Institute of Arthritis and Musculoskeletal and Skin Diseases (R01AR059847). The content is solely the responsibility of the authors and does not necessarily represent the official views of the National Institutes of Health.

REFERENCES

Adams, J. M. 2nd, Pratipanawatr, T., Berria, R., Wang, E., Defronzo, R. A., Sullards, M. C., et al. (2004). Ceramide content is increased in skeletal muscle from obese insulin-resistant humans. *Diabetes* 53, 25–31. doi: 10.2337/diabetes.53.1.25

Allen, D. L., Cleary, A. S., Hanson, A. M., Lindsay, S. F., and Reed, J. M. (2010). CCAAT/enhancer binding protein-delta expression is increased in fast skeletal muscle by food deprivation and regulates myostatin transcription *in vitro*. *Am. J. Physiol. Regul. Integr. Comp. Physiol.* 299, R1592–R1601. doi: 10.1152/ajpregu.00247.2010

Allen, D. L., Cleary, A. S., Speaker, K. J., Lindsay, S. F., Uyenishi, J., Reed, J. M., et al. (2008). Myostatin, activin receptor IIb, and follistatin-like-3 gene expression are altered in adipose tissue and skeletal muscle of obese mice. *Am. J. Physiol. Endocrinol. Metab.* 294, E918–E927. doi: 10.1152/ajpendo.00798.2007

Allen, D. L., Hittel, D. S., and McPherron, A. C. (2011). Expression and function of myostatin in obesity, diabetes, and exercise adaptation. *Med. Sci. Sports Exerc.* 43, 1828–1835. doi: 10.1249/MSS.0b013e3182178bb4

Allen, D. L., and Loh, A. S. (2011). Posttranscriptional mechanisms involving microRNA-27a and b contribute to fast-specific and glucocorticoid-mediated myostatin expression in skeletal muscle. *Am. J. Physiol. Cell Physiol.* 300, C124–C137. doi: 10.1152/ajpcell.00142.2010

Allen, D. L., and Unterman, T. G. (2007). Regulation of myostatin expression and myoblast differentiation by FoxO and SMAD transcription factors. *Am. J. Physiol. Cell Physiol.* 292, C188–C199. doi: 10.1152/ajpcell.00542.2005

Anagnostis, P., Athyros, V. G., Tziomalos, K., Karagiannis, A., and Mikhailidis, D. P. (2009). Clinical review: the pathogenetic role of cortisol in the metabolic syndrome: a hypothesis. *J. Clin. Endocrinol. Metab.* 94, 2692–2701. doi: 10.1210/jc.2009-0370

Arnold, L., Henry, A., Poron, F., Baba-Amer, Y., Van Rooijen, N., Plonquet, A., et al. (2007). Inflammatory monocytes recruited after skeletal muscle injury switch into antiinflammatory macrophages to support myogenesis. *J. Exp. Med.* 204, 1057–1069. doi: 10.1084/jem.20070075

Arounleut, P., Bowser, M., Upadhyay, S., Shi, X. M., Fulzele, S., Johnson, M. H., et al. (2013). Absence of functional leptin receptor isoforms in the POUND (Lepr(db/lb)) mouse is associated with muscle atrophy and altered myoblast proliferation and differentiation. *PLoS ONE* 8:e72330. doi: 10.1371/annotation/3a7d6e24-137c-4603-93ca-879bec7fab80

Arsic, N., Zacchigna, S., Zentilin, L., Ramirez-Correa, G., Pattarini, L., Salvi, A., et al. (2004). Vascular endothelial growth factor stimulates skeletal muscle regeneration *in vivo*. *Mol. Ther.* 10, 844–854. doi: 10.1016/j.ymthe.2004.08.007

Bikman, B. T., and Summers, S. A. (2011). Ceramides as modulators of cellular and whole-body metabolism. *J. Clin. Invest.* 121, 4222–4230. doi: 10.1172/JCI57144

Billington, L. (1997). Reinnervation and regeneration of denervated rat soleus muscles. *Muscle Nerve* 20, 744–746. doi: 10.1002/(SICI)1097-4598(199706)20:6<744::AID-MUS13>3.0.CO;2-U

Bloemberg, D., and Quadrilatero, J. (2012). Rapid determination of myosin heavy chain expression in rat, mouse, and human skeletal muscle using multi-color immunofluorescence analysis. *PLoS ONE* 7:e35273. doi: 10.1371/journal.pone.0035273

Bodell, P. W., Kodesh, E., Haddad, F., Zaldivar, F. P., Cooper, D. M., and Adams, G. R. (2009). Skeletal muscle growth in young rats is inhibited by chronic exposure to IL-6 but preserved by concurrent voluntary endurance exercise. *J. Appl. Physiol.* 106, 443–453. doi: 10.1152/japplphysiol.90831.2008

Boden, G., and Shulman, G. I. (2002). Free fatty acids in obesity and type 2 diabetes: defining their role in the development of insulin resistance and beta-cell dysfunction. *Eur. J. Clin. Invest.* 32(Suppl. 3), 14–23. doi: 10.1046/j.1365-2362.32.s3.3.x

Bodine, S. C. (2006). mTOR signaling and the molecular adaptation to resistance exercise. *Med. Sci. Sports Exerc.* 38, 1950–1957. doi: 10.1249/01.mss.0000233797.24035.35

Bodine, S. C., Stitt, T. N., Gonzalez, M., Kline, W. O., Stover, G. L., Bauerlein, R., et al. (2001). Akt/mTOR pathway is a crucial regulator of skeletal muscle hypertrophy and can prevent muscle atrophy *in vivo*. *Nat. Cell Biol.* 3, 1014–1019. doi: 10.1038/ncb1101-1014

Boesch, C., Machann, J., Vermathen, P., and Schick, F. (2006). Role of proton MR for the study of muscle lipid metabolism. *NMR Biomed.* 19, 968–988. doi: 10.1002/nbm.1096

Bonen, A., Parolin, M. L., Steinberg, G. R., Calles-Escandon, J., Tandon, N. N., Glatz, J. F., et al. (2004). Triacylglycerol accumulation in human obesity and type 2 diabetes is associated with increased rates of skeletal muscle fatty acid transport and increased sarcolemmal FAT/CD36. *FASEB J.* 18, 1144–1146. doi: 10.1096/fj.03-1065fje

Bonnard, C., Durand, A., Peyrol, S., Chanseaume, E., Chauvin, M. A., Morio, B., et al. (2008). Mitochondrial dysfunction results from oxidative stress in the skeletal muscle of diet-induced insulin-resistant mice. *J. Clin. Invest.* 118, 789–800. doi: 10.1172/JCI32601

Bosma, M., Kersten, S., Hesselink, M. K., and Schrauwen, P. (2012). Re-evaluating lipotoxic triggers in skeletal muscle: relating intramyocellular lipid metabolism to insulin sensitivity. *Prog. Lipid Res.* 51, 36–49. doi: 10.1016/j.plipres.2011.11.003

Broussard, S. R., McCusker, R. H., Novakofski, J. E., Strle, K., Shen, W. H., Johnson, R. W., et al. (2004). IL-1beta impairs insulin-like growth factor i-induced differentiation and downstream activation signals of the insulin-like growth factor i receptor in myoblasts. *J. Immunol.* 172, 7713–7720. doi: 10.1210/en.2003-0087

Broussard, S. R., McCusker, R. H., Novakofski, J. E., Strle, K., Shen, W. H., Johnson, R. W., et al. (2003). Cytokine-hormone interactions: tumor necrosis factor alpha impairs biologic activity and downstream activation signals of the insulin-like growth factor I receptor in myoblasts. *Endocrinology* 144, 2988–2996. doi: 10.1210/en.2003-0087

Bruce, C. R., Hoy, A. J., Turner, N., Watt, M. J., Allen, T. L., Carpenter, K., et al. (2009). Overexpression of carnitine palmitoyltransferase-1 in skeletal muscle is sufficient to enhance fatty acid oxidation and improve high-fat diet-induced insulin resistance. *Diabetes* 58, 550–558. doi: 10.2337/db08-1078

Bruusgaard, J. C., Johansen, I. B., Egner, I. M., Rana, Z. A., and Gundersen, K. (2010). Myonuclei acquired by overload exercise precede hypertrophy and are not lost on detraining. *Proc. Natl. Acad. Sci. U.S.A.* 107, 15111-15116. doi: 10.1073/pnas.0913935107

Cantini, M., Massimino, M. L., Bruson, A., Catani, C., Dalla Libera, L., and Carraro, U. (1994). Macrophages regulate proliferation and differentiation of satellite cells. *Biochem. Biophys. Res. Commun.* 202, 1688–1696. doi: 10.1006/bbrc.1994.2129

Cazzolli, R., Carpenter, L., Biden, T. J., and Schmitz-Peiffer, C. (2001). A role for protein phosphatase 2A-like activity, but not atypical protein kinase Czeta, in the inhibition of protein kinase B/Akt and glycogen synthesis by palmitate. *Diabetes* 50, 2210–2218. doi: 10.2337/diabetes.50.10.2210

Cerletti, M., Jang, Y. C., Finley, L. W., Haigis, M. C., and Wagers, A. J. (2012). Short-term calorie restriction enhances skeletal muscle stem cell function. *Cell Stem Cell* 10, 515–519. doi: 10.1016/j.stem.2012.04.002

Charge, S. B., and Rudnicki, M. A. (2004). Cellular and molecular regulation of muscle regeneration. *Physiol Rev.* 84, 209–238. doi: 10.1152/physrev.00019.2003

Chavez, J. A., Knotts, T. A., Wang, L. P., Li, G., Dobrowsky, R. T., Florant, G. L., et al. (2003). A role for ceramide, but not diacylglycerol, in the antagonism of insulin signal transduction by saturated fatty acids. *J. Biol. Chem.* 278, 10297–10303. doi: 10.1074/jbc.M212307200

Coen, P. M., and Goodpaster, B. H. (2012). Role of intramyocelluar lipids in human health. *Trends Endocrinol. Metab.* 23, 391–398. doi: 10.1016/j.tem.2012.05.009

d'Albis, A., Couteaux, R., Janmot, C., Roulet, A., and Mira, J. C. (1988). Regeneration after cardiotoxin injury of innervated and denervated slow and fast muscles of mammals. Myosin isoform analysis. *Eur. J. Biochem.* 174, 103–110. doi: 10.1111/j.1432-1033.1988.tb14068.x

De Larichaudy, J., Zufferli, A., Serra, F., Isidori, A. M., Naro, F., Dessalle, K., et al. (2012). TNF-alpha- and tumor-induced skeletal muscle atrophy involves sphingolipid metabolism. *Skelet. Muscle* 2, 2. doi: 10.1186/2044-5040-2-2

Deasy, B. M., Feduska, J. M., Payne, T. R., Li, Y., Ambrosio, F., and Huard, J. (2009). Effect of VEGF on the regenerative capacity of muscle stem cells in dystrophic skeletal muscle. *Mol. Ther.* 17, 1788–1798. doi: 10.1038/mt.2009.136

Deng, B., Wehling-Henricks, M., Villalta, S. A., Wang, Y., and Tidball, J. G. (2012). IL-10 triggers changes in macrophage phenotype that promote muscle growth and regeneration. *J. Immunol.* 189, 3669–3680. doi: 10.4049/jimmunol.1103180

Fissoune, R., Janier, M., Briguet, A., and Hiba, B. (2009). *In vivo* assessment of mouse hindleg intramyocellular lipids by 1H-MR spectroscopy. *Acad. Radiol.* 16, 890–896. doi: 10.1016/j.acra.2008.12.007

Frost, R. A., Lang, C. H., and Gelato, M. C. (1997). Transient exposure of human myoblasts to tumor necrosis factor-alpha inhibits serum and insulin-like growth factor-I stimulated protein synthesis. *Endocrinology* 138, 4153–4159. doi: 10.1210/en.138.10.4153

Fujimoto, T., Ohsaki, Y., Cheng, J., Suzuki, M., and Shinohara, Y. (2008). Lipid droplets: a classic organelle with new outfits. *Histochem. Cell. Biol.* 130, 263–279. doi: 10.1007/s00418-008-0449-0

Fulco, M., Cen, Y., Zhao, P., Hoffman, E. P., McBurney, M. W., Sauve, A. A., et al. (2008). Glucose restriction inhibits skeletal myoblast differentiation by activating SIRT1 through AMPK-mediated regulation of Nampt. *Dev. Cell.* 14, 661–673. doi: 10.1016/j.devcel.2008.02.004

Fulco, M., Schiltz, R. L., Iezzi, S., King, M. T., Zhao, P., Kashiwaya, Y., et al. (2003). Sir2 regulates skeletal muscle differentiation as a potential sensor of the redox state. *Mol. Cell.* 12, 51–62. doi: 10.1016/S1097-2765(03)00226-0

Gibson, M. C., and Schultz, E. (1983). Age-related differences in absolute numbers of skeletal muscle satellite cells. *Muscle Nerve* 6, 574–580. doi: 10.1002/mus.880060807

Glass, D., and Roubenoff, R. (2010). Recent advances in the biology and therapy of muscle wasting. *Ann. N.Y. Acad. Sci.* 1211, 25–36. doi: 10.1111/j.1749-6632.2010.05809.x

Glass, D. J. (2010). PI3 kinase regulation of skeletal muscle hypertrophy and atrophy. *Curr. Top. Microbiol. Immunol.* 346, 267–278. doi: 10.1007/82_2010_78

Goodpaster, B. H., Thaete, F. L., and Kelley, D. E. (2000a). Thigh adipose tissue distribution is associated with insulin resistance in obesity and in type 2 diabetes mellitus. *Am. J. Clin. Nutr.* 71, 885–892.

Goodpaster, B. H., Theriault, R., Watkins, S. C., and Kelley, D. E. (2000b). Intramuscular lipid content is increased in obesity and decreased by weight loss. *Metabolism* 49, 467–472. doi: 10.1016/S0026-0495(00)80010-4

Goodpaster, B. H., and Wolf, D. (2004). Skeletal muscle lipid accumulation in obesity, insulin resistance, and type 2 diabetes. *Pediatr. Diabetes* 5, 219–226. doi: 10.1111/j.1399-543X.2004.00071.x

Greenhalgh, D. G. (2003). Wound healing and diabetes mellitus. *Clin. Plast. Surg.* 30, 37–45. doi: 10.1016/S0094-1298(02)00066-4

Gregor, M. F., and Hotamisligil, G. S. (2011). Inflammatory mechanisms in obesity. *Annu. Rev. Immunol.* 29, 415–445. doi: 10.1146/annurev-immunol-031210-101322

Gunther, S., Kim, J., Kostin, S., Lepper, C., Fan, C. M., and Braun, T. (2013). Myf5-Positive Satellite Cells Contribute to Pax7-Dependent Long-Term Maintenance of Adult Muscle Stem Cells. *Cell Stem Cell.* 13, 590–601. doi: 10.1016/j.stem.2013.07.016

Hajduch, E., Balendran, A., Batty, I. H., Litherland, G. J., Blair, A. S., Downes, C. P., et al. (2001). Ceramide impairs the insulin-dependent membrane recruitment of protein kinase B leading to a loss in downstream signalling in L6 skeletal muscle cells. *Diabetologia* 44, 173–183. doi: 10.1007/s001250051596

Han, D. S., Huang, H. P., Wang, T. G., Hung, M. Y., Ke, J. Y., Chang, K. T., et al. (2010). Transcription activation of myostatin by trichostatin A in differentiated C2C12 myocytes via ASK1-MKK3/4/6-JNK and p38 mitogen-activated protein kinase pathways. *J. Cell. Biochem.* 111, 564–573. doi: 10.1002/jcb.22740

Henique, C., Mansouri, A., Fumey, G., Lenoir, V., Girard, J., Bouillaud, F., et al. (2010). Increased mitochondrial fatty acid oxidation is sufficient to protect skeletal muscle cells from palmitate-induced apoptosis. *J. Biol. Chem.* 285, 36818–36827. doi: 10.1074/jbc.M110.170431

Heredia, J. E., Mukundan, L., Chen, F. M., Mueller, A. A., Deo, R. C., Locksley, R. M., et al. (2013). Type 2 innate signals stimulate fibro/adipogenic progenitors to facilitate muscle regeneration. *Cell* 153, 376–388. doi: 10.1016/j.cell.2013.02.053

Hilton, T. N., Tuttle, L. J., Bohnert, K. L., Mueller, M. J., and Sinacore, D. R. (2008). Excessive adipose tissue infiltration in skeletal muscle in individuals with obesity, diabetes mellitus, and peripheral neuropathy: association with performance and function. *Phys. Ther.* 88, 1336–1344. doi: 10.2522/ptj.20080079

Hittel, D. S., Berggren, J. R., Shearer, J., Boyle, K., and Houmard, J. A. (2009). Increased secretion and expression of myostatin in skeletal muscle from extremely obese women. *Diabetes* 58, 30–38. doi: 10.2337/db08-0943

Holland, W. L., Brozinick, J. T., Wang, L. P., Hawkins, E. D., Sargent, K. M., Liu, Y., et al. (2007). Inhibition of ceramide synthesis ameliorates glucocorticoid-, saturated-fat-, and obesity-induced insulin resistance. *Cell Metab.* 5, 167–179. doi: 10.1016/j.cmet.2007.01.002

Hu, Z., Wang, H., Lee, I. H., Modi, S., Wang, X., Du, J., et al. (2010). PTEN inhibition improves muscle regeneration in mice fed a high-fat diet. *Diabetes* 59, 1312–1320. doi: 10.2337/db09-1155

Hulver, M. W., Berggren, J. R., Cortright, R. N., Dudek, R. W., Thompson, R. P., Pories, W. J., et al. (2003). Skeletal muscle lipid metabolism with obesity. *Am. J. Physiol. Endocrinol. Metab.* 284, E741–E747. doi: 10.1152/ajpendo.00514.2002

Hyde, R., Hajduch, E., Powell, D. J., Taylor, P. M., and Hundal, H. S. (2005). Ceramide down-regulates System A amino acid transport and protein synthesis in rat skeletal muscle cells. *FASEB J.* 19, 461–463. doi: 10.1096/fj.04-2284fje

Jackson, J. R., Mula, J., Kirby, T. J., Fry, C. S., Lee, J. D., Ubele, M. F., et al. (2012). Satellite cell depletion does not inhibit adult skeletal muscle regrowth following unloading-induced atrophy. *Am. J. Physiol. Cell. Physiol.* 303, C854–C861. doi: 10.1152/ajpcell.00207.2012

Jang, Y. C., Sinha, M., Cerletti, M., Dall'osso, C., and Wagers, A. J. (2011). Skeletal muscle stem cells: effects of aging and metabolism on muscle regenerative function. *Cold Spring Harb. Symp. Quant. Biol.* 76, 101–111. doi: 10.1101/sqb.2011.76.010652

Joe, A. W., Yi, L., Natarajan, A., Le Grand, F., So, L., Wang, J., Rudnicki, M. A., et al. (2010). Muscle injury activates resident fibro/adipogenic progenitors that facilitate myogenesis. *Nat. Cell. Biol.* 12, 153–163. doi: 10.1038/ncb2015

Joulia-Ekaza, D., and Cabello, G. (2006). Myostatin regulation of muscle development: molecular basis, natural mutations, physiopathological aspects. *Exp. Cell. Res.* 312, 2401–2414. doi: 10.1016/j.yexcr.2006.04.012

Joulia, D., Bernardi, H., Garandel, V., Rabenoelina, F., Vernus, B., and Cabello, G. (2003). Mechanisms involved in the inhibition of myoblast proliferation and differentiation by myostatin. *Exp. Cell. Res.* 286, 263–275. doi: 10.1016/S0014-4827(03)00074-0

Kadi, F., Schjerling, P., Andersen, L. L., Charifi, N., Madsen, J. L., Christensen, L. R., et al. (2004). The effects of heavy resistance training and detraining on satellite cells in human skeletal muscles. *J. Physiol.* 558, 1005–1012. doi: 10.1113/jphysiol.2004.065904

Kahn, S. E., Hull, R. L., and Utzschneider, K. M. (2006). Mechanisms linking obesity to insulin resistance and type 2 diabetes. *Nature* 444, 840–846. doi: 10.1038/nature05482

Kellerer, M., Koch, M., Metzinger, E., Mushack, J., Capp, E., and Haring, H. U. (1997). Leptin activates PI-3 kinase in C2C12 myotubes via janus kinase-2 (JAK-2) and insulin receptor substrate-2 (IRS-2) dependent pathways. *Diabetologia* 40, 1358–1362. doi: 10.1007/s001250050832

Kharraz, Y., Guerra, J., Mann, C. J., Serrano, A. L., and Munoz-Canoves, P. (2013). Macrophage plasticity and the role of inflammation in skeletal muscle repair. *Mediators Inflamm.* 2013, 491497. doi: 10.1155/2013/491497

Kim, Y. B., Uotani, S., Pierroz, D. D., Flier, J. S., and Kahn, B. B. (2000). *In vivo* administration of leptin activates signal transduction directly in insulin-sensitive tissues: overlapping but distinct pathways from insulin. *Endocrinology* 141, 2328–2339. doi: 10.1210/en.141.7.2328

Kollias, H. D., and McDermott, J. C. (2008). Transforming growth factor-beta and myostatin signaling in skeletal muscle. *J. Appl. Physiol.* 104, 579-587. doi: 10.1152/japplphysiol.01091.2007

Kuhlmann, J., Neumann-Haefelin, C., Belz, U., Kalisch, J., Juretschke, H. P., Stein, M., et al. (2003). Intramyocellular lipid and insulin resistance: a longitudinal *in vivo* 1H-spectroscopic study in Zucker diabetic fatty rats. *Diabetes* 52, 138–144. doi: 10.2337/diabetes.52.1.138

Kurtz, T. W., Morris, R. C., and Pershadsingh, H. A. (1989). The Zucker fatty rat as a genetic model of obesity and hypertension. *Hypertension* 13, 896–901. doi: 10.1161/01.HYP.13.6.896

Kusminski, C. M., Shetty, S., Orci, L., Unger, R. H., and Scherer, P. E. (2009). Diabetes and apoptosis: lipotoxicity. *Apoptosis* 14, 1484–1495. doi: 10.1007/s10495-009-0352-8

Langen, R. C., Schols, A. M., Kelders, M. C., Van Der Velden, J. L., Wouters, E. F., and Janssen-Heininger, Y. M. (2006). Muscle wasting and impaired muscle regeneration in a murine model of chronic pulmonary inflammation. *Am. J. Respir. Cell Mol. Biol.* 35, 689–696. doi: 10.1165/rcmb.2006-0103OC

Langen, R. C., Schols, A. M., Kelders, M. C., Wouters, E. F., and Janssen-Heininger, Y. M. (2001). Inflammatory cytokines inhibit myogenic differentiation through activation of nuclear factor-kappaB. *FASEB J.* 15, 1169–1180. doi: 10.1096/fj.00-0463

Langley, B., Thomas, M., Bishop, A., Sharma, M., Gilmour, S., and Kambadur, R. (2002). Myostatin inhibits myoblast differentiation by down-regulating MyoD expression. *J. Biol. Chem.* 277, 49831–49840. doi: 10.1074/jbc.M204291200

Lavie, C. J., Milani, R. V., and Ventura, H. O. (2009). Obesity and cardiovascular disease: risk factor, paradox, and impact of weight loss. *J. Am. Coll. Cardiol.* 53, 1925–1932. doi: 10.1016/j.jacc.2008.12.068

Layne, M. D., and Farmer, S. R. (1999). Tumor necrosis factor-alpha and basic fibroblast growth factor differentially inhibit the insulin-like growth factor-I induced expression of myogenin in C2C12 myoblasts. *Exp. Cell Res.* 249, 177–187. doi: 10.1006/excr.1999.4465

Lee, S., Kim, Y., White, D. A., Kuk, J. L., and Arslanian, S. (2012a). Relationships between insulin sensitivity, skeletal muscle mass and muscle quality in obese adolescent boys. *Eur. J. Clin. Nutr.* 66, 1366–1368. doi: 10.1038/ejcn.2012.142

Lee, S. J., Huynh, T. V., Lee, Y. S., Sebald, S. M., Wilcox-Adelman, S. A., Iwamori, N., et al. (2012b). Role of satellite cells versus myofibers in muscle hypertrophy induced by inhibition of the myostatin/activin signaling pathway. *Proc. Natl. Acad. Sci. U.S.A.* 109, E2353–E2360. doi: 10.1073/pnas.1206410109

Lee, S. Y., Kim, J. R., Ha, M. Y., Shim, S. M., and Park, T. S. (2013). Measurements of diacylglycerols in skeletal muscle by atmospheric pressure chemical ionization mass spectrometry. *Lipids* 48, 287–296. doi: 10.1007/s11745-013-3766-6

Lelliott, C., and Vidal-Puig, A. J. (2004). Lipotoxicity, an imbalance between lipogenesis de novo and fatty acid oxidation. *Int. J. Obes. Relat. Metab. Disord.* 28(Suppl. 4), S22–S28. doi: 10.1038/sj.ijo.0802854

Lepper, C., Partridge, T. A., and Fan, C. M. (2011). An absolute requirement for Pax7-positive satellite cells in acute injury-induced skeletal muscle regeneration. *Development* 138, 3639–3646. doi: 10.1242/dev.067595

Lesault, P. F., Theret, M., Magnan, M., Cuvellier, S., Niu, Y., Gherardi, R. K., et al. (2012). Macrophages improve survival, proliferation and migration of engrafted myogenic precursor cells into MDX skeletal muscle. *PLoS ONE* 7:e46698. doi: 10.1371/journal.pone.0046698

Levak-Frank, S., Radner, H., Walsh, A., Stollberger, R., Knipping, G., Hoefler, G., et al. (1995). Muscle-specific overexpression of lipoprotein lipase causes a severe myopathy characterized by proliferation of mitochondria and peroxisomes in transgenic mice. *J. Clin. Invest.* 96, 976–986. doi: 10.1172/JCI118145

Li, Y., Soos, T. J., Li, X., Wu, J., Degennaro, M., Sun, X., et al. (2004). Protein kinase C Theta inhibits insulin signaling by phosphorylating IRS1 at Ser(1101). *J. Biol. Chem.* 279, 45304–45307. doi: 10.1074/jbc.C400186200

Li, Y. P. (2003). TNF-alpha is a mitogen in skeletal muscle. *Am. J. Physiol. Cell Physiol.* 285, C370–C376. doi: 10.1152/ajpcell.00453.2002

Liu, D., Black, B. L., and Derynck, R. (2001). TGF-beta inhibits muscle differentiation through functional repression of myogenic transcription factors by Smad3. *Genes Dev.* 15, 2950–2966. doi: 10.1101/gad.925901

Madaro, L., Pelle, A., Nicoletti, C., Crupi, A., Marrocco, V., Bossi, G., et al. (2012). PKC theta ablation improves healing in a mouse model of muscular dystrophy. *PLoS ONE* 7:e31515. doi: 10.1371/journal.pone.0031515

Maffei, M., Halaas, J., Ravussin, E., Pratley, R. E., Lee, G. H., Zhang, Y., et al. (1995). Leptin levels in human and rodent: measurement of plasma leptin and ob RNA in obese and weight-reduced subjects. *Nat. Med.* 1, 1155–1161. doi: 10.1038/nm1195-1155

Magnusson, Y. K., Friberg, P., Sjovall, P., Malm, J., and Chen, Y. (2008). TOF-SIMS analysis of lipid accumulation in the skeletal muscle of ob/ob mice. *Obesity (Silver Spring)* 16, 2745–2753. doi: 10.1038/oby.2008.424

Malenfant, P., Joanisse, D. R., Theriault, R., Goodpaster, B. H., Kelley, D. E., and Simoneau, J. A. (2001). Fat content in individual muscle fibers of lean and obese subjects. *Int. J. Obes. Relat. Metab. Disord.* 25, 1316–1321. doi: 10.1038/sj.ijo.0801733

Mann, C. J., Perdiguero, E., Kharraz, Y., Aguilar, S., Pessina, P., Serrano, A. L., et al. (2011). Aberrant repair and fibrosis development in skeletal muscle. *Skelet. Muscle* 1, 21. doi: 10.1186/2044-5040-1-21

Marino, J. S., Hinds, T. D. Jr., Potter, R. A., Ondrus, E., Onion, J. L., Dowling, A., et al. (2013). Suppression of protein kinase C theta contributes to enhanced myogenesis *in vitro* via IRS1 and ERK1/2 phosphorylation. *BMC Cell Biol.* 14:39. doi: 10.1186/1471-2121-14-39

Maroni, P., Bendinelli, P., and Piccoletti, R. (2003). Early intracellular events induced by *in vivo* leptin treatment in mouse skeletal muscle. *Mol. Cell Endocrinol.* 201, 109–121. doi: 10.1016/S0303-7207(02)00427-6

Maroni, P., Bendinelli, P., and Piccoletti, R. (2005). Intracellular signal transduction pathways induced by leptin in C2C12 cells. *Cell. Biol. Int.* 29, 542–550. doi: 10.1016/j.cellbi.2005.03.008

Marotta, M., Ferrer-Martnez, A., Parnau, J., Turini, M., Mace, K., and Gomez Foix, A. M. (2004). Fiber type- and fatty acid composition-dependent effects of high-fat diets on rat muscle triacylglyceride and fatty acid transporter protein-1 content. *Metabolism* 53, 1032–1036. doi: 10.1016/j.metabol.2004.03.011

Martin, S. S., Qasim, A., and Reilly, M. P. (2008). Leptin resistance: a possible interface of inflammation and metabolism in obesity-related cardiovascular disease. *J. Am. Coll. Cardiol.* 52, 1201–1210. doi: 10.1016/j.jacc.2008.05.060

Massimino, M. L., Rapizzi, E., Cantini, M., Libera, L. D., Mazzoleni, F., Arslan, P., et al. (1997). ED2+ macrophages increase selectively myoblast proliferation in muscle cultures. *Biochem. Biophys. Res. Commun.* 235, 754–759. doi: 10.1006/bbrc.1997.6823

McCarthy, J. J., Mula, J., Miyazaki, M., Erfani, R., Garrison, K., Farooqui, A. B., et al. (2011). Effective fiber hypertrophy in satellite cell-depleted skeletal muscle. *Development* 138, 3657–3666. doi: 10.1242/dev.068858

McCroskery, S., Thomas, M., Maxwell, L., Sharma, M., and Kambadur, R. (2003). Myostatin negatively regulates satellite cell activation and self-renewal. *J. Cell. Biol.* 162, 1135–1147. doi: 10.1083/jcb.200207056

Mebarek, S., Komati, H., Naro, F., Zeiller, C., Alvisi, M., Lagarde, M., et al. (2007). Inhibition of de novo ceramide synthesis upregulates phospholipase D and enhances myogenic differentiation. *J. Cell. Sci.* 120, 407–416. doi: 10.1242/jcs.03331

Merly, F., Lescaudron, L., Rouaud, T., Crossin, F., and Gardahaut, M. F. (1999). Macrophages enhance muscle satellite cell proliferation and delay their differentiation. *Muscle Nerve* 22, 724–732. doi: 10.1002/(SICI)1097-4598(199906)22:6<724::AID-MUS9>3.0.CO;2-O

Messina, S., Mazzeo, A., Bitto, A., Aguennouz, M., Migliorato, A., De Pasquale, M. G., et al. (2007). VEGF overexpression via adeno-associated virus gene transfer promotes skeletal muscle regeneration and enhances muscle function in mdx mice. *FASEB J.* 21, 3737–3746. doi: 10.1096/fj.07-8459com

Miller, S. C., Ito, H., Blau, H. M., and Torti, F. M. (1988). Tumor necrosis factor inhibits human myogenesis *in vitro*. *Mol. Cell Biol.* 8, 2295–2301.

Mittendorfer, B., Magkos, F., Fabbrini, E., Mohammed, B. S., and Klein, S. (2009). Relationship between body fat mass and free fatty acid kinetics in men and women. *Obesity (Silver Spring)* 17, 1872–1877. doi: 10.1038/oby.2009.224

Nguyen, M. H., Cheng, M., and Koh, T. J. (2011). Impaired muscle regeneration in ob/ob and db/db mice. *ScientificWorldJournal* 11, 1525–1535. doi: 10.1100/tsw.2011.137

Ochoa, O., Sun, D., Reyes-Reyna, S. M., Waite, L. L., Michalek, J. E., McManus, L. M., et al. (2007). Delayed angiogenesis and VEGF production in CCR2-/- mice during impaired skeletal muscle regeneration. *Am. J. Physiol. Regul. Integr. Comp. Physiol.* 293, R651–R661. doi: 10.1152/ajpregu.00069.2007

Paturi, S., Gutta, A. K., Kakarla, S. K., Katta, A., Arnold, E. C., Wu, M., et al. (2010). Impaired overload-induced hypertrophy in obese Zucker rat slow-twitch skeletal muscle. *J. Appl. Physiol.* 108, 7–13. doi: 10.1152/japplphysiol.00330.2009

Penton, C. M., Thomas-Ahner, J. M., Johnson, E. K., McAllister, C., and Montanaro, F. (2013). Muscle side population cells from dystrophic or injured muscle adopt a fibro-adipogenic fate. *PLOS ONE* 8:e54553. doi: 10.1371/journal.pone.0054553

Peterson, J. M., Bryner, R. W., and Alway, S. E. (2008a). Satellite cell proliferation is reduced in muscles of obese Zucker rats but restored with loading. *Am. J. Physiol. Cell Physiol.* 295, C521–C528. doi: 10.1152/ajpcell.00073.2008

Peterson, J. M., Wang, Y., Bryner, R. W., Williamson, D. L., and Alway, S. E. (2008b). Bax signaling regulates palmitate-mediated apoptosis in C(2)C(12) myotubes. *Am. J. Physiol. Endocrinol. Metab.* 295, E1307–E1314. doi: 10.1152/ajpendo.00738.2007

Petrella, J. K., Kim, J. S., Mayhew, D. L., Cross, J. M., and Bamman, M. M. (2008). Potent myofiber hypertrophy during resistance training in humans is associated with satellite cell-mediated myonuclear addition: a cluster analysis. *J. Appl. Physiol. (1985)* 104, 1736-1742. doi: 10.1152/japplphysiol.01215.2007

Pijet, M., Pijet, B., Litwiniuk, A., Pajak, B., Gajkowska, B., and Orzechowski, A. (2013). Leptin impairs myogenesis in C2C12 cells through JAK/STAT and MEK signaling pathways. *Cytokine* 61, 445–454. doi: 10.1016/j.cyto.2012.11.002

Powell, D. J., Hajduch, E., Kular, G., and Hundal, H. S. (2003). Ceramide disables 3-phosphoinositide binding to the pleckstrin homology domain of protein kinase B (PKB)/Akt by a PKCzeta-dependent mechanism. *Mol. Cell Biol.* 23, 7794–7808. doi: 10.1128/MCB.23.21.7794-7808.2003

Powell, D. J., Turban, S., Gray, A., Hajduch, E., and Hundal, H. S. (2004). Intracellular ceramide synthesis and protein kinase Czeta activation play an essential role in palmitate-induced insulin resistance in rat L6 skeletal muscle cells. *Biochem. J.* 382, 619–629. doi: 10.1042/BJ20040139

Purchas, R. W., Romsos, D. R., Allen, R. E., and Merkel, R. A. (1985). Muscle growth and satellite cell proliferative activity in obese (OB/OB) mice. *J. Anim. Sci.* 60, 644–651.

Rachek, L. I., Musiyenko, S. I., Ledoux, S. P., and Wilson, G. L. (2007). Palmitate induced mitochondrial deoxyribonucleic acid damage and apoptosis in l6 rat skeletal muscle cells. *Endocrinology* 148, 293–299. doi: 10.1210/en.2006-0998

Radley, H. G., De Luca, A., Lynch, G. S., and Grounds, M. D. (2007). Duchenne muscular dystrophy: focus on pharmaceutical and nutritional interventions. *Int. J. Biochem. Cell Biol.* 39, 469–477. doi: 10.1016/j.biocel.2006.09.009

Raso, G. M., Pacilio, M., Esposito, E., Coppola, A., Di Carlo, R., and Meli, R. (2002). Leptin potentiates IFN-gamma-induced expression of nitric oxide synthase and cyclo-oxygenase-2 in murine macrophage J774A.1. *Br. J. Pharmacol.* 137, 799–804. doi: 10.1038/sj.bjp.0704903

Rodrigues Ade, C., and Schmalbruch, H. (1995). Satellite cells and myonuclei in long-term denervated rat muscles. *Anat. Rec.* 243, 430–437. doi: 10.1002/ar.1092430405

Rosenblatt, J. D., Yong, D., and Parry, D. J. (1994). Satellite cell activity is required for hypertrophy of overloaded adult rat muscle. *Muscle Nerve* 17, 608–613. doi: 10.1002/mus.880170607

Ryall, J. G. (2012). The role of sirtuins in the regulation of metabolic homeostasis in skeletal muscle. *Curr. Opin. Clin. Nutr. Metab. Care* 15, 561–566. doi: 10.1097/MCO.0b013e3283590914

Ryall, J. G. (2013). Metabolic reprogramming as a novel regulator of skeletal muscle development and regeneration. *FEBS J* 280, 4004–4013. doi: 10.1111/febs.12189

Sainz, N., Rodriguez, A., Catalan, V., Becerril, S., Ramirez, B., Gomez-Ambrosi, J., et al. (2009). Leptin administration favors muscle mass accretion by decreasing FoxO3a and increasing PGC-1alpha in ob/ob mice. *PLoS ONE* 4:e6808. doi: 10.1371/journal.pone.0006808

Salehian, B., Mahabadi, V., Bilas, J., Taylor, W. E., and Ma, K. (2006). The effect of glutamine on prevention of glucocorticoid-induced skeletal muscle atrophy is associated with myostatin suppression. *Metabolism* 55, 1239–1247. doi: 10.1016/j.metabol.2006.05.009

Salinas, M., Lopez-Valdaliso, R., Martin, D., Alvarez, A., and Cuadrado, A. (2000). Inhibition of PKB/Akt1 by C2-ceramide involves activation of ceramide-activated protein phosphatase in PC12 cells. *Mol. Cell. Neurosci.* 15, 156–169. doi: 10.1006/mcne.1999.0813

Samuel, V. T., Petersen, K. F., and Shulman, G. I. (2010). Lipid-induced insulin resistance: unravelling the mechanism. *Lancet* 375, 2267–2277. doi: 10.1016/S0140-6736(10)60408-4

Samuel, V. T., and Shulman, G. I. (2012). Mechanisms for insulin resistance: common threads and missing links. *Cell* 148, 852–871. doi: 10.1016/j.cell.2012.02.017

Santos-Alvarez, J., Goberna, R., and Sanchez-Margalet, V. (1999). Human leptin stimulates proliferation and activation of human circulating monocytes. *Cell. Immunol.* 194, 6–11. doi: 10.1006/cimm.1999.1490

Sartorelli, V., and Fulco, M. (2004). Molecular and cellular determinants of skeletal muscle atrophy and hypertrophy. *Sci. STKE* 2004, re11. doi: 10.1126/stke.2442004re11

Simoneau, J. A., Colberg, S. R., Thaete, F. L., and Kelley, D. E. (1995). Skeletal muscle glycolytic and oxidative enzyme capacities are determinants of insulin sensitivity and muscle composition in obese women. *FASEB J.* 9, 273–278.

Sinha, R., Dufour, S., Petersen, K. F., Lebon, V., Enoksson, S., Ma, Y. Z., et al. (2002). Assessment of skeletal muscle triglyceride content by (1)H nuclear magnetic resonance spectroscopy in lean and obese adolescents: relationships to insulin sensitivity, total body fat, and central adiposity. *Diabetes* 51, 1022–1027. doi: 10.2337/diabetes.51.4.1022

Sishi, B., Loos, B., Ellis, B., Smith, W., Du Toit, E. F., and Engelbrecht, A. M. (2011). Diet-induced obesity alters signalling pathways and induces atrophy and apoptosis in skeletal muscle in a prediabetic rat model. *Exp. Physiol.* 96, 179–193. doi: 10.1113/expphysiol.2010.054189

Sitnick, M., Bodine, S. C., and Rutledge, J. C. (2009). Chronic high fat feeding attenuates load-induced hypertrophy in mice. *J. Physiol.* 587, 5753–5765. doi: 10.1113/jphysiol.2009.180174

Spiller, M. P., Kambadur, R., Jeanplong, F., Thomas, M., Martyn, J. K., Bass, J. J., et al. (2002). The myostatin gene is a downstream target gene of basic helix-loop-helix transcription factor MyoD. *Mol. Cell Biol.* 22, 7066–7082. doi: 10.1128/MCB.22.20.7066-7082.2002

Stratford, S., Hoehn, K. L., Liu, F., and Summers, S. A. (2004). Regulation of insulin action by ceramide: dual mechanisms linking ceramide accumulation to the inhibition of Akt/protein kinase B. *J. Biol. Chem.* 279, 36608–36615. doi: 10.1074/jbc.M406499200

Strle, K., Broussard, S. R., McCusker, R. H., Shen, W. H., Johnson, R. W., Freund, G. G., et al. (2004). Proinflammatory cytokine impairment of insulin-like growth factor I-induced protein synthesis in skeletal muscle myoblasts requires ceramide. *Endocrinology* 145, 4592–4602. doi: 10.1210/en.2003-1749

Tamilarasan, K. P., Temmel, H., Das, S. K., Al Zoughbi, W., Schauer, S., Vesely, P. W., et al. (2012). Skeletal muscle damage and impaired regeneration due to LPL-mediated lipotoxicity. *Cell Death Dis.* 3, e354. doi: 10.1038/cddis.2012.91

Taylor, W. E., Bhasin, S., Artaza, J., Byhower, F., Azam, M., Willard, D. H. Jr., et al. (2001). Myostatin inhibits cell proliferation and protein synthesis in C2C12 muscle cells. *Am. J. Physiol. Endocrinol. Metab.* 280, E221–E228.

Thiele, C., and Spandl, J. (2008). Cell biology of lipid droplets. *Curr. Opin. Cell Biol.* 20, 378–385. doi: 10.1016/j.ceb.2008.05.009

Thomas, M., Langley, B., Berry, C., Sharma, M., Kirk, S., Bass, J., et al. (2000). Myostatin, a negative regulator of muscle growth, functions by inhibiting myoblast proliferation. *J. Biol. Chem.* 275, 40235–40243. doi: 10.1074/jbc.M004356200

Timmers, S., Schrauwen, P., and De Vogel, J. (2008). Muscular diacylglycerol metabolism and insulin resistance. *Physiol. Behav.* 94, 242–251. doi: 10.1016/j.physbeh.2007.12.002

Torrente, Y., El Fahime, E., Caron, N. J., Del Bo, R., Belicchi, M., Pisati, F., et al. (2003). Tumor necrosis factor-alpha (TNF-alpha) stimulates chemotactic response in mouse myogenic cells. *Cell Transplant.* 12, 91–100. doi: 10.3727/000000003783985115

Toth, K. G., McKay, B. R., De Lisio, M., Little, J. P., Tarnopolsky, M. A., and Parise, G. (2011). IL-6 induced STAT3 signalling is associated with the proliferation of human muscle satellite cells following acute muscle damage. *PLoS ONE* 6:e17392. doi: 10.1371/journal.pone.0017392

Trendelenburg, A. U., Meyer, A., Jacobi, C., Feige, J. N., and Glass, D. J. (2012). TAK-1/p38/nNFkappaB signaling inhibits myoblast differentiation by increasing levels of Activin A. *Skelet. Muscle* 2, 3. doi: 10.1186/2044-5040-2-3

Tschop, M., and Heiman, M. L. (2001). Rodent obesity models: an overview. *Exp. Clin. Endocrinol. Diabetes* 109, 307–319. doi: 10.1055/s-2001-17297

Turban, S., and Hajduch, E. (2011). Protein kinase C isoforms: mediators of reactive lipid metabolites in the development of insulin resistance. *FEBS Lett.* 585, 269–274. doi: 10.1016/j.febslet.2010.12.022

Turinsky, J., Bayly, B. P., and O'Sullivan, D. M. (1990). 1,2-Diacylglycerol and ceramide levels in rat skeletal muscle and liver *in vivo*. Studies with insulin, exercise, muscle denervation, and vasopressin. *J. Biol. Chem.* 265, 7933–7938.

Turner, N., Kowalski, G. M., Leslie, S. J., Risis, S., Yang, C., Lee-Young, R. S., et al. (2013). Distinct patterns of tissue-specific lipid accumulation during the induction of insulin resistance in mice by high-fat feeding. *Diabetologia* 56, 1638–1648. doi: 10.1007/s00125-013-2913-1

Turpin, S. M., Lancaster, G. I., Darby, I., Febbraio, M. A., and Watt, M. J. (2006). Apoptosis in skeletal muscle myotubes is induced by ceramides and is positively related to insulin resistance. *Am. J. Physiol. Endocrinol. Metab.* 291, E1341–E1350. doi: 10.1152/ajpendo.00095.2006

Turpin, S. M., Ryall, J. G., Southgate, R., Darby, I., Hevener, A. L., Febbraio, M. A., et al. (2009). Examination of 'lipotoxicity' in skeletal muscle of high-fat fed and ob/ob mice. *J. Physiol.* 587, 1593–1605. doi: 10.1113/jphysiol.2008.166033

Uezumi, A., Fukada, S., Yamamoto, N., Takeda, S., and Tsuchida, K. (2010). Mesenchymal progenitors distinct from satellite cells contribute to ectopic fat cell formation in skeletal muscle. *Nat. Cell Biol.* 12, 143–152. doi: 10.1038/ncb2014

Unger, R. H. (2003). Minireview: weapons of lean body mass destruction: the role of ectopic lipids in the metabolic syndrome. *Endocrinology* 144, 5159–5165. doi: 10.1210/en.2003-0870

Unger, R. H., Clark, G. O., Scherer, P. E., and Orci, L. (2010). Lipid homeostasis, lipotoxicity and the metabolic syndrome. *Biochim. Biophys. Acta* 1801, 209–214. doi: 10.1016/j.bbalip.2009.10.006

Ussher, J. R., Koves, T. R., Cadete, V. J., Zhang, L., Jaswal, J. S., Swyrd, S. J., et al. (2010). Inhibition of de novo ceramide synthesis reverses diet-induced insulin resistance and enhances whole-body oxygen consumption. *Diabetes* 59, 2453–2464. doi: 10.2337/db09-1293

Van Herpen, N. A., and Schrauwen-Hinderling, V. B. (2008). Lipid accumulation in non-adipose tissue and lipotoxicity. *Physiol. Behav.* 94, 231–241. doi: 10.1016/j.physbeh.2007.11.049

Vincent, A. M., Callaghan, B. C., Smith, A. L., and Feldman, E. L. (2011). Diabetic neuropathy: cellular mechanisms as therapeutic targets. *Nat. Rev. Neurol.* 7, 573–583. doi: 10.1038/nrneurol.2011.137

Wang, X., Wu, H., Zhang, Z., Liu, S., Yang, J., Chen, X., et al. (2008). Effects of interleukin-6, leukemia inhibitory factor, and ciliary neurotrophic factor on the proliferation and differentiation of adult human myoblasts. *Cell Mol. Neurobiol.* 28, 113–124. doi: 10.1007/s10571-007-9247-9

Wang, Y. X., and Rudnicki, M. A. (2012). Satellite cells, the engines of muscle repair. *Nat. Rev. Mol. Cell Biol.* 13, 127–133. doi: 10.1038/nrm3265

Warren, G. L., Hulderman, T., Mishra, D., Gao, X., Millecchia, L., O'Farrell, L., et al. (2005). Chemokine receptor CCR2 involvement in skeletal muscle regeneration. *FASEB J.* 19, 413–415. doi: 10.1096/fj.04-2421fje

Warren, G. L., Summan, M., Gao, X., Chapman, R., Hulderman, T., and Simeonova, P. P. (2007). Mechanisms of skeletal muscle injury and repair revealed by gene expression studies in mouse models. *J. Physiol.* 582, 825–841. doi: 10.1113/jphysiol.2007.132373

Watts, R., McAinch, A. J., Dixon, J. B., O'Brien, P. E., and Cameron-Smith, D. (2013). Increased Smad signaling and reduced MRF expression in skeletal muscle from obese subjects. *Obesity (Silver Spring)* 21, 525–528. doi: 10.1002/oby.20070

Wellen, K. E., and Hotamisligil, G. S. (2005). Inflammation, stress, and diabetes. *J. Clin. Invest.* 115, 1111–1119. doi: 10.1172/JCI200525102

Will, K., Kalbe, C., Kuzinski, J., Losel, D., Viergutz, T., Palin, M. F., et al. (2012). Effects of leptin and adiponectin on proliferation and protein metabolism of porcine myoblasts. *Histochem. Cell Biol.* 138, 271–287. doi: 10.1007/s00418-012-0949-9

Woo, M., Isganaitis, E., Cerletti, M., Fitzpatrick, C., Wagers, A. J., Jimenez-Chillaron, J., et al. (2011). Early life nutrition modulates muscle stem cell number: implications for muscle mass and repair. *Stem Cells Dev.* 20, 1763–1769. doi: 10.1089/scd.2010.0349

World Health Organization. (2013). Obesity and overweight Fact Sheet N°311. WHO Media Centre. Geneva, Switzerland.

Ye, Q., Danzer, C. F., Fuchs, A., Krek, W., Mueggler, T., Baltes, C., et al. (2011). Longitudinal evaluation of intramyocellular lipids (IMCLs) in tibialis anterior muscle of ob/ob and ob/+ control mice using a cryogenic surface coil at 9.4 T. *NMR Biomed.* 24, 1295–1301. doi: 10.1002/nbm.1691

Ylitalo, K. R., Sowers, M., and Heeringa, S. (2011). Peripheral vascular disease and peripheral neuropathy in individuals with cardiometabolic clustering and obesity: National Health and Nutrition Examination Survey 2001–2004. *Diabetes Care* 34, 1642–1647. doi: 10.2337/dc10-2150

Yu, C., Chen, Y., Cline, G. W., Zhang, D., Zong, H., Wang, Y., et al. (2002). Mechanism by which fatty acids inhibit insulin activation of insulin receptor substrate-1 (IRS-1)-associated phosphatidylinositol 3-kinase activity in muscle. *J. Biol. Chem.* 277, 50230–50236. doi: 10.1074/jbc.M200958200

Yuzefovych, L., Wilson, G., and Rachek, L. (2010). Different effects of oleate vs. palmitate on mitochondrial function, apoptosis, and insulin signaling in L6 skeletal muscle cells: role of oxidative stress. *Am. J. Physiol. Endocrinol. Metab.* 299, E1096–E1105. doi: 10.1152/ajpendo.00238.2010

2

New roles for old enzymes: Killer caspases as the engine of cell behavior changes

Patrick F. Connolly[1], Richard Jäger[2] and Howard O. Fearnhead[1]*

[1] *Pharmacology and Therapeutics, National University of Ireland Galway, Galway, Ireland*
[2] *Department of Natural Sciences, Bonn-Rhein-Sieg University of Applied Sciences, Rheinbach, Germany*

Correspondence:
Howard O. Fearnhead, National University of Ireland Galway, Biological Sciences Building, University Road, Galway, Ireland
e-mail: howard.fearnhead@nuigalway.ie

It has become increasingly clear that caspases, far from being merely cell death effectors, have a much wider range of functions within the cell. These functions are as diverse as signal transduction and cytoskeletal remodeling, and caspases are now known to have an essential role in cell proliferation, migration, and differentiation. There is also evidence that apoptotic cells themselves can direct the behavior of nearby cells through the caspase-dependent secretion of paracrine signaling factors. In some processes, including the differentiation of skeletal muscle myoblasts, both caspase activation in differentiating cells as well as signaling from apoptotic cells has been reported. Here, we review the non-apoptotic outcomes of caspase activity in a range of different model systems and attempt to integrate this knowledge.

Keywords: caspase, apoptosis, myogenesis, proliferation, differentiation, non-apoptotic roles

INTRODUCTION

Caspases are intracellular cysteine proteases that cut after specific aspartic acid residues. In mammals, 18 caspases have been characterized (**Table 1**), the majority of them playing roles in mediating apoptotic cell-demolition (Cohen, 1997). During apoptosis, these "killer caspases" cleave numerous cellular proteins, and they are the primary effectors responsible for taking apart the cell during apoptosis, playing a major proteolytic role in the disassembly of the nucleus and the cytoskeletal structure (Lüthi and Martin, 2007).

Caspases are present in all cells as inactive zymogens, called procaspases. They are activated through cleavage to generate the subunits that form an active caspase (Pop and Salvesen, 2009). At the apex of the activation cascade are the so-called initiator caspases (**Table 1**). Upon exposure to an apoptotic stimulus they become recruited to specific adaptor proteins which then assemble into activation platforms, which are large multimeric protein complexes mediating activation of the initiator caspases (reviewed in Mace and Riedl, 2010). Initiators activate downstream effectors which rapidly disassemble the cell. The ability of these caspases to kill cells is controlled, in part, by the inhibitor of apoptosis proteins (IAPs) which bind to active caspases and either inhibit proteolytic activity or induce ubiquitin-mediated caspase degradation (Mace et al., 2010).

Different activation platforms classify the main apoptotic pathways. The extrinsic pathway is initiated at the cell membrane by ligands of receptors of the tumor necrosis factor (TNF) receptor family. Ligand-binding leads to assembly of the death-inducing signaling complex (DISC) containing these receptors. Caspase-8 and -10 are recruited to the DISC and then activated, in a process that requires the adaptor protein FADD. The intrinsic pathway is initiated by mitochondria, whose outer membranes become permeable to cytochrome *c* upon certain cellular stresses. Released cytochrome *c* then binds to the adaptor protein APAF-1 which subsequently assembles into a large heptameric protein complex, the so-called apoptosome, which is the activation platform for caspase-9. The release of cytochrome *c* is controlled by proteins of the Bcl-2 family (Tait and Green, 2010). Concomitant with release of cytochrome *c*, other small proteins may be released, some of which block IAPs allowing for unrestrained caspase activation.

The majority of studies of caspases have focused on their roles as cell killers. There were some notable exceptions describing caspase-dependent cellular differentiation processes that involve denucleation or other degenerative events (Fernando and Megeney, 2007), but these appear to represent a limited or frustrated apoptosis, rather than a fundamentally different process. More recently, the study of apoptotic caspases has broadened to include caspase-dependent paracrine signaling from apoptotic cells to explain how apoptotic cells alter the behavior of surrounding cells (Li et al., 2010a).

However, it has also emerged that apoptosis-associated caspases play non-apoptotic roles and that they are not simply destructive. Examples of these are cell differentiation (Fernando and Kelly, 2002), embryonic development (Miura, 2012; Suzanne and Steller, 2013), motility (Barbero et al., 2009), and compensatory proliferation (Fan and Bergmann, 2008). Within these processes, the "killer" caspases clearly do not cause cell demolition. This gives caspases an entirely new role in determining the fate or behavior of cells. Thus, caspases drive in a far wider range of cellular behaviors than previously known.

There are several theories to explain how apoptotic caspases can lead to non-apoptotic outcomes (**Figure 1**). In one mechanism, the "cell-autonomous" or "direct" model, caspase activity leads to altered cell behavior through the modulation of regulatory networks, such as through cleavage of cell cycle repressors to alter cell proliferation (Schwerk and Schulze-Osthoff, 2003; Woo et al., 2003), activation of gene transcription to induce skeletal

Table 1 | Roles of caspases.

Caspase	Conventional role	Other roles
Caspase-1	Inflammatory response (Kuranaga and Miura, 2007)	Unknown
Caspase-2	Apoptosis (Initiator) (Inoue et al., 2009)	DNA damage response (Fava et al., 2012)
Caspase-3	Apoptosis (Executioner) (Kuranaga and Miura, 2007)	Differentiation of many cell types (see **Table 2**)
Caspase-5	Inflammatory response (Fuchs and Steller, 2011)	Possibly tumor suppression (Soung et al., 2008)
Caspase-6	Apoptosis (Initiator) (Inoue et al., 2009)	Unknown
Caspase-7	Apoptosis (Executioner) (Inoue et al., 2009)	Unknown
Caspase-8	Apoptosis (Executioner) (Fuchs and Steller, 2011)	Embryonic development (Suzanne and Steller, 2013), motility (Helfer et al., 2006), tumor metastasis (Barbero et al., 2009), T-cell proliferation (Kennedy et al., 1999), cell cycle regulation (Zhang et al., 2001; Hashimoto et al., 2011), bacterial infection response (Kayagaki et al., 2011)
Caspase-9	Apoptosis (Initiator) (Cohen, 1997)	Differentiation of many cell types (see **Table 2**)
Caspase-10	Apoptosis (Initiator) (Inoue et al., 2009)	Immune response to dsRNA (Takahashi et al., 2006), possible tumor suppressor (Park et al., 2002)
Caspase-11	Inflammatory response (Li et al., 2007)	Cell migration (Li et al., 2007)
Caspase-12	Inflammatory response (Leulier et al., 2000)	Unknown
Caspase-14	Keratinocyte differentiation (Zermati et al., 2001)	Unknown
Caspase-15	Apoptosis (Initiator) (Eckhart et al., 2005)	Unknown
Caspase-16	Unknown, phylogenetic association with caspase-14 (Eckhart et al., 2008)	Unknown
Caspase-17	Unknown, phylogenetic association with caspase-3 (Eckhart et al., 2008)	Unknown
Caspase-18	Unknown, phylogenetic association with caspase-8 (Eckhart et al., 2008)	Unknown

The majority of caspases are primarily involved in programmed cell death, and the minority are primarily involved in the generation of immune responses. Most have been discovered to play other roles as well.

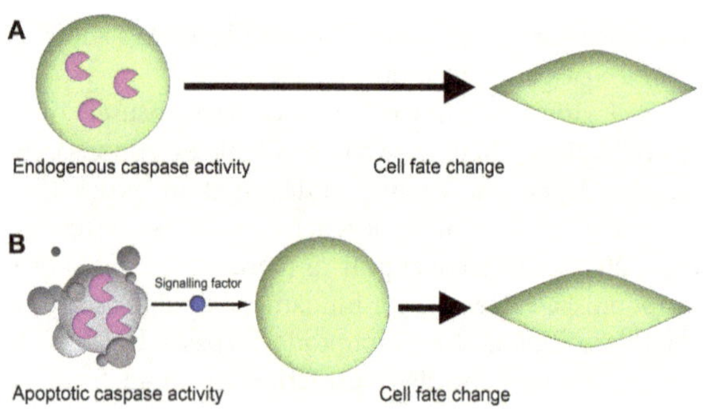

FIGURE 1 | Cell-autonomous vs. non-cell-autonomous models of caspase signaling. (A) Cell-autonomous model. In the proliferating cell, a non-apoptotic caspase signaling pathway leads to a change in cell behavior through modulation of gene expression, cytoskeletal restructuring, or other means. This signaling is endogenous to the proliferating cell itself, and no apoptotic cell signaling is involved. **(B)** Non-cell-autonomous model. In this model, caspase activity within apoptotic cells lead to the generation of signaling factors which stimulate the cell behavior change of nearby cells in a paracrine fashion.

muscle differentiation (Larsen and Megeney, 2010) or cleavage of cytoskeletal proteins to influence cell motility (Helfer et al., 2006). In these cases the caspase activity is "autonomous" in that the entire process of caspase activation, cleavage of substrates, and downstream effects on cell behavior all occur within the same cell.

In this cell autonomous model, it is as yet unclear how apoptotic caspase activity is harnessed for non-apoptotic purposes without killing the cell, although work in *Drosophila melanogaster* has begun to unravel this problem. For example, a recent report of caspase activation in *Drosophila* proposes a model in which both the magnitude and rate of caspase activation is controlled, which can give rise to high (apoptotic) levels of caspase activity as well as low (non-apoptotic) levels of activity (Florentin and Arama, 2012). It is also possible that, unlike the traditional model where executioner caspases are only activated upon receipt of a cell stress signal, there is a constant basal level of activated caspases within the cell, but these are normally held in check by inhibitory mechanisms. Such basal levels of caspase activity have been found in the context of cell behavior changes in glioblastoma cells, where low levels of constitutively-active caspase-8 and -3 are found to be necessary for cell migration and invasion (Gdynia et al., 2007). Along with this, relatively high levels of caspases activity may be tolerated if they can be sequestered within their target organelle or sub-cellular region, as is observed in the dendritic pruning of neurons (Williams et al., 2006), in spermatid individualization in Drosophila (Arama et al., 2007; Kaplan et al., 2010), and in the nuclear degradation of keratinocytes (Weil et al., 1999).

In the "non-autonomous" or "indirect" model to explain the role of caspases in non-apoptotic processes, the caspase activity is localized within apoptotic cells, catalyzing the generation of secretory paracrine signaling factors or enabling cell surface-mediated signaling (Hochreiter-Hufford et al., 2013). This model is indirect in that the caspase activity is associated with one cell, while the downstream effect is induced in another cell by an intercellular signaling event. In this model the caspase-mediated non-apoptotic effects do not necessarily require the survival of the "caspase-active" cell, as apoptotic cells are still quite capable of signaling to their environment (Jäger and Fearnhead, 2012).

Here, we review the major non-apoptotic roles of caspases discovered to date, and discuss these findings in light of the direct and indirect theories of caspase signaling, with a particular focus on skeletal muscle. This is a rapidly advancing field of study, and a summation of the current state of the field is necessary.

TISSUE REPAIR AND REGENERATION

Caspases are key players in the homeostatic balance between apoptosis and regeneration used to maintain tissue structure and function. In response to injury, dead cells engage in a signaling behavior which drives the proliferation of cells at the periphery of the site of injury until damaged portion of tissue is replaced with a new section of the same size and shape (**Figure 2**) (Bergmann and Steller, 2010). The role of caspases in repair and regeneration has been demonstrated in several different experimental models.

In the simple metazoan Hydra, surgical-induced injury produces an apoptotic response which stimulates a compensatory proliferative mechanism in surrounding progenitor cells. Treatment with pan-caspase inhibitors abolishes this regenerative response (Cikala et al., 1999; Chera et al., 2009). Regeneration in the amphibian *Xenopus* requires caspase-mediated events (Tseng et al., 2007), as does tissue regeneration in planaria (Fuchs and Steller, 2011), and the regeneration of newt forelimbs (Vlaskalin et al., 2004).

Regeneration of mammalian tissue is never so dramatic but some tissues, like the liver, can undergo remarkable regeneration after injury (Taub, 2004). Liver regeneration and the healing of skin wounds is impaired in caspase-3 and -7 deficient mice, showing that the role of caspases in regenerative processes is conserved in mammals (Li et al., 2010a).

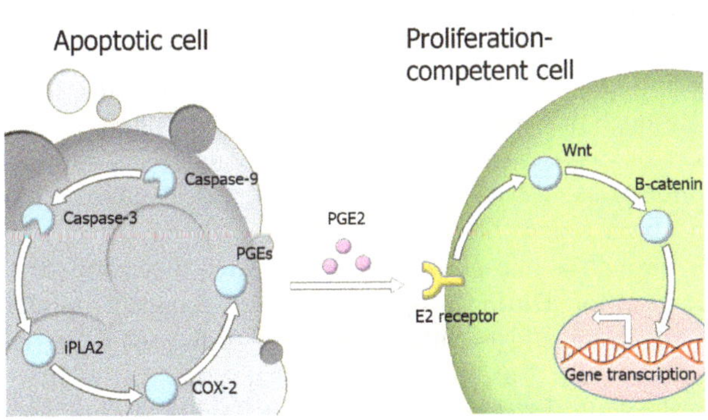

FIGURE 2 | Model of compensatory proliferation. Caspase activity within apoptotic cells leads to the activation of the prostaglandin E2-synthesis pathway. Secreted prostaglandin E2 binds to E2 receptors on proliferation-competent cells, leading to changes in gene expression which trigger proliferation. Abbreviations: iPLA2, Phospholipase A2; COX-2, Cyclooxygenase-2; PGEs, Prostaglandin E synthase; PGE2, Prostaglandin E2.

Paracrine molecules secreted by the apoptotic cells appear to be important in caspase-dependent regeneration. Prostaglandin E2 is one such a molecule, as its production pathway is directly controlled by caspase-3 (Boland et al., 2013), and has a wide number of roles in regeneration and proliferation (Castellone et al., 2005; Goessling et al., 2009; Morata et al., 2011; Beaulieu et al., 2012; Boland et al., 2013). This effect is exerted through transient activation of the Wnt-β-catenin pathway via binding to members of the EP receptor family (Goessling et al., 2009).

Lysophosphatidylcholine (LPC) is another molecule which mediates caspase-activity-induced regenerative responses. It is produced by apoptotic cells, and its presence in the interstitial medium acts as an attraction signal to phagocytes (Lauber et al., 2003). Moreover, LPC induces the differentiation of keratinocytes, which is a necessary step in the wound healing response in skin (Ryborg et al., 2004).

Sphingosine-1-phosphate is another molecule that is secreted by apoptotic cells and is a chemoattractant signal for immune cells (Brecht et al., 2011). It is produced by the enzyme ceramidase, and is a signal that drives growth arrest and differentiation, as well as cell migration and adhesion (Mao and Obeid, 2008), all of which are involved in wound-healing responses.

Fractalkine (CX3CL1) is a large peptide that engages in prosurvival functions in many cell types (White and Greaves, 2012) and is released from apoptotic cells in a caspase-dependant process (Truman et al., 2008). Fractalkine is normally associated with immune cell chemotaxis (Chazaud et al., 2003), but it is also known that soluble fractalkine promotes both migration of endothelial cells and differentiation of osteoblasts (Koizumi et al., 2009). This makes it another potential paracrine signaling factor released by apoptotic cells to modulate tissue regeneration.

From the examples described, it is seen that caspase activity in a dying cell can indirectly induce compensatory proliferation of neighboring cells as part of the regenerative response to injury. Thus, regenerative processes conform to the indirect, apoptotic cell-driven model of caspase function in non-apoptotic processes. However, caspases can also regulate cell proliferation in a cell-autonomous manner through the cleavage of cell cycle regulators.

LYMPHOCYTE PROLIFERATION

There are hundreds of confirmed caspase substrates (Lüthi and Martin, 2007; Johnson and Kornbluth, 2008), although the functional significance of cleavage is often uncertain. Among this large group there are several key cell cycle regulators (Hashimoto et al., 2011) and a series of studies have implicated both initiator and effector caspases in the control of the cell cycle of lymphocytes. Because of this, abnormal caspase activity can lead to either depressed or hyperactive cell proliferation.

Through the DISC adaptor protein FADD, caspases-8 and -10 play a role in cell proliferation (Imtiyaz et al., 2009). Peripheral T-cells from FADD deficient mice show a profound impairment of proliferation once they are activated by mitogens or antigens, leading to a reduced number of mature T-cells (Zhang et al., 1998). This inhibition of proliferation results from a failure to enter the cell cycle at the beginning of S-phase due to abnormal expression of cyclin-dependent kinases (Zhang et al., 2001).

Pharmacological inhibition of caspases prevents T-cell proliferation *in vitro* supporting the idea that caspase activity is required for proliferation (Kennedy et al., 1999). The cell cycle role for caspases may not be limited to T-cells as impaired T-cell, B-cell, and NK-cell proliferation is seen in immune-deficient humans with caspase-8 defects (Chun et al., 2002).

As well as caspases-8 and -10, caspase-3 has also been found to play a role in regulating cell proliferation. Proliferative brain cells were found to contain active caspase-3, localized in the nucleus (Oomman et al., 2005). In lymphoid cells, caspase-3 supports the proliferation through cleavage of the CDK inhibitor p27 (Frost et al., 2001). In these examples, caspase-mediated stimulation of proliferation appears to be a cell-autonomous event. On the other hand, proliferating cells utilize caspases in a non-apoptotic capacity to downregulate cell cycle inhibitors which normally keep the cell in a quiescent state (Zhang et al., 2001; Woo et al., 2003; Lamkanfi et al., 2007). For example, caspase-3 can exert a strongly anti-proliferative effect in B-cells through cleavage of p21 and caspase-3 knockout mice show a hyperproliferative phenotype in their B-cells (Woo et al., 2003). Thus, killer caspases seem to be able to exert both positive and negative regulation of cell proliferation through selective cleavage of cell cycle regulators without necessarily inducing apoptosis.

Caspase-1, which is involved in toxin-sensing (Li et al., 1995; Franchi et al., 2009), and caspase-11, involved in the production of inflammatory factors (Kayagaki et al., 2011) have long been associated with inflammation and immunity and are not central to cell death processes. However, it has more recently been discovered that apoptotic caspases also have roles in immunity. This can be through their role in the differentiation programs of immune cells, such as with caspase-8 paralog Dredd (Leulier et al., 2000), or through the modulation of the immune response itself, such as with caspase-12 (Saleh et al., 2004) and caspase-3 paralog ced-3 (Aballay and Ausubel, 2001). Such modulation may occur through the generation of inflammatory and anti-inflammatory factors (Kuranaga and Miura, 2007) or through their role in the apoptosis of infected cells.

DIFFERENTIATION

Caspases engage in irreversible signal transduction (Kuranaga, 2012). Such irreversible signaling mechanisms are suitable for guiding cell fate choices, such as differentiation. Indeed, such caspase signaling has been found to play important roles in the terminal differentiation programs of several cell types, both in early development, and in tissue regeneration.

The first cell types in which caspases were found to have a direct role in differentiation had one feature in common: their differentiation programs bore a strong resemblance to apoptosis. For example, during terminal differentiation of the lens fiber cells degenerative processes including organelle degradation, chromatin condensation, and DNA fragmentation all occur, and are mediated by the activity of caspases (Ishizaki et al., 1998). The time required for this apoptosis-like process is much longer than that required for caspase-driven cell death, suggesting a more controlled and meticulous version of the same general procedure. Soon after this, erythrocytes and keratinocytes were also found to utilize caspase activity in their terminal differentiation programs (Eckhart et al., 2000; Zermati et al., 2001).

Subsequently, it was found that caspases also play roles in differentiation programs that bore no major similarity to apoptosis. An example of this is the differentiation of peripheral blood monocytes into macrophages, which requires the activation of the caspases-3, -8, and -9 for differentiation (Sordet et al., 2002). Deletion of caspase-3 limits the cytokine-induced differentiation of hematopoietic stem cells (Janzen et al., 2008) and the differentiation ability of iPSCs is enhanced by transient induction of caspase activity (Li et al., 2010b). Several other caspase-dependent cell differentiation programs have been discovered, including those of skeletal myoblasts, osteoblasts, spermatids, placental trophoblast, and embryonic and neural stem cells (**Table 2**).

A well-studied example of caspase-stimulated *in vitro* differentiation is that of mouse muscle myoblasts into multinucleated myotubes (Fernando and Kelly, 2002; Murray et al., 2008; Larsen et al., 2010). In this model capase-3-mediates activation in differentiating mouse myoblasts of a specific DNase called CAD (Larsen et al., 2010). Normally CAD (DFF40 in humans) is bound to a chaperone called ICAD (DFF45) that inhibits the nuclease activity of CAD. Caspase-3 mediated cleavage of ICAD releases CAD, allowing it to cleave DNA. This is a key step in the generation of oligonucleosomal DNA fragments seen in apoptosis. Perhaps surprisingly, activation of CAD occurs in differentiating myoblasts and RNAi directed against CAD causes profound inhibition of myoblast differentiation. Larsen et al. propose that CAD-dependent activation of p21 expression is the key event explaining this defect as p21 expression is an early and necessary event in myoblast differentiation (Larsen et al., 2010). In other words, it is proposed that caspase-3 drives non-apoptotic outcomes by inducing expression of specific genes. In addition, Fernando et al. showed that microinjection of active caspase-3 induced expression of muscle specific genes (Fernando and Kelly, 2002). These two reports support the idea that caspase activity is present in the differentiating myoblast (the direct/autonomous model). Caspase-3 activation during differentiation requires caspase-9 and is blocked by overexpression of Bcl-XL (Murray et al., 2008), which implicates the intrinsic or mitochondrial apoptotic pathway, although the role of cytochrome *c* release or Apaf-1 in this differentiation has not been conclusively demonstrated.

Although this seems like strong evidence for cell-autonomous model of caspase action, there are also data to support non-autonoumous roles for caspase activity in muscle differentiation. It has been found that myoblast fusion is driven by apoptotic cells through a phosphatidylserine-mediated activation of the BAI1 receptor. During apoptosis, caspase-dependent presentation of phosphatidylserine (PS) on the surface of dying cells is an important "eat me" signal for phagocytes and so plays a central role in the clearance of apoptotic bodies. Adding apoptotic cells to cultures where caspase activity has been abolished with pharmacological inhibitors restores myoblast fusion, and adding annexin V, a PS-binding protein, blocks myoblast fusion (Hochreiter-Hufford et al., 2013). This finding thus supports the non-cell-autonomous model, in that fusion is driven by caspase-mediated presentation of cell-surface signaling factors on apoptotic cells. It may be that both cell autonomous and

Table 2 | Caspase involvement in the differentiation programs of several cell types.

Differentiation morphology	Cell type	Caspase(s)	References
Apoptosis-like	Erythrocyte	Caspase-2, -3, -9	Zermati et al., 2001
	Keratinocyte	Caspase-3, -14	Weil et al., 1999; Eckhart et al., 2000
	Epithelial lens	Caspase-3	Ishizaki et al., 1998
	Megakaryocyte	Caspase-3, -9	De Botton et al., 2002
Non-apoptosis-like	Macrophage	Caspase-3, -8, -9	Sordet et al., 2002; Kang and Ben-Moshe, 2004
	Skeletal myoblast	Caspase-3, -9	Fernando and Kelly, 2002; Murray et al., 2008; Larsen et al., 2010
	Neuron	Caspase-3, -1	Fernando et al., 2005; Vaisid et al., 2005
	Glial cell	Caspase-3	Oomman et al., 2006
	Osteoblast	Caspase-2, -3, -8	Mogi and Togari, 2003
	Placental trophoblast	Caspase-8	Black et al., 2004
	Embryonic stem cell	Caspase-3	Fujita et al., 2008
	Hematopoietic stem cell	Caspase-3	Janzen et al., 2008
	Spermatid	Drice (Caspase-3), Dredd (Caspase-8), Dronc (Caspase-9)	Arama et al., 2003, 2007; Huh et al., 2004; Kaplan et al., 2010
	Odontoblast	Caspase-7	Matalova et al., 2013

Some programs follow a "frustrated apoptosis" phenotype, while others have a distinctly non-apoptotic-like morphology.

non-autonomous roles for caspases are important in myoblast differentiation.

A question that arises with the cell-autonomous model of caspase activity; how is this activity prevented from progressing to apoptosis? The convention is that activation of apoptotic caspases is an irreversible threshold event, leading to a runaway process of proteolytic cleavage, culminating in apoptotic cell death. If caspases truly are activated within differentiating cells themselves, there must be some mechanism for restraining, sequestering, or otherwise preventing this activity from killing the cell. Members of the IAP family are important caspase regulators (Mace et al., 2010), but there is so far little evidence that any of these proteins regulates caspase activity during muscle differentiation. Kaplan et al. showed that in spermatids there is a gradient of the giant IAP protein, dBRUCE, that establishes a gradient of caspase activity during the process of spermatid individualization in *Drosophila* (Kaplan et al., 2010). There is also other evidence for caspase localization being important during differentiation (**Table 3**). Interestingly, myogenin expressing satellite cells from young donors display active caspase-3 only at the nucleus, whereas myogenin expressing satellite cells from aged donors contain active caspase-3 both at the nucleus and at the cytoplasm. The satellite cells from aged donors also show a higher level of apoptotic cell death and together these data suggest a model in which the failure to properly localize active caspase-3 leads to satellite cell death and impaired muscle regeneration as we age (Fulle et al., 2013).

Moving to *in vivo* models of muscle differentiation, the role of caspases in regeneration becomes less clear. In caspase-9 (Hakem et al., 1998; Kuida et al., 1998) and caspase-3 (Kuida et al., 1996) knock-out mice embryonic myogenesis appears normal so the role of caspase-9 and caspase-3 in muscle differentiation *in vivo* at first appears unlikely. However, besides prenatal myogenesis, there is a distinct postnatal muscle development process as well as repair and regeneration processes in adult muscle that have not been evaluated in the caspase knock-out mice. Defects in these processes underlie a range of muscular dystrophies and age-related sarcopenia. In some instances, defects that have profound effects on muscle regeneration do not affect embryonic muscle development. For example, mice lacking caveolin-3 or expressing a Pro104Leu mutation in caveolin-3 (a model for human Limb Girdle Muscular Dystrophy 1C) show normal muscle development but muscle degeneration after 8 weeks of age (Hagiwara et al., 2000; Sunada et al., 2001). It is therefore possible that caspase-driven processes are important primarily in regeneration of adult muscle rather than muscle development but defects have not been observed in caspase deficient mice because of the perinatal lethality associated with these knock outs.

Table 3 | Compartmentalization of caspases has been found to be used in the differentiation programs of several cell types.

Cell type	Caspase	Form of compartmentalization
Platelet	Caspase-3	During platelet formation, caspase activity is localized in punctate bodies within the cytoplasm (De Botton et al., 2002)
Lens cell	Caspase-3	Partial localization to equatorial epithelium (Weber and Menko, 2005)
Spermatid	Drice (Caspase-3)	Localized within the cystic bulge of the cytoplasm (Kaplan et al., 2010)
Keratinocyte	Caspase-3	Probable localization in the nucleus during enucleation (Okuyama et al., 2004)
Glia	Caspase-3	Active caspase localized to the nucleus (Oomman et al., 2005, 2006)

Activation of caspase-8 by TNF induces apoptosis and blocks muscle regeneration in *in vivo* models of cachexia (Moresi et al., 2008, 2009), data that also appears inconsistent with a model in which caspase activity is required for differentiation. The conflicting reports of the role of caspases in muscle differentiation may be reconciled by a model in which caspase-8 induces high levels of effector caspase activity that kill cells while differentiation is associated with lower effector caspase activity. Just such a switch between death and differentiation has been reported in Drosophila models (Florentin and Arama, 2012). Alternatively, TNF-dependent caspase activation may result in a different localization of active caspases compared to caspase activation associated with differentiation as discussed above for young and aged satellite cells (Fulle et al., 2013).

It is also possible that a particular cellular differentiation process involves more than one caspase-driven step. Muscle differentiation may represent an example of this, with caspase signaling from apoptotic cells as well as caspase activity in the differentiating cells. Differentiating myoblasts may even rely on their caspase activity to drive more than one process during differentiation. Larsen et al. present compelling evidence that caspase-3 mediated DNA damage drives changes in gene expression that are required for myoblast differentiation (Larsen et al., 2010). Others have argued that primary consequence of preventing caspase activation in differentiation is a failure of myoblast fusion (Murray et al., 2008). It is possible that caspases contribute to myoblast fusion by influencing cell motility, as this is required for both muscle development (Brand-Saberi et al., 1996; Molkentin and Olson, 1996) and regeneration (Seale and Rudnicki, 2000).

MOTILITY AND METASTASIS

Cellular locomotion essentially involves the continuous deformation and manipulation of the cytoskeleton to achieve movement. Caspases are the major manipulators of cytoskeletal structure during apoptosis, so it is conceivable that caspases could also have a role in enabling cell motility. In support of this model, *in vitro* studies have shown that caspase-8-knockout mouse embryonic fibroblasts are both motility-defective, and unable to form proper lamellipodia (Helfer et al., 2006). It is thought that caspase-8 engages in a multiprotein complex with calpain to cleave focal adhesion substrates (Helfer et al., 2006).

Additionally, the embryonic lethality of caspase-8 homozygous knockout mice has been attributed to the failure to develop a functional circulatory system through a defect in endothelial cell migration (Kang and Ben-Moshe, 2004). It is as yet unknown how caspase-8 mediates migration. It could be mediated through activation of downstream effector caspases like caspase-3, leading to modification of the cytoskeleton, or it could act through a separate pathway that does not involve executioner caspases. There is even evidence suggesting that the catalytic activity of caspase-8 is not required for its effects on cell motility (Senft et al., 2007). In addition to caspase-8, caspase-3 has also been implicated in cell motility. Pharmacological inhibition of caspase-3 activity reduces cancer cell motility and invasiveness (Gdynia et al., 2007).

Metastasis of tumor cells involves cellular migration and invasion of tissues, and the subsequent growth of secondary tumors at distant sites. Normally, cells are unable to escape into systemic circulation, as detachment from their basement matrix induces cell death through anoikis or amorphosis (Mehlen and Puisieux, 2006). However, when apoptosis is compromised through silencing of the downstream effector caspase-3, caspase-8 can act to promote metastasis. In this state, caspase-8 enters into a complex with FAK and CPN2, engaging a signaling pathway which induces cell migration (Barbero et al., 2009).

In a *Drosophila* model of tumor invasion, a non-apoptotic effector caspase pathway is utilized to activate the key invasion protein Mmp1 via JNK signaling (Rudrapatna et al., 2013) (**Figure 3**). It has been proposed that this cell invasion is achieved through co-opting functions of apoptotic caspase such as cytoskeletal modification. This could be extrapolated as a general feature of non-apoptotic caspase activities in different processes. Together, this suggests a new way of thinking about caspases. Perhaps it is more constructive to think of caspases as cell-structure modifying enzymes rather than as just cell death effectors. This idea is consistent with emerging data showing the role of caspases in neuronal plasticity.

NEURAL SIGNALING AND POTENTIATION

During early development, live imaging of caspase activity in the brain shows a complex pattern of expression and subcellular localization, occurring in discrete waves (Oomman et al., 2006). These waves of activity correspond to specific periods of brain maturation. Here, we look at the roles of this non-apoptotic caspase activity in neuronal network pruning, synaptic plasticity, signal modulation, and axonal guidance (Hyman and Yuan, 2012).

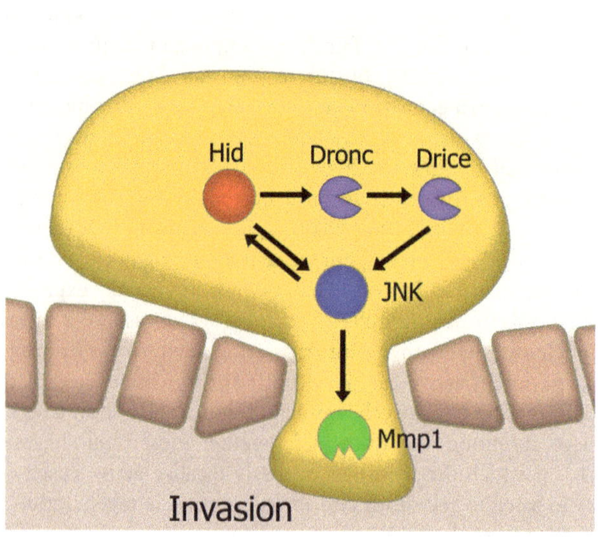

FIGURE 3 | Model of caspase-mediated tissue invasion based on *Drosophila* studies. A sub-apoptotic level of caspase activation leads to the activation, via JNK signaling, of matrix metalloproteases. This metalloprotease activity is a necessary step in the invasion of tissues. Abbreviations: JNK, Jun kinase; Mmp1, Matrix metalloprotease 1; Hid, *head involution defective*; Dronc, Drosophila Nedd2-like caspase; Drice, Drosophila ICE.

Pruning of axons and dendrites are the mechanisms through which undesired neural connections are removed. Neural network pruning during larval development in *Drosophila* is carried out through severing the connection between the outgrowth and the cell body, by means of localized executioner caspase activity, which is mediated by the spatially-restricted degradation of IAP proteins through caspase-3-like activity. An essential step in the process is degradation of DIAP1, a key inhibitor of caspase activity. Inhibition of the caspase-3-ortholog Dronc prevents this pruning process (Kuo et al., 2006) (**Figure 4**).

In mammals, caspases were found to modulate synaptic plasticity through localized activation within synaptic terminals and neurites in response to stressors. Caspase-3 activity leads to dephosphorylation and internalization of AMPA-type receptors. The loss of these receptors causes degradation of the local dendritic spine. This leads to overall modulation of glutamate signaling. Consequentially, caspases have a role in long-term depression (LTD) of neurons, and overexpression of the anti-apoptotic proteins XIAP or Bcl-xL prevent this LTD (Li et al., 2010c).

Axonal guidance is carried out through the diffusion of molecular signals by the target site, generating a chemotrophic gradient for the axon. Caspases also contribute to this chemotrophic migration by regulating the growth of neurites, through localized proteolytic activity within growth cone structures. Caspase-3 activation is required for this response, as LPA-induced growth cone collapse and netrin-1-induced growth cone attraction are both blocked by caspase-3 inhibitors (Campbell and Holt, 2003). This caspase-3-mediated effect does not require caspase-9 activation, suggesting a distinct, non-canonical activation pathway. It has been speculated that caspase-3 mediated modulation of growth cones is carried out through degradation of cytoskeletal structural elements such as actin and gelsolin (Campbell and Holt, 2003) and rock-1 (Riento and Ridley, 2003).

Such caspase-mediated modulation of synaptic plasticity, axon pruning, and growth cone mobility appear to be cell-autonomous events, in that all utilize localized caspase activity within the target cell, likely through spatially-restricted degradation of inhibitors of caspase activity.

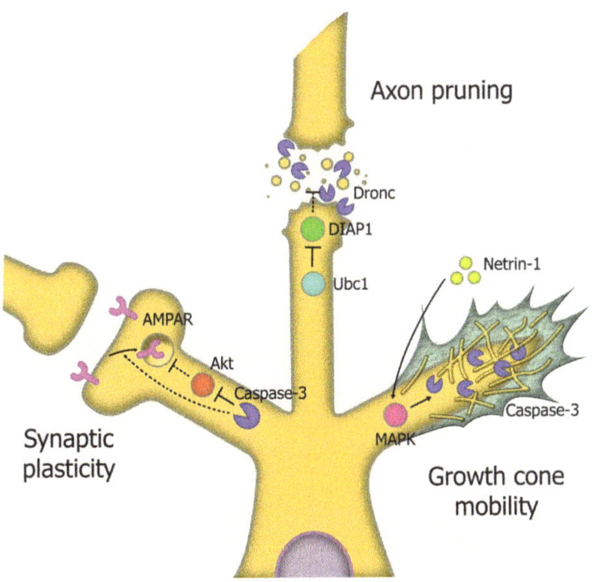

FIGURE 4 | Caspases in neuronal restructuring and signaling. *Synaptic plasticity*: Through cleavage of Akt, caspase-3 is involved in the endocytosis of AMPA receptors, leading to Long-Term Depression (LTD) of synaptic signaling. *Axonal pruning:* Localized proteosomal degradation of Inhibitor of Apoptosis proteins (IAPs) within axons lead to a localized caspase activity which shears the axon from the cell body. This process does not kill the parent neuron. *Growth cone mobility:* Netrin-1 acts as a chemoattractant, signaling MAP Kinase-mediated activation of caspase-3, which remodels the cytoskeletal structure within the growth cone, allowing axonal migration down the chemotrophic gradient. Abbreviations: AMPAR, AMPA receptor; Ubc1, Ubiquitin-conjugating enzyme E2 1; DIAP1, Drosophila Inhibitor of Apoptosis 1; MAPK, Mitogen-activated protein kinase.

CONCLUSION

Here, we reviewed the major non-apoptotic roles of caspases discovered to date. We discussed such roles in terms of different cell behaviors such as differentiation, migration, and cell signaling, and presented evidence for the cell autonomous and non-cell-autonomous models of caspase signaling.

In some systems, it seems rather clear that a cell autonomous event is occurring. This is the case in, for example, axonal pruning, where a defined cell autonomous pathway of caspase activation has been elucidated. Other systems appear to be examples of the non-cell-autonomous model. An example of this is the process of compensatory proliferation, whereby caspase-generated signals from apoptotic cells stimulate the proliferation of nearby cells in an intercellular, receptor mediated fashion. Finally, there are systems where the evidence is conflicting. This includes the process of myoblast differentiation, in which there appears to be an essential role for both cell membrane contact with apoptotic, PS exposing cells, and for the cell autonomous caspase activation of nucleases to enable the transcription of myogenic genes. Some further approaches that may prove fruitful for this field include the live imaging of caspase activity in individual cells undergoing differentiation, the identification of soluble mitogenic signaling factors from apoptotic cells, and investigation of the interplay between caspase signaling pathways and other signaling pathways.

Regardless of how caspases are regulated in these models, it seems clear that caspases do indeed have roles other than as effectors of cell death. This new understanding suggests unexpected complications in situations where caspase-dependent cell death is considered desitable, such as in response to cancer chemotherapy. The newfound alternative roles of caspases present the possibility that chemotherapy drugs may induce a wide range of cell behaviors such as increased migration and compensatory proliferation of cancer cells (Jäger and Zwacka, 2010) that are both unexpected and unwanted.

REFERENCES

Aballay, A., and Ausubel, F. M. (2001). Programmed cell death mediated by ced-3 and ced-4 protects Caenorhabditis elegans from Salmonella typhimurium-mediated killing. *Proc. Natl. Acad. Sci. U.S.A.* 98, 2735–2739. doi: 10.1073/pnas.041613098

Arama, E., Agapite, J., and Steller, H. (2003). Caspase activity and a specific cytochrome C are required for sperm differentiation in Drosophila. *Dev. Cell* 4, 687–697. doi: 10.1016/S1534-5807(03)00120-5

Arama, E., Bader, M., Rieckhof, G. E., and Steller, H. (2007). A ubiquitin ligase complex regulates caspase activation during sperm differentiation in Drosophila. *PLoS Biol.* 5:e251. doi: 10.1371/journal.pbio.0050251

Barbero, S., Mielgo, A., Torres, V., and Teitz, T. (2009). Caspase-8 association with the focal adhesion complex promotes tumor cell migration and metastasis. *Cancer Res.* 69, 3755–3763. doi: 10.1158/0008-5472.CAN-08-3937

Beaulieu, D., Thebault, P., Pelletier, R., Chapdelaine, P., Tarnopolsky, M., Furling, D., et al. (2012). Abnormal prostaglandin E2 production blocks myogenic differentiation in myotonic dystrophy. *Neurobiol. Dis.* 45, 122–129. doi: 10.1016/j.nbd.2011.06.014

Bergmann, A., and Steller, H. (2010). Apoptosis, stem cells, and tissue regeneration. *Sci. Signal.* 3, 1–16. doi: 10.1126/scisignal.3145re8.Apoptosis

Black, S., Kadyrov, M., Kaufmann, P., Ugele, B., Emans, N., and Huppertz, B. (2004). Syncytial fusion of human trophoblast depends on caspase 8. *Cell Death Differ.* 11, 90–98. doi: 10.1038/sj.cdd.4401307

Boland, K., Flanagan, L., and Prehn, J. (2013). Paracrine control of tissue regeneration and cell proliferation by Caspase-3. *Cell Death Dis.* 4, e725. doi: 10.1038/cddis.2013.250

Brand-Saberi, B., Müller, T. S., Wilting, J., Christ, B., and Birchmeier, C. (1996). Scatter factor/hepatocyte growth factor (SF/HGF) induces emigration of myogenic cells at interlimb level *in vivo*. *Dev. Biol.* 179, 303–308. doi: 10.1006/dbio.1996.0260

Brecht, K., Weigert, A., Hu, J., Popp, R., Fisslthaler, B., Korff, T., et al. (2011). Macrophages programmed by apoptotic cells promote angiogenesis via prostaglandin E2. *FASEB J.* 25, 2408–2417. doi: 10.1096/fj.10-179473

Campbell, D. S., and Holt, C. E. (2003). Apoptotic pathway and MAPKs differentially regulate chemotropic responses of retinal growth cones. *Neuron* 37, 939–952. doi: 10.1016/S0896-6273(03)00158-2

Castellone, M. D., Teramoto, H., Williams, B. O., Druey, K. M., and Gutkind, J. S. (2005). Prostaglandin E2 promotes colon cancer cell growth through a Gs-axin-beta-catenin signaling axis. *Science* 310, 1504–1510. doi: 10.1126/science.1116221

Chazaud, B., Sonnet, C., Lafuste, P., Bassez, G., Rimaniol, A. C., Poron, F., et al. (2003). Satellite cells attract monocytes and use macrophages as a support to escape apoptosis and enhance muscle growth. *J. Cell Biol.* 163, 1133–1143. doi: 10.1083/jcb.200212046

Chera, S., Ghila, L., Dobretz, K., Wenger, Y., Bauer, C., Buzgariu, W., et al. (2009). Apoptotic cells provide an unexpected source of Wnt3 signaling to drive hydra head regeneration. *Dev. Cell* 17, 279–289. doi: 10.1016/j.devcel.2009.07.014

Chun, H. J., Zheng, L., Ahmad, M., Wang, J., Speirs, C. K., Siegel, R. M., et al. (2002). Pleiotropic defects in lymphocyte activation caused by caspase-8 mutations lead to human immunodeficiency. *Nature* 419, 395–399. doi: 10.1038/nature01063

Cikala, M., Wilm, B., Hobmayer, E., Böttger, A., and David, C. N. (1999). Identification of caspases and apoptosis in the simple metazoan Hydra. *Curr. Biol.* 9, 959–962. doi: 10.1016/S0960-9822(99)80423-0

Cohen, G. M. (1997). Caspases: the executioners of apoptosis. *Biochem. J.* 326, 1–16.

De Botton, S., Sabri, S., Daugas, E., Zermati, Y., Guidotti, J. E., Hermine, O., et al. (2002). Platelet formation is the consequence of caspase activation within megakaryocytes. *Blood* 100, 1310–1317. doi: 10.1182/blood-2002-03-0686

Eckhart, L., Ballaun, C., Hermann, M., Vandeberg, J. L., Sipos, W., Uthman, A., et al. (2008). Identification of novel mammalian caspases reveals an important role of gene loss in shaping the human caspase repertoire. *Mol. Biol. Evol.* 25, 831–841. doi: 10.1093/molbev/msn012

Eckhart, L., Ballaun, C., Uthman, A., Kittel, C., Stichenwirth, M., Buchberger, M., et al. (2005). Identification and characterization of a novel mammalian caspase with proapoptotic activity. *J. Biol. Chem.* 280, 35077–35080. doi: 10.1074/jbc.C500282200

Eckhart, L., Declercq, W., Ban, J., Rendl, M., Lengauer, B., Mayer, C., et al. (2000). Terminal differentiation of human keratinocytes and stratum corneum formation is associated with caspase-14 activation. *J. Invest. Dermatol.* 115, 1148–1151. doi: 10.1046/j.1523-1747.2000.00205.x

Fan, Y., and Bergmann, A. (2008). Apoptosis-induced compensatory proliferation. The Cell is dead. Long live the Cell! *Trends Cell Biol.* 18, 467–473. doi: 10.1016/j.tcb.2008.08.001

Fava, L. L., Bock, F. J., Geley, S., and Villunger, A. (2012). Caspase-2 at a glance. *J. Cell Sci.* 125, 5911–5915. doi: 10.1242/jcs.115105.95

Fernando, P., Brunette, S., and Megeney, L. A. (2005). Neural stem cell differentiation is dependent upon endogenous caspase 3 activity. *FASEB J.* 19, 1671–1673. doi: 10.1096/fj.04-2981fje

Fernando, P., and Kelly, J. (2002). Caspase 3 activity is required for skeletal muscle differentiation. *Proc. Natl. Acad. Sci. U.S.A.* 99, 11025–11030. doi: 10.1073/pnas.162172899

Fernando, P., and Megeney, L. A. (2007). Is caspase-dependent apoptosis only cell differentiation taken to the extreme? *FASEB J.* 21, 8–17. doi: 10.1096/fj.06-5912hyp

Florentin, A., and Arama, E. (2012). Caspase levels and execution efficiencies determine the apoptotic potential of the cell. *J. Cell Biol.* 196, 513–527. doi: 10.1083/jcb.201107133

Franchi, L., Eigenbrod, T., Muñoz-Planillo, R., and Nuñez, G. (2009). The inflammasome: a caspase-1-activation platform that regulates immune responses and disease pathogenesis. *Nat. Immunol.* 10, 241–247. doi: 10.1038/ni.1703

Frost, V., Al-Mehairi, S., and Sinclair, A. J. (2001). Exploitation of a non-apoptotic caspase to regulate the abundance of the cdkI p27(KIP1) in transformed lymphoid cells. *Oncogene* 20, 2737–2748. doi: 10.1038/sj.onc.1204367

Fuchs, Y., and Steller, H. (2011). Programmed cell death in animal development and disease. *Cell* 147, 742–758. doi: 10.1016/j.cell.2011.10.033

Fujita, J., Crane, A. M., Souza, M. K., Dejosez, M., Kyba, M., Flavell, R. A., et al. (2008). Caspase activity mediates the differentiation of embryonic stem cells. *Cell Stem Cell* 2, 595–601. doi: 10.1016/j.stem.2008.04.001

Fulle, S., Sancilio, S., Mancinelli, R., Gatta, V., and Di Pietro, R. (2013). Dual role of the caspase enzymes in satellite cells from aged and young subjects. *Cell Death Dis.* 4, e955. doi: 10.1038/cddis.2013.472

Gdynia, G., Grund, K., Eckert, A., Böck, B. C., Funke, B., Macher-Goeppinger, S., et al. (2007). Basal caspase activity promotes migration and invasiveness in glioblastoma cells. *Mol. Cancer Res.* 5, 1232–1240. doi: 10.1158/1541-7786.MCR-07-0343

Goessling, W., North T. E., Loewer, S., Lord, A. M., Lee, S., Stoick-Cooper, C. L., et al. (2009). Genetic interaction of PGE2 and Wnt signaling regulates developmental specification of stem cells and regeneration *Cell* 136, 1136–1147. doi: 10.1016/j.cell.2009.01.015

Hagiwara, Y., Sasaoka, T., Araishi, K., Imamura, M., Yorifuji, H., Nonaka, I., et al. (2000). Caveolin-3 deficiency causes muscle degeneration in mice. *Hum. Mol. Genet.* 9, 3047–3054. doi: 10.1093/hmg/9.20.3047

Hakem, R., Hakem, A., Duncan, G. S., Henderson, J. T., Woo, M., Soengas, M. S., et al. (1998). Differential requirement for caspase 9 in apoptotic pathways *in vivo*. *Cell* 94, 339–352. doi: 10.1016/S0092-8674(00)81477-4

Hashimoto, T., Kikkawa, U., and Kamada, S. (2011). Contribution of caspase(s) to the cell cycle regulation at mitotic phase. *PLoS ONE* 6:e18449. doi: 10.1371/journal.pone.0018449

Helfer, B., Boswell, B. C., Finlay, D., Cipres, A., Vuori, K., Bong Kang, T., et al. (2006). Caspase-8 promotes cell motility and calpain activity under nonapoptotic conditions. *Cancer Res.* 66, 4273–4278. doi: 10.1158/0008-5472.CAN-05-4183

Hochreiter-Hufford, A. E., Lee, C. S., Kinchen, J. M., Sokolowski, J. D., Arandjelovic, S., Call, J. A., et al. (2013). Phosphatidylserine receptor BAI1 and apoptotic cells as new promoters of myoblast fusion. *Nature* 497, 263–267. doi: 10.1038/nature12135

Huh, J. R., Vernooy, S. Y., Yu, H., Yan, N., Shi, Y., Guo, M., et al. (2004). Multiple apoptotic caspase cascades are required in nonapoptotic roles for Drosophila spermatid individualization. *PLoS Biol.* 2:E15. doi: 10.1371/journal.pbio.0020015

Hyman, B. T., and Yuan, J. (2012). Apoptotic and non-apoptotic roles of caspases in neuronal physiology and pathophysiology. *Nat. Rev. Neurosci.* 13, 395–406. doi: 10.1038/nrn3228

Imtiyaz, H. Z., Zhou, X., Zhang, H., Chen, D., Hu, T., and Zhang, J. (2009). The death domain of FADD is essential for embryogenesis, lymphocyte development, and proliferation. *J. Biol. Chem.* 284, 9917–9926. doi: 10.1074/jbc.M900249200

Inoue, S., Browne, G., Melino, G., and Cohen, G. M. (2009). Ordering of caspases in cells undergoing apoptosis by the intrinsic pathway. *Cell Death Differ.* 16, 1053–1061. doi: 10.1038/cdd.2009.29

Ishizaki, Y., Jacobson, M. D., and Raff, M. C. (1998). A role for caspases in lens fiber differentiation. *J. Cell Biol.* 140, 153–158.

Jäger, R., and Fearnhead, H. O. (2012). "Dead Cells Talking": the silent form of cell death is not so quiet. *Biochem. Res. Int.* 2012:453838. doi: 10.1155/2012/453838

Jäger, R., and Zwacka, R. M. (2010). The enigmatic roles of caspases in tumor development. *Cancers (Basel)* 2, 1952–1979. doi: 10.3390/cancers2041952

Janzen, V., Fleming, H. E., Riedt, T., Karlsson, G., Riese, M. J., Lo Celso, C., et al. (2008). Hematopoietic stem cell responsiveness to exogenous signals is limited by caspase-3. *Cell Stem Cell* 2, 584–594. doi: 10.1016/j.stem.2008.03.012

Johnson, C. E., and Kornbluth, S. (2008). Caspase cleavage is not for everyone. *Cell* 134, 720–721. doi: 10.1016/j.cell.2008.08.019

Kang, T., and Ben-Moshe, T. (2004). Caspase-8 serves both apoptotic and non-apoptotic roles. *J. Immunol.* 173, 2976–2984.

Kaplan, Y., Gibbs-Bar, L., Kalifa, Y., Feinstein-Rotkopf, Y., and Arama, E. (2010). Gradients of a ubiquitin E3 ligase inhibitor and a caspase inhibitor determine differentiation or death in spermatids. *Dev. Cell* 19, 160–173. doi: 10.1016/j.devcel.2010.06.009

Kayagaki, N., Warming, S., Lamkanfi, M., Vande Walle, L., Louie, S., Dong, J., et al. (2011). Non-canonical inflammasome activation targets caspase-11. *Nature* 479, 117–121. doi: 10.1038/nature10558

Kennedy, N. J., Kataoka, T., Tschopp, J., and Budd, R. C. (1999). Caspase activation is required for T cell proliferation. *J. Exp. Med.* 190, 1891–1896. doi: 10.1084/jem.190.12.1891

Koizumi, K., Saitoh, Y., Minami, T., Takeno, N., Tsuneyama, K., Miyahara, T., et al. (2009). Role of CX3CL1/fractalkine in osteoclast differentiation and bone resorption. *J. Immunol.* 183, 7825–7831. doi: 10.4049/jimmunol.0803627

Kuida, K., Haydar, T. F., Kuan, C. Y., Gu, Y., Taya, C., Karasuyama, H., et al. (1998). Reduced apoptosis and cytochrome c-mediated caspase activation in mice lacking caspase 9. *Cell* 94, 325–337. doi: 10.1016/S0092-8674(00)81476-2

Kuida, K., Zheng, T. S., Na, S., Kuan, C., Yang, D., Karasuyama, H., et al. (1996). Decreased apoptosis in the brain and premature lethality in CPP32-deficient mice. *Nature* 384, 368–372.

Kuo, C. T., Zhu, S., Younger, S., Jan, L. Y., and Jan, Y. N. (2006). Identification of E2/E3 ubiquitinating enzymes and caspase activity regulating Drosophila sensory neuron dendrite pruning. *Neuron* 51, 283–290. doi: 10.1016/j.neuron.2006.07.014

Kuranaga, E. (2012). Beyond apoptosis: caspase regulatory mechanisms and functions *in vivo*. *Genes Cells* 17, 83–97. doi: 10.1111/j.1365-2443.2011.01579.x

Kuranaga, E., and Miura, M. (2007). Nonapoptotic functions of caspases: caspases as regulatory molecules for immunity and cell-fate determination. *Trends Cell Biol.* 17, 135–144. doi: 10.1016/j.tcb.2007.01.001

Lamkanfi, M., Festjens, N., Declercq, W., Vanden-Berghe, T., and Vandenabeele, P. (2007). Caspases in cell survival, proliferation and differentiation. *Cell Death Differ.* 14, 44–55. doi: 10.1038/sj.cdd.4402047

Larsen, B. D., and Megeney, L. A. (2010). Parole terms for a killer: directing caspase3/CAD induced DNA strand breaks to coordinate changes in gene expression. *Cell Cycle* 9, 2940–2945. doi: 10.4161/cc.9.15.12335

Larsen, B. D., Rampalli, S., Burns, L. E., Brunette, S., Dilworth, F. J., and Megeney, L. A. (2010). Caspase 3/caspase-activated DNase promotes cell differentiation by inducing DNA strand breaks. *Proc. Natl. Acad. Sci. U.S.A.* 107, 4230–4235. doi: 10.1073/pnas.0913089107

Lauber, K., Bohn, E., Kröber, S., and Xiao, Y. (2003). Apoptotic cells induce migration of phagocytes via caspase-3-mediated release of a lipid attraction signal. *Cell* 113, 717–730. doi: 10.1016/S0092-8674(03)00422-7

Leulier, F., Rodriguez, A., Khush, R. S., Abrams, J. M., and Lemaitre, B. (2000). The Drosophila caspase Dredd is required to resist gram-negative bacterial infection. *EMBO Rep.* 1, 353–358. doi: 10.1093/embo-reports/kvd073

Li, F., He, Z., Shen, J., Huang, Q., Li, W., Liu, X., et al. (2010b). Apoptotic caspases regulate induction of iPSCs from human fibroblasts. *Cell Stem Cell* 7, 508–520. doi: 10.1016/j.stem.2010.09.003

Li, F., Huang, Q., Chen, J., Peng, Y., Roop, D. R., and Bedford, J. S. (2010a). Apoptotic cells activate the "phoenix rising" pathway to promote wound healing and tissue regeneration. *Sci. Signal.* 3, 13. doi: 10.1126/scisignal.2000634

Li, J., Brieher, W. M., Scimone, M. L., Kang, S. J., Zhu, H., Yin, H., et al. (2007). Caspase-11 regulates cell migration by promoting Aip1-Cofilin-mediated actin depolymerization. *Nat. Cell Biol.* 9, 276–286. doi: 10.1038/ncb1541

Li, P., Allen, H., Banerjee, S., Frankli, S., Herzog, L., Johnston, C., et al. (1995). Mice deficient in IL-1 beta-converting enzyme are defective in production of mature IL-1 beta and resistant to endotoxic shock. *Cell* 80, 401–411.

Li, Z., Jo, J., Jia, J. M., Lo, S. C., Whitcomb, D. J., Jiao, S., et al. (2010c). Caspase-3 activation via mitochondria is required for long-term depression and AMPA receptor internalization. *Cell* 141, 859–871. doi: 10.1016/j.cell.2010.03.053

Lüthi, A. U., and Martin, S. J. (2007). The CASBAH: a searchable database of caspase substrates. *Cell Death Differ.* 14, 641–650. doi: 10.1038/sj.cdd.4402103

Mace, P. D., and Riedl, S. J. (2010). Molecular cell death platforms and assemblies. *Curr. Opin. Cell Biol.* 22, 828–836. doi: 10.1016/j.ceb.2010.08.004

Mace, P. D., Shirley, S., and Day, C. L. (2010). Assembling the building blocks: structure and function of inhibitor of apoptosis proteins. *Cell Death Differ.* 17, 46–53. doi: 10.1038/cdd.2009.45

Mao, C., and Obeid, L. M. (2008). Ceramidases: regulators of cellular responses mediated by ceramide, sphingosine, and sphingosine-1-phosphate. *Biochim. Biophys. Acta* 1781, 424–434. doi: 10.1016/j.bbalip.2008.06.002

Matalova, E., Lesot, H., Svandova, E., Vanden Berghe, T., Sharpe, P. T., Healy, C., et al. (2013). Caspase-7 participates in differentiation of cells forming dental hard tissues. *Dev. Growth Differ.* 55, 615–621. doi: 10.1111/dgd.12066

Mehlen, P., and Puisieux, A. (2006). Metastasis: a question of life or death. *Nat. Rev. Cancer* 6, 449–458. doi: 10.1038/nrc1886

Miura, M. (2012). Apoptotic and nonapoptotic caspase functions in animal development. *Cold Spring Harb. Perspect. Biol.* 4, 1–16. doi: 10.1101/cshperspect.a008664

Mogi, M., and Togari, A. (2003). Activation of caspases is required for osteoblastic differentiation. *J. Biol. Chem.* 278, 47477–47482. doi: 10.1074/jbc.M307055200

Molkentin, J. D., and Olson, E. N. (1996). Defining the regulatory networks for muscle development. *Curr. Opin. Genet. Dev.* 6, 445–453. doi: 10.1016/S0959-437X(96)80066-9

Morata, G., Shlevkov, E., and Pérez-Garijo, A. (2011). Mitogenic signaling from apoptotic cells in Drosophila. *Dev. Growth Differ.* 53, 168–176. doi: 10.1111/j.1440-169X.2010.01225.x

Moresi, V., Garcia-Alvarez, G., Pristerà, A., Rizzuto, E., Albertini, M. C., Rocchi, M., et al. (2009). Modulation of caspase activity regulates skeletal muscle regeneration and function in response to vasopressin and tumor necrosis factor. *PLoS ONE* 4:e5570. doi: 10.1371/journal.pone.0005570

Moresi, V., Pristerà, A., Scicchitano, B. M., Molinaro, M., Teodori, L., Sassoon, D., et al. (2008). Tumor necrosis factor-alpha inhibition of skeletal muscle regeneration is mediated by a caspase-dependent stem cell response. *Stem Cells* 26, 997–1008. doi: 10.1634/stemcells.2007-0493

Murray, T. V., McMahon, J. M., Howley, B. H., Stanley, A., Ritter, T., Mohr, A., et al. (2008). A non-apoptotic role for caspase-9 in muscle differentiation. *J. Cell Sci.* 121, 3786–3793. doi: 10.1242/jcs.024547

Okuyama, R., Nguyen, B. C., Talora, C., Ogawa, E., Tommasi di Vignano, A., Lioumi, M., et al. (2004). High commitment of embryonic keratinocytes to terminal differentiation through a Notch1-caspase 3 regulatory mechanism. *Dev. Cell* 6, 551–562. doi: 10.1016/S1534-5807(04)00098-X

Oomman, S., Strahlendorf, H., Dertien, J., and Strahlendorf, J. (2006). Bergmann glia utilize active caspase-3 for differentiation. *Brain Res.* 1078, 19–34. doi: 10.1016/j.brainres.2006.01.041

Oomman, S., Strahlendorf, H., Finckbone, V., and Strahlendorf, J. (2005). Non-lethal active caspase-3 expression in Bergmann glia of postnatal rat cerebellum. *Brain Res. Dev. Brain Res.* 160, 130–145. doi: 10.1016/j.devbrainres.2005.07.010

Park, W. S., Lee, J. H., Shin, M. S., Park, J. Y., Kim, H. S., Lee, J. H., et al. (2002). Inactivating mutations of the caspase-10 gene in gastric cancer. *Oncogene* 21, 2919–2925. doi: 10.1038/sj.onc.1205394

Pop, C., and Salvesen, G. S. (2009). Human caspases: activation, specificity, and regulation. *J. Biol. Chem.* 284, 21777–21781. doi: 10.1074/jbc.R800084200

Riento, K., and Ridley, A. J. (2003). Rocks: multifunctional kinases in cell behaviour. *Nat. Rev. Mol. Cell Biol.* 4, 446–456. doi: 10.1038/nrm1128

Rudrapatna, V. A., Bangi, E., and Cagan, R. L. (2013). Caspase signalling in the absence of apoptosis drives Jnk-dependent invasion. *EMBO Rep.* 14, 172–177. doi: 10.1038/embor.2012.217

Ryborg, A. K., Johansen, C., Iversen, L., and Kragballe, K. (2004). Lysophosphatidylcholine induces keratinocyte differentiation and upregulation of AP-1- and NF-kappaB DNA-binding activity. *Acta Derm. Venereol.* 84, 433–438. doi: 10.1080/00015550410016930

Saleh, M., Vaillancourt, J. P., Graham, R. K., and Huyck, M. (2004). Differential modulation of endotoxin responsiveness by human caspase-12 polymorphisms. *Nature* 429, 75–79. doi: 10.1038/nature02502.1

Schwerk, C., and Schulze-Osthoff, K. (2003). Non-apoptotic functions of caspases in cellular proliferation and differentiation. *Biochem. Pharmacol.* 66, 1453–1458. doi: 10.1016/S0006-2952(03)00497-0

Seale, P., and Rudnicki, M. A. (2000). A new look at the origin, function, and "stem-cell" status of muscle satellite cells. *Dev. Biol.* 218, 115–124. doi: 10.1006/dbio.1999.9565

Senft, J., Helfer, B., and Frisch, S. M. (2007). Caspase-8 interacts with the p85 subunit of phosphatidylinositol 3-kinase to regulate cell adhesion and motility. *Cancer Res.* 67, 11505–11509. doi: 10.1158/0008-5472.CAN-07-5755

Sordet, O., Rébé, C., Plenchette, S., Zermati, Y., Hermine, O., Vainchenker, W., et al. (2002). Specific involvement of caspases in the differentiation of monocytes into macrophages. *Blood* 100, 4446–4453. doi: 10.1182/blood-2002-06-1778

Soung, Y. H., Jeong, E. G., Ahn, C. H., Kim, S. S., Song, S. Y., Yoo, N. J., et al. (2008). Mutational analysis of caspase 1, 4, and 5 genes in common human cancers. *Hum. Pathol.* 39, 895–900. doi: 10.1016/j.humpath.2007.10.015

Sunada, Y., Ohi, H., Hase, A., Ohi, H., Hosono, T., Arata, S., et al. (2001). Transgenic mice expressing mutant caveolin-3 show severe myopathy associated with increased nNOS activity. *Hum. Mol. Genet.* 10, 173–178. doi: 10.1093/hmg/10.3.173

Suzanne, M., and Steller, H. (2013). Shaping organisms with apoptosis. *Cell Death Differ.* 20, 669–675. doi: 10.1038/cdd.2013.11

Tait, S. W. G., and Green, D. R. (2010). Mitochondria and cell death: outer membrane permeabilization and beyond. *Nat. Rev. Mol. Cell Biol.* 11, 621–632. doi: 10.1038/nrm2952

Takahashi, K., Kawai, T., Kumar, H., Sato, S., Yonehara, S., and Akira, S. J. (2006). Roles of caspase-8 and caspase-10 in innate immune responses to double-stranded RNA. *J. Immunol.* 176, 4520–4524.

Taub, R. (2004). Liver regeneration: from myth to mechanism. *Nat. Rev. Mol. Cell Biol.* 5, 836–847. doi: 10.1038/nrm1489

Truman, L. A., Ford, C. A., Pasikowska, M., Pound, J. D., Wilkinson, S. J., Dumitriu, I. E., et al. (2008). CX3CL1/fractalkine is released from apoptotic lymphocytes to stimulate macrophage chemotaxis. *Blood* 112, 5026–5036. doi: 10.1182/blood-2008-06-162404

Tseng, A. S., Adams, D. S., Qiu, D., Koustubhan, P., and Levin, M. (2007). Apoptosis is required during early stages of tail regeneration in Xenopus laevis. *Dev. Biol.* 301, 62–69. doi: 10.1016/j.ydbio.2006.10.048

Vaisid, T., Kosower, N. S., and Barnoy, S. (2005). Caspase-1 activity is required for neuronal differentiation of PC12 cells: cross-talk between the caspase and calpain systems. *Biochim. Biophys. Acta* 1743, 223–230. doi: 10.1016/j.bbamcr.2005.01.001

Vlaskalin, T., Wong, C. J., and Tsilfidis, C. (2004). Growth and apoptosis during larval forelimb development and adult forelimb regeneration in the newt (Notophthalmus viridescens). *Dev. Genes Evol.* 214, 423–431. doi: 10.1007/s00427-004-0417-1

Weber, G. F., and Menko, A. S. (2005). The canonical intrinsic mitochondrial death pathway has a non-apoptotic role in signaling lens cell differentiation. *J. Biol. Chem.* 280, 22135–22145. doi: 10.1074/jbc.M414270200

Weil, M., Raff, M. C., and Braga, V. M. (1999). Caspase activation in the terminal differentiation of human epidermal keratinocytes. *Curr. Biol.* 9, 361–364. doi: 10.1016/S0960-9822(99)80162-6

White, G. E., and Greaves, D. R. (2012). Fractalkine: a survivor's guide: chemokines as antiapoptotic mediators. *Arterioscler. Thromb. Vasc. Biol.* 32, 589–594. doi: 10.1161/ATVBAHA.111.237412

Williams, D. W., Kondo, S., Krzyzanowska, A., Hiromi, Y., and Truman, J. W. (2006). Local caspase activity directs engulfment of dendrites during pruning. *Nat. Neurosci.* 9, 1234–1236. doi: 10.1038/nn1774

Woo, M., Hakem, R., Furlonger, C., Hakem, A., Duncan, G. S., Sasaki, T., et al. (2003). Caspase-3 regulates cell cycle in B cells: a consequence of substrate specificity. *Nat. Immunol.* 4, 1016–1022. doi: 10.1038/ni976

Zermati, Y., Garrido, C., Amsellem, S., Fishelson, S., Bouscary, D., Valensi, F., et al. (2001). Caspase activation is required for terminal erythroid differentiation. *J. Exp. Med.* 193, 247–254. doi: 10.1084/jem.193.2.247

Zhang, J., Cado, D., Chen, A., Kabra, N., and Winoto, A. (1998). Fas-mediated apoptosis and activation-induced T-cell proliferation are defective in mice lacking FADD/Mort1. *Nature* 392, 296–300. doi: 10.1038/32681

Zhang, J., Kabra, N. H., Cado, D., Kang, C., and Winoto, A. (2001). FADD-deficient T cells exhibit a disaccord in regulation of the cell cycle machinery. *J. Biol. Chem.* 276, 29815–29818. doi: 10.1074/jbc.M103838200

3

Novel excitation-contraction coupling related genes reveal aspects of muscle weakness beyond atrophy—New hopes for treatment of musculoskeletal diseases

Heather Manring[1], Eduardo Abreu[2], Leticia Brotto[2], Noah Weisleder[1] and Marco Brotto[2,3,4]*

[1] *Department of Physiology and Cell Biology, Davis Heart and Lung Research Institute, The Ohio State University Wexner Medical Center, Columbus, OH, USA*
[2] *Muscle Biology Research Group, School of Nursing and Health Studies, University of Missouri-Kansas City, Kansas City, MO, USA*
[3] *Basic Medical Sciences Pharmacology, School of Medicine, University of Missouri-Kansas City, Kansas City, MO, USA*
[4] *Basic Medical Sciences Pharmacology, School of Pharmacy, University of Missouri-Kansas City, Kansas City, MO, USA*

***Correspondence:**
Marco Brotto, Muscle Biology Research Group-MUBIG, School of Nursing and Health Studies, School of Medicine, School of Pharmacy, 2464 Charlotte St., Health Sciences Building Suite 2246, Kansas City, 64108 MO, USA
e-mail: brottom@umkc.edu

Research over the last decade strengthened the understanding that skeletal muscles are not only the major tissue in the body from a volume point of view but also function as a master regulator contributing to optimal organismal health. These new contributions to the available body of knowledge triggered great interest in the roles of skeletal muscle beyond contraction. The World Health Organization, through its Global Burden of Disease (GBD) report, recently raised further awareness about the key importance of skeletal muscles as the GDB reported musculoskeletal (MSK) diseases have become the second greatest cause of disability, with more than 1.7 billion people in the globe affected by a diversity of MSK conditions. Besides their role in MSK disorders, skeletal muscles are also seen as principal metabolic organs with essential contributions to metabolic disorders, especially those linked to physical inactivity. In this review, we have focused on the unique function of new genes/proteins (i.e., MTMR14, MG29, sarcalumenin, KLF15) that during the last few years have helped provide novel insights about muscle function in health and disease, muscle fatigue, muscle metabolism, and muscle aging. Next, we provide an in depth discussion of how these genes/proteins converge into a common function of acting as regulators of intracellular calcium homeostasis. A clear link between dysfunctional calcium homeostasis is established and the special role of store-operated calcium entry is analyzed. The new knowledge that has been generated by the understanding of the roles of previously unknown modulatory genes of the skeletal muscle excitation-contraction coupling (ECC) process brings exciting new possibilities for treatment of MSK diseases, muscle regeneration, and skeletal muscle tissue engineering. The next decade of skeletal muscle and MSK research is bound to bring to fruition applied knowledge that will hopefully offset the current heavy and sad burden of MSK diseases on the planet.

Keywords: musculoskeletal diseases, MG29, MTMR14, sarcalumenin, KLF15, calcium homeostasis, sarcopenia, aging

INTRODUCTION TO THE GLOBAL PROBLEM

The Global Burden of Disease Study (GBD) of 2010 estimates 1.7 billion people worldwide are affected by musculoskeletal disorders (MSDs). Among the almost 300 diseases and injuries evaluated in the GBD study of 2010, MSDs rank as the second greatest cause of disability according to the calculated years lived with disability (YLDs) for affected individuals. This equates to roughly 21.3% of all YLDs. MSDs only rank below mental and behavioral disorders with respect to this measure. Between 1990 and 2010, a 44.7% increase in the YLDs of musculoskeletal disorders was observed (Vos et al., 2010). When disorders are evaluated in terms of disability-adjusted life years (DALYs), MSDs ranked fourth below cardiovascular diseases, neoplasms, and mental disorders. DALYs give a more accurate representation of the drivers of poor health by accounting for both disability and death associated with a disorder rather than basing the impact solely on the number of deaths over time. In 2010, MSDs accounted for roughly 6.8% of total DALYs globally which increased from the estimated 4.7% in 1990 (Murray et al., 2010). The distribution and impact of MSDs is relatively equal globally as these conditions are not considered indigenous to a specific region. The GBD of 2010 suggests that healthcare systems need to focus on developing a policy to deal with the increasing burden caused by MSDs (Murray et al., 2010; Vos et al., 2010).

Musculoskeletal disorders include a variety of conditions that affect muscles, bones, and joints throughout the body. The impact of MSDs on daily life ranges from minimal discomfort to debilitating pain that considerably affects the performance of simple everyday activities. In terms of severity, MSDs encompass a broad spectrum of symptoms ranging from minor conditions to major disorders, including arthritis, back and neck pain, and muscle wasting disorders. In this review we will focus on some of the most severe of these disorders, specifically skeletal muscle wasting disorders that have the broadest impact on human health and patient outcomes. The increased prevalence of muscle wasting disorders appears to be in part due to the increasing life span of humans with age as a contributing factor in approximately one-third of documented MSDs (561 million people). A 49.9% increase in DALYs between 1990 and 2010 was observed for all types of muscle wasting disorders, which is slightly larger than the change observed for MSDs in general (Murray et al., 2010). Muscle wasting is a comorbidity of the ever increasing conditions of heart failure and cancer in addition to its association with skeletal muscle disorders. With its rise in prevalence, muscle wasting disorders and their underlying mechanisms are of great importance in an effort to provide appropriate treatments (Teixeira Vde et al., 2012). While multiple MSDs contribute to changes in human health, skeletal muscle wasting will be the major focus of this review.

MUSCLE WASTING DISORDERS

MUSCLE WASTING IS MUCH MORE THAN MUSCLE LOSS

In skeletal muscle, the number of cells (muscle fibers) present in an anatomical muscle stabilizes early in life and remains constant into adulthood, after which time increased muscle mass and strength is dependent on an increase in the size of muscle fibers (hypertrophy). Injured muscle fibers can be repaired or replaced by activation of neighboring satellite cells that will proliferate and repair damaged muscle fibers. A decrease in muscle fiber size is a factor contributing to muscle weakness. While muscle weakness is a shared characteristic of many skeletal muscle wasting disorders including atrophy, sarcopenia, myopathy, and others, the long term outcome of these disorders in addition to the biochemical and molecular processes driving them can be distinct (Romanick et al., 2013). For this reason, further research on the mechanisms behind each disorder and evaluation of possible therapeutic interventions for the associated muscle weakness is of vital importance.

Atrophy is the loss of myofiber size and quantity most commonly due to disuse of muscles (Lexell, 1993; Brooks and Faulkner, 1994; Schakman et al., 2013). While the pathophysiological effects of atrophy caused by inactivity can typically be restored by physical activity, these effects are not easily reversed in situations such as sarcopenia and other muscle wasting disorders (Faulkner et al., 1995; Bortz and Bortz, 1996; Gonzalez et al., 2000; Zahn et al., 2006; Romero-Suarez et al., 2010). In these conditions, recovery of muscle strength caused by the functional and physical loss of muscle fibers is very difficult. This continued and irreversible detrimental effect on muscle fibers leads to fragility and eventually hinders the quality of life and independence of individuals. Sarcopenia has been specifically referred to as muscle atrophy and wasting that accompanies aging. A variety of molecular targets and processes proposed to be involved in sarcopenia include muscle proteolysis, increased cellular autophagy, aberrant activation of Ca^{2+}-activated proteases and proteasomes, and dysfunction or loss of satellite cells (Teixeira Vde et al., 2012; Romanick et al., 2013). While sarcopenia is considered a normal part of healthy aging, studies suggest that the progression of sarcopenia can be slowed if the specific molecular process responsible for its pathophysiological effects can be determined and specifically targeted (Romanick et al., 2013). In fact, the complexity of these diseases associated with muscle wasting is further compounded by an intriguing signature where muscle mass does not necessarily match functional status (i.e. muscle contractile force and muscle power) (Lowe et al., 2002, 2004; Romero-Suarez et al., 2010; Manini and Clark, 2012; Russ et al., 2012). Multiple factors contribute to this phenomenon, including increased fatty infiltration and an increased prevalence of myosin type I expression in aging skeletal muscle. While the loss of muscle mass itself is detrimental to health because of its obvious metabolic consequences, the loss of functional capacity surpasses the muscle content loss and aggravates these conditions (Lowe et al., 2002, 2004; Mitchell et al., 2012; Romanick et al., 2013).

It is important to distinguish between muscle wasting and muscle weakness that can be two distinct processes involving loss of muscle mass or loss of functional muscle output respectively. Muscle weakness itself is a major contributor to morbidity, risk of falls, and mortality (Brotto and Abreu, 2012). Our research groups have proposed since the early 2000's that the definition of sarcopenia for example must not be limited to "loss of muscle mass." It is still puzzling that despite many recent efforts sarcopenia is not defined as a disease; an International Disease Code (IDC) still does not exist for sarcopenia, which should be defined as a disease of aging characterized by a loss of muscle strength that surpasses the loss of muscle mass. Muscle fatigue is another essential characteristic of muscle that is commonly affected in muscle wasting disorders and in the aging process. In general, muscle fatigue is defined as a reversible decline in the ability of a muscle to create force either due to repetitive or continued activity. Muscle fatigue is thought to be a biological process to minimize damage to muscles that is produced by overexertion; however, the exact cellular mechanisms contributing to muscle fatigue remain to be fully clarified (Bruton et al., 1998; Nagaraj et al., 2000; de Paula Brotto et al., 2001; Brotto et al., 2002). A better understanding of muscle weakness, atrophy and fatigue are necessary to be able to develop medical interventions to restore muscle strength and reduce the fatigability of muscles, which are essential for effective treatment of muscle wasting disorders (Romanick et al., 2013).

MUSCLE MYOPATHIES

A GENERAL DEFINITION

Myopathies are a distinct group of muscle wasting disorders. Myopathies are neuromuscular disorders in which the main symptom is muscle weakness caused by dysfunction of muscle fibers (Chawla, 2011). There are many types of myopathies including inherited myopathies such as muscular dystrophies and acquired myopathies (Sewry, 2008). The distinct biochemical and cellular mechanisms underlying the pathology of these myopathies lead to greatly varied prognoses and treatments. Only palliative care is currently available for many of these disorders due to the limited understanding of their pathology.

THE SPECIAL CASE OF ETHANOL-INDUCED MYOPATHY

Ethanol-induced myopathy is acquired following excessive and/or chronic consumption of alcohol and is roughly five times more common than alcoholic cirrhosis (Estruch et al., 1993). Multiple studies have confirmed the prevalence of this myopathy and determined that loss of muscle bulk as well as weakness is the result. Abstinence and nutritional support facilitates recovery of these patients but muscle strength does not revert to baseline values suggesting this is an irreversible process (Urbano-Marquez and Fernandez-Sola, 2004). While the causative agent of this myopathy has been known, the steps leading to its development are unknown. Over the past 30 years progress has been made in understanding of this disease entity. The mechanisms underlying this multi-factorial disease include disruption of protein metabolism, signal transduction, and improper gene regulation (Urbano-Marquez and Fernandez-Sola, 2004; Noordzij et al., 2007; Gonzalez-Reimers et al., 2010; Chawla, 2011). *In vivo* and *in vitro* studies using models for alcohol-induced myopathy observed a decrease in muscle mass specifically fast twitch (Type II) fibers with multiple possible contributory mechanisms identified. Protein synthesis of myofibrillar proteins is impaired at the initiation step of translation by alcohol (Preedy and Peters, 1988; Urbano-Marquez et al., 1995; Lang et al., 1999). Analysis of mRNA and protein expression following chronic and acute alcohol exposure determined multiple pathways and processes are modified by alcohol including the ATP-dependent multi-catalytic proteasome pathway. In skeletal muscles, alcohol induced apoptosis and changed expression and activity of the mTOR pathway (Lang et al., 2003; Nakahara et al., 2003, 2006; Hong-Brown et al., 2006). An additional contributory mechanism being evaluated in this disease is oxidative damage due to increased reactive oxygen species or changes in prevalence of antioxidants (Hofer et al., 2005; Fernandez-Sola et al., 2007). Recently, corollary studies by Preedy et al. have firmly established that ethanol-induced myopathies could account for more than 50% of all cases of myopathies (Preedy et al., 2001a,b). Despite the prevalence of this syndrome, effective treatments to either prevent or to cure this condition remain unavailable.

MUSCULAR DYSTROPHY

Muscular dystrophies encompass another group of degenerative myopathies which involve progressive muscle weakness that often presents at birth or starting in early childhood However, there are many types of muscular dystrophy that vary in their underlying genetic foundation, the severity of disease including the body regions affected, the time of onset, and the rate of disease progression. These distinct types are associated with perturbations of various genes including *DYSF* (dysferlin), *DUX4* (double homeobox 4), *LMN* (Lamin), and the *DMD* gene that encodes the dystrophin protein (Rahimov and Kunkel, 2013). Disruption of these genes and several others lead to muscle damage partially attributed to defects in sarcolemmal membrane stability and repair. This damage is associated with progressive muscle weakness, which appears to have a greater functional consequence than loss of muscle mass.

Duchenne muscular dystrophy (DMD) is a recessive X-linked form of muscular dystrophy that affects approximately 1 in 3600 boys. Symptoms of DMD tend to appear at or before six years of age with muscle weakness in the legs and pelvis followed by other body regions as the disorder progresses. Muscle deterioration and immobility eventually lead to paralysis with an average lifespan of around 25 years. The observed muscle degeneration is associated with mutations in the dystrophin gene. Dystrophin is an important structural component of the dystroglycan complex of the cell membrane that contributes to maintaining muscle fiber strength, preventing muscle injury, and retaining the mechanical stability of muscle cells (Rahimov and Kunkel, 2013). Absence of functional dystrophin protein leads to increased membrane fragility, myocyte death, fibrosis, and progressive loss of muscle strength. While more is known regarding the genetic perturbations underlying DMD, available treatments to counteract or prevent debilitating muscle weakness are still limited and lack efficacy for this and other muscular dystrophies (Rahimov and Kunkel, 2013).

CENTRONUCLEAR MUSCLE MYOPATHIES

Centronuclear myopathies (CNMs) are inherited neuromuscular disorders with features of congenital myopathy that are characterized by a high proportion of myofibers with centrally located nuclei (Wallgren-Pettersson et al., 1995; Pierson et al., 2005; Tosch et al., 2006). Normally, the nucleus is found along the edges of rod-shaped muscle cells but in people with CNM the nucleus is located in the center of these cells. It is unclear exactly how the change in the location of the nucleus directly affects muscle cells. It is likely that absence of the cellular mechanism responsible for moving nuclei to the periphery, which could involve defects in the cytoskeleton, is involved in the etiology of this myopathy (Jungbluth et al., 2008). Centronuclear myopathies are divided into forms based on their proposed pattern of inheritance, associated symptoms and muscle pathology. Mutations to the dynamin 2 gene (*DNM2*) were recently associated with the autosomal dominant form of CNM while X-linked CNMs were associated with mutations in *DNM2*, *AMPH* (amphiphysin), *MTM1* (myotubularin) and most recently *MTMR14* (myotubularin-related protein-14) genes (Laporte et al., 1996, 2003; Jungbluth et al., 2008; Romero, 2010; Romero and Bitoun, 2011). How mutations to these genes lead to the observed muscle weakness and other specific features of these myopathies is unclear but it is suggested that intracellular trafficking of essential molecules is disrupted. The functional impact of the observed progressive muscle weakness in CNMs is much greater than would be expected if based simply on the loss of muscle mass leading to interest in exploring other aspects of muscle physiology including muscle strength and fatigue.

A LOOK AT KEY GENETIC PERTURBATIONS UNDERLYING MUSCLE WASTING DISORDERS

Many genes have been proposed to be associated with various muscle wasting disorders but the mechanisms by which these perturbations cause the observed pathology is complex and remains unclear (Sewry, 2008). These proposed genes are involved in a multitude of biochemical processes that are essential for proper functioning of skeletal muscles including but not limited to stabilizing cell membranes, Ca^{2+} handling required for proper contraction and relaxation of muscles, and proper ubiquitin-mediated degradation of proteins (Teixeira Vde et al., 2012). While the loss of muscle mass is a critical part of these disorders, ultimately it is the progressive muscle weakness that increases the morbidity and mortality associated with musculoskeletal disorders. By understanding the biochemical processes leading to the observed phenotypes, treatments and therapeutics can be designed to reduce the functional impact of muscle weakness and slow its progression.

Skeletal muscle serves many functions throughout the human body beyond controlling muscle contraction including the more recent focus on its role in body metabolism and in metabolic and physical inactivity disorders. In this section, the unique key functions of specific genes, including *MTMR14*, *SAR* (sarcalumenin), *MG29*, and *KLF15*, will be discussed. Over the past few years, these genes have provided novel insights about muscle function in health and disease including muscle fatigue, muscle metabolism, and muscle aging (see **Figure 1**). These are major health issues as indicated by the large global impact of musculoskeletal disorders on both morbidity and mortality.

MTMR14 PLAYS A KEY ROLE IN CALCIUM HOMEOSTASIS AND REGULATION OF AUTOPHAGY IN SKELETAL MUSCLE CELLS

Myotubularin (MTM) and myotubularin-related (MTMR) genes belong to a family of genes that encode dual-specificity phosphatases that modify phosphoinositides and regulate membrane traffic (Dowling et al., 2009, 2010). Genes in this family are shown to be important in muscle cell differentiation and mutations to *MTM* and *MTMR* genes are observed in patients with specific centronuclear myopathies (Laporte et al., 1996, 2003; Wishart and Dixon, 2002; Dowling et al., 2009, 2010). In 2010, multiple research groups identified mutations to *MTMR14*, one member of this gene family, in several patients with CNMs and in sarcopenia (Tosch et al., 2006; Dowling et al., 2009; Romero-Suarez et al., 2010). The MTMR14 gene was first identified as a cytoplasmic localized phosphatase specific to skeletal and cardiac muscle (Tosch et al., 2006; Vergne et al., 2009). Initially, this gene was named as muscle-specific inositol phosphatase (MIP) or Jumpy but when this gene was found to have high homology to the catalytic motif of myotubularin family proteins, it was renamed MTMR14 (Alonso et al., 2004; Tosch et al., 2006; Shen et al., 2009). MTMR14 specifically targets 1-O-(3-sn-phosphatidyl)-1D-myo-inositol 3-(dihydrogen phosphate) (phosphatidylinositol 3-phosphate (PtdIns(3)P)) and L-alpha-phosphatidyl-D-myo-inositol 3,5 bisphosphate, dipalmitoyl (phosphatidylinositol 3,5-diphosphate (PtdIns(3,5)P) substrates (Tosch et al., 2006; Dowling et al., 2009; Gibbs et al., 2010; Romero-Suarez et al., 2010). The products of this reaction are PtdIns and PtdIns(5)P, which are involved in cytoskeletal dynamics and intracellular membrane trafficking.

Using *MTMR14* specific knockout mice, a number of research groups explored the function of *MTMR14* and identified MTMR14 as a contributory factor in sarcopenia. Initial studies in these mice found excess PtdIns(3,5)P in skeletal muscle cells confirming this as a substrate of MTMR14 and suggesting this substrate plays an active role downstream (Shen et al., 2009; Romero-Suarez et al., 2010). Altered abundance of this phosphoinositide substrate and other phosphoinositides can cause defects in Ca^{2+} homeostasis thus creating a possible link for MTMR14 function in skeletal muscle pathophysiology.

Brotto and collaborators observed young *MTMR14* knockout (KO) mice exhibited impaired Ca^{2+} homeostasis, decreased muscle contractile force, and loss of muscle mass, all of which are reminiscent of aging (**Figure 1**). In comparing muscles of young and old wild type mice, levels of MTMR14 protein were reduced in older wild type mice (Romero-Suarez et al., 2010). Similarly, Shen et al. found *mtmr14*$^{-/-}$ mice were prone to greater skeletal muscle fatigue and these mice showed decreased motor function including decreased walking speed and decreased running time prior to exhaustion. Extensor digitorum longus (EDL) muscles of these knockout mice had a 60% decrease in force-generating capacity and a prolonged relaxation profile post-muscle contraction compared to wild type mice of the same age. When the fatigue-resistant, slow-twitch soleus muscles of these KO mice were examined, they showed a shift toward higher frequencies while exhibiting greater fatigue and diminished recovery post-fatigue (Shen et al., 2009). This shift may reflect lesser Ca^{2+} release from the SR, therefore at higher frequencies of stimulation more calcium can be released. These defects could be explained by the alterations in calcium homeostasis, particularly the reduced availability of calcium for effective calcium release during contraction/relaxation cycles.

Knockout mice also exhibited defects in the regulation of Ca^{2+} levels including elevated resting Ca^{2+} concentrations, decreased Ca^{2+} content in the sarcoplasmic reticulum (SR), and prolonged release or defective Ca^{2+} clearance in these muscles. While store-operated calcium entry (SOCE) was functional in these mutant muscles, it was severely blunted and associated with muscle weakness and impairment of muscle relaxation. The findings from *MTMR14* knockout mice point to a role of the MTMR14 phosphatase in regulating Ca^{2+} essential for excitation-contraction coupling and SOCE function. Defects in these processes result in muscle fibers that are more susceptible to exercise-induced muscle damage and will lead to muscle weakness, both of which are trademarks of muscle wasting especially in sarcopenia (Zhao et al., 2008; Romero-Suarez et al., 2010) (**Figure 1**). For example, elevated levels of Ca^{2+} can lead to activation of proteolytic enzymes and dysfunctional autophagy. Dowling et al. (2010) determined that while MTMR14 is required for motor function, it is not essential for myocyte homeostasis or normal embryonic development. Morpholino-mediated knockdown of MTMR14 in zebrafish resulted in morphological abnormalities and a developmental motor phenotype characterized by diminished spontaneous contractions and impaired excitation-contraction coupling. Unlike knockdown of another member of this gene family, MTM1, in this model, knockdown of *MTMR14* did not affect muscle ultrastructure (Shen et al., 2009). MTMR14 appeared to act in concert with MTM1 in the development of muscle pathology since simultaneous knockdown of both genes impaired motor function and muscle ultrastructure (Dowling et al., 2009). The resulting phenotype was more severe than that observed with knockdown of either gene alone. Analysis following the knockdown of both of these genes suggested the phenotype observed is likely mediated by an increase in autophagy (Dowling et al., 2010). Defects in Ca^{2+} homeostasis observed in *mtmr14*$^{-/-}$ mice may be an initiator of this observed autophagy.

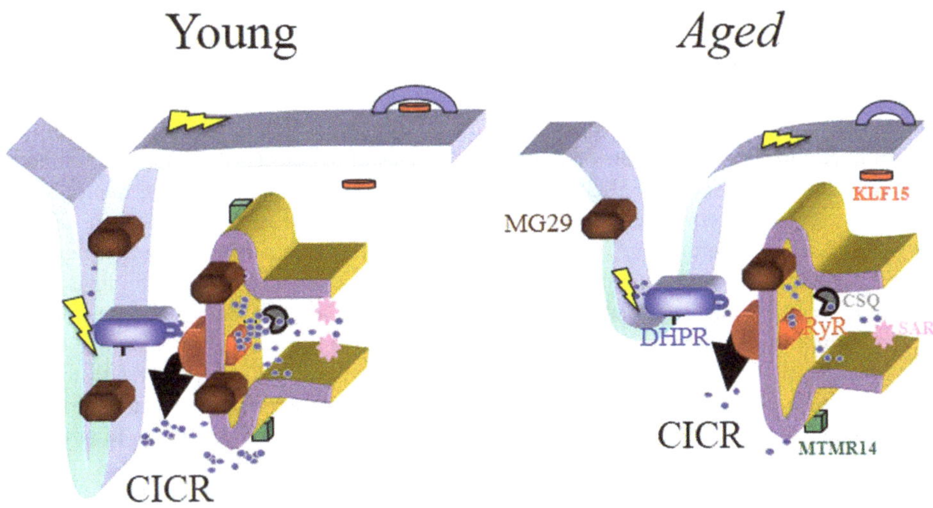

FIGURE 1 | Schematic drawing of the triad junction, the chief site of the E-C coupling process in skeletal muscles. The predicted localization of the four genes/proteins emphasized in this review article is shown and they are represented in different colors along with the Dihydropyridine Receptor (DHPR), the Ryanodine Receptor type 1 (RyR1) and Calsequestrin (CSQ). In young muscles E-C coupling is effectively maintained through coordinated actions of the E-C coupling machinery and the optimal participation of MG29, MTMR14, SAR, and KLF15. Their concentration and/or effectiveness is reduced with aging, which associates with structural changes of the triad junction itself. Together these biochemical and morphological changes contribute to the reduced coupling between depolarization of the sarcolemma and contraction due to the reduced calcium release capacity of aged muscles. In summary, "E-C coupling quality" is reduced in aged muscles, and becomes a key factor to reduced muscle quality during aging. The steps of the E-C coupling process are described in detail in the text. In skeletal muscles, depolarization of the sarcolemma and its invaginations (t-tubules) represented by the lightning bolt in yellow color alters the configuration of the DHPR, which modifies its interaction with RyR1, leading to the dominant type of calcium release in skeletal muscle (depolarization-induced calcium release, DICR). This initial release phase can be further amplified by a secondary mechanism, calcium-induced calcium release (CICR), the main release mechanism in cardiac muscles. The structural deformation as well as the lack of organized triads is a hallmark of aged muscles and also common in other diseases covered in this article. Not detailed in this figure is the process of calcium entry or re-entry, store-operated calcium entry (SOCE), responsible for continual refilling of the sarcoplasmic reticulum (SR). SOCE is also reduced with aging, which we have postulated contributes to sarcopenia and to the un-matching between muscle mass and muscle contractile force during aging, since force/power decrease significantly more than the observed decrease in muscle mass. We foresee that new generations of drugs could be developed to specifically target the different steps of E-C coupling in disease states to increase efficiency of Ca^{2+} handling.

The role of MTMR14 as a negative regulator of autophagy was further evaluated by Gibbs et al. who observed several mutations in the *MTMR14* gene in cases of CNM (Gibbs et al., 2010). In these studies, knockdown of MTMR14 *in vitro* and *in vivo* significantly changed muscle function especially in embryos where decreased developmental motor activity and pronounced fatigability were observed. Knockdown also increased basal and starvation-induced autophagy of muscle cells demonstrated by increased LC3-II levels (Vergne et al., 2009; Dowling et al., 2010). During autophagy, the cytoplasmic form of LC3 (LC3-I) is processed to create LC3-II, which is recruited to autophagosomes. This conversion is used to monitor autophagic activity and LC3-II is considered an autophagic marker. A possibility that MTMR14 may act as a modifier of disease rather than direct cause has been raised. While function-altering MTMR14 mutations have been found in sporadic cases of centronuclear myopathy, one of these patients also carried a disease-associated mutation in *DNM2*. A more severe phenotype was observed in this patient than patients with only the *DNM2* mutation suggesting MTMR14 was not the primary cause of disease but did have a role in exacerbating the phenotype (Bitoun et al., 2005; Dowling et al., 2010).

The mutation of *MTMR14* in cases of CNM and the decreased presence of MTMR14 protein in muscles from aged mice suggest the importance of MTMR14 in muscle physiology and pathophysiology. MTMR14 studies have identified its roles in regulating the abundance of phosphatidylinositol phosphates, which observably alters Ca^{2+} homeostasis. Changes in Ca^{2+} concentrations are a known inducer of autophagy supporting the increased levels of autophagy observed following MTMR14 knockdown (Bonaldo and Sandri, 2013; Smaili et al., 2013). Functionally, MTMR14 affected muscle performance specifically muscle fatigue and muscle weakness.

One key message from these MTMR14 studies is that finely controlled levels of phosphoinositides in muscle cells is essential for maintaining Ca^{2+} homeostasis and enabling effective muscle performance. Improper regulation of Ca^{2+} concentrations by any means, including that observed with these MTMR14 studies, interferes with excitation-contraction (E-C) coupling, which is another physiological process fundamental to muscle pathology. E-C coupling, the conversion of an electrical stimulus by cells to a mechanical response, is aberrantly regulated in various pathologies including muscle wasting disorders (Yoshida et al., 2005; Rossi and Dirksen, 2006). In skeletal muscle, E-C coupling requires two specific proteins, the sarcoplasmic reticulum Ca^{2+} release channel (known as the ryandonine receptor or RyR) and voltage-gated Ca^{2+} channels (known as dihydropyridine receptors or DHPRs). Depolarization of the membrane potential of these cells by an action potential activates voltage-gated DHPRs.

This activates RyR type 1 via physical linkage and conformational changes. As RyRs open, Ca^{2+} is released from the SR into the junctional space then diffuses into the cytoplasm to cause a Ca^{2+} transient (Bellinger et al., 2008; Andersson et al., 2011). Ca^{2+} released into the cytoplasm binds to Troponin C on actin filaments to produce force or contraction of the cell. The sarco/endoplasmic reticulum Ca^{2+} ATPase (SERCA) pumps Ca^{2+} back into the SR and with this the force begins to decline and relaxation occurs. The SR is the dynamic Ca^{2+} governor in muscle cells that receives feedback allowing it to maintain SR and cytoplasmic Ca^{2+} levels. The SR contains an elaborate set of Ca^{2+} regulating proteins including luminal Ca^{2+} binding proteins involved in Ca^{2+} storage, SR Ca^{2+} release channels, and SERCA pumps for Ca^{2+} reuptake. Spatial and temporal control of Ca^{2+} uptake, Ca^{2+} buffering, and Ca^{2+} release is maintained by these highly organized Ca^{2+} regulatory proteins in the SR (O'Connell et al., 2008) (**Figure 1**).

SARCALUMENIN FUNCTIONS IN CALCIUM HANDLING

Another gene related to E-C coupling with a role in muscle pathology is sarcalumenin (*SAR*). Similar to calsequestrin, sarcalumenin is a Ca^{2+} binding protein localized to the sarcoplasmic reticulum of the intracellular Ca^{2+} store of striated muscle cells. While calsequestrin and sarcalumenin are both Ca^{2+} binding proteins of the SR, they are located in different regions of the SR. Sarcalumenin observably colocalizes with SERCA. Two isoforms of SAR, a 160 kDa and a 35 kDa glycoprotein are formed as the products of alternative splicing of the primary transcript (Leberer et al., 1989, 1990). The SAR luminal protein binds Ca^{2+} with high capacity but low affinity (Zhao et al., 2005). Increased SAR expression during muscle development suggests its role in proper functioning of mature SR (Yoshida et al., 2005). Currently, sarcalumenin is considered to be important in the release and uptake of Ca^{2+}, which is the essential second messenger of the excitation-contraction-relaxation cycle in skeletal muscle cells (Yoshida et al., 2005; Rossi and Dirksen, 2006; O'Connell et al., 2008). Using a *SAR* knockout mouse, Yoshida et al. determined that while SAR is not essential for fundamental muscle function, it does play a role in improving Ca^{2+} handling functions of the SR in striated muscle. Muscle from *sar*$^{-/-}$ mice exhibited weakened Ca^{2+} uptake in isolated SR vesicles. In mutant muscles, expression of SERCA protein was decreased while levels of the mRNA remained consistent with wild type muscles. Sarcalumenin unlike most proteins of the SR lacks the four amino acid (KDEL) ER/SR retention signal so it is likely that the direct interaction of SAR with SERCA serves this function (Leberer et al., 1990; Yoshida et al., 2005; Dowling et al., 2009). This is suggestive of SAR acting as a chaperone of SERCA and its involvement in SERCA turnover since the absence of SAR directly impacts the abundance of SERCA protein. Together these findings suggest SAR contributes to Ca^{2+} buffering and the maintenance of Ca^{2+} pump proteins, both of which are essential for E-C coupling and retaining muscle strength. From current research, it remains inconclusive whether SERCA content or a combination of SERCA content and buffering capacity is responsible for the observed effects linked to sarcalumenin expression.

Reduced levels of SAR protein were detected in the dystrophin deficient *mdx* mouse model of muscular dystrophy leading Zhao et al. to further evaluate its role in muscle wasting (Dowling et al., 2004; Zhao et al., 2005). The *sar*$^{-/-}$ mouse model exhibited enhanced fatigue resistance. This finding was determined by evaluating the Ca^{2+} ion storage function of the contractile machinery using single, mechanically skinned muscle fibers loaded with two calcium dyes, one that specifically reported t-tubule calcium and the other that reported SR calcium (Zhao et al., 2005). A number of key findings were obtained using this method for comparison of wild type and *sar*$^{-/-}$ mice. Muscle fibers from SAR deficient mice showed elevated SOCE activity as previously observed and reduced fatigability. Putting the findings from these studies together suggests the fatigue resistant phenotype of *sar*$^{-/-}$ mice is likely due to more effective E-C coupling and SOCE observed in these muscles.

While ATP is thought to play a major role in fatigue, it is typically associated with long-term fatigue under specific conditions. It has been demonstrated by many laboratories that a major culprit in the muscle fatigue process is dysfunctional intracellular calcium homeostasis, specifically impaired Ca^{2+} release from the SR. In normal muscles, calcium stores are more easily depleted than ATP stores and normal muscle function is directly related to Ca^{2+} availability. As less Ca^{2+} becomes available with each contraction/relaxation cycle, fatigue will develop if SOCE is reduced (Brotto et al., 2002; Weisleder et al., 2006; Allen et al., 2008; Place et al., 2009). The studies discussed here concluded the role of sarcalumenin in SOCE function may be useful in reducing or reversing weakness associated with various muscle wasting disorders. Additionally, these studies raised the possibility that the reduced levels of SAR protein observed in *mdx* mice could be interpreted as a compensatory mechanism of adaptation in muscles from these mice in an effort to improve muscle function (Zhao et al., 2005). Further studies suggested that another gene Mitsugumin-29 (*MG29*), might be involved with the compensation observed in the *sar*$^{-/-}$ muscle.

MG29 FUNCTIONS IN MUSCLE FATIGUE AND STORE-OPERATED CALCIUM ENTRY

MG29 is another protein of interest for its identified role in muscle physiology and pathology. Over the last ten years, research has evaluated the role of MG29 in muscle fatigue and SOCE. Using an extensive proteoimmunologic library of antibodies that targeted proteins of the triad junctional membrane structures of skeletal muscle, MG29 was one of the most significant proteins identified (Takeshima et al., 1998). Mitsugumin-29 (MG29) is a member of the synaptophysin family of transmembrane proteins that has been extensively evaluated for their role in muscles. MG29 is almost exclusively expressed in skeletal muscle fibers (Takeshima et al., 1998). MG29 contains four transmembrane domains with a cytoplasmic amino and carboxy terminus. The transmembrane domains allow MG29 to localize at both the transverse (t-) tubular membrane and the SR membrane of the triad junction, which suggests a possible role of MG29 in mediating communication between t-tubular and junctional SR membranes (Thomas et al., 1988, 1998; Thomas and Betz, 1990).

Besides the homologous amino acid sequence, MG29 also shares other characteristic structural features with members of the synaptophysin family of neurotransmitters. Synaptophysin was identified as an abundant immunogenic membrane protein of small synaptic vesicles and is also found in neurosecretory granules (Thomas et al., 1988, 1998; Thomas and Betz, 1990). The structural role of synaptophysin in synaptic vesicle biogenesis and its tight interaction with other proteins of the synaptic vesicle membrane contribute to its essential role in neurotransmitter secretion (Thiele et al., 2000). Similarities between the structure and localization patterns of MG29 to synaptophysin suggest MG29 has an important role in modulating membrane structures in skeletal muscle. Skeletal muscle is one of the most plastic tissues in the human body and since normal muscle physiology requires the formation and maintenance of complex membrane structures, it has been proposed that MG29 may be the structural counterpart of synaptophysin in skeletal muscle biogenesis and maintenance (Booth et al., 2000; Booth and Vyas, 2001).

Mutations of *MG29* have not been observed in specific skeletal muscle wasting disorders; however, its expression and abundance are observed to vary under certain conditions. For example, MG29 expression is known to decrease in aging mouse skeletal muscle (Weisleder et al., 2006). To determine the physiological role of MG29 in normal muscle function and possibly in muscle pathology, an *MG29* knockout mouse was established. The MG29 null mouse was the first experimental indication of the role MG29 plays in muscle membrane integrity. Skeletal muscle from these mice showed multiple abnormalities in membrane structure specifically around the triad junction. Within the triad junction, t-tubules appeared swollen and the SR networks were poorly formed with fragmented structures (Nishi et al., 1999; Thiele et al., 2000). Based on what is known regarding synaptophysin, these findings suggest MG29 functions in membrane fusion associated with the creation and maintenance of membrane structures in the triad junction.

Considering the extent of malformation of the triad junction membrane ultrastructure, the lack of a functional impact of *MG29* knockout was surprising so the phenotype was further evaluated under conditions of physiological stress (Nagaraj et al., 2000). During treadmill running, MG29 knockout mice ran significantly less and were unable to sustain physical activity for the extended period of time compared to littermate controls suggesting a direct role of MG29 in muscle performance specifically during increased physical activity. Additional *ex vivo* muscle contractility assays confirmed increased fatigability in isolated *mg29*$^{-/-}$ muscles. *MG29* null muscles fatigued to a greater extent while also recovering less after fatigue. These muscles also produced less force than wild type control mice even with the addition of caffeine. These findings continue to suggest that E-C coupling in MG29 ablated skeletal muscles is disrupted since muscle fatigue was reduced in *mg29*$^{-/-}$ muscles when Ca^{2+} was removed from the extracellular medium and by pharmacologically blocking extracellular Ca^{2+} entry (Nagaraj et al., 2000). It is clear that the inability of humans to sustain physical activity may lead to chronic degenerative diseases, reduced muscle function, and muscle wasting (Booth et al., 2000). However, the contribution of changes in fatigability to sarcopenia and age related frailty has not been fully resolved as some reports indicate some degree of fatigue resistance develops during muscle aging (Gonzalez and Delbono, 2001a,b). Given that MG29 levels decrease in aging skeletal muscle these findings show that muscle aging is a multivariate situation where changes in multiple factors contribute to the development of aging phenotypes, and emphasize the need for additional studies in this important area of investigation (Weisleder et al., 2006).

The implication of extracellular Ca^{2+} entry as a major factor in muscle fatigue in *mg29*$^{-/-}$ muscle lead to investigation of whether store-operated calcium entry (SOCE) is altered in these muscles compared to wild type control muscles. SOCE is an extracellular calcium entry pathway. In SOCE, reduced Ca^{2+} concentration in the intracellular stores of the sarcoplasmic reticulum induces influx of Ca^{2+} from the extracellular space to replenish the diminished Ca^{2+} stores. While SOCE functions in many different cell types, it is extremely important in the physiology of excitable cells such as muscles and neurons (Albert and Large, 2003; Ma and Pan, 2003; Nilius, 2004; Targos et al., 2005; Ma et al., 2006; Lewis, 2007). Disruption of SOCE activity results in various physiological pathologies (Nilius, 2004; Targos et al., 2005). Its impairment can lead to numerous disorders including cancer and primary immunodeficiency and is being continually researched for its possible role in Alzheimer disease and age-related muscle weakness (sarcopenia) (Nilius, 2004; Targos et al., 2005; Lewis, 2007). The diverse pathologies linked to SOCE is likely due to the wide ranging importance of Ca^{2+} as a second messenger in controlling cellular functions including contraction, secretion, gene expression, and cell cycle.

SOCE is important in long term maintenance of Ca^{2+} homeostasis since it is the mechanism by which additional Ca^{2+} is provided for muscle contraction under conditions where SR Ca^{2+} is depleted such as fatigue, intense exercise, and some pathologies (Zhu and Birnbaumer, 1998; Elliott, 2001; Putney et al., 2001; Parekh and Putney, 2005; Yoshida et al., 2005; Zhao et al., 2005, 2008). Elevated SOCE can also be detrimental as increased resting intracellular Ca^{2+} concentrations potentially underlies development and progression of the muscle injury observed with muscular dystrophy (Brotto et al., 2002). Together, these differential effects of aberrant SOCE suggest its fine-tuned modulation is essential for overall skeletal muscle health. Reduced SOCE was displayed in *MG29* null muscles supporting a role of Ca^{2+} entry in the observed phenotypic changes (Pan et al., 2002). *mg29*$^{-/-}$ muscles fatigued to a greater extent when blockers of SOCE were employed which suggests that the main problem in Ca^{2+} handling is due to reduced SOCE leading to reduced SR calcium storage. Additional studies using more specific SOCE antagonists and genetically silencing players in SOCE will shed more light on this mechanism. Aberrant reduction of SOCE was mirrored in aged skeletal muscles, which also demonstrated decreased expression of MG29 protein resulting in a direct correlation of MG29 protein levels and fatiguing of skeletal muscles.

Additional evidence to support the role of MG29 in SOCE and muscle fatigue stems from the sarcalumenin knockout mouse previously discussed (Yoshida et al., 2005). Muscles isolated from *sar*$^{-/-}$ mice exhibited reduced fatigability and elevated SOCE activity compared to wild type mice. These observed features correlated with increased abundance of MG29 (Zhao et al., 2005). Based on the increased susceptibility of MG29 null muscles to fatigue, it is proposed that the increased presence of MG29 in *sar*$^{-/-}$ mice may be compensatory for the loss of SAR. The compensatory mechanism would contribute to enhanced Ca^{2+} release from the SR and more efficient SR coupling in these muscles. This finding further supports the role of both MG29 and sarcalumenin in maintenance of Ca^{2+} homeostasis and suggests both genes as targets for restoring muscle strength. Putting all these findings together, MG29 may function as a sentinel against age related dysfunction in skeletal muscle by its likely role in regulation of SOCE. MG29 and SAR may serve as therapeutic targets for pathophysiologic muscle conditions including aging and dystrophy where muscle fatigue and strength are impacted. The two main physiologic effects on skeletal muscle by muscle wasting disorders are the physical loss of muscle mass and increased muscle weakness. Both are important processes in the effort to maintain proper functioning of skeletal muscles especially with age. The genes covered above, *MTMR14*, *SAR*, and *MG29*, are being heavily researched for their role in muscle weakness and the induction of fatigue in these disorders. On the other hand, KLF15 has been evaluated for its role in the loss of muscle mass and its possible role in muscle weakness.

KRUPPEL-LIKE FACTOR 15

Kruppel-Like Factor 15 (*KLF15*) belongs to the Kruppel-like factor (KLF) family of transcription factors in a zinc-finger class of DNA binding transcriptional factors. Their transcriptional activity makes their function critical in muscle physiology and muscle pathophysiology. KLFs include three Cys_2/His_2 containing zinc fingers, all of which are located at the extreme c-terminus of the protein. The seven residues separating these zinc fingers are also highly conserved but the non-DNA binding regions of these factors are highly divergent allowing modulation of transactivation or transrepression and mediating protein-protein interactions (Bieker, 1996; Turner and Crossley, 1999; Haldar et al., 2007, 2012; Pearson et al., 2008) This sequence variation likely contributes to the varied expression patterns and functions of the family members. KLFs are differentially expressed in development as well as in response to physiological stresses and are found to play critical roles in cardiovascular biology and in muscle biology, including skeletal muscle (Yamamoto et al., 2004; Haldar et al., 2007). Of specific interest in skeletal muscle biology is KLF15. KLF15 is expressed in all three types of muscle and is known to be a negative regulator of hypertrophic remodeling within the heart by repressing key features required for the hypertrophic process (Fisch et al., 2007; Haldar et al., 2007, 2012).

Research over the past ten years has discovered the importance of KLF15 in skeletal muscle metabolism for both amino acid catabolism and lipid utilization. Its role in metabolism may contribute to its association with muscle atrophy. In two separate studies, KLF15 was evaluated for its function in muscle atrophy and hypertrophy. Schakman et al. researched KLF15 expression in response to glucocorticoids (GC). Long term administration of glucocorticoids as treatment for specific diseases results in debilitating muscle atrophy (Schakman et al., 2013). Biochemically, glucocorticoids were found to increase the rate of protein breakdown and decrease the rate of protein synthesis thus contributing to a loss of muscle mass (Tomas et al., 1979; Goldberg et al., 1980; Lofberg et al., 2002; Drummond and Rasmussen, 2008; Schakman et al., 2013). It was determined that mTORC1 signaling is repressed in the presence of increased GCs through enhanced transcription of *REDD1* and *KLF15*. The mechanism by which KLF15 contributes to protein catabolism is not completely understood but KLF15 appears to activate branched-chain amino acid aminotransferases (BCAT) that are responsible for the degradation of branched chain amino acids (BCAAs). Accelerated BCAA degradation leads to the observed decrease in mTORC1 activity (Chaillou et al., 1985; Bodine et al., 2001; Shimizu et al., 2011; Atherton and Smith, 2012). Further analysis showed that KLF15 in coordination with FOXO1 upregulates E3 ubiquitin ligases Atrogin-1 and MURF1 (Schakman et al., 2013). KLF15 appears to contribute to muscle atrophy by altering the ratio of protein catabolism and synthesis.

While studying the development of muscle hypertrophy, Chaillou et al. recently discovered that KLF15 expression is downregulated in response to overload induced hypertrophy. Decreased KLF15 expression in skeletal muscle resulted in greater protein accretion possibly through decreased degradation of BCAAs leading to increased availability of BCAAs and maintained synthesis of proteins (Chaillou et al., 1985). The mechanism by which KLF15 affects protein synthesis through altered BCAA degradation remains unclear due to the complex nature of this process. Protein synthesis depends on specific roles of the liver and constant crosstalk between the liver and skeletal muscles as well as the commonly ignored function of insulin, which also stimulates skeletal muscle utilization of amino acids/proteins, besides its more readily, attributed effect on glucose uptake. In a parallel study, increased concentrations of BCAAs prolonged activation of mTORC1, which is vital to the process of muscle hypertrophy by enhancing protein synthesis. For this reason, KLF15 may be a target of future studies for controlling skeletal muscle hypertrophy and more specifically skeletal muscle atrophy associated with certain conditions. It appears repression of KLF15 may beneficially impact skeletal muscle by restoring muscle cell loss.

While the role of KLF15 in protein synthesis and catabolism has been researched, KLF15 has also been shown to have a role in lipid utilization in skeletal muscles. With its regulation of amino acid catabolism and its role in fasting gluconeogenesis, KLF15 is proposed to have a role in metabolic adaptation in conditions of physiologic stress such as endurance exercise and fasting (Gray et al., 2007; Shimizu et al., 2011; Haldar et al., 2012). In the lack of sufficient glucose, which is vital for brain function, skeletal muscle resorts to proteins and lipids for its fuel. Specifically, abnormalities of lipid flux impact energetic failure and tolerance to exercise. Studies by Haldar et al. propose that KLF15 and its signaling interaction with glucocorticoids are important in the physiological response to exercise based on its role in both protein and lipid metabolism (Haldar et al., 2012). Yamamoto et al. observed that fasting elevated levels of KLF15 and this lead to increased expression of the mitochondrial acetyl-CoA synthetase gene AceCS2 in skeletal muscle (Fujino et al., 2001; Yamamoto et al., 2004). This enzyme is vital during periods of insufficient glucose and under ketogenic conditions for providing an energy source for muscles (Yamamoto et al., 2004; Gray et al., 2007). The exact role of KLF15 in metabolic lipid flux in skeletal muscle remains unknown but research is focused on understanding the role of KLF15 in defective lipid flux and protein catabolism, both of which can contribute to detrimental changes in muscle cells. Atrophy can be a result of these defects as muscles try to adapt to metabolic changes. In addition to its evaluation in atrophy, KLF15 has been linked to facioscapulohumeral dystrophy (FSHD). For FSHD, KLF15 activated the D4Z4 enhancer element leading to overexpression of DUX4 while this effect was abolished with silencing of *KLF15*. DUX4 is known to be overexpressed in this type of muscular dystrophy (Dmitriev et al., 2011). KLF15 appears to be a promising research target in understanding how metabolism of proteins and lipids may contribute to muscle atrophy as well as its possible role in muscle wasting disorders such as types of muscular dystrophy (Chaillou et al., 1985).

CONCLUSIONS AND FUTURE DIRECTIONS

The available research on MTMR14, sarcalumenin, MG29, and KLF15 in skeletal muscle biology has provided new information toward the better understanding of muscle physiology and pathophysiology. Specific interest is focused on these genes and their possible roles in muscle weakness including that observed during the natural aging process (**Figure 1**). In aging, the most debilitating effects of sarcopenia are the increased muscle weakness and fatigue. This is the case for many other muscle wasting disorders. Muscle wasting disorders display a loss of muscle mass but of greater functional importance is the increased muscle weakness. Muscle weakness is the pathophysiological condition that has the greatest effect on quality of life, independence, and outcome for individuals affected by these disorders. The genes reviewed here are observed to affect key processes in muscle function including SOCE and E-C coupling, which both have proposed roles in muscle fatigue and weakness. While the underlying mechanisms behind these genes and other genes in the loss of muscle strength are finally coming to light, hope is that with additional research, these genes will provide new avenues in finding a therapeutic target in the fight against muscle wasting disorders. We foresee that a new generation of drugs that specifically modulate E-C coupling and calcium homeostasis would be great assets in this fight that is currently being won by the diseases.

AUTHOR CONTRIBUTIONS

Dr. Manring drafted and organized the entire review. Drs. Weisleder and Brotto have had substantial contributions to the conception or design of the work, the acquisition, analysis, and interpretation of data on the genes presented in this review. Dr. Leticia Brotto has contributed during more than one decade in conducting a large amount of the many experiments that led to characterization of the knockout animal models discussed in this article. Dr. Abreu critically revised the initial draft for intellectual and organization content. Dr. Brotto conducted the final approval of the version to be published in agreement with all the authors and he is accountable for all aspects of the work in ensuring that questions related to the accuracy or integrity of any part of the work are appropriately investigated and resolved.

ACKNOWLEDGMENTS

The work summarized in this review article was partially supported by NIH-National Cancer Institute TREC Award U54-116867, American Heart Association Grant (N5505355), NIH-National Institutes of Aging Program Project Grant P01 AG039355-01-A1 and the Thompson Endowment Fund (Marco Brotto). In addition, the work was support by the NIH-NIAMS grant R01AR063084 to Dr. Noah Weisleder and by a NIH Training Grant T32 (T32HL098039) Fellowship.

REFERENCES

Albert, A. P., and Large, W. A. (2003). Store-operated Ca2+-permeable nonselective cation channels in smooth muscle cells. *Cell Calcium* 33, 345–356. doi: 10.1016/S0143-4160(03)00048-4

Allen, D. G., Lamb, G. D., and Westerblad, H. (2008). Skeletal muscle fatigue: cellular mechanisms. *Physiol. Rev.* 88, 287–332. doi: 10.1152/physrev.00015.2007

Alonso, A., Sasin, J., Bottini, N., Friedberg, I., Osterman, A., Godzik, A., et al. (2004). Protein tyrosine phosphatases in the human genome. *Cell* 117, 699–711. doi: 10.1016/j.cell.2004.05.018

Andersson, D. C., Betzenhauser, M. J., Reiken, S., Meli, A. C., Umanskaya, A., Xie, W., et al. (2011). Ryanodine receptor oxidation causes intracellular calcium leak and muscle weakness in aging. *Cell Metab.* 14, 196–207. doi: 10.1016/j.cmet.2011.05.014

Atherton, P. J., and Smith, K. (2012). Muscle protein synthesis in response to nutrition and exercise. *J. Physiol.* 590(Pt 5), 1049–1057. doi: 10.1113/jphysiol.2011.225003

Bellinger, A. M., Reiken, S., Dura, M., Murphy, P. W., Deng, S. X., Landry, D. W., et al. (2008). Remodeling of ryanodine receptor complex causes "leaky" channels: a molecular mechanism for decreased exercise capacity. *Proc. Natl. Acad. Sci. U.S.A.* 105, 2198–2202. doi: 10.1073/pnas.0711074105

Bieker, J. J. (1996). Isolation, genomic structure, and expression of human erythroid Kruppel-like factor (EKLF). *DNA Cell Biol.* 15, 347–352. doi: 10.1089/dna.1996.15.347

Bitoun, M., Maugenre, S., Jeannet, P. Y., Lacene, E., Ferrer, X., Laforet, P., et al. (2005). Mutations in dynamin 2 cause dominant centronuclear myopathy. *Nat. Genet.* 37, 1207–1209. doi: 10.1038/ng1657

Bodine, S. C., Stitt, T. N., Gonzalez, M., Kline, W. O., Stover, G. L., Bauerlein, R., et al. (2001). Akt/mTOR pathway is a crucial regulator of skeletal muscle hypertrophy and can prevent muscle atrophy *in vivo*. *Nat. Cell Biol.* 3, 1014–1019. doi: 10.1038/ncb1101-1014

Bonaldo, P., and Sandri, M. (2013). Cellular and molecular mechanisms of muscle atrophy. *Dis. Model. Mech.* 6, 25–39. doi: 10.1242/dmm.010389

Booth, F. W., Gordon, S. E., Carlson, C. J., and Hamilton, M. T. (2000). Waging war on modern chronic diseases: primary prevention through exercise biology. *J. Appl. Physiol.* 88, 774–787.

Booth, F. W., and Vyas, D. R. (2001). Genes, environment, and exercise. *Adv. Exp. Med. Biol.* 502, 13–20. doi: 10.1007/978-1-4757-3401-0_3

Bortz, W. M. T., and Bortz, W. M. 2nd. (1996). How fast do we age? Exercise performance over time as a biomarker. *J. Gerontol. A Biol. Sci. Med. Sci.* 51, M223–M225. doi: 10.1093/gerona/51A.5.M223

Brooks, S. V., and Faulkner, J. A. (1994). Skeletal muscle weakness in old age: underlying mechanisms. *Med. Sci. Sports Exerc.* 26, 432–439. doi: 10.1249/00005768-199404000-00006

Brotto, M., and Abreu, E. L. (2012). Sarcopenia: pharmacology of today and tomorrow. *J. Pharmacol. Exp. Ther.* 343, 540–546. doi: 10.1124/jpet.112.191759

Brotto, M. A., Nosek, T. M., and Kolbeck, R. C. (2002). Influence of ageing on the fatigability of isolated mouse skeletal muscles from mature and aged mice. *Exp. Physiol.* 87, 77–82. doi: 10.1113/eph8702224

Bruton, J. D., Lannergren, J., and Westerblad, H. (1998). Mechanisms underlying the slow recovery of force after fatigue: importance of intracellular calcium. *Acta Physiol. Scand.* 162, 285–293. doi: 10.1046/j.1365-201X.1998.0292f.x

Chaillou, T., Lee, J. D., England, J. H., Esser, K. A., and McCarthy, J. J. (1985). Time course of gene expression during mouse skeletal muscle hypertrophy. *J. Appl. Physiol.* 115, 1065–1074. doi: 10.1152/japplphysiol.00611.2013

Chawla, J. (2011). Stepwise approach to myopathy in systemic disease. *Front. Neurol.* 2:49. doi: 10.3389/fneur.2011.00049

de Paula Brotto, M., van Leyen, S. A., Brotto, L. S., Jin, J. P., Nosek, C. M., and Nosek, T. M. (2001). Hypoxia/fatigue-induced degradation of troponin I and troponin C: new insights into physiologic muscle fatigue. *Pflugers Arch.* 442, 738–744. doi: 10.1007/s004240100587

Dmitriev, P., Petrov, A., Ansseau, E., Stankevicins, L., Charron, S., Kim, E., et al. (2011). The Kruppel-like factor 15 as a molecular link between myogenic factors and a chromosome 4q transcriptional enhancer implicated in facioscapulohumeral dystrophy. *J. Biol. Chem.* 286, 44620–44631. doi: 10.1074/jbc.M111.254052

Dowling, J. J., Low, S. E., Busta, A. S., and Feldman, E. L. (2010). Zebrafish MTMR14 is required for excitation-contraction coupling, developmental motor function and the regulation of autophagy. *Hum. Mol. Genet.* 19, 2668–2681. doi: 10.1093/hmg/ddq153

Dowling, J. J., Vreede, A. P., Low, S. E., Gibbs, E. M., Kuwada, J. Y., Bonnemann, C. G., et al. (2009). Loss of myotubularin function results in T-tubule disorganization in zebrafish and human myotubular myopathy. *PLoS Genet.* 5:e1000372. doi: 10.1371/journal.pgen.1000372

Dowling, P., Doran, P., and Ohlendieck, K. (2004). Drastic reduction of sarcalumenin in Dp427 (dystrophin of 427 kDa)-deficient fibres indicates that abnormal calcium handling plays a key role in muscular dystrophy. *Biochem. J.* 379, 479–488. doi: 10.1042/BJ20031311

Drummond, M. J., and Rasmussen, B. B. (2008). Leucine-enriched nutrients and the regulation of mammalian target of rapamycin signalling and human skeletal muscle protein synthesis. *Curr. Opin. Clin. Nutr. Metab. Care* 11, 222–226. doi: 10.1097/MCO.0b013e3282fa17fb

Elliott, A. C. (2001). Recent developments in non-excitable cell calcium entry. *Cell Calcium* 30, 73–93. doi: 10.1054/ceca.2001.0215

Estruch, R., Nicolas, J. M., Villegas, E., Junque, A., and Urbano-Marquez, A. (1993). Relationship between ethanol-related diseases and nutritional status in chronically alcoholic men. *Alcohol Alcohol.* 28, 543–550.

Faulkner, J. A., Brooks, S. V., and Zerba, E. (1995). Muscle atrophy and weakness with aging: contraction-induced injury as an underlying mechanism. *J. Gerontol. A Biol. Sci. Med. Sci.* 50(Spec No), 124–129.

Fernandez-Sola, J., Preedy, V. R., Lang, C. H., Gonzalez-Reimers, E., Arno, M., Lin, J. C., et al. (2007). Molecular and cellular events in alcohol-induced muscle disease. *Alcohol. Clin. Exp. Res.* 31, 1953–1962. doi: 10.1111/j.1530-0277.2007.00530.x

Fisch, S., Gray, S., Heymans, S., Haldar, S. M., Wang, B., Pfister, O., et al. (2007). Kruppel-like factor 15 is a regulator of cardiomyocyte hypertrophy. *Proc. Natl. Acad. Sci. U.S.A.* 104, 7074–7079. doi: 10.1073/pnas.0701981104

Fujino, T., Kondo, J., Ishikawa, M., Morikawa, K., and Yamamoto, T. T. (2001). Acetyl-CoA synthetase 2, a mitochondrial matrix enzyme involved in the oxidation of acetate. *J. Biol. Chem.* 276, 11420–11426. doi: 10.1074/jbc.M008782200

Gibbs, E. M., Feldman, E. L., and Dowling, J. J. (2010). The role of MTMR14 in autophagy and in muscle disease. *Autophagy* 6, 819–820. doi: 10.4161/auto.6.6.12624

Goldberg, A. L., Tischler, M., DeMartino, G., and Griffin, G. (1980). Hormonal regulation of protein degradation and synthesis in skeletal muscle. *Fed. Proc.* 39, 31–36.

Gonzalez, E., and Delbono, O. (2001a). Age-dependent fatigue in single intact fast- and slow fibers from mouse EDL and soleus skeletal muscles. *Mech. Ageing Dev.* 122, 1019–1032. doi: 10.1016/S0047-6374(01)00229-9

Gonzalez, E., and Delbono, O. (2001b). Recovery from fatigue in fast and slow single intact skeletal muscle fibers from aging mouse. *Muscle Nerve* 24, 1219–1224. doi: 10.1002/mus.1135

Gonzalez, E., Messi, M. L., and Delbono, O. (2000). The specific force of single intact extensor digitorum longus and soleus mouse muscle fibers declines with aging. *J. Membr. Biol.* 178, 175–183. doi: 10.1007/s002320010025

Gonzalez-Reimers, E., Duran-Castellon, M. C., Lopez-Lirola, A., Santolaria-Fernandez, F., Abreu-Gonzalez, P., Alvisa-Negrin, J., et al. (2010). Alcoholic myopathy: vitamin D deficiency is related to muscle fibre atrophy in a murine model. *Alcohol Alcohol.* 45, 223–230. doi: 10.1093/alcalc/agq010

Gray, S., Wang, B., Orihuela, Y., Hong, E. G., Fisch, S., Haldar, S., et al. (2007). Regulation of gluconeogenesis by Kruppel-like factor 15. *Cell Metab.* 5, 305–312. doi: 10.1016/j.cmet.2007.03.002

Haldar, S. M., Ibrahim, O. A., and Jain, M. K. (2007). Kruppel-like Factors (KLFs) in muscle biology. *J. Mol. Cell. Cardiol.* 43, 1–10. doi: 10.1016/j.yjmcc.2007.04.005

Haldar, S. M., Jeyaraj, D., Anand, P., Zhu, H., Lu, Y., Prosdocimo, D. A., et al. (2012). Kruppel-like factor 15 regulates skeletal muscle lipid flux and exercise adaptation. *Proc. Natl. Acad. Sci. U.S.A.* 109, 6739–6744. doi: 10.1073/pnas.1121060109

Hofer, T., Badouard, C., Bajak, E., Ravanat, J. L., Mattsson, A., and Cotgreave, I. A. (2005). Hydrogen peroxide causes greater oxidation in cellular RNA than in DNA. *Biol. Chem.* 386, 333–337. doi: 10.1515/BC.2005.040

Hong-Brown, L. Q., Brown, C. R., Huber, D. S., and Lang, C. H. (2006). Alcohol and indinavir adversely affect protein synthesis and phosphorylation of MAPK and mTOR signaling pathways in C2C12 myocytes. *Alcohol. Clin. Exp. Res.* 30, 1297–1307. doi: 10.1111/j.1530-0277.2006.00157.x

Jungbluth, H., Wallgren-Pettersson, C., and Laporte, J. (2008). Centronuclear (myotubular) myopathy. *Orphanet J. Rare Dis.* 3, 26. doi: 10.1186/1750-1172-3-26

Lang, C. H., Frost, R. A., Deshpande, N., Kumar, V., Vary, T. C., Jefferson, L. S., et al. (2003). Alcohol impairs leucine-mediated phosphorylation of 4E-BP1, S6K1, eIF4G, and mTOR in skeletal muscle. *Am. J. Physiol. Endocrinol. Metab.* 285, E1205–E1215. doi: 10.1152/ajpendo.00177.2003

Lang, C. H., Wu, D., Frost, R. A., Jefferson, L. S., Kimball, S. R., and Vary, T. C. (1999). Inhibition of muscle protein synthesis by alcohol is associated with modulation of eIF2B and eIF4E. *Am. J. Physiol.* 277(2 Pt 1), E268–E276.

Laporte, J., Bedez, F., Bolino, A., and Mandel, J. L. (2003). Myotubularins, a large disease-associated family of cooperating catalytically active and inactive phosphoinositides phosphatases. *Hum. Mol. Genet.* 12(Spec No 2), R285–R292. doi: 10.1093/hmg/ddg273

Laporte, J., Hu, L. J., Kretz, C., Mandel, J. L., Kioschis, P., Coy, J. F., et al. (1996). A gene mutated in X-linked myotubular myopathy defines a new putative tyrosine phosphatase family conserved in yeast. *Nat. Genet.* 13, 175–182. doi: 10.1038/ng0696-175

Leberer, E., Charuk, J. H., Green, N. M., and MacLennan, D. H. (1989). Molecular cloning and expression of cDNA encoding a lumenal calcium binding glycoprotein from sarcoplasmic reticulum. *Proc. Natl. Acad. Sci. U.S.A.* 86, 6047–6051. doi: 10.1073/pnas.86.16.6047

Leberer, E., Timms, B. G., Campbell, K. P., and MacLennan, D. H. (1990). Purification, calcium binding properties, and ultrastructural localization of the 53, 000- and 160, 000 (sarcalumenin)-dalton glycoproteins of the sarcoplasmic reticulum. *J. Biol. Chem.* 265, 10118–10124.

Lewis, R. S. (2007). The molecular choreography of a store-operated calcium channel. *Nature* 446, 284–287. doi: 10.1038/nature05637

Lexell, J. (1993). Ageing and human muscle: observations from Sweden. *Can. J. Appl. Physiol.* 18, 2–18. doi: 10.1139/h93-002

Lofberg, E., Gutierrez, A., Wernerman, J., Anderstam, B., Mitch, W. E., Price, S. R., et al. (2002). Effects of high doses of glucocorticoids on free amino acids, ribosomes and protein turnover in human muscle. *Eur. J. Clin. Invest.* 32, 345–353. doi: 10.1046/j.1365-2362.2002.00993.x

Lowe, D. A., Husom, A. D., Ferrington, D. A., and Thompson, L. V. (2004). Myofibrillar myosin ATPase activity in hindlimb muscles from young and aged rats. *Mech. Ageing Dev.* 125, 619–627. doi: 10.1016/j.mad.2004.07.002

Lowe, D. A., Thomas, D. D., and Thompson, L. V. (2002). Force generation, but not myosin ATPase activity, declines with age in rat muscle fibers. *Am. J. Physiol. Cell Physiol.* 283, C187–C192. doi: 10.1152/ajpcell.00008.2002

Ma, J., and Pan, Z. (2003). Retrograde activation of store-operated calcium channel. *Cell Calcium* 33, 375–384. doi: 10.1016/S0143-4160(03)00050-2

Ma, R., Du, J., Sours, S., and Ding, M. (2006). Store-operated Ca2+ channel in renal microcirculation and glomeruli. *Exp. Biol. Med. (Maywood)* 231, 145–153.

Manini, T. M., and Clark, B. C. (2012). Dynapenia and aging: an update. *J. Gerontol. A Biol. Sci. Med. Sci.* 67, 28–40. doi: 10.1093/gerona/glr010

Mitchell, W. K., Williams, J., Atherton, P., Larvin, M., Lund, J., and Narici, M. (2012). Sarcopenia, dynapenia, and the impact of advancing age on human skeletal muscle size and strength; a quantitative review. *Front. Physiol.* 3:260. doi: 10.3389/fphys.2012.00260

Murray, C. J., Vos, T., Lozano, R., Naghavi, M., Flaxman, A. D., Michaud, C., et al. (2010). Disability-adjusted life years (DALYs) for 291 diseases and injuries in 21 regions, 1990-2010, a systematic analysis for the Global Burden of Disease Study. *Lancet* 380, 2197–2223. doi: 10.1016/S0140-6736(12)61689-4

Nagaraj, R. Y., Nosek, C. M., Brotto, M. A., Nishi, M., Takeshima, H., Nosek, T. M., et al. (2000). Increased susceptibility to fatigue of slow- and fast-twitch muscles from mice lacking the MG29 gene. *Physiol. Genomics* 4, 43–49.

Nakahara, T., Hashimoto, K., Hirano, M., Koll, M., Martin, C. R., and Preedy, V. R. (2003). Acute and chronic effects of alcohol exposure on skeletal muscle c-myc, p53, and Bcl-2 mRNA expression. *Am. J. Physiol. Endocrinol. Metab.* 285, E1273–E1281. doi: 10.1152/ajpendo.00019.2003

Nakahara, T., Hunter, R., Hirano, M., Uchimura, H., McArdle, A., Broome, C. S., et al. (2006). Alcohol alters skeletal muscle heat shock protein gene expression in rats: these effects are moderated by sex, raised endogenous acetaldehyde, and starvation. *Metabolism* 55, 843–851. doi: 10.1016/j.metabol.2006.02.009

Nilius, B. (2004). Store-operated Ca2+ entry channels: still elusive! *Sci. STKE* 2004, pe36. doi: 10.1126/stke.2342004pe36

Nishi, M., Komazaki, S., Kurebayashi, N., Ogawa, Y., Noda, T., Iino, M., et al. (1999). Abnormal features in skeletal muscle from mice lacking mitsugumin29. *J. Cell Biol.* 147, 1473–1480. doi: 10.1083/jcb.147.7.1473

Noordzij, M., Boeschoten, E. W., Bos, W. J., Dekker, F. W., Bossuyt, P. M., Krediet, R. T., et al. (2007). Disturbed mineral metabolism is associated with muscle and skin complaints in a prospective cohort of dialysis patients. *Nephrol. Dial. Transplant* 22, 2944–2949. doi: 10.1093/ndt/gfm319

O'Connell, K., Gannon, J., Doran, P., and Ohlendieck, K. (2008). Reduced expression of sarcalumenin and related Ca2+ -regulatory proteins in aged rat skeletal muscle. *Exp. Gerontol.* 43, 958–961. doi: 10.1016/j.exger.2008.07.006

Pan, Z., Yang, D., Nagaraj, R. Y., Nosek, T. A., Nishi, M., Takeshima, H., et al. (2002). Dysfunction of store-operated calcium channel in muscle cells lacking mg29. *Nat. Cell Biol.* 4, 379–383. doi: 10.1038/ncb788

Parekh, A. B., and Putney, J. W. Jr. (2005). Store-operated calcium channels. *Physiol. Rev.* 85, 757–810. doi: 10.1152/physrev.00057.2003

Pearson, R., Fleetwood, J., Eaton, S., Crossley, M., and Bao, S. (2008). Kruppel-like transcription factors: a functional family. *Int. J. Biochem. Cell Biol.* 40, 1996–2001. doi: 10.1016/j.biocel.2007.07.018

Pierson, C. R., Tomczak, K., Agrawal, P., Moghadaszadeh, B., and Beggs, A. H. (2005). X-linked myotubular and centronuclear myopathies. *J. Neuropathol. Exp. Neurol.* 64, 555–564. doi: 10.1097/01.jnen.0000171653.17213.2e

Place, N., Bruton, J. D., and Westerblad, H. (2009). Mechanisms of fatigue induced by isometric contractions in exercising humans and in mouse isolated single muscle fibres. *Clin. Exp. Pharmacol. Physiol.* 36, 334–339. doi: 10.1111/j.1440-1681.2008.05021.x

Preedy, V. R., Adachi, J., Ueno, Y., Ahmed, S., Mantle, D., Mullatti, N., et al. (2001a). Alcoholic skeletal muscle myopathy: definitions, features, contribution of neuropathy, impact and diagnosis. *Eur. J. Neurol.* 8, 677–687. doi: 10.1046/j.1468-1331.2001.00303.x

Preedy, V. R., Paice, A., Mantle, D., Dhillon, A. S., Palmer, T. N., and Peters, T. J. (2001b). Alcoholic myopathy: biochemical mechanisms. *Drug Alcohol Depend.* 63, 199–205. doi: 10.1016/S0376-8716(00)00219-2

Preedy, V. R., and Peters, T. J. (1988). The effect of chronic ethanol ingestion on protein metabolism in type-I- and type-II-fibre-rich skeletal muscles of the rat. *Biochem. J.* 254, 631–639.

Putney, J. W. Jr., Broad, L. M., Braun, F. J., Lievremont, J. P., and Bird, G. S. (2001). Mechanisms of capacitative calcium entry. *J. Cell Sci.* 114(Pt 12), 2223–2229.

Rahimov, F., and Kunkel, L. M. (2013). The cell biology of disease: cellular and molecular mechanisms underlying muscular dystrophy. *J. Cell Biol.* 201, 499–510. doi: 10.1083/jcb.201212142

Romanick, M., Thompson, L. V., and Brown-Borg, H. M. (2013). Murine models of atrophy, cachexia, and sarcopenia in skeletal muscle. *Biochim. Biophys. Acta* 1832, 1410–1420. doi: 10.1016/j.bbadis.2013.03.011

Romero, N. B. (2010). Centronuclear myopathies: a widening concept. *Neuromuscul. Disord.* 20, 223–228. doi: 10.1016/j.nmd.2010.01.014

Romero, N. B., and Bitoun, M. (2011). Centronuclear myopathies. *Semin. Pediatr. Neurol.* 18, 250–256. doi: 10.1016/j.spen.2011.10.006

Romero-Suarez, S., Shen, J., Brotto, L., Hall, T., Mo, C., Valdivia, H. H., et al. (2010). Muscle-specific inositide phosphatase (MIP/MTMR14) is reduced with age and its loss accelerates skeletal muscle aging process by altering calcium homeostasis. *Aging (Albany NY).* 2, 504–513.

Rossi, A. E., and Dirksen, R. T. (2006). Sarcoplasmic reticulum: the dynamic calcium governor of muscle. *Muscle Nerve* 33, 715–731. doi: 10.1002/mus.20512

Russ, D. W., Gregg-Cornell, K., Conaway, M. J., and Clark, B. C. (2012) Evolving concepts on the age-related changes in "muscle quality." *J. Cachexia Sarcopenia Muscle* 3, 95–109. doi: 10.1007/s13539-011-0054-2

Schakman, O., Kalista, S., Barbe, C., Loumaye, A., and Thissen, J. P. (2013). Glucocorticoid-induced skeletal muscle atrophy. *Int. J. Biochem. Cell Biol.* 45, 2163–2172. doi: 10.1016/j.biocel.2013.05.036

Sewry, C. A. (2008). Pathological defects in congenital myopathies. *J. Muscle Res. Cell Motil.* 29, 231–238. doi: 10.1007/s10974-008-9155-8

Shen, J., Yu, W. M., Brotto, M., Scherman, J. A., Guo, C., Stoddard, C., et al. (2009). Deficiency of MIP/MTMR14 phosphatase induces a muscle disorder by disrupting Ca(2+) homeostasis. *Nat. Cell Biol.* 11, 769–776. doi: 10.1038/ncb1884

Shimizu, N., Yoshikawa, N., Ito, N., Maruyama, T., Suzuki, Y., Takeda, S., et al. (2011). Crosstalk between glucocorticoid receptor and nutritional sensor mTOR in skeletal muscle. *Cell Metab.* 13, 170–182. doi: 10.1016/j.cmet.2011.01.001

Smaili, S. S., Pereira, G. J., Costa, M. M., Rocha, K. K., Rodrigues, L., do Carmo, L. G., et al. (2013). The role of calcium stores in apoptosis and autophagy. *Curr. Mol. Med.* 13, 252–265. doi: 10.2174/156652413804810772

Takeshima, H., Shimuta, M., Komazaki, S., Ohmi, K., Nishi, M., Iino, M., et al. (1998). Mitsugumin29, a novel synaptophysin family member from the triad junction in skeletal muscle. *Biochem. J.* 331(Pt 1), 317–322.

Targos, B., Baranska, J., and Pomorski, P. (2005). Store-operated calcium entry in physiology and pathology of mammalian cells. *Acta Biochim. Pol.* 52, 397–409.

Teixeira Vde, O., Filippin, L. I., and Xavier, R. M. (2012). Mechanisms of muscle wasting in sarcopenia. *Rev. Bras. Reumatol.* 52, 252–259. doi: 10.1590/S0482-50042012000200009

Thiele, C., Hannah, M. J., Fahrenholz, F., and Huttner, W. B. (2000). Cholesterol binds to synaptophysin and is required for biogenesis of synaptic vesicles. *Nat. Cell Biol.* 2, 42–49. doi: 10.1038/71366

Thomas, L., and Betz, H. (1990). Synaptophysin binds to physophilin, a putative synaptic plasma membrane protein. *J. Cell Biol.* 111(5 Pt 1), 2041–2052. doi: 10.1083/jcb.111.5.2041

Thomas, L., Hartung, K., Langosch, D., Rehm, H., Bamberg, E., Franke, W. W., et al. (1988). Identification of synaptophysin as a hexameric channel protein of the synaptic vesicle membrane. *Science* 242, 1050–1053. doi: 10.1126/science.2461586

Thomas, S. G., Takahashi, M., Neill, J. D., and Clarke, I. J. (1998). Components of the neuronal exocytotic machinery in the anterior pituitary of the ovariectomised ewe and the effects of oestrogen in gonadotropes as studied with confocal microscopy. *Neuroendocrinology* 67, 244–259. doi: 10.1159/000054320

Tomas, F. M., Munro, H. N., and Young, V. R. (1979). Effect of glucocorticoid administration on the rate of muscle protein breakdown *in vivo* in rats, as measured by urinary excretion of N tau-methylhistidine. *Biochem. J.* 178, 139–146.

Tosch, V., Rohde, H. M., Tronchere, H., Zanoteli, E., Monroy, N., Kretz, C., et al. (2006). A novel PtdIns3P and PtdIns(3, 5)P2 phosphatase with an inactivating variant in centronuclear myopathy. *Hum. Mol. Genet.* 15, 3098–3106. doi: 10.1093/hmg/ddl250

Turner, J., and Crossley, M. (1999). Basic Kruppel-like factor functions within a network of interacting haematopoietic transcription factors. *Int. J. Biochem. Cell Biol.* 31, 1169–1174. doi: 10.1016/S1357-2725(99)00067-9

Urbano-Marquez, A., Estruch, R., Fernandez-Sola, J., Nicolas, J. M., Pare, J. C., and Rubin, E. (1995). The greater risk of alcoholic cardiomyopathy and myopathy in women compared with men. *JAMA* 274, 149–154. doi: 10.1001/jama.1995.03530020067034

Urbano-Marquez, A., and Fernandez-Sola, J. (2004). Effects of alcohol on skeletal and cardiac muscle. *Muscle Nerve* 30, 689–707. doi: 10.1002/mus.20168

Vergne, I., Roberts, E., Elmaoued, R. A., Tosch, V., Delgado, M. A., Proikas-Cezanne, T., et al. (2009). Control of autophagy initiation by phosphoinositide 3-phosphatase Jumpy. *EMBO J.* 28, 2244–2258. doi: 10.1038/emboj.2009.159

Vos, T., Flaxman, A. D., Naghavi, M., Lozano, R., Michaud, C., Ezzati, M., et al. (2010). Years lived with disability (YLDs) for 1160 sequelae of 289 diseases and injuries 1990-2010, a systematic analysis for the Global Burden of Disease Study. *Lancet* 380, 2163–2196. doi: 10.1016/S0140-6736(12)61729-2

Wallgren-Pettersson, C., Clarke, A., Samson, F., Fardeau, M., Dubowitz, V., Moser, H., et al. (1995). The myotubular myopathies: differential diagnosis of the X linked recessive, autosomal dominant, and autosomal recessive forms and present state of DNA studies. *J. Med. Genet.* 32, 673–679. doi: 10.1136/jmg.32.9.673

Weisleder, N., Brotto, M., Komazaki, S., Pan, Z., Zhao, X., Nosek, T., et al. (2006). Muscle aging is associated with compromised Ca2+ spark signaling and segregated intracellular Ca2+ release. *J. Cell Biol.* 174, 639–645. doi: 10.1083/jcb.200604166

Wishart, M. J., and Dixon, J. E. (2002). PTEN and myotubularin phosphatases: from 3-phosphoinositide dephosphorylation to disease. *Trends Cell Biol.* 12, 579–585. doi: 10.1016/S0962-8924(02)02412-1

Yamamoto, J., Ikeda, Y., Iguchi, H., Fujino, T., Tanaka, T., Asaba, H., et al. (2004). A Kruppel-like factor KLF15 contributes fasting-induced transcriptional activation of mitochondrial acetyl-CoA synthetase gene AceCS2. *J. Biol. Chem.* 279, 16954–16962. doi: 10.1074/jbc.M312079200

Yoshida, M., Minamisawa, S., Shimura, M., Komazaki, S., Kume, H., Zhang, M., et al. (2005). Impaired Ca2+ store functions in skeletal and cardiac muscle cells from sarcalumenin-deficient mice. *J. Biol. Chem.* 280, 3500–3506. doi: 10.1074/jbc.M406618200

Zahn, J. M., Sonu, R., Vogel, H., Crane, E., Mazan-Mamczarz, K., Rabkin, R., et al. (2006). Transcriptional profiling of aging in human muscle reveals a common aging signature. *PLoS Genet.* 2:e115. doi: 10.1371/journal.pgen.0020115

Zhao, X., Weisleder, N., Thornton, A., Oppong, Y., Campbell, R., Ma, J., et al. (2008). Compromised store-operated Ca2+ entry in aged skeletal muscle. *Aging Cell* 7, 561–568. doi: 10.1111/j.1474-9726.2008.00408.x

Zhao, X., Yoshida, M., Brotto, L., Takeshima, H., Weisleder, N., Hirata, Y., et al. (2005). Enhanced resistance to fatigue and altered calcium handling properties of sarcalumenin knockout mice. *Physiol. Genomics* 23, 72–78. doi: 10.1152/physiolgenomics.00020.2005

Zhu, X., and Birnbaumer, L. (1998). Calcium channels formed by mammalian Trp homologues. *News Physiol. Sci.* 13, 211–217.

4

Nuclear positioning in muscle development and disease

Eric S. Folker*[1] *and Mary K. Baylies*[2]

[1] *Department of Biology, Boston College, Chestnut Hill, MA, USA*
[2] *Department of Developmental Biology, Sloan-Kettering Institute, New York, NY, USA*

Correspondence:
Mary K. Baylies, Department of Developmental Biology, Sloan Kettering Institute, Box 310 430 East 67th Street, NY 10065, USA
e-mail: m-baylies@ski.mskcc.org

Muscle disease as a group is characterized by muscle weakness, muscle loss, and impaired muscle function. Although the phenotype is the same, the underlying cellular pathologies, and the molecular causes of these pathologies, are diverse. One common feature of many muscle disorders is the mispositioning of myonuclei. In unaffected individuals, myonuclei are spaced throughout the periphery of the muscle fiber such that the distance between nuclei is maximized. However, in diseased muscles, the nuclei are often clustered within the center of the muscle cell. Although this phenotype has been acknowledged for several decades, it is often ignored as a contributor to muscle weakness. Rather, these nuclei are taken only as a sign of muscle repair. Here we review the evidence that mispositioned myonuclei are not merely a symptom of muscle disease but also a cause. Additionally, we review the working models for how myonuclei move from two different perspectives: from that of the nuclei and from that of the cytoskeleton. We further compare and contrast these mechanisms with the mechanisms of nuclear movement in other cell types both to draw general themes for nuclear movement and to identify muscle-specific considerations. Finally, we focus on factors that can be linked to muscle disease and find that genes that regulate myonuclear movement and positioning have been linked to muscular dystrophy. Although the cause-effect relationship is largely speculative, recent data indicate that the position of nuclei should no longer be considered only a means to diagnose muscle disease.

Keywords: Nuclear movement, muscle disease, nucleoskeleton, cytoskeleton

HISTORY

Myofibers are the cellular units of mature skeletal muscles. The structure of myofibers, and the basic principles that govern the development of myofibers, are conserved from *Drosophila* to humans. Skeletal muscle accounts for nearly 50% of adult body mass, and the organization of the myofibers is repetitive and striking. This repetitive structure is most notably illustrated by the myofibril network, the linear and repetitive arrangement of sarcomeres and associated proteins that enable muscle contraction. The myofibril network of skeletal muscle garnered much early attention and has been studied in detail since the early 1940s, when Ramsey and Street published their observations that the length of the sarcomere corresponded to the physical output of the muscle (Ramsey and Street, 1940). With improved electron microscopy techniques to better understand subcellular organization, the structure of the myofibrils was examined in more depth, culminating in development of the sarcomeric sliding filament model described in 1954 (Huxley and Hanson, 1954; Huxley and Niedergerke, 1954). Importantly, work in the field of muscle biology maintained its focus on correlating the structure of the muscle with the function, or physical output, of the muscle cell. Moving forward, the feature that the functional output of muscle can be easily assessed makes muscle an ideal tissue in which to understand additional aspects of cellular structure and organization and how they impact function.

With the contractile myofibrillary network described, and the development of more sophisticated imaging techniques, further definition of the myofiber structure and how that structure impacts function has gained traction. Coincident with the ability to more precisely examine muscle structure, advancements in sequencing and gene identification have made it evident that sarcomere assembly and myofibril organization are not sufficient for full muscle function. In fact, many mutations that cause muscle disease do not appear to directly affect sarcomere structure. For example, Emery-Dreifuss Muscular Dystrophy (EDMD) is characterized by progressive muscle weakness, but the genes that are mutated in patients with EDMD encode proteins that localize to the nucleus rather than the sarcomere. Furthermore, at least a subset of EDMD causing mutations do not impact the assembly of the sarcomere (Gueneau et al., 2009). This makes clear that sarcomere assembly on its own is not sufficient for muscle cells to generate maximal force and indicates that additional aspects of cellular organization impact muscle physiology and likely underlie many muscle diseases. Thus, to fully understand general muscle biology, and muscle disease pathogenesis specifically, we must determine how muscle cells become organized and the relative contributions of each aspect of organization to muscle function.

Like all eukaryotic cells, myofibers require several organelles that compartmentalize different cellular functions. For example, mitochondria compartmentalize energy production, the nuclei compartmentalize gene regulation, the sarcoplasmic reticulum compartmentalizes calcium storage and release, and the Golgi apparatus compartmentalizes protein sorting. Each of these organelles is essential to proper muscle function. This fact is illustrated by the identification of mutations in genes related to each organelle that cause muscle disease (Cohen et al., 2013; Gazzerro et al., 2013; Schreiber and Kennedy, 2013). Although the metabolic importance of muscle has been recognized for decades, and significant information regarding the relationship between mutations in metabolic enzymes and muscle disease exists (Muntoni et al., 2011; Bonaldo and Sandri, 2013), the role of general muscle architecture in muscle function is less clear. Little is known regarding the aspects of organization that are essential, how each organelle contributes to muscle function, and whether the positioning of different organelles are linked or occur independently.

These are overarching questions that will require years of work to understand as only recently have researchers begun studying the positioning of organelles in muscle. This review will focus on the organization of nuclei within the myofiber. Specifically, we will explore the mechanisms by which nuclei are positioned, and the evidence that the precise positioning of nuclei is essential for proper muscle function.

NUCLEAR POSITIONING IN MUSCLE

Nuclei in muscle are positioned at the periphery of each myofiber. Furthermore, these peripheral nuclei are positioned to maximize the distance between adjacent nuclei (Bruusgaard et al., 2003). Although it is not known why nuclei are positioned in this way, there are intuitive and compelling possibilities to explain both aspects of nuclear position. The myodomains theory states that each nucleus nourishes a discrete portion of the muscle (Pavlath et al., 1989) and provides a logical explanation for the maximizing of internuclear distances. If nuclei were clustered rather than spaced evenly, different regions of the muscle would lack the transcription and translation necessary to maintain the myofiber. Regarding the positioning of the nuclei at the periphery of the myofiber, rather than within the myofiber, it is intuitive that nuclei in the center of the myofiber could act as physical obstacles to contraction and therefore impede muscle output. Alternatively, maintaining nuclei at the muscle periphery may be a means to protect nuclei from the force of contraction that they would need to withstand in the central portion of the muscle. Importantly, these options are not mutually exclusive.

Consistent with these potential functions for myonuclear positioning, biopsies of the muscles from patients with several different muscle disorders display large numbers of myofibers with centrally positioned nuclei (>25% compared to <3% in unaffected individuals). Mispositioned nuclei were originally noted with respect to muscle disease by Dr. Spiro (Spiro et al., 1966) regarding a patient with Myotubular Myopathy, one of a subset of muscle diseases that would become collectively referred to as Central Nuclear Myopathies (CNM). However, centrally positioned nuclei are not unique to CNM and have been noted, and are prominent, in many distinct muscle disorders. Moreover, central nuclei have been routinely used for nearly 50 years as a pathological marker for differentiating muscle disorders from neurological disorders (Dubowitz et al., 2007). Indeed, muscle biopsies from patients with most muscle disorders, including relatively common disorders such as Duchenne Muscular Dystrophy (DMD) (Wang et al., 2000), Becker Muscular Dystrophy (BMD), and EDMD (Gueneau et al., 2009), show nuclei prominently within the center of individual muscle fibers.

However, despite the prevalence of centrally positioned nuclei in the myofibers of patients suffering from disparate muscle diseases, the importance of nuclear positioning to disease pathogenesis and muscle weakness is not clear. Moreover, there is little to be found in the scientific literature exploring the role of nuclear positioning in muscle function or disease. This is in part explained by the prevailing hypothesis that is used to explain centrally positioned nuclei: central nuclei are considered to be merely a marker of ongoing myofiber repair. This assumption is well supported by the general mechanisms of muscle development and repair during which all muscle nuclei undergo at least three dramatic movements.

Multinucleate muscle fibers form from the fusion of mononucleated myoblasts rather than through nuclear divisions in the absence of cytokinesis as was once thought (Capers, 1960). Upon fusion, each newly incorporated nucleus is actively moved to the center of the immature myotube (Kelly and Zacks, 1969; Cadot et al., 2012) (**Figure 1**). Following many fusion events, the myotube will mature into a myofiber. Historically, this maturation process is identified by the development of a dense myofibril network throughout the cell. However, this maturation process also correlates with the second type of nuclear movement during which nuclei are moved from the center of the myofiber to the periphery (Capers, 1960) and the third movement in which the distance between adjacent nuclei is maximized (Bruusgaard et al., 2003) (**Figure 1**). It is not clear whether the movement of the nuclei to the periphery and the assembly of the myofibril network are functionally linked and/or whether one process is dependent on the other. Yet, the coincident nature of these two events and the prevalence of aberrant nuclear positioning in individuals with muscle disease, suggest that the peripheral localization of nuclei and the maximizing of internuclear distance are important factors in muscle development.

Following the movement of nuclei to the muscle periphery, a small subset of muscle nuclei will undergo an additional movement. These myonuclei can move as either individuals or as clusters to the Neuromuscular Junction (NMJ) and stably localize there as clusters of between 3 and 8 nuclei (Englander and Rubin, 1987). This last movement to the NMJ is an active process, and these nuclei have unique transcriptional profiles and different levels of nuclear membrane proteins compared to the majority of the muscle nuclei (Sanes et al., 1991; Moscoso et al., 1995). Furthermore, it has been demonstrated that the positioning of these nuclei is essential for synaptic transmission (Jevsek et al., 2006) and that the absence of nuclei clustered at the NMJ correlate with neuro-muscular disease (Grady et al., 2005; Zhang et al., 2007).

Similar nuclear movements are seen during myofiber repair (**Figure 1**). First, activated satellite cells fuse with the damaged myofiber (Yin et al., 2013). However, rather than maintaining its position at the myofiber periphery where it fused, a newly

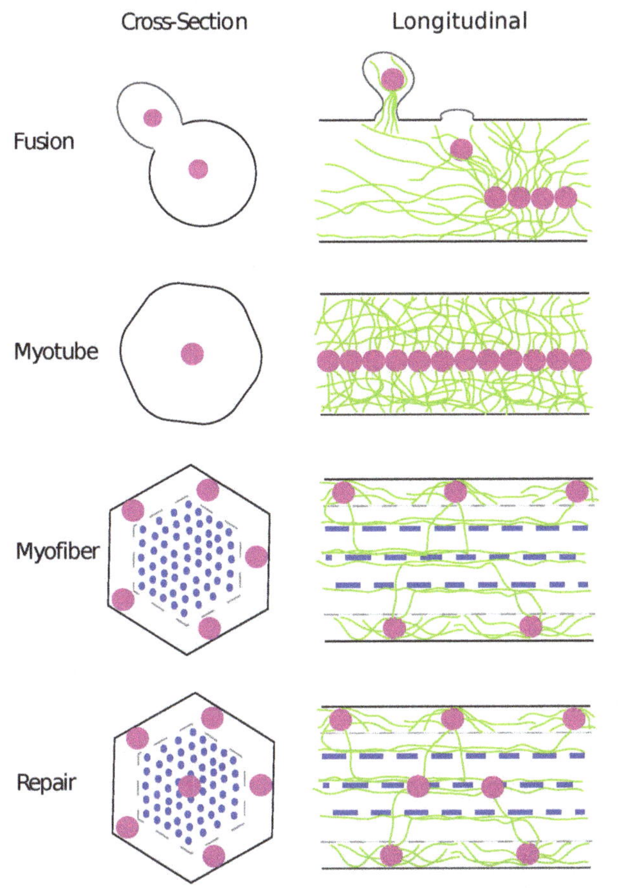

FIGURE 1 | Position of nuclei during muscle development as seen in cross-section (left) and longitudinal samples (right). As new nuclei (pink) are incorporated from myoblasts during fusion, they are rapidly moved to the center of the myotube by a process that requires the microtubule cytoskeleton (green). Thus, in the myotube, the nuclei are aligned in the center of the cell. As the myotube matures into a myofiber with the assembly of the sarcomere (blue), the nuclei move to the periphery of the muscle and reside directly above the sarcolemna (gray) and space to maximize the internuclear distance. Coincident with these nuclear movements, the microtubule cytoskeleton becomes highly ordered. Microtubules are nucleated at or near the nuclear envelope with some overlap of microtubules emanating from adjacent nuclei. Additionally, microtubules extend to the sarcomeres and run parallel to these highly ordered actin-myosin based structures. During repair, newly incorporated nuclei undergo movements similar to the movements of nuclei in the developing muscle. New nuclei are incorporated into the myofiber as myotubes fuse with the myofiber. The newly incorporated nuclei move to the center of the myofiber before moving out to the myofiber periphery in two separate microtubule-dependent processes.

incorporated nucleus is moved to the center of the myofiber before being moved back out to the cell periphery (Dubowitz et al., 2007). The reason for these long-range nuclear movements is not known. However, cross-sectional analysis reveals that many more myofibers will have centrally positioned nuclei when a muscle is undergoing repair compared to steady-state muscles. Thus, centrally positioned nuclei provide an easy assay to determine which myofibers are undergoing repair in response to either disease or physical insult (Dubowitz et al., 2007).

For all of these reasons, it has been presumed that centrally positioned nuclei are a consequence of continual myofiber repair in patients with muscle disease. Therefore, the possibility that mispositioned nuclei contribute to muscle weakness and disease have been ignored. However, that both nuclear movements are maintained in already mature myofibers suggests that there is a biological necessity to these movements. Significant energy is spent moving nuclei to the center of the myofiber and back to the periphery indicating that nuclear movement in muscle is necessary for proper muscle function. It is therefore essential to understand the mechanisms that drive these nuclear movements and the biological significance of these nuclear movements to fully understand and treat muscle disease.

Furthermore, many genes that are mutated in patients with muscle disease encode proteins that localize to the nucleus. The first identified proteins that localize to the nucleus and cause muscle disease have known roles in regulating gene expression (Maraldi et al., 2002; Tsukahara et al., 2002). Therefore, the initial, and still enticing, hypothesis was that muscle diseases associated with these mutations resulted from aberrant gene regulation. However, proteins that localize exclusively in the outer nuclear envelope and regulate the interactions between the nucleus and the cytoskeleton have recently been identified as mutated in patients with muscle disease (Wheeler et al., 2007; Zhang et al., 2007; Puckelwartz et al., 2009). Because these genes do not directly interact with the genome, these data raise the possibility that the nucleus may have a role in muscle development and function independent of its general role in gene regulation and might suggest a role for nucleus-cytoskeleton interactions and nuclear positioning in muscle development and disease pathogenesis.

We will review the mechanisms of nuclear positioning, specifically in muscle, from the perspective of both the nucleus and the cytoskeleton. Although we will discuss the mechanisms of nuclear movement in broad strokes, we will further focus the discussion toward genes known to be mutated in patients with muscle disease.

THE NUCLEUS

It is intuitive that proteins of the nuclear envelope will participate in the movement and positioning of nuclei. With few exceptions in which nuclei are moved by bulk movement of the cytoplasm (Ramos-García et al., 2009), nuclear envelope proteins are required for the nucleus to interact with the cytoskeleton. In turn, the cytoskeleton provides the force to move nuclei, but requires specific and often highly regulated interactions with the nuclei (Gundersen and Worman, 2013). This is true in muscle also. Both the LINC complex (Linker of nucleoskeleton and cytoskeleton; reviewed Tapley and Starr, 2013), and the nucleoskeleton, which is a filamentous network of proteins that provides structure to the nucleus, are essential for nuclear movement and positioning in muscle cells. Moreover, mutations in several of these proteins have been identified in patients with muscle disease, specifically EDMD (Stewart et al., 2007).

THE LINC COMPLEX

The LINC complex is composed of Nesprin proteins (also known as Klarsicht, Anc, and Syne Homology (KASH) proteins) that span the outer nuclear envelope and SUN proteins that span the inner nuclear envelope. Nesprin proteins come in many isoforms. Mammals have at least four different Nesprin genes and each of these genes is differentially spliced to form in total dozens of Nesprin proteins. Similarly, SUN proteins exist in at least two different varieties from two different genes termed Sun1 and Sun2. The LINC complex and its general roles in nuclear positioning have been reviewed (Tapley and Starr, 2013), but we will focus here in greater detail on the data from muscle systems and its impact on muscle function.

Capitalizing on work in *C. elegans* (Starr et al., 2001; Starr and Han, 2002), the role of the Nesprin protein, Syne-1, was examined in mouse muscles. Expression of a dominant negative Syne-1 protein, which can localize to the nucleus but cannot interact with the cytoskeleton, displaced endogenous Syne-1 from the nucleus without generally disrupting nuclear structure. The disruption of endogenous Syne-1 localization did not appear to dramatically impact the peripheral localization of nuclei nor did it affect their general spacing. However, the clustering of nuclei at the NMJ was lost (Grady et al., 2005). Further analysis found that genetic deletion of the Syne-1 KASH domain, the domain that enables localization to the nuclear envelope, caused both synaptic and non-synaptic nuclei to be mispositioned (Zhang et al., 2007; Puckelwartz et al., 2009). Similarly, deletion of both SUN proteins, Sun-1 and Sun-2, resulted in fewer nuclei at the NMJ and the clustering of nuclei throughout the muscle fiber (Lei et al., 2009). Finally, although disruption of Syne-1 did not impact Sun-1 or Sun-2 localization (Grady et al., 2005), the deletion of Sun1/2 decreased the localization of Syne-1 to the nucleus. However, neither Sun1/2 deletion nor Syne-1/Syne-2 deletion impacted the organization of the nucleoskeleton (Lei et al., 2009). This indicates that the localization of proteins necessary for nuclear movement in muscle proceeds in a unidirectional manner from the nucleoplasm to the cytoskeleton.

The role of the LINC complex in positioning muscle nuclei is not confined to *in vivo* mouse muscles. The same proteins have been shown to be essential for moving nuclei in the mouse cell culture system of C2C12 myotubes. Specifically, it has been demonstrated that disruption of the LINC complex by expression of a dominant negative Syne-1 protein, similar to the experiment carried out *in vivo*, causes nuclei *in vitro* to move less dynamically and therefore to cluster (Wilson and Holzbaur, 2012). Similarly, in developing *Drosophila* larvae, deletion of the KASH domain from either of two KASH domain proteins in the genome (Klarsicht and Msp-300) results in clustered nuclei in the larval muscles (Elhanany-Tamir et al., 2012). Furthermore, mutation of the *Drosophila* SUN protein Klaroid, affected the position of nuclei in the embryonic musculature (Elhanany-Tamir et al., 2012).

The precise role of these LINC complex proteins during nuclear movement in muscles is not known. However, in a general sense, they enable the nucleus to interact with the cytoskeleton, which provides the force to move nuclei. For example in the C2C12 culture system, it has been demonstrated that KASH proteins enable the microtubule motors Kinesin-1 and cytoplasmic Dynein to interact with and move nuclei (Wilson and Holzbaur, 2012). This is consistent with data from several other systems including *C. elegans* (Meyerzon et al., 2009; Fridolfsson et al., 2010) and mammalian neurons (Zhang et al., 2009; Yu et al., 2011). But the data from *Drosophila* larval muscles suggest an alternative mechanism in which the KASH proteins are necessary to maintain microtubule-nucleus interactions (Elhanany-Tamir et al., 2012). Supporting this hypothesis, many KASH domain-containing proteins harbor domains that can directly interact with the cytoskeleton. However, despite the dramatic effect that the loss of KASH proteins have on microtubule organization, the effect could be indirect and result from inefficient recruitment of the aforementioned microtubule motors. Further work is necessary to distinguish these mechanisms and/or demonstrate how the two mechanisms are coordinated.

Another confounding issue in these data is that the initial study in mouse, in which Syne-1 and Syne-2 were displaced from the nuclear envelope by the expression of the Syne-2 KASH domain, only affected the positioning of the synaptic nuclei. It is not clear why the displacement of the endogenous protein from the nuclear envelope causes a different phenotype than does the expression of a KASH-less protein. A simple interpretation of these data is that a portion of the endogenous protein remains localized to the nucleus even in the presence of the dominant negative, and that the synaptic nuclei are more sensitive to levels of endogenous Syne-1 and Syne-2. However, further work is necessary to fully understand these data.

THE NUCLEOSKELETON

The nucleoskeleton is a meshwork of proteins contained within the nucleus and adjacent to the inner nuclear membrane that provides the nucleus with its shape and its ability to withstand mechanical stresses. The primary components of the nucleoskeleton are the nuclear lamin proteins which exist in several varieties. There are two B-type lamins that originate from two genes, *LMNB1* and *LMNB2*. The A-type lamins, Lamin A and Lamin C, are, respectively, the immature and fully processed gene products of the *LMNA* gene and will be the forms discussed here; it is these proteins that directly contribute to nuclear positioning in muscles, and mutations in the *LMNA* gene result in the autosomal dominant form of EDMD (Stewart et al., 2007).

Work in cell culture has demonstrated that in the absence of Lamin A/C, nuclear movement is inhibited (Lee et al., 2007; Hale et al., 2008; Houben et al., 2009; Folker et al., 2011), the ability of the nucleus to withstand physical stress is limited (Broers et al., 2004; Lammerding et al., 2004), and the ability of the cell to organize its genome is compromised (Gnocchi et al., 2011; Mattout et al., 2011). Each of these biological functions has been, and continues to be, explored as possible pathogenic mechanisms of *LMNA* mutations and significant data support each of these hypotheses.

The first *Lmna*$^{-/-}$ mouse study was published in 1999 and changes in both nuclear structure and nuclear localization were noted. Moreover, mice lacking Lamin A/C were described as dystrophic (Sullivan et al., 1999). All of these characteristics were similar to those described in human EDMD patients carrying *LMNA* mutations (Bonne et al., 2000). Similarly, larval muscles in *Drosophila* which lack Lamin C (the only A-type lamin in *Drosophila*) have nuclei with variable and distorted structures that are commonly mispositioned (Dialynas et al., 2010; Zwerger et al., 2013). Yet, none of these studies have been able to clarify the relative contributions of distorted nuclear structure and aberrant nuclear positions to muscle disease.

Attempts to clarify this question using cell culture based systems have added support for each possibility. For example, more detailed rheological analysis has clearly demonstrated that not only does the loss of Lamin A/C make cells and their nuclei more sensitive to mechanical stress, but that mutations which cause EDMD have the same effect (Zwerger et al., 2013). Similarly, *LMNA* mutations that when heterozygous in humans cause EDMD inhibit nuclear movement when expressed in fibroblasts suggesting a dominant negative role for these mutations. Interestingly, *LMNA* mutations that cause Dunnigan Type 2 Familial-Partial Lipodystrophy, also in a dominant negative manner, have no effect on nuclear movement, suggesting that mediating nuclear positioning or nuclear-cytoskeletal interactions are a function of Lamin A/C that is particularly important in muscle (Folker et al., 2011).

Finally, although the experiments in *Drosophila* do not differentiate between effects on nuclear structure, gene regulation, and nuclear position, they do provide insight toward the relevance of nuclear position. As noted previously, the consensus has been that the mispositioned nuclei in patients with muscle disease are merely a result of ongoing myofiber repair. However, there is no evidence that *Drosophila* larval muscles undergo repair. Yet, the nuclei in *Drosophila* larval muscles are dramatically mispositioned when Lamin C is absent or when disease causing variants of Lamin C are expressed only in the muscle (Dialynas et al., 2010). This suggests that myonuclear positioning is an active and critically maintained process and that all nuclear mispositioning is not merely a marker of ongoing muscle repair.

Taken together, these data make clear that Lamin A/C is essential for proper nuclear positioning in muscle. Additionally, and most importantly for this discussion, is that the contribution of Lamin A/C to nuclear position is inhibited by mutations that cause muscle disease. This correlation suggests that the role of Lamin A/C in positioning nuclei may contribute to muscle weakness and disease. More generally, these data further suggest that the positioning of the nucleus within the muscle may be fundamentally important and that aberrant nuclear positioning may contribute to disease pathogenesis.

Proteins that interact with the Lamin A/C also cause muscle disease and have also been implicated in regulating nuclear structure, gene expression and nuclear position (Zhong et al., 2010). Emerin (*EMD*) is among the best described Lamin-interacting proteins; it was identified as a gene mutated in patients with X-linked EDMD prior to the identification of *LMNA* as the gene responsible for the autosomal dominant form of EDMD (Bione et al., 1994). Emerin null fibroblasts are similar to Lamin null fibroblasts in that they fail polarize and instead form inefficient nucleus-cytoskeleton interactions (Chang et al., 2013; Ho et al., 2013). However, the analysis of Emerin and its functions *in vivo* are limited when compared to Lamin A/C. Analysis of the Emerin null mouse has likely lagged relative to the Lamin null mouse due to the lack of phenotype. Although the Emerin null mouse does have delayed muscle regeneration (Melcon et al., 2006), there are no overt dystrophic phenotypes (Melcon et al., 2006; Ozawa et al., 2006). The reason for this discrepancy requires further examination, but perhaps Emerin is involved in enhancing or specifying a specific Lamin A/C function. If Lamin A/C is contributing to muscle function through multiple pathways, one might reason that the effects of mutating each individual regulating protein would be diminished relative to loss of Lamin A/C itself.

Unfortunately, it is not clear how mutations in *EMD* and *LMNA* cause muscle disease. However, both genes are necessary to maintain the structure of individual nuclei, to position nuclei, and to maintain proper gene regulation as discussed above. Perhaps these three aspects of nuclear biology in muscle are critically linked.

Indeed, it has been argued that improper gene regulation in *Lmna* null mice causes the clustering of nuclei. This clustering is particularly evident near the NMJ, and nuclei in this location vary from levels of almost no acetylated histone H3 to high levels of acetylated histone H3. This is contrasted by the nuclei in WT muscles which have consistent and moderate levels of acetylated histone H3 (Gnocchi et al., 2011). However, it is equally plausible that improper positioning leads to the change in gene expression. There is in fact clear evidence that nuclear position can influence gene expression. For example, nuclei at the NMJ have a unique transcriptional profile relative to the non-synaptic nuclei (Jevsek et al., 2006). Perhaps nuclei being in close proximity can communicate and coordinate their transcriptional output such that individual nuclei down-regulate transcription. Alternatively, nuclei may sense the proximity of other nuclei and up-regulate transcription in an effort to repair or remodel the muscle. Although the cause-effect relationship is not clear, that both phenotypes are common and can be caused by mutations in the nucleoskeleton highlights the need to better understand how these processes relate to muscle function. The ability to affect the position of nuclei without directly affecting their transcriptional profile, and vice versa, is essential to gaining a full understanding of this relationship.

THE CYTOSKELETON

Movement of nuclei by the cytoskeleton is seen in eukaryotes ranging from yeast to mammals and is relevant to processes ranging from DNA segregation during mitosis to cellular locomotion (Gundersen and Worman, 2013). In the next several paragraphs we will consider how the cytoskeleton moves nuclei and will focus on mechanisms determined in muscle systems.

Two different cytoskeletal networks have been demonstrated to drive nuclear movements. Most nuclear movements, in both muscles and other tissues, are driven by microtubules and their associated proteins and motors. Other nuclear movements and positioning events require the action of the actin cytoskeleton and its associated factors. In most cellular contexts the actin network and the microtubule network are intimately connected, often co-regulated, and can directly impinge on the activity of the other, making it difficult to discern the specific effects of either network (Rodriguez et al., 2003). Still, several mechanisms of either nuclear movement or nuclear positioning have been elucidated and attributed to one cytoskeletal network or the other.

MICROTUBULES

The organization of the microtubule network in muscle cells is different from that in most other cell types. Most eukaryotic cells have a single microtubule organizing center (MTOC) from which most microtubules emanate and at which microtubule minus-ends are anchored. In higher eukaryotes this is accomplished by the centrosome and in many lower eukaryotes such as yeast, this is accomplished by an analogous structure called the spindle pole body. Muscle cells do not have a single MTOC. This is not merely a result of having many nuclei because each nucleus has several associated MTOCs. In culture, after myoblasts fuse to a growing myotube they disassemble their centrosome and redistribute their pericentriolar material and γ-tubulin around the entire nuclear envelope (Tassin et al., 1985) and in smaller quantities to the Golgi apparatus (Ralston et al., 2001). Similar organization is seen *in vivo*, where each nuclear envelope and Golgi apparatus thus serves as a MTOC with microtubules emanating from many locations on both the nucleus and the Golgi apparatus (Oddoux et al., 2013). Given that there are often tens to hundreds of nuclei in a given muscle, mature muscles have microtubules that originate from many distinct locations.

Except for the number of MTOCs, the microtubules emanating from the nuclei behave similarly to those in other cell types. Microtubules grow in all directions with equal probabilities and have similar dynamics to microtubules in standard cell culture experiments (Wilson and Holzbaur, 2012) and *in vivo* (Oddoux et al., 2013; Folker et al., 2014). However, this is not the only microtubule network in muscle cells. In the mature muscles of mammals and flies, a second microtubule network is present within the myofibril network and is characterized by a significantly different population of microtubules. Microtubules in this region are less dense and are oriented such that they run along the length of the myofibrils, with occasional microtubules running transversely between the myofibrils (Kano et al., 1991; Metzger et al., 2012). Additionally, it appears that many of the microtubules that exist in this central portion of the muscle originate from perinuclear regions near the muscle periphery (Kano et al., 1991). Thus, it is likely that the nuclei serve as the MTOC for both microtubule networks that are observed within skeletal muscle. Furthermore, given that microtubules are directly interacting with nuclei in muscles, the organization and activity of the microtubule cytoskeleton will inevitably impact the spatial distribution of nuclei.

The role of microtubules in positioning muscle nuclei dates back to early studies using explants from chick embryos which demonstrated that nuclei moved, rotated and eventually became fixed in position (Capers, 1960). Subsequent analysis using cultures derived from mice and rats found that nuclei underwent similar movements and further demonstrated that the dynamic movements required microtubules. Specifically, it was shown that if microtubules were depolymerized with colchicine, nuclear movements and rotations stopped (Englander and Rubin, 1987).

Remarkably, little more was learned regarding how the microtubule cytoskeleton moves muscle nuclei until recently. New work has confirmed a role for microtubules in moving muscle nuclei and expanded the mechanistic understanding of the process. Generally, the proteins that move nuclei in other systems (Gundersen and Worman, 2013) contribute to the movement of nuclei in muscle systems.

The two factors that generate most of the force that moves nuclei in muscles are the two microtubule motors, Kinesin-1 that moves toward microtubule plus-ends, and cytoplasmic Dynein that moves toward microtubule minus-ends. These two motors are also essential for microtubule based nuclear movement in virtually every other system (Tapley and Starr, 2013), suggesting that the basic mechanisms are conserved among cell types and species. However, there are several unique aspects to nuclear movements in muscle. Furthermore, recent analyses have described distinct mechanisms that contribute to different types of nuclear movements in muscle both *in vivo* during embryonic *Drosophila* development and in mouse culture systems (Cadot et al., 2012; Folker et al., 2012; Metzger et al., 2012; Wilson and Holzbaur, 2012).

One of the most striking aspects of nuclear movement in muscle is that the nuclei dynamically rotate in three dimensions during translocation. This aspect was also first noted in cultures derived from chick embryos (Capers, 1960) but has recently been described in mammalian culture systems (Wilson and Holzbaur, 2012) and developing *Drosophila* embryos (Folker et al., 2014). Furthermore, moving myonuclei in the developing *Drosophila* embryo have a defined leading and lagging edge which enables rapid changes in nuclear shape. These shape changes require the coordinated actions of Kinesin and Dynein at the nucleus, an aspect of nuclear movement that has to date only been described in developing muscle (Folker et al., 2014).

The role of these rotations and shape changes are not clear. However, each of these reports hypothesizes that these behaviors provide nuclei with a unique ability to maximize movement velocity in dense cellular and embryonic environments. Similar rotations of translocating nuclei have been noted in *C. elegans* where rotations were also proposed as a means to navigate the dense cellular environment (Fridolfsson and Starr, 2010). Additionally, dramatic changes in nuclear shape have been noted in neurons (Tsai et al., 2007) where they seem to be essential to move through spatially restricted environments.

Although similar behaviors have been noted in other systems, the mechanisms and persistence of these behaviors in muscle are different. For example, the nuclear rotations in *C. elegans* appear to occur only to navigate past blockages whereas in muscle, nuclear rotations are common and are not strictly correlated with defined translocation (Wilson and Holzbaur, 2012; Folker et al., 2014). Additionally, the changes in nuclear shape during translocation in neurons are dependent only on the activity of Dynein from a position distant from the nucleus (Tsai et al., 2007), whereas the analogous behavior in muscle requires the spatially segregated activities of Dynein and Kinesin (Folker et al., 2014). These distinctions may be driven by the multinucleate nature of muscle and may reveal information regarding interactions between nuclei. If nuclei do indeed interact with one another, it is likely that nuclear position affects these interactions. Altered interactions between nuclei could greatly influence the maintenance of myodomains as well as the transcriptional profile of individual nuclei, and thus have dramatic effects on muscle structure and function.

Kinesin and Dynein move nuclei in muscle systems but they contribute to different types of movement using different arrays of regulators/accessory proteins. Consider again the types of nuclear movement in the muscle. In simple terms, there is (1) movement to the center of the myotube/myofiber following fusion, (2) movement of each nucleus to the muscle periphery, (3) equidistant spacing of nuclei, and (4) movement of nuclei to the NMJ. Experiments using mouse culture systems have identified the small GTPase Cdc42, and the polarity proteins Par6 and Par3, as necessary for newly fused nuclei to move toward the center of the myotube (Cadot et al., 2012). Each of these proteins contributes to nuclear movement in other systems by enabling Dynein anchored at the cell cortex to pull nuclei that are attached to microtubule minus-ends toward itself (Kotak and Gönczy, 2013). Nuclei in muscle are moved by a similar mechanism, but the details may be slightly different. In immature myotubes, Dynein, Par3, and Par6 localize to the already incorporated nuclei. From the central cluster of nuclei, Dynein pulls the new nuclei to the myotube center (Cadot et al., 2012). *In vivo* experiments looking at embryonic muscle development in *Drosophila* suggest mechanisms more analgous to those in *C. elegans*. Specifically, Dynein is anchored at the muscle cortex by Pins and pulls microtubule minus-ends and the attached myonuclei toward the end of the muscle dependent on the microtubule plus-end tracking protein, CLIP-190 (Folker et al., 2012). The difference between the data in mammalian cell culture and that in developing *Drosophila* embryos may result from *in vitro/in vivo* differences or because different types of nuclear movement are being analyzed. That other mechanisms seem to be conserved between the two systems suggests that the latter may be the case.

The study of nuclear movement in muscle has revealed novel behaviors of moving nuclei (Wilson and Holzbaur, 2012; Folker et al., 2014), and has also identified proteins with novel roles in nuclear movement. MAP7/Ensconsin was long ago identified as a microtubule associated protein (Bulinski and Bossler, 1994), but a cellular role for this protein had not been identified. Work in both the developing muscles of the *Drosophila* embryo and mammalian cell culture have found MAP7/Ensconsin to be essential for nuclear movement in muscle (Metzger et al., 2012). Additionally, unlike Cdc42, Par6, Par3, and Dynein, MAP7/Ensconsin does not affect the movement of nuclei toward the muscle center, but is essential only for the spacing of nuclei throughout the muscle by a mechanism identified in both developing *Drosophila* and mammalian culture systems further illustrating that different types of nuclear movement in muscle are driven by distinct mechanisms (Cadot et al., 2012; Metzger et al., 2012). The mechanism by which MAP7 contributes to nuclear movement is not known. However, MAP7 can physically interact with Kinesin (Metzger et al., 2012), and the *Drosophila* homolog of MAP7, Ensconsin, can increase Kinesin-microtubule interactions, thus resulting in increased Kinesin motility (Sung et al., 2008). Finally, a fusion protein containing the MAP7 microtubule binding domain and the Kinesin motor domain can move nuclei (Metzger et al., 2012). These data have all been used to suggest that MAP7/Ensconsin helps spread and maintain the spacing between nuclei by enabling Kinesin to slide antiparallel microtubules which emanate from neighboring nuclei, similar to the way in which Kinesin and Ensconsin transport microtubules in neurons (Barlan et al., 2013). The result of this sliding is the pushing apart of adjacent nuclei similar to the mechanism by which mitotic spindles are elongated in cell divisions (Metzger et al., 2012).

To date, mutations in Dynein and its regulatory proteins, Kinesin and its regulatory proteins, and MAP7/Ensconsin have not been identified in patients with muscle disease. That is likely due to the very fundamental roles each of these proteins play in all cells. Thus, if the ability of Dynein and/or Kinesin to move nuclei is eliminated, its ability to move other cargos throughout the cell are also likely compromised. However, these analyses have provided insight to the relevance of nuclear positioning in muscle. Tissue specific depletions of these proteins in *Drosophila* have confirmed that these proteins have a muscle autonomous effect on nuclear positioning without affects on nuclear morphology (Folker et al., 2012; Metzger et al., 2012). Yet, the ability of *Drosophila* lacking these proteins specifically in the muscle to move is inhibited (Folker et al., 2012; Metzger et al., 2012). This is not to suggest that nuclear morphology and gene regulation are not essential and relevant contributions to disease. Instead these data makes evident that the clustering of nuclei, in the absence of other obvious defects in muscle architecture, does inhibit muscle function.

ACTIN

There are far fewer examples of actin-dependent nuclear movement compared to microtubule-dependent nuclear movement throughout biology. Furthermore, there is no evidence of actin-dependent nuclear movement in muscle. However, there is evidence that actin contributes to the anchoring of nuclei in different locations (Zhang et al., 2002, 2010; Puckelwartz et al., 2009). Additionally, there is substantial evidence from experiments in cell culture that nuclear proteins interact with actin and that these interactions can influence nuclear structure (Nikolova et al., 2004; Lüke et al., 2008; Khatau et al., 2009), cellular rheology (Maniotis et al., 1997; Lammerding et al., 2004), and nuclear movement and positioning (Luxton et al., 2010).

In fibroblasts, actin moves the nucleus as an initial step in cell migration (Gomes et al., 2005). Furthermore, this movement requires the same LINC complex components that are mutated in patients with muscle disease. As in muscle, the LINC complex enables the direct interaction between the nucleus and the cytoskeleton, but in this case the nucleus interacts with the actin cytoskeleton rather than the microtubule cytoskeleton (Luxton et al., 2010). Similarly, Lamin A/C is necessary for nuclear movement in this system and contributes by serving as an anchor for the LINC complex so that it can couple the movement of actin to the nucleus. Essential to this review, mutations in Lamin A/C that cause muscle disease also inhibit the ability of the nuclear lamina to anchor the LINC complex (Folker et al., 2011). This raises the possibility that the ability of Lamin A/C to anchor the LINC complex so that force can be transmitted from the cytoskeleton to the nucleus is fundamental to muscle biology and muscle disease pathogenesis.

Only one report has suggested even indirect roles for actin in regulating the position of myonuclei *in vivo*. It was demonstrated that the KASH domain containing protein, Msp-300, was essential for nuclear positioning in larval muscles. Although most of this work focused on the effects that the loss of Msp-300 had on the organization of microtubules, it also found Msp-300 to be localized to the Z-disks suggesting a role in sarcomere organization (Elhanany-Tamir et al., 2012). Furthermore, although Msp-300 did not interact directly with actin, it did interact with actin via the thick filament protein, Titin and these interactions may be necessary for proper nuclear positioning.

Although there is limited evidence for actin dependent nuclear movement in muscle, the fact that genes identified as causes of EDMD are essential for actin-dependent nuclear movement in other systems is compelling. Furthermore, it has been reported that mutations in each of these genes in addition to having effects on the nucleus as discussed throughout this review, also affect actin organization (Ho et al., 2013). And work in *Drosophila* and mice has found that the genetic disruptions that cause nuclear mispositioning (along with other effects) also impact the organization of the actin cytoskeleton (Dialynas et al., 2010). Thus, despite far less evidence for actin dependent nuclear movement, further exploration of this possibility is necessary.

CONCLUSION

The subcellular structure and organization of muscle has been studied since the advent of microscopes. Although, the assembly and organization of myofibrils which dominated early research is still being examined, new avenues of research have emerged. In general, the questions of where the different organelles are located, why they are located in such a manner, how they become localized, and whether the organization of different organelles are linked have garnered increased focus. Yet, the complex organization of individual muscle cells, the multinucleate nature of individual muscle cells, and the bundling and further bundling of these cells have provided many obstacles to detailed understanding of muscle development.

Nevertheless the technology and systems to address these questions are becoming available (Oddoux et al., 2013). Although this review focused on how nuclei move and the correlations between nuclear positioning and muscle disease, similar analyses have been performed with respect to mitochondria (Pathi et al., 2012), t-tubules (Flucher et al., 1994) and other organelles. We have highlighted some of the data regarding the mechanisms of nuclear movement in muscle and indicated that the basic principles of nuclear movement are conserved between species and between cell types. The conservation of the proteins used to move nuclei provides a list of proteins to examine in systems of muscle development. Furthermore, it expands the list of targets that we should evaluate in patients suffering from muscle disease.

Indeed, many of the proteins that are necessary to move nuclei are mutated in individuals with muscle disease. However, this is almost exclusively true of those proteins that localize to the nucleus and contribute from that location by regulating the interactions between the nucleus and the cytoskeleton. The cytoskeletal proteins that contribute to nuclear movement in muscle have not yet been linked to muscle disease. This is likely because mutations that would affect the ability of the cytoskeleton to move nuclei would also cause general developmental defects as has been demonstrated for Kinesin (Wang et al., 2013). But it is important that the contribution of these proteins to nuclear movement not be ignored on grounds that they do not cause disease. With regards to basic biology, these genes can provide a means to study nuclear position in the absence of global effects on nuclear architecture and gene regulation. More therapeutically relevant, they are essential for a process that is highly correlated with disease. Thus, with sufficient understanding it may be possible to circumvent the disease causing mutations by targeting the cytoskeleton.

Despite the high correlation between aberrant nuclear positioning and muscle disease the idea that nuclear position in muscle is essential for muscle function will likely remain controversial. Recent analyses in *Drosophila* which demonstrated reduced muscle output when nuclei were mispositioned without additional underlying defects (Metzger et al., 2012) may convince some, but not all. However, reconsidering the process of muscle repair may provide the most compelling evidence that nuclear movement is important and essential, even if mispositioned nuclei do not cause disease. Organisms, and cells, in general optimize their energy usage. With that premise, it is unlikely that nuclei would move to the center and then back out to the periphery of an already mature myofiber. Energetically speaking it would be far more efficient to incorporate a new nucleus at the point of entry at which point the nuclei could undergo slight movements to space along the myofiber. Nuclear movement to the center and then back to the periphery of a muscle must be essential to muscle development and repair. With newly found focus we may soon understand the biological necessity of these long range nuclear movements in muscle.

Finally, nuclear position is almost certainly not the final answer with regards to muscle disease. But with the evidence that nuclear positioning is essential to muscle function is increased, making it time that the muscle biology community begin to consider centrally localized nuclei as more than merely a marker of ongoing muscle repair and as a phenotype that may influence muscle function and health.

ACKNOWLEDGMENTS

We thank the members of the Baylies lab for discussions. Our work is supported by the Muscular Dystrophy Association (MDA) and National Institute of Health (NIH) (GM078318 to Mary K. Baylies).

REFERENCES

Barlan, K., Lu, W., and Gelfand, V. I. (2013). The microtubule-binding protein ensconsin is an essential cofactor of kinesin-1. *Curr. Biol.* 23, 317–322. doi: 10.1016/j.cub.2013.01.008

Bione, S., Maestrini, E., Rivella, S., Mancini, M., Regis, S., Romeo, G., et al. (1994). Identification of a novel X-linked gene responsible for Emery-Dreifuss muscular dystrophy. *Nat. Genet.* 8, 323–327. doi: 10.1038/ng1294-323

Bonaldo, P., and Sandri, M. (2013). Cellular and molecular mechanisms of muscle atrophy. *Dis. Model. Mech.* 6, 25–39. doi: 10.1242/dmm.010389

Bonne, G., Mercuri, E., Muchir, A., Urtizberea, A., Bécane, H. M., Recan, D., et al. (2000). Clinical and molecular genetic spectrum of autosomal dominant Emery-Dreifuss muscular dystrophy due to mutations of the lamin A/C gene. *Ann. Neurol.* 48, 170–180. doi: 10.1002/1531-8249(200008)48:2<170::AID-ANA6>3.3.CO;2-A

Broers, J. L. V., Peeters, E. A. G., Kuijpers, H. J. H., Endert, J., Bouten, C. V. C., Oomens, C. W. J., et al. (2004). Decreased mechanical stiffness in LMNA$^{-/-}$ cells is caused by defective nucleo-cytoskeletal integrity: implications for the development of laminopathies. *Hum. Mol. Genet.* 13, 2567–2580. doi: 10.1093/hmg/ddh295

Bruusgaard, J. C., Liestøl, K., Ekmark, M., Kollstad, K., and Gundersen, K. (2003). Number and spatial distribution of nuclei in the muscle fibres of normal mice studied *in vivo*. *J. Physiol.* 551, 467–478. doi: 10.1113/jphysiol.2003.045328

Bulinski, J. C., and Bossler, A. (1994). Purification and characterization of ensconsin, a novel microtubule stabilizing protein. *J. Cell. Sci.* 107(Pt 10), 2839–2849.

Cadot, B., Gache, V., Vasyutina, E., Falcone, S., Birchmeier, C., and Gomes, E. R. (2012). Nuclear movement during myotube formation is microtubule and dynein dependent and is regulated by Cdc42, Par6 and Par3. *EMBO Rep.* 13, 741–749. doi: 10.1038/embor.2012.89

Capers, C. R. (1960). Multinucleation of skeletal muscle *in vitro*. *J. Biophys. Biochem. Cytol.* 7, 559–566. doi: 10.1083/jcb.7.3.559

Chang, W., Folker, E., Worman, H., and Gundersen, G. (2013). Emerin organizes actin flow for nuclear movement and centrosome organization in migrating fibroblasts. *MBoC*. (in press).

Cohen, T. V., Gnocchi, V. F., Cohen, J. E., Phadke, A., Liu, H., Ellis, J. A., et al. (2013). Defective skeletal muscle growth in lamin A/C-deficient mice is rescued by loss of Lap2. *Hum. Mol. Genet.* 22, 2852–2869. doi: 10.1093/hmg/ddt135

Dialynas, G., Speese, S., Budnik, V., Geyer, P. K., and Wallrath, L. L. (2010). The role of Drosophila Lamin C in muscle function and gene expression. *Development* 137, 3067–3077. doi: 10.1242/dev.048231

Dubowitz, V., Sewry, C. A., and Lane, R. (2007). *Muscle Biopsy: A Practical Approach*. Philadephia, PA: Elsevier Limited.

Elhanany-Tamir, H., Yu, Y. V., Shnayder, M., Jain, A., Welte, M., and Volk, T. (2012). Organelle positioning in muscles requires cooperation between two KASH proteins and microtubules. *J. Cell Biol.* 198, 833–846. doi: 10.1083/jcb.201204102

Englander, L. L., and Rubin, L. L. (1987). Acetylcholine receptor clustering and nuclear movement in muscle fibers in culture. *J. Cell Biol.* 104, 87–95. doi: 10.1083/jcb.104.1.87

Flucher, B. E., Andrews, S. B., and Daniels, M. P. (1994). Molecular organization of transverse tubule/sarcoplasmic reticulum junctions during development of excitation-contraction coupling in skeletal muscle. *Mol. Biol. Cell* 5, 1105–1118. doi: 10.1091/mbc.5.10.1105

Folker, E. S., Ostlund, C., Luxton, G. W. G., Worman, H. J., and Gundersen, G. G. (2011). Lamin A variants that cause striated muscle disease are defective in anchoring transmembrane actin-associated nuclear lines for nuclear movement. *Proc. Natl. Acad. Sci. U.S.A.* 108, 131–136. doi: 10.1073/pnas.1000824108

Folker, E. S., Schulman, V. K., and Baylies, M. K. (2012). Muscle length and myonuclear position are independently regulated by distinct Dynein pathways. *Development* 139, 3827–3837. doi: 10.1242/dev.079178

Folker, E. S., Schulman, V. K., and Baylies, M. K. (2014). Translocating myonuclei have distinct leading and lagging edges which require Kinesin and Dynein. *Development*. (in press).

Fridolfsson, H. N., Ly, N., Meyerzon, M., and Starr, D. A. (2010). UNC-83 coordinates kinesin-1 and dynein activities at the nuclear envelope during nuclear migration. *Dev. Biol.* 338, 237–250. doi: 10.1016/j.ydbio.2009.12.004

Fridolfsson, H. N., and Starr, D. A. (2010). Kinesin-1 and dynein at the nuclear envelope mediate the bidirectional migrations of nuclei. *J. Cell Biol.* 191, 115–128. doi: 10.1083/jcb.201004118

Gazzerro, E., Andreu, A. L., and Bruno, C. (2013). Neuromuscular disorders of glycogen metabolism. *Curr. Neurol. Neurosci. Rep.* 13, 333–340. doi: 10.1007/s11910-012-0333-0

Gnocchi, V. F., Scharner, J., Huang, Z., Brady, K., Lee, J. S., White, R. B., et al. (2011). Uncoordinated transcription and compromised muscle function in the lmna-null mouse model of Emery- Emery-Dreyfuss muscular dystrophy. *PLoS ONE* 6:e16651. doi: 10.1371/journal.pone.0016651

Gomes, E. R., Jani, S., and Gundersen, G. G. (2005). Nuclear movement regulated by Cdc42, MRCK, myosin, and actin flow establishes MTOC polarization in migrating cells. *Cell* 121, 451–463. doi: 10.1016/j.cell.2005.02.022

Grady, R. M., Starr, D. A., Ackerman, G. L., Sanes, J. R., and Han, M. (2005). Syne proteins anchor muscle nuclei at the neuromuscular junction. *Proc. Natl. Acad. Sci. U.S.A.* 102, 4359–4364. doi: 10.1073/pnas.0500711102

Gueneau, L., Bertrand, A. T., Jais, J.-P., Salih, M. A., Stojkovic, T., Wehnert, M., et al. (2009). Mutations of the FHL1 gene cause Emery-Dreifuss muscular dystrophy. *Am. J. Hum. Genet.* 85, 338–353. doi: 10.1016/j.ajhg.2009.07.015

Gundersen, G. G., and Worman, H. J. (2013). Nuclear positioning. *Cell* 152, 1376–1389. doi: 10.1016/j.cell.2013.02.031

Hale, C. M., Shrestha, A. L., Khatau, S. B., Stewart-Hutchinson, P. J., Hernandez, L., Stewart, C. L., et al. (2008). Dysfunctional connections between the nucleus and the actin and microtubule networks in laminopathic models. *Biophys. J.* 95, 5462–5475. doi: 10.1529/biophysj.108.139428

Ho, C. Y., Jaalouk, D. E., Vartiainen, M. K., and Lammerding, J. (2013). Lamin A/C and emerin regulate MKL1-SRF activity by modulating actin dynamics. *Nature* 497, 507–511. doi: 10.1038/nature12105

Houben, F., Willems, C. H., Declercq, I. L., Hochstenbach, K., Kamps, M. A., Snoeckx, L. H., et al. (2009). Disturbed nuclear orientation and cellular migration in A-type lamin deficient cells. *Biochim. Biophys. Acta* 1793, 312–324. doi: 10.1016/j.bbamcr.2008.10.003

Huxley, A. F., and Niedergerke, R. (1954). Structural changes in muscle during contraction. *Nature* 173, 971–973. doi: 10.1038/173971a0

Huxley, H., and Hanson, J. (1954). Changes in the cross-striations of muscle during contraction and stretch and their structural interpretation. *Nature* 173, 973–976. doi: 10.1038/173973a0

Jevsek, M., Jaworski, A., Polo-Parada, L., Kim, N., Fan, J., Landmesser, L. T., et al. (2006). CD24 is expressed by myofiber synaptic nuclei and regulates synaptic transmission. *Proc. Natl. Acad. Sci. U.S.A.* 103, 6374–6379. doi: 10.1073/pnas.0601468103

Kano, Y., Fujimaki, N., and Ishikawa, H. (1991). The distribution and arrangement of microtubules in mammalian skeletal muscle fibers. *Cell Struct. Funct.* 3, 251–261. doi: 10.1247/csf.16.251

Kelly, A. M., and Zacks, S. I. (1969). The histogenesis of rat intercostal muscle. *J. Cell Biol.* 42, 135–153. doi: 10.1083/jcb.42.1.135

Khatau, S. B., Hale, C. M., Stewart-Hutchinson, P. J., Patel, M. S., Stewart, C. L., Searson, P. C., et al. (2009). A perinuclear actin cap regulates nuclear shape. *Proc. Natl. Acad. Sci. U.S.A.* 106, 19017–19022. doi: 10.1073/pnas.0908686106

Kotak, S., and Gönczy, P. (2013). Mechanisms of spindle positioning: cortical force generators in the limelight. *Curr. Opin. Cell Biol.* 213, 1–8. doi: 10.1016/j.ceb.2013.07.008

Lammerding, J., Schulze, P. C., Takahashi, T., Kozlov, S., Sullivan, T., Kamm, R. D., et al. (2004). Lamin A/C deficiency causes defective nuclear mechanics and mechanotransduction. *J. Clin. Invest.* 113, 370–378. doi: 10.1172/JCI200419670

Lee, J. S. H., Hale, C. M., Panorchan, P., Khatau, S. B., George, J. P., Tseng, Y., et al. (2007). Nuclear lamin A/C deficiency induces defects in cell mechanics, polarization, and migration. *Biophys. J.* 93, 2542–2552. doi: 10.1529/biophysj.106.102426

Lei, K., Zhang, X., Ding, X., Guo, X., Chen, M., Zhu, B., et al. (2009). SUN1 and SUN2 play critical but partially redundant roles in anchoring nuclei in skeletal muscle cells in mice. *Proc. Natl. Acad. Sci. U.S.A.* 106, 10207–10212. doi: 10.1073/pnas.0812037106

Lüke, Y., Zaim, H., Karakesisoglou, I., Jaeger, V. M., Sellin, L., Lu, W., et al. (2008). Nesprin-2 Giant (NUANCE) maintains nuclear envelope architecture and composition in skin. *J. Cell. Sci.* 121, 1887–1898. doi: 10.1242/jcs.019075

Luxton, G. W. G., Gomes, E. R., Folker, E. S., Vintinner, E., and Gundersen, G. G. (2010). Linear arrays of nuclear envelope proteins harness retrograde actin flow for nuclear movement. *Science* 329, 956–959. doi: 10.1126/science.1189072

Maniotis, A. J., Chen, C. S., and Ingber, D. E. (1997). Demonstration of mechanical connections between integrins, cytoskeletal filaments, and nucleoplasm that stabilize nuclear structure. *Proc. Natl. Acad. Sci. U.S.A.* 94, 849–854. doi: 10.1073/pnas.94.3.849

Maraldi, N. M., Lattanzi, G., Sabatelli, P., Ognibene, A., and Squarzoni, S. (2002). Functional domains of the nucleus: implications for Emery-Dreifuss muscular dystrophy. *Neuromuscul. Disord.* 12, 815–823. doi: 10.1016/S0960-8966(02)00067-6

Mattout, A., Pike, B. L., Towbin, B. D., Bank, E. M., Gonzalez-Sandoval, A., Stadler, M. B., et al. (2011). An EDMD mutation in C. elegans lamin blocks muscle-specific gene relocation and compromises muscle integrity. *Curr. Biol.* 21, 1603–1614. doi: 10.1016/j.cub.2011.08.030

Melcon, G., Kozlov, S., Cutler, D. A., Sullivan, T., Hernandez, L., Zhao, P., et al. (2006). Loss of emerin at the nuclear envelope disrupts the Rb1/E2F and MyoD pathways during muscle regeneration. *Hum. Mol. Genet.* 15, 637–651. doi: 10.1093/hmg/ddi479

Metzger, T., Gache, V., Xu, M., Cadot, B., Folker, E. S., Richardson, B. E., et al. (2012). MAP and kinesin-dependent nuclear positioning is required for skeletal muscle function. *Nature* 484, 120–124. doi: 10.1038/nature10914

Meyerzon, M., Fridolfsson, H. N., Ly, N., McNally, F. J., and Starr, D. A. (2009). UNC-83 is a nuclear-specific cargo adaptor for kinesin-1-mediated nuclear migration. *Development* 136, 2725–2733. doi: 10.1242/dev.038596

Moscoso, L. M., Chu, G. C., Gautam, M., Noakes, P. G., Merlie, J. P., and Sanes, J. R. (1995). Synapse-associated expression of an acetylcholine receptor-inducing protein, ARIA/heregulin, and its putative receptors, ErbB2 and ErbB3, in developing mammalian muscle. *Dev. Biol.* 172, 158–169. doi: 10.1006/dbio.1995.0012

Muntoni, F., Torelli, S., Wells, D. J., and Brown, S. C. (2011). Muscular dystrophies due to glycosylation defects: diagnosis and therapeutic strategies. *Curr. Opin. Neurol.* 24, 437–442. doi: 10.1097/WCO.0b013e32834a95e3

Nikolova, V., Leimena, C., McMahon, A. C., Tan, J. C., Chandar, S., Jogia, D., et al. (2004). Defects in nuclear structure and function promote dilated cardiomyopathy in lamin A/C–deficient mice. *J. Clin. Invest.* 113, 357–369. doi: 10.1172/JCI200419448

Oddoux, S., Zaal, K. J., Tate, V., Kenea, A., Nandkeolyar, S. A., Reid, E., et al. (2013). Microtubules that form the stationary lattice of muscle fibers are dynamic and nucleated at Golgi elements. *J. Cell Biol.* 203, 205–213. doi: 10.1083/jcb.201304063

Ozawa, R., Hayashi, Y. K., Ogawa, M., Kurokawa, R., Matsumoto, H., Noguchi, S., et al. (2006). Emerin-lacking mice show minimal motor and cardiac dysfunctions with nuclear-associated vacuoles. *Am. J. Pathol.* 168, 907–917. doi: 10.2353/ajpath.2006.050564

Pathi, B., Kinsey, S. T., Howdeshell, M. E., Priester, C., McNeill, R. S., and Locke, B. R. (2012). The formation and functional consequences of heterogeneous mitochondrial distributions in skeletal muscle. *J. Exp. Biol.* 215, 1871–1883. doi: 10.1242/jeb.067207

Pavlath, G. K., Rich, K., Webster, S. G., and Blau, H. M. (1989). Localization of muscle gene products in nuclear domains. *Nature* 337, 570–573. doi: 10.1038/337570a0

Puckelwartz, M. J., Kessler, E., Zhang, Y., Hodzic, D., Randles, K. N., Morris, G., et al. (2009). Disruption of nesprin-1 produces an Emery Dreifuss muscular dystrophy-like phenotype in mice. *Hum. Mol. Genet.* 18, 607–620. doi: 10.1093/hmg/ddn386

Ralston, E., Ploug, T., Kalhovde, J., and Lomo, T. (2001). Golgi complex, endoplasmic reticulum exit sites, and microtubules in skeletal muscle fibers are organized by patterned activity. *J. Neurosci.* 21, 875–883.

Ramos-García, S. L., Roberson, R. W., Freitag, M., Bartnicki-García, S., and Mouriño-Pérez, R. R. (2009). Cytoplasmic bulk flow propels nuclei in mature hyphae of Neurospora crassa. *Eukaryotic Cell* 8, 1880–1890. doi: 10.1128/EC.00062-09

Ramsey, R. W., and Street, S. F. (1940). The isometric length-tension diagram of isolated skeletal muscle fibers of the frog. *J. Cell. Physiol.* 15, 11–34. doi: 10.1002/jcp.1030150103

Rodriguez, O. C., Schaefer, A. W., and Mandato, C. A. (2003). Conserved microtubule–actin interactions in cell movement and morphogenesis. *Nat. Cell Biol.* 5, 599–609. doi: 10.1038/ncb0703-599

Sanes, J. R., Johnson, Y. R., Kotzbauer, P. T., Mudd, J., Hanley, T., Martinou, J. C., et al. (1991). Selective expression of an acetylcholine receptor-lacZ transgene in synaptic nuclei of adult muscle fibers. *Development* 113, 1181–1191.

Schreiber, K. H., and Kennedy, B. K. (2013). When lamins go bad: nuclear structure and disease. *Cell* 152, 1365–1375. doi: 10.1016/j.cell.2013.02.015

Spiro, A. J., Shy, G. M., and Gonatas, N. K. (1966). Myotubular myopathy. Persistence of fetal muscle in an adolescent boy. *Arch. Neurol.* 14, 1–14. doi: 10.1001/archneur.1966.00470070005001

Starr, D. A., and Han, M. (2002). Role of ANC-1 in tethering nuclei to the actin cytoskeleton. *Science* 298, 406–409. doi: 10.1126/science.1075119

Starr, D. A., Hermann, G. J., Malone, C. J., Fixsen, W., Priess, J. R., Horvitz, H. R., et al. (2001). unc-83 encodes a novel component of the nuclear envelope and is essential for proper nuclear migration. *Development* 128, 5039–5050.

Stewart, C. L., Roux, K. J., and Burke, B. (2007). Blurring the boundary: the nuclear envelope extends its reach. *Science* 318, 1408–1412. doi: 10.1126/science.1142034

Sullivan, T., Escalante-Alcalde, D., Bhatt, H., Anver, M., Bhat, N., Nagashima, K., et al. (1999). Loss of A-type lamin expression compromises nuclear envelope integrity leading to muscular dystrophy. *J. Cell Biol.* 147, 913–920. doi: 10.1083/jcb.147.5.913

Sung, H.-H., Telley, I. A., Papadaki, P., Ephrussi, A., Surrey, T., and Rørth, P. (2008). Drosophila ensconsin promotes productive recruitment of Kinesin-1 to microtubules. *Dev. Cell* 15, 866–876. doi: 10.1016/j.devcel.2008.10.006

Tapley, E. C., and Starr, D. A. (2013). Connecting the nucleus to the cytoskeleton by SUN-KASH bridges across the nuclear envelope. *Curr. Opin. Cell Biol.* 25, 57–62. doi: 10.1016/j.ceb.2012.10.014

Tassin, A. M., Maro, B., and Bornens, M. (1985). Fate of microtubule-organizing centers during myogenesis *in vitro*. *J. Cell Biol.* 100, 35–46. doi: 10.1083/jcb.100.1.35

Tsai, J.-W., Bremner, K. H., and Vallee, R. B. (2007). Dual subcellular roles for LIS1 and dynein in radial neuronal migration in live brain tissue. *Nat. Neurosci.* 10, 970–979. doi: 10.1038/nn1934

Tsukahara, T., Tsujino, S., and Arahata, K. (2002). CDNA microarray analysis of gene expression in fibroblasts of patients with X-linked Emery-Dreifuss muscular dystrophy. *Muscle Nerve* 25, 898–901. doi: 10.1002/mus.10085

Wang, B., Li, J., and Xiao, X. (2000). Adeno-associated virus vector carrying human minidystrophin genes effectively ameliorates muscular dystrophy in mdx mouse model. *Proc. Natl. Acad. Sci. U.S.A.* 97, 13714–13719. doi: 10.1073/pnas.240335297

Wang, Z., Cui, J., Wong, W. M., Li, X., Xue, W., Lin, R., et al. (2013). Kif5b controls the localization of myofibril components for their assembly and linkage to the myotendinous junctions. *Development* 140, 617–626. doi: 10.1242/dev.085969

Wheeler, M. A., Davies, J. D., Zhang, Q., Emerson, L. J., Hunt, J., Shanahan, C. M., et al. (2007). Distinct functional domains in nesprin-1alpha and nesprin-2beta bind directly to emerin and both interactions are disrupted in X-linked Emery-Dreifuss muscular dystrophy. *Exp. Cell Res.* 313, 2845–2857. doi: 10.1016/j.yexcr.2007.03.025

Wilson, M. H., and Holzbaur, E. L. F. (2012). Opposing microtubule motors drive robust nuclear dynamics in developing muscle cells. *J. Cell. Sci.* 125, 4158–4169. doi: 10.1242/jcs.108688

Yin, H., Price, F., and Rudnicki, M. A. (2013). Satellite cells and the muscle stem cell niche. *Physiol. Rev.* 93, 23–67. doi: 10.1152/physrev.00043.2011

Yu, J., Lei, K., Zhou, M., Craft, C. M., Xu, G., Xu, T., et al. (2011). KASH protein Syne-2/Nesprin-2 and SUN proteins SUN1/2 mediate nuclear migration during mammalian retinal development. *Hum. Mol. Genet.* 20, 1061–1073. doi: 10.1093/hmg/ddq549

Zhang, J., Felder, A., Liu, Y., Guo, L. T., Lange, S., Dalton, N. D., et al. (2010). Nesprin 1 is critical for nuclear positioning and anchorage. *Hum. Mol. Genet.* 19, 329–341. doi: 10.1093/hmg/ddp499

Zhang, Q., Bethmann, C., Worth, N. F., Davies, J. D., Wasner, C., Feuer, A., et al. (2007). Nesprin-1 and -2 are involved in the pathogenesis of Emery Dreifuss muscular dystrophy and are critical for nuclear envelope integrity. *Hum. Mol. Genet.* 16, 2816–2833. doi: 10.1093/hmg/ddm238

Zhang, Q., Ragnauth, C., Greener, M. J., Shanahan, C. M., and Roberts, R. G. (2002). The nesprins are giant actin-binding proteins, orthologous to *Drosophila melanogaster* muscle protein MSP-300. *Genomics* 80, 473–481. doi: 10.1006/geno.2002.6859

Zhang, X., Lei, K., Yuan, X., Wu, X., Zhuang, Y., Xu, T., et al. (2009). SUN1/2 and Syne/Nesprin-1/2 complexes connect centrosome to the nucleus during neurogenesis and neuronal migration in mice. *Neuron* 64, 173–187. doi: 10.1016/j.neuron.2009.08.018

Zhong, Z., Wilson, K. L., and Dahl, K. N. (2010). Beyond lamins other structural components of the nucleoskeleton. *Methods Cell Biol.* 98, 97–119. doi: 10.1016/S0091-679X(10)98005-9

Zwerger, M., Jaalouk, D. E., Lombardi, M. L., Isermann, P., Mauermann, M., Dialynas, G., et al. (2013). Myopathic lamin mutations impair nuclear stability in cells and tissue and disrupt nucleo-cytoskeletal coupling. *Hum. Mol. Genet.* 22, 2335–2349. doi: 10.1093/hmg/ddt079

5

Skeletal muscle as a regulator of the longevity protein, Klotho

Keith G. Avin[1,2], Paul M. Coen[3,4], Wan Huang[1], Donna B. Stolz[5], Gwendolyn A. Sowa[1], John J. Dubé[3], Bret H. Goodpaster[3], Robert M. O'Doherty[3] and Fabrisia Ambrosio[1,6]*

[1] Department of Physical Medicine and Rehabilitation, University of Pittsburgh, Pittsburgh, PA, USA
[2] Division of Geriatric Medicine, Department of Medicine, University of Pittsburgh, PA, USA
[3] Division of Endocrinology and Metabolism, Department of Medicine, University of Pittsburgh, Pittsburgh, PA, USA
[4] Department of Health and Physical Education, University of Pittsburgh, Pittsburgh, PA, USA
[5] Department of Cell Biology and Physiology, University of Pittsburgh, Pittsburgh, PA, USA
[6] McGowan Institute for Regenerative Medicine, University of Pittsburgh, Pittsburgh, PA, USA

Correspondence:
Fabrisia Ambrosio, Department of Physical Medicine and Rehabilitation, McGowan Institute for Regenerative Medicine, Suite 308, Bridgeside Point Building II, 450 Technology Drive, Pittsburgh, PA 15219, USA
e-mail: ambrosiof@upmc.edu

Klotho is a powerful longevity protein that has been linked to the prevention of muscle atrophy, osteopenia, and cardiovascular disease. Similar anti-aging effects have also been ascribed to exercise and physical activity. While an association between muscle function and Klotho expression has been previously suggested from longitudinal cohort studies, a direct relationship between circulating Klotho and skeletal muscle has not been investigated. In this paper, we present a review of the literature and preliminary evidence that, together, suggests Klotho expression may be modulated by skeletal muscle activity. Our pilot clinical findings performed in young and aged individuals suggest that circulating Klotho levels are upregulated in response to an acute exercise bout, but that the response may be dependent on fitness level. A similar upregulation of circulating Klotho is also observed in response to an acute exercise in young and old mice, suggesting that this may be a good model for mechanistically probing the role of physical activity on Klotho expression. Finally, we highlight overlapping signaling pathways that are modulated by both Klotho and skeletal muscle and propose potential mechanisms for cross-talk between the two. It is hoped that this review will stimulate further consideration of the relationship between skeletal muscle activity and Klotho expression, potentially leading to important insights into the well-documented systemic anti-aging effects of exercise.

Keywords: skeletal muscle, Klotho, aging, regeneration, exercise

INTRODUCTION

Mankind has long sought means to extend longevity and counteract the effects of aging on physical functioning. Modern day scientific discoveries have made considerable strides in our biological understanding of contributing factors in the aging process. Such discoveries are critical for the development of therapeutic strategies to prevent, delay or reverse age-related declines.

Skeletal muscle is the largest organ of the human body, and it comprises over 40% of the body's mass in non obese individuals. It is therefore not surprising that alterations to the skeletal muscle contractile unit have profound effects on overall organismal health. Age-related declines are manifest by a decreased ability for aged skeletal muscle to respond to physiological stimuli such as muscle loading or acute injury. Indeed, older adults often exhibit an age-related reduction in the number and size of muscle fibers, known as sarcopenia (Lexell, 1995). The subsequent sarcopenia-related muscle weakening and atrophy soon leads to the onset of decreased mobility. Secondary effects of sarcopenia include an increased risk for falls (Tinetti, 1987), declines in physical functioning (Rantanen et al., 1997) and a decreased participation in activities of daily living (Tinetti, 1987; Szulc et al., 2005; Reid et al., 2008). Macro-level deficits are, at least partially, the result of age-related molecular and cellular alterations. These alterations include impaired metabolic pathways (i.e., insulin/IGF, forkhead transcription factor, and mTOR signaling) and altered muscle maintenance systems (i.e., ubiquitin-proteasome system, autophagy-lysosome system) (Sandri et al., 2013). In addition, muscle stem (satellite) cells (MuSCs), responsible for dictating skeletal muscle regenerative capacity, display impaired functioning with increasing age (reviewed in Conboy and Rando, 2012). With age, these cells demonstrate a decline in regenerative potential owing to altered cellular proliferation and myogenic differentiation (reviewed in Mann et al., 2011; Conboy and Rando, 2012). As the number of elderly individuals in the United States grows, functional detriments resulting from these age-related declines in skeletal muscle maintenance and healing capacity will increasingly represent an important public health burden. The development of methods to promote healthy aging has, therefore, become more important than ever.

There is abundant evidence that exercise may be effective in preventing, delaying or reversing the effect of age on tissue health and functioning. The anti-aging physiological benefits of physical activity/exercise have been well documented and include the prevention of muscle wasting, cardiovascular diseases, and hypertension (see **Table 1**). Accordingly, physical fitness level is an important predictor of both being able to live independently

Table 1 | Summary depicting overlapping physiological and functional responses to Klotho expression and exercise/physical activity.

Age-related phenotype	Klotho	Exercise
Gait function	Positive association: gait dysfunction observed in *Kl* mice; in humans, higher klotho levels are associated with improved scores on tests of lower extremity strength and functioning (Kuro-o et al., 1997; Crasto et al., 2012)	Positive association: improved fitness is associated with greater walking capacity (Peeters and Mets, 1996; Newman et al., 2006; Simonsick et al., 2006)
Cardiovascular disease (CVD)	Negative association: *Kl* mice demonstrate arteriosclerosis (Kuro-o et al., 1997). In humans, higher klotho levels were associated with lower likelihood of CVD (Semba et al., 2011)	Negative association: sedentary behavior is positively associated with mortality and CVD (Matthews et al., 2008; Warren et al., 2010; Chomistek et al., 2013)
Osteoporosis	Negative association: decreased Klotho levels are associated with decreased bone mineral density of hindlimb bones, primarily as a result of decreased cortical bone thickness (Kuro-o et al., 1997)	Negative association: lower physical activity is associated with decreased bone mineral density (Martyn-St James and Carroll, 2009; Hamilton et al., 2010)
Cognitive function	Positive association: *Kl* mice display impaired novel-object recognition and associative memory (Nagai et al., 2003; Kuang et al., 2014). Klotho levels have been shown to be lower in those with Alzheimer's disease (Semba et al., 2014)	Positive association: exercise promotes brain plasticity and has been shown to halt, delay and/or reverse the effects of aging on cognitive function (reviewed in Foster et al., 2011)
Angiogenesis	Positive association: *Kl* mice demonstrate significantly decreased skeletal muscle capillary density and evidence of angiogenesis following an ischemic injury (Fukino et al., 2002; Shimada et al., 2004)	Positive association: muscle loading results in a significantly increased skeletal muscle capillary density and the promotion of angiogenesis (Hoier et al., 2012)
Resistance to stress	Positive association: Klotho protects cells from apoptosis induced by oxidative stress (Yamamoto et al., 2005)	Positive association: whereas acute stress may induce oxidative stress and reactive oxygen species accumulation, chronic training has been shown to promote upregulation of antioxidants (Gomez-Cabrera et al., 2008; Mangner et al., 2013)
Tissue regeneration	Positive association: *Kl* mice display increase Wnt signaling, decreased stem cell numbers and an impaired regenerative response (Liu et al., 2007)	Positive association: muscle loading enhances the participation of stem cells in muscle regeneration (Ambrosio et al., 2010; Distefano et al., 2013). An acute bout of exercise results in increased satellite cell number (Dreyer et al., 2006; Kosek et al., 2006; Cermak et al., 2012), while chronic, repeated bouts mRNA expression of myogenic markers and reduces mRNA expression for inhibitors of myogenesis (Carey, 2007; Costa et al., 2007). Endurance exercise increases satellite cell content by 30–58% (Charifi et al., 2003; Verney et al., 2008)

into old age and all-cause mortality (Myers et al., 2002; Gulati et al., 2003; Myers, 2003). Studies have suggested that improving physical fitness may decrease the risk of death by up to 44% (Blair et al., 1995). Inherent to physical activity or exercise is skeletal muscle contractile activity. While other benefits of exercise, such as improved cardiovascular health, may not be discounted, adequate skeletal muscle functioning is likely a *sine qua non* in the anti-aging effects of exercise (Castillo-Garzon et al., 2006). Indeed, handgrip strength, a surrogate measure for total body muscle strength (Rantanen et al., 2003), has been shown in previous studies to be a reliable marker of wellbeing (Lord et al., 2003; Chang et al., 2004; Hulsmann et al., 2004) and is a potent predictor of both the expectancy to live independently and mortality (Castillo-Garzon et al., 2006). Perhaps even more compelling are findings that grip strength in healthy, middle aged men is predictive of functional limitations and disability 25 years later (Rantanen et al., 1999). Based on this and other studies, Rantanen and colleagues suggested that muscle strength may serve as a marker of "physiological reserve" even in midlife, and that the extent of this reserve may be indicative of vulnerability to disease and disability into old age (Rantanen et al., 2012).

What is the biological basis underlying the relationship between skeletal muscle contractile activity and tissue declines? The systemic anti-aging benefits of exercise suggest that humoral factors may play a role. Indeed, a potential relationship between the circulating longevity protein, Klotho, and the pathogenesis of sarcopenia was recently suggested by a large, population-based study of aging by Semba et al. (2011). Klotho has been called an "aging suppressor gene" and has been suggested to delay age-related declines in physiological functioning (Kuro-o et al., 1997). The protein product of this gene has been detected in the circulatory system of both animals and humans (Kuro-o et al., 1997; Xiao et al., 2004), although its serum concentration gradually declines with increasing age (Xiao et al., 2004). In two studies, a strong association between plasma Klotho expression and skeletal muscle strength (Semba et al., 2012) and functioning (Crasto et al., 2012) were revealed. As summarized in **Table 1**, there are many parallels between age-related processes/pathologies that are regulated by Klotho and those regulated by exercise/or physical activity. Given these parallels, we were driven by a curiosity as to whether there may be a cross-talk between skeletal muscle activity and expression of this longevity protein. The purpose of this "Hypothesis and Theory" style manuscript is to present a literature review and preliminary results from our laboratory in support of our novel hypothesis that biochemical events originating within skeletal muscle are important triggers of Klotho expression. Specifically, we hypothesize that skeletal muscle contractile activity modulates circulating Klotho expression and that this regulation may play a role in the well-documented systemic anti-aging effects of exercise. Moreover, we propose that Klotho may participate in the skeletal muscle regenerative cascade and that age-related declines in Klotho levels may contribute to the decreased ability of aged skeletal muscle to heal after injury.

THE REGULATION AND ROLES OF KLOTHO

Klotho is present in both membrane-bound and secreted forms. The secreted form is generated through alternative splicing or through shedding of the extracellular domain of the transmembrane protein by membrane-anchored proteases (Kuro-o et al., 1997), including A disintegrin and metalloproteinase domain–containing protein 10 (ADAM10), ADAM metallopeptidase domain 17 (ADAM17) and Beta-secretase 1 (BACE 1) (Chen et al., 2007). The secreted form of Klotho has been shown to exert biological effects throughout the body, indicating its potential as a humoral factor. The membrane-bound version serves as an obligate co-receptor for fibroblast growth factor-23 (FGF23) signaling (Kurosu et al., 2006), whereas the secreted protein functions independently of FGF23. Since its original discovery in 1997, two homologs of Klotho, α and β, have been identified, with β-Klotho sharing 41% amino acid identity with α-Klotho. Throughout this paper, the term "Klotho" refers to the α-Klotho homolog.

Klotho is most highly expressed in the kidney, brain and pituitary gland, and is present in lower levels within skeletal muscle, the urinary bladder, the ovary and the testes (Kuro-o et al., 1997). Trace amounts of Klotho are also observed in the placenta, aorta, colon, and the thyroid gland (Kuro-o et al., 1997) (See **Figure 1**, reprinted from Kuro-o et al., 1997). β-Klotho is expressed in adipose tissue, as well as the liver and pancreas (Ito et al., 2000).

The intriguing role for Klotho in age-related declines was first identified through the serendipitous discovery of the *Klotho* knockout mouse (*kl* mouse). *Kl* mice display limited membrane-bound and secreted Klotho protein expression as a result of an ectopic DNA insertion into the Klotho gene. This mutation results in lifespans approximately 5–6% that of their wild type counterparts (10–12 weeks and 2.5–3 years, respectively) (Kuro-o et al., 1997). Although the exact cause of death is unknown, within their short lifespan, the decreased longevity of *kl* mice is consistent with a myriad of aging phenotypes, including decreased activity levels, hypokinesis, gait disturbance, atherosclerosis, cognitive impairment, sarcopenia and an impaired wound repair process. Importantly, genetic up-regulation of Klotho in mice reverses age-related declines in the physiological functioning of various tissues and extends lifespan by 20–30% beyond the normal lifespan of wild type mice (Kurosu et al., 2005).

THE EFFECT OF EXERCISE AND TRAINING ON PLASMA KLOTHO EXPRESSION

There is limited data exploring the relationship between parameters of physical health/fitness and Klotho. Analyses obtained from the Invecchiare in Chianti "Aging in the Chianti Area" (InCHIANTI) study, a population-based longitudinal study, revealed that low plasma levels of Klotho are associated with decreased activities of daily living in older individuals (Crasto et al., 2012). Low plasma Klotho levels have also been associated with a lower score on the Short Physical Performance Battery (a test of lower extremity strength and functioning) (Crasto et al., 2012), as well as poor muscle strength in older, community dwelling adults (Semba et al., 2012). Like poor handgrip strength (Rantanen et al., 1999), low plasma Klotho levels were also shown to be an independent predictor of all-cause mortality (Semba et al., 2011). While reports failed to observe any direct relationship between "physical activity" and circulating Klotho levels, in these studies, physical activity was a self-reported measure of behavior [ranked on a progression scale from 0 (inactive) to 7 (intense exercise several times/week)] and may not necessarily be indicative of physical fitness levels, *per se*.

Clinical correlations between Klotho expression and skeletal muscle strength are consistent with a pre-clinical study where grip strength and running endurance were compared among *kl* mice, Klotho overexpressing mice (*EFmKL46*) and wild-type (WT) control mice (Phelps et al., 2013). *Kl* mice were significantly weaker, and displayed strength of ~50% less than both *EFmKL46* and WT-controls (there was no difference between *EFmKL46* and WT-controls). Interestingly, *kl* mice ran on a running wheel at the same speed as the other two groups, but they demonstrated an endurance capacity ~60% less than that of *EFmKL46* and WT-controls.

As a first step to probe the relationship between physical activity, age and Klotho expression, we quantified the effect of an acute exercise bout on circulating Klotho levels in both young (3–4 months) and aged (22–24 months) C57Bl6/J mice. The acute exercise consisted of 45-min of treadmill running at a 0° incline, performed at approximately 70% maximal aerobic capacity (VO_2max) (Schefer and Talan, 1996). Immediately after exercise, we observed a significant increase in circulating Klotho levels in both young and aged mice, although the response was blunted in aged animals when compared to young counterparts (**Figure 2**, unpublished results).

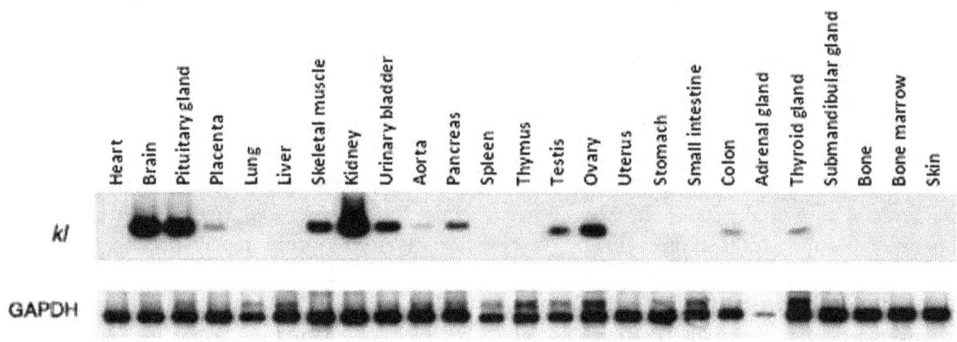

FIGURE 1 | Klotho gene expression in multiple tissues. Kuro-o and colleagues quantified Klotho gene expression of multiple tissues using RT-PCR. The kidney, brain and pituitary gland demonstrate the greatest expression, whereas skeletal muscle, ovaries and testes express Klotho to a relatively lesser extent. (Reproduced from Kuro-o et al., 1997).

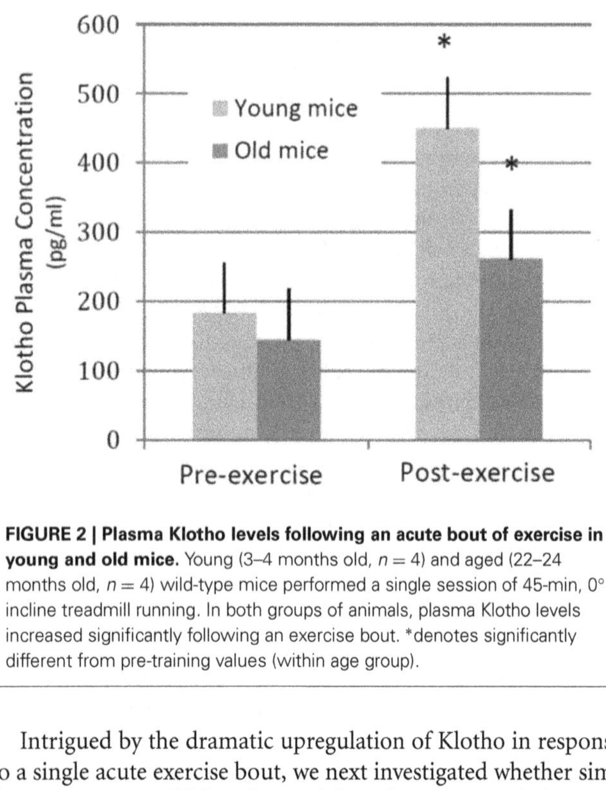

FIGURE 2 | Plasma Klotho levels following an acute bout of exercise in young and old mice. Young (3–4 months old, $n = 4$) and aged (22–24 months old, $n = 4$) wild-type mice performed a single session of 45-min, 0° incline treadmill running. In both groups of animals, plasma Klotho levels increased significantly following an exercise bout. *denotes significantly different from pre-training values (within age group).

Intrigued by the dramatic upregulation of Klotho in response to a single acute exercise bout, we next investigated whether similar responses could be observed in a human population. We utilized a convenience sample of banked serum from "young" (age 36.0 ± 7.0 *SD* years; $n = 12$ females) and "older" (age 68.3 ± 3.0 SD years; $n = 7$ females) sedentary (exercised $\leq 1\times$/week) individuals to evaluate the change in circulating Klotho levels before and after completion of an acute exercise bout. In addition, we investigated whether completion of an exercise training protocol may affect the Klotho response to an acute exercise bout. Young women were mildly obese (BMI 30–38 kg/m^2); older women varied between a BMI of 22–34 kg/m^2. Exclusionary criteria included diagnosis of type 2 diabetes, coronary heart disease, peripheral vascular disease, or clinically significant hyperlipidemia. Individuals with treated or untreated hypertension were also excluded. The protocol was approved by the University of Pittsburgh Institutional Review Board, and written informed consent was obtained from each subject prior to participation.

The acute exercise bout for the young group consisted of one hour of treadmill walking at 55% VO_2max, as determined using a standard incremental protocol (Swain and American College of Sports Medicine, 2014). Subjects were given a standard meal consisting of 10 kcal/kg of 50% carbohydrate- 30% fat-20% protein and then fasted overnight until the completion of the exercise bout (~10:00 am). Additionally, they were instructed to avoid strenuous physical activity for two days before the test. The young group then completed a 16-week progressive exercise training protocol consisting of four to six exercise sessions weekly, which primarily included cycling on a stationary bicycle, rowing or walking/jogging. At least one exercise session per week was supervised for each participant to assure that the target exercise intensity and duration was achieved. Following the 16-week training protocol, the young group completed the acute exercise bout again. The study protocol for the "older" group was essentially the same with the exception that the acute exercise bout was conducted on a cycle ergometer at 45% of VO_2max and the exercise training protocol was for 12 weeks, and not 16 weeks as was performed for the young group. The fact that serum was collected from a banked convenience sample precluded matching training protocols exactly across age groups. For both young and older groups, blood was drawn a total of 4 times: before and after acute exercise both at baseline (ie. pre-training) and again post-training. Circulating Klotho levels were measured using a human soluble α-Klotho enzyme-linked immunosorbent assay Kit (Immuno-Biological Laboratories Co., Ltd., Takasaki, Japan).

Prior to training, we observed no significant changes in the circulating levels of Klotho in response to an acute exercise bout [average change in circulating Klotho (pg/ml) pre-to-post acute exercise in young: −1.9% ± 9.53 *SE* and older: 7.06% ± 2.68 *SE*; **Figure 3**, unpublished results]. However, completion of a 16-week training program resulted in a significant increase in circulating Klotho levels in response to an acute exercise bout in young individuals [change in circulating Klotho (pg/ml): 30.08 ± 11.94%; $p < 0.05$, **Figure 3**]. Following training, older individuals also demonstrated an increase in circulating Klotho in response to acute exercise, although the effect of training was

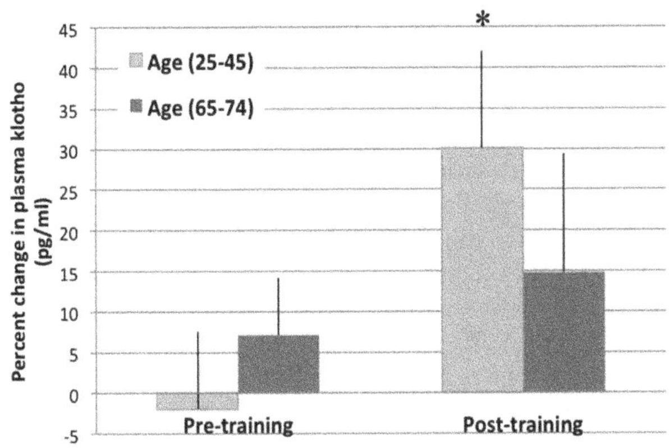

FIGURE 3 | Plasma Klotho levels following an acute bout of exercise in young and older individuals. The change in plasma Klotho levels are depicted at baseline and immediately following an acute exercise bout (pre- and post-training). There was no change in circulating Klotho levels pre-training. However, post-training, there was a significant increase in circulating Klotho levels in the young (age 25–45 years) cohort after an acute bout of exercise. This response was blunted in the older cohort (age 65–74). *denotes significantly different than pre-training values (within age group).

attenuated when compared to young counterparts [change in circulating Klotho (pg/ml): 15.25% ± 6.56 *SE*; $p = 0.07$ **Figure 3**, unpublished results].

Taken together, these findings in murine and human models suggest that exercise is a potent stimulus to increase plasma Klotho levels, but that the response may be dependent on physical fitness level as well as age. While this response to an acute exercise bout and training appears, from the current results, to be attenuated in older individuals, it should be noted that the training protocol for the aged individuals was slightly less intense and of a shorter duration than that of the young individuals. These differences in training intensity may confound the age-related differences in the response of Klotho to acute exercise and further clinical studies are warranted. However, in our murine studies, where the exercise intensity was matched across age groups, a similar age-related decline in the Klotho response following an acute exercise bout was also observed. Another intriguing observation came from the fact that individuals included in the pilot clinical study were overweight-obese. Interestingly, when the young participants were stratified according to BMI (<30 or >30 kg/m^2) individuals with a lower BMI demonstrated significantly higher circulating Klotho levels after acute exercise (Average change = 10 ± 2.7% *SE*; $p < 0.05$), whereas those individuals in the higher BMI group demonstrated no change in circulating Klotho levels following acute exercise at baseline (−3.2% ± 7.5 *SE*; $p = 0.40$). However, following completion of a training program, individuals in the higher BMI group trended toward a significant increase in Klotho levels following an acute exercise bout (~30% increase; $p = 0.06$). These findings further support the hypothesis that the effect of an acute exercise bout on Klotho expression may be dependent on fitness levels. Future studies should investigate the effect of exercise intensity or duration on circulating Klotho levels.

Our findings in humans and mice that demonstrate an upregulation of Klotho expression in response to acute activity demands are consistent with previous reports suggesting that Klotho plays an important role in energy metabolism. Recent studies have focused on the relationship between Klotho and peroxisome proliferator-activated receptor (PPAR) family members, which have been shown to act as lipid sensors to regulate energy metabolism. Specifically, PPAR-ϒ induces expression of the β-Klotho homolog (Zhang et al., 2008) and, conversely, β-Klotho upregulates PPAR-ϒ synthesis (Chihara et al., 2006), implicating the Klotho family of proteins as playing a role in lipid metabolism. Within the context of lipid oxidation, elderly individuals oxidize less fat during exercise when compared to young counterparts (Sial et al., 1996). However, training may be effective in reversing the age-related alterations in exercise response, and it is well established that, in both young and aged individuals, intramuscular fat oxidation during exercise is increased dramatically after training, an effect primarily attributed to an increased muscle respiratory capacity (Coggan et al., 1992; Proctor et al., 1995). One explanation for this benefit may come from the fact that training results in increased mitochondrial content, which thereby increases muscle respiratory capacity and promotes the utilization of fat over that of carbohydrate. Although excessive lipid accumulation is clearly detrimental to organismal health, maintenance of an adequate amount of lipid is clearly critical for maintaining physiological energy balance (Razzaque, 2012), and it is possible that the role of Klotho in maintaining this balance is mediated, at least in part, by skeletal muscle contractile activity. It would be interesting to investigate whether exercise-induced increases in Klotho may be a response to increased intramuscular fat oxidation as a feedback mechanism to maintain tissue lipid supplies under conditions of increased utilization. However, it should be noted that the role of Klotho in lipid metabolism has been linked to the β-Klotho homolog (reviewed in Kurosu and Kuro, 2009), whereas we specifically measured circulating α-Klotho levels in the current pilot studies. Further studies are needed to investigate how our observed exercise-induced changes in α-Klotho may be concomitant with alterations in β-Klotho. Alternatively, it is possible that increased skeletal muscle contractile activity induces a shift in calcium metabolism through Klotho-mediated FGF signaling, and that alterations in lipid metabolism may be a secondary effect of altered calcium homeostasis and mitochondrial biogenesis after exercise. Although further studies are needed to confirm the similarities between murine and clinical responses, the parallels observed in these preliminary studies suggest that pre-clinical investigations may serve as a good model for future mechanistic studies designed to interrogate the effect of physical fitness and skeletal muscle activity on the modulation of this potent longevity protein.

REGULATION OF KLOTHO IN RESPONSE TO SKELETAL MUSCLE INJURY

In addition to sarcopenia, increasing age typically results in a decreased overall skeletal muscle regeneration in response to damage (Jarvinen et al., 1983; Carlson and Faulkner, 1989; Brooks and Faulkner, 1990). Following injury, aged skeletal muscle demonstrates a shift from functional myofiber repair, as is typically seen in young individuals, to a "quick-fix" default toward fibrosis formation (Brack et al., 2007). This impaired response initiates a devastating cascade of muscle atrophy and weakness (Carlson and Faulkner, 1989), increased susceptibility to recurrent muscle injury (Croisier, 2004), and a prolonged recovery (McBride et al., 1995).

In young, healthy skeletal muscle, MuSCs are readily activated from a quiescent state in order to repair damaged myofibers (Mauro, 1961). While MuSC activation in young skeletal muscle often restores the original architecture and function of the damaged fibers, there is an age-related decrease in MuSC responses, as evidenced by MuSC differentiation toward a fibrogenic lineage (Brack et al., 2007), increased apoptosis (Ryall et al., 2008) and a decreased proliferation (Conboy et al., 2003). Declines in the activation of myogenic molecular pathways, including phosphatidylinositol 3-kinase (PI3K/Akt) signaling pathway, which directs cellular apoptosis, as well as Notch signaling, indispensable for MuSC proliferation immediately following injury (Conboy et al., 2003), have been implicated as culprits in age-related MuSC dysfunction. The mitogen activated protein kinase (MAPK) pathway, a positive regulator of Notch, is similarly age-responsive (Carlson et al., 2009a). Finally, it appears that decreased signaling for myogenesis is concomitant with increased activation of fibrogenic pathways owing to an age-related increased activation of the canonical Wnt signaling pathway, which contributes to a myogenic-to-fibrogenic conversion of MuSCs (Brack et al., 2007).

Fortunately, age-related changes in skeletal muscle regenerative potential are reversible, and several murine experiments have shown that rejuvenation of the systemic skeletal muscle microenvironment largely restores healing potential in aged mice (Carlson and Faulkner, 1989; Conboy et al., 2005; Brack et al., 2007). *In vivo,* heterochronic muscle transplantation experiments (Carlson and Faulkner, 1989) and parabiotic pairings, in which young and aged animals are surgically joined such that they share a common blood circulation, significantly enhances myofiber regeneration and decreases fibrosis formation of aged muscle following injury (Conboy et al., 2005; Brack et al., 2008). This enhanced tissue healing is concomitant with an inhibition of the Wnt signaling pathway and a decreased fibrogenic conversion of aged MuSCs (Brack et al., 2007). Importantly, it has been shown that the improved muscle healing of aged parabiotic partners is not the result of a physical contribution of the young cells within the circulation (Conboy et al., 2005). Taken together, these studies suggest that systemic niche factors play a critical role in dictating skeletal muscle regenerative potential, perhaps even more so than the intrinsic characteristics of the stem cells themselves. It has been hypothesized that the introduction of youthful factors into the circulation of aged partners inhibits, or functionally neutralizes, deleterious factors typically found in old animals (Carlson et al., 2009b).

There is precedence to suggest a relationship between Klotho expression and tissue regenerative capacity. In the skin, stomach, small intestine and kidney, the impaired tissue regenerative response of *kl* mice has been associated with a decreased stem cell frequency (Liu et al., 2007; Izbeki et al., 2010) and proliferation (Liu et al., 2007), impaired angiogenesis (Fukino et al., 2002), and decreased cellular resistance to stress (Yamamoto et al., 2005; Izbeki et al., 2010). In addition, the subcutaneous transplantation of bone marrow mesenchymal stem cells results in an attenuation of age-related degenerative processes and a concomitant lifespan extension of recipient mice, effects that were associated with an increased Klotho expression (Yamaza et al., 2009). Liu et al demonstrated that Klotho enhances stem cell regenerative potential and promotes tissue-healing through an inhibition of Wnt signaling activation (Liu et al., 2007). These latter findings were confirmed in recent studies demonstrating that, within the kidney, Klotho is able to directly bind to Wnt ligands extracellularly (Zhou et al., 2013). In the case of renal fibrosis, decreased Klotho expression was associated with an increased Wnt signaling activation and subsequent activation of fibrogenic signaling pathways (Zhou et al., 2013). Whether age-related declines in Klotho expression may contribute to the increased skeletal muscle Wnt signaling in aged animals, and thereby increased fibrosis deposition after injury, has not, to the best of our knowledge, been previously investigated.

Another potential mechanism by which Klotho may play be implicated as a potential regulator of skeletal muscle regeneration is through inhibition of Transforming Growth Factor-beta1 (TGF-β1) signaling. TGF-β1 is regarded as "master switch" for promoting mesenchymal transition toward a fibroblastic lineage in several tissues, including the kidney and lung (Willis and Borok, 2007; Doi et al., 2011). TGF-β1 ligands may be transported through the blood and bind to their specific receptors to initiate TGF-β-pSMAD signaling. With aging, circulating TGF-β1 expression in both mice and humans is increased, as is expression of the TGF-β1 receptors (Carlson et al., 2009b). It has been suggested that this may play a role in the increased fibrosis formation after injury of aged skeletal muscle (Li et al., 2004; Carlson et al., 2009b). Of note, physiological levels of TGF-β1 in young mice were predicted, based on *in vitro* investigations, to be inhibitory of MuSC myogenesis, suggesting that young sera may contain either a natural decoy of TGF-β1or a competitor to TGF-β1 signaling that inhibits the fibrotic cascade, and that the level of this decoy is decreased with increased age (Carlson et al., 2009b). Could Klotho act as such a decoy?

In a recent study by Doi et al., it was shown in the kidney that Klotho is indeed capable of interfering with TGF-β1signaling, but not TGF-β1 expression, in order to decrease myofibroblast infiltration and decrease fibrosis formation (Doi et al., 2011). Specifically, Klotho was shown to bind to the TGF-β1 receptor to inhibit TGF-β1 binding. Whereas Klotho depletion resulted in increased renal fibrosis, Klotho replacement therapy significantly alleviated the pathology, suggesting that decreased Klotho levels may contribute to the pathogenesis of renal fibrosis (Doi et al., 2011). Accordingly, systemic administration of a TGF-β1 receptor 1 (R1) kinase inhibitor effectively enhanced myofiber regeneration after injury, whereas application of a TGF-β1 neutralizing antibody had no effect (Carlson et al., 2009b). These findings support the above stated hypothesis that a natural decoy of TGF-β1 signaling may minimize activation of fibrogenic pathways in young animals following skeletal muscle injury, but that this suppression is lost in aged animals. Given the interactions between Klotho expression and TGF-β1 signaling, it is possible that age-related declines in circulating

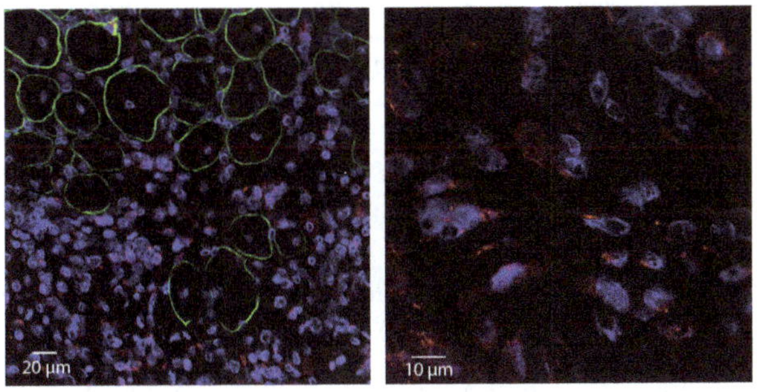

FIGURE 4 | Acute injury increases local Klotho expression within skeletal muscle. Young (3–4 months old) wild type animals were exposed to a cardiotoxin injury to the tibialis anterior muscle. Two weeks after injury, TAs were harvested, cryosectioned and incubated with anti-Klotho (red), anti-Dystrophin (green) and nuclear (blue) antibodies (**left image**; 20× magnification). Corresponding high magnification image (**right image**; 100× magnification). Note that Klotho is undetectable in areas of more mature, regenerating myofibers. In contrast, strong expression of Klotho is observed in the area of cellular infiltrate.

Klotho may result in a decreased opposition of TGF-β1 signaling, ultimately promoting fibrosis formation and impairing myofiber regeneration after injury. Moreover, it has been suggested in the kidney that Klotho effectively inhibits TGF-β1 activation of β-catenin, a downstream target of Wnt signaling, in tubular epithelial cells (Zhou et al., 2013). Future studies should explore the ability of Klotho to modulate Wnt signaling, potentially via inhibition of TGF-β1, in aged skeletal muscle models.

Our preliminary studies support a potential contribution of Klotho to the skeletal muscle regenerative response. Two weeks following administration of an acute muscle injury to the tibialis anterior muscle of young wild type mice, we observed a dramatic increase in local Klotho expression (**Figure 4**, unpublished results). Importantly, Klotho was only expressed in the regions of cellular infiltrate and nascent myotubes, and not in the more mature regenerating myofibers (**Figure 4**). An important question is whether aged muscle displays an impaired Klotho response to injury as compared to young counterparts, and whether this decline contributes to the decreased regenerative capacity characterizing aged skeletal muscle. Future investigations should perform quantitative analysis of the response of Klotho to an acute injury event.

CONCLUSIONS

History is replete with evidence demonstrating man's quest for a universal panacea to reverse the effects of aging in order to maintain and/or restore youthfulness. While a single "fountain of youth" remedy that counteracts all of the effects of time on organismal functioning is unlikely, an improved mechanistic understanding of tissue responses to the aging process and modifiable factors that may promote rejuvenation of these responses is desirable. Among such modifiable factors, physical activity has long been acknowledged for its anti-aging effects and the impact of skeletal muscle health on physical functioning and longevity is undeniable.

Indeed, systemic influences of skeletal muscle have been a growing topic of investigation and increased attention has been paid in recent years to the capacity of skeletal muscle to function as an endocrine organ capable of communicating with and dictating the behavior of distant organs. Modulation of Klotho expression through skeletal muscle contraction represents an intriguing relationship that may help explain the anti-aging effects of physical activity, and, as highlighted in this review, there is emerging evidence to suggest that such a relationship exists. Still unknown is whether skeletal muscle contractile activity itself results in the local production and secretion of Klotho into the bloodstream, or whether some myokine (a cytokine of skeletal muscle origin) is responsible for inducing Klotho expression in the kidney or brain, for example. This would be an interesting topic for future investigations. An improved mechanistic understanding of the potential role of skeletal muscle as a regulator of Klotho expression is important, as it may lead to the development of targeted and specific rehabilitation programs designed to counteract the effect of aging on organismal health.

ACKNOWLEDGMENTS

Support was provided by grant K01AG039477 (Fabrisia Ambrosio) from the National Institute on Aging, National Institutes of Health, the Pittsburgh Claude D. Pepper Older Americans Independence Center (P30 AG024827, T32 Training Program) and the University of Pittsburgh Institute on Aging.

REFERENCES

Ambrosio, F., Ferrari, R. J., Distefano, G., Plassmeyer, J. M., Carvell, G. E., Deasy, B. M., et al. (2010). The synergistic effect of treadmill running on stem-cell transplantation to heal injured skeletal muscle. *Tissue Eng. A* 16, 839–849. doi: 10.1089/ten.tea.2009.0113

Blair, S. N., Kohl, H. W. 3rd., Barlow, C. E., Paffenbarger, R. S. Jr., Gibbons, L. W., and Macera, C. A. (1995). Changes in physical fitness and all-cause mortality. A prospective study of healthy and unhealthy men. *JAMA* 273, 1093–1108. doi: 10.1001/jama.1995.03520380029031

Brack, S., Conboy, I. M., Conboy, M. J., Shen, J., and Rando, T. A. (2008). A temporal switch from notch to Wnt signaling in muscle stem cells is necessary for normal adult myogenesis. *Cell Stem Cell* 2, 50–59. doi: 10.1016/j.stem.2007.10.006

Brack, S., Conboy, M. J., Roy, S., Lee, M., Kuo, C. J., Keller, C., et al. (2007). Increased Wnt signaling during aging alters muscle stem cell fate and increases fibrosis. *Science* 317, 807–810. doi: 10.1126/science.1144090

Brooks, S. V., and Faulkner, J. A. (1990). Contraction-induced injury: recovery of skeletal muscles in young and old mice. *Am. J. Physiol.* 258(3 Pt 1), C436–C442.

Carey, J. R. (2007). Invited commentary. *Phys. Ther.* 87, 1603–1605. author reply: 1605–1607. doi: 10.2522/ptj.20060310.ic

Carlson, B. M., and Faulkner, J. A. (1989). Muscle transplantation between young and old rats: age of host determines recovery. *Am. J. Physiol.* 256(6 Pt 1), C1262–C1266.

Carlson, M. E., Conboy, M. J., Hsu, M., Barchas, L., Jeong, J., Agrawal, A., et al. (2009b). Relative roles of TGF-beta1 and Wnt in the systemic regulation and aging of satellite cell responses. *Aging Cell* 8, 676–689. doi: 10.1111/j.1474-9726.2009.00517.x

Carlson, M. E., Suetta, C., Conboy, M. J., Aagaard, P., Mackey, A., Kjaer, M., et al. (2009a). Molecular aging and rejuvenation of human muscle stem cells. *EMBO Mol. Med.* 1, 381–391. doi: 10.1002/emmm.200900045

Castillo-Garzon, M. J., Ruiz, J. R., Ortega, F. B., and Gutierrez, A. (2006). Anti-aging therapy through fitness enhancement. *Clin. Interv. Aging* 1, 213–220. doi: 10.2147/ciia.2006.1.3.213

Cermak, N. M., Noseworthy, M. D., Bourgeois, J. M., Tarnopolsky, M. A., and Gibala, M. J. (2012). Diffusion tensor MRI to assess skeletal muscle disruption following eccentric exercise. *Muscle Nerve* 46, 42–50. doi: 10.1002/mus.23276

Chang, J. T., Morton, S. C., Rubenstein, L. Z., Mojica, W. A., Maglione, M., Suttorp, M. J., et al. (2004). Interventions for the prevention of falls in older adults: systematic review and meta-analysis of randomised clinical trials. *BMJ* 328:680. doi: 10.1136/bmj.328.7441.680

Charifi, N., Kadi, F., Feasson, L., and Denis, C. (2003). Effects of endurance training on satellite cell frequency in skeletal muscle of old men. *Muscle Nerve* 28, 87–92. doi: 10.1002/mus.10394

Chen, C. D., Podvin, S., Gillespie, E., Leeman, S. E., and Abraham, C. R. (2007). Insulin stimulates the cleavage and release of the extracellular domain of Klotho by ADAM10 and ADAM17. *Proc. Natl. Acad. Sci. U.S.A.* 104, 19796–19801. doi: 10.1073/pnas.0709805104

Chihara, Y., Rakugi, H., Ishikawa, K., Ikushima, M., Maekawa, Y., Ohta, J., et al. (2006). Klotho protein promotes adipocyte differentiation. *Endocrinology* 147, 3835–3842. doi: 10.1210/en.2005-1529

Chomistek, K., Manson, J. E., Stefanick, M. L., Lu, B., Sands-Lincoln, M., Going, S. B., et al. (2013). Relationship of sedentary behavior and physical activity to incident cardiovascular disease: results from the Women's Health Initiative. *J. Am. Coll. Cardiol.* 61, 2346–2354. doi: 10.1016/j.jacc.2013.03.031

Coggan, R., Spina, R. J., King, D. S., Rogers, M. A., Brown, M., Nemeth, P. M., et al. (1992). Skeletal muscle adaptations to endurance training in 60- to 70-yr-old men and women. *J. Appl. Physiol.* 72, 1780–1176.

Conboy, M., Conboy, M. J., Smythe, G. M., and Rando, T. A. (2003). Notch-mediated restoration of regenerative potential to aged muscle. *Science* 302, 1575–1577. doi: 10.1126/science.1087573

Conboy, M., Conboy, M. J., Wagers, A. J., Girma, E. R., Weissman, I. L., and Rando, T. A. (2005). Rejuvenation of aged progenitor cells by exposure to a young systemic environment. *Nature* 433, 760–764. doi: 10.1038/nature 03260

Conboy, M., and Rando, T. A. (2012). Heterochronic parabiosis for the study of the effects of aging on stem cells and their niches. *Cell Cycle* 11, 2260–2267. doi: 10.4161/cc.20437

Costa, A., Dalloul, H., Hegyesi, H., Apor, P., Csende, Z., Racz, M., et al. (2007). Impact of repeated bouts of eccentric exercise on myogenic gene expression. *Eur. J. Appl. Physiol.* 101, 427–436. doi: 10.1007/s00421-007-0510-z

Crasto, C. L., Semba, R. D., Sun, K., Cappola, A. R., Bandinelli, S., and Ferrucci, L. (2012). Relationship of low-circulating "anti-agingll" klotho hormone with disability in activities of daily living among older community-dwelling adults. *Rejuvenation Res.* 15, 295–301. doi: 10.1089/rej.2011.1268

Croisier, J. L. (2004). Factors associated with recurrent hamstring injuries. *Sports Med.* 34, 681–695. doi: 10.2165/00007256-200434100-00005

Distefano, G., Ferrari, R. J., Weiss, C., Deasy, B. M., Boninger, M. L., Fitzgerald, G. K., et al. (2013). Neuromuscular electrical stimulation as a method to maximize the beneficial effects of muscle stem cells transplanted into dystrophic skeletal muscle. *PLoS ONE* 8:e54922. doi: 10.1371/journal.pone.0054922

Doi, S., Zou, Y., Togao, O., Pastor, J. V., John, G. B., Wang, L., et al. (2011). Klotho inhibits transforming growth factor-beta1 (TGF-beta1) signaling and suppresses renal fibrosis and cancer metastasis in mice. *J. Biol. Chem.* 286, 8655–8665. doi: 10.1074/jbc.M110.174037

Dreyer, H. C., Blanco, C. E., Sattler, F. R., Schroeder, E. T., and Wiswell, R. A. (2006). Satellite cell numbers in young and older men 24 hours after eccentric exercise. *Muscle Nerve* 33, 242–253. doi: 10.1002/mus.20461

Foster, P. P., Rosenblatt, K. P., and Kuljis, R. O. (2011). Exercise-induced cognitive plasticity, implications for mild cognitive impairment and Alzheimer's disease. *Front. Neurol.* 2:28. doi: 10.3389/fneur.2011.00028

Fukino, K., Suzuki, T., Saito, Y., Shindo, T., Amaki, T., Kurabayashi, M., et al. (2002). Regulation of angiogenesis by the aging suppressor gene klotho. *Biochem. Biophys. Res. Commun.* 293, 332–337. doi: 10.1016/S0006-291X(02) 00216-4

Gomez-Cabrera, M. C., Domenech, E., and Vina, J. (2008). Moderate exercise is an antioxidant: upregulation of antioxidant genes by training. *Free Radic. Biol. Med.* 44, 126–131. doi: 10.1016/j.freeradbiomed.2007.02.001

Gulati, M., Pandey, D. K., Arnsdorf, M. F., Lauderdale, D. S., Thisted, R. A., Wicklund, R. H., et al. (2003). Exercise capacity and the risk of death in women: the St James Women Take Heart Project. *Circulation* 108, 1554–1559. doi: 10.1161/01.CIR.0000091080.57509.E9

Hamilton, C. J., Swan, V. J., and Jamal, S. A. (2010). The effects of exercise and physical activity participation on bone mass and geometry in postmenopausal women: a systematic review of pQCT studies. *Osteoporos. Int.* 21, 11–23. doi: 10.1007/s00198-009-0967-1

Hoier, B., Nordsborg, N., Andersen, S., Jensen, L., Nybo, L., Bangsbo, J., et al. (2012). Pro- and anti-angiogenic factors in human skeletal muscle in response to acute exercise and training. *J. Physiol.* 590(Pt 3), 595–606. doi: 10.1113/jphysiol.2011.216135

Hulsmann, M., Quittan, M., Berger, R., Crevenna, R., Springer, C., Nuhr, M., et al. (2004). Muscle strength as a predictor of long-term survival in severe congestive heart failure. *Eur. J. Heart Fail.* 6, 101–107. doi: 10.1016/j.ejheart.2003.07.008

Ito, S., Kinoshita, S., Shiraishi, N., Nakagawa, S., Sekine, S., Fujimori, T., et al. (2000). Molecular cloning and expression analyses of mouse betaklotho, which encodes a novel Klotho family protein. *Mech. Dev.* 98, 115–119. doi: 10.1016/S0925-4773(00)00439-1

Izbeki, F., Asuzu, D. T., Lorincz, A., Bardsley, M. R., Popko, L. N., Choi, K. M., et al. (2010). Loss of Kitlow progenitors, reduced stem cell factor and high oxidative stress underlie gastric dysfunction in progeric mice. *J. Physiol.* 588(Pt 16), 3101–3117. doi: 10.1113/jphysiol.2010.191023

Jarvinen, M., Aho, A. J., Lehto, M., and Toivonen, H. (1983). Age dependent repair of muscle rupture. A histological and microangiographical study in rats. *Acta Orthop. Scand.* 54, 64–74. doi: 10.3109/17453678308992871

Kosek, D. J., Kim, J. S., Petrella, J. K., Cross, J. M., and Bamman, M. M. (2006). Efficacy of 3 days/wk resistance training on myofiber hypertrophy and myogenic mechanisms in young vs. older adults. *J. Appl. Physiol.* 101, 531–544. doi: 10.1152/japplphysiol.01474.2005

Kuang, X., Chen, Y. S., Wang, L. F., Li, Y. J., Liu, K., Zhang, M. X., et al. (2014). Klotho upregulation contributes to the neuroprotection of ligustilide in an Alzheimer's disease mouse model. *Neurobiol. Aging* 35, 169–178. doi: 10.1016/j.neurobiolaging.2013.07.019

Kuro-o, M., Matsumura, Y., Aizawa, H., Kawaguchi, H., Suga, T., Utsugi, T., et al. (1997). Mutation of the mouse klotho gene leads to a syndrome resembling ageing. *Nature* 390, 45–51. doi: 10.1038/36285

Kurosu, H., and Kuro, O. M. (2009). The Klotho gene family as a regulator of endocrine fibroblast growth factors. *Mol. Cell. Endocrinol.* 299, 72–78. doi: 10.1016/j.mce.2008.10.052

Kurosu, H., Ogawa, Y., Miyoshi, M., Yamamoto, M., Nandi, A., Rosenblatt, K. P., et al. (2006). Regulation of fibroblast growth factor-23 signaling by klotho. *J. Biol. Chem.* 281, 6120–6123. doi: 10.1074/jbc.C500457200

Kurosu, H., Yamamoto, M., Clark, J. D., Pastor, J. V., Nandi, A., Gurnani, P., et al. (2005). Suppression of aging in mice by the hormone Klotho. *Science* 309, 1829–1833. doi: 10.1126/science.1112766

Lexell, J. (1995). Human aging, muscle mass, and fiber type composition. *J. Gerontol. A Biol. Sci. Med. Sci.* 50.Spec.No, 11–16.

Li, Y., Foster, W., Deasy, B. M., Chan, Y., Prisk, V., Tang, Y., et al. (2004). Transforming growth factor-beta1 induces the differentiation of myogenic cells into fibrotic cells in injured skeletal muscle: a key event in muscle fibrogenesis. *Am. J. Pathol.* 164, 1007–119. doi: 10.1016/S0002-9440(10)63188-4

Liu, H., Fergusson, M. M., Castilho, R. M., Liu, J., Cao, L., Chen, J., et al. (2007). Augmented Wnt signaling in a mammalian model of accelerated aging. *Science* 317, 803–806. doi: 10.1126/science.1143578

Lord, S. R., Castell, S., Corcoran, J., Dayhew, J., Matters, B., Shan, A., et al. (2003). The effect of group exercise on physical functioning and falls in frail older people living in retirement villages: a randomized, controlled trial. *J. Am. Geriatr. Soc.* 51, 1685–1192. doi: 10.1046/j.1532-5415.2003.51551.x

Mangner, N., Linke, A., Oberbach, A., Kullnick, Y., Gielen, S., Sandri, M., et al. (2013). Exercise training prevents TNF-alpha induced loss of force in the diaphragm of mice. *PLoS ONE* 8:e52274. doi: 10.1371/journal.pone.0052274

Mann, C. J., Perdiguero, E., Kharraz, Y., Aguilar, S., Pessina, P., Serrano, A. L., et al. (2011). Aberrant repair and fibrosis development in skeletal muscle. *Skelet. Muscle* 1:21. doi: 10.1186/2044-5040-1-21

Martyn-St James, M., and Carroll, S. (2009). A meta-analysis of impact exercise on postmenopausal bone loss: the case for mixed loading exercise programmes. *Br. J. Sports Med.* 43, 898–908. doi: 10.1136/bjsm.2008.052704

Matthews, E., Chen, K. Y., Freedson, P. S., Buchowski, M. S., Beech, B. M., Pate, R. R., et al. (2008). Amount of time spent in sedentary behaviors in the United States, 2003-(2004). *Am. J. Epidemiol.* 167, 875–881. doi: 10.1093/aje/kwm390

Mauro, A. (1961). Satellite cell of skeletal muscle fibers. *J. Biophys. Biochem. Cytol.* 9, 493–445. doi: 10.1083/jcb.9.2.493

McBride, T. A., Gorin, F. A., and Carlsen, R. C. (1995). Prolonged recovery and reduced adaptation in aged rat muscle following eccentric exercise. *Mech. Ageing Dev.* 83, 185–200. doi: 10.1016/0047-6374(95)01629-E

Myers, J. (2003). Cardiology patient pages. Exercise and cardiovascular health. *Circulation* 107, e2–e5. doi: 10.1161/01.CIR.0000048890.59383.8D

Myers, J., Prakash, M., Froelicher, V., Do, D., Partington, S., and Atwood, J. E. (2002). Exercise capacity and mortality among men referred for exercise testing. *N. Engl. J. Med.* 346, 793–801. doi: 10.1056/NEJMoa011858

Nagai, T., Yamada, K., Kim, H. C., Kim, Y. S., Noda, Y., Imura, A., et al. (2003). Cognition impairment in the genetic model of aging klotho gene mutant mice: a role of oxidative stress. *FASEB J.* 17, 50–52. doi: 10.1096/fj.02-0448fje

Newman, B., Simonsick, E. M., Naydeck, B. L., Boudreau, R. M., Kritchevsky, S. B., Nevitt, M. C., et al. (2006). Association of long-distance corridor walk performance with mortality, cardiovascular disease, mobility limitation, and disability. *JAMA* 295, 2018–2026. doi: 10.1001/jama.295.17.2018

Peeters, P., and Mets, T. (1996). The 6-minute walk as an appropriate exercise test in elderly patients with chronic heart failure. *J. Gerontol. A Biol. Sci. Med. Sci.* 51, M147–M151. doi: 10.1093/gerona/51A.4.M147

Phelps, M., Pettan-Brewer, C., Ladiges, W., and Yablonka-Reuveni, Z. (2013). Decline in muscle strength and running endurance in klotho deficient C57BL/6 mice. *Biogerontology* 14, 729–739. doi: 10.1007/s10522-013-9447-2

Proctor, D. N., Sinning, W. E., Walro, J. M., Sieck, G. C., and Lemon, P. W. (1995). Oxidative capacity of human muscle fiber types: effects of age and training status. *J. Appl. Physiol.* 78, 2033–2208.

Rantanen, T., Era, P., and Heikkinen, E. (1997). Physical activity and the changes in maximal isometric strength in men and women from the age of 75 to 80 years. *J. Am. Geriatr. Soc.* 45, 1439–145.

Rantanen, T., Guralnik, J. M., Foley, D., Masaki, K., Leveille, S., Curb, J. D., et al. (1999). Midlife hand grip strength as a predictor of old age disability. *JAMA* 281, 558–560. doi: 10.1001/jama.281.6.558

Rantanen, T., Masaki, K., He, Q., Ross, G. W., Willcox, B. J., and White, L. (2012). Midlife muscle strength and human longevity up to age 100 years: a 44-year prospective study among a decedent cohort. *Age* 34, 563–570. doi: 10.1007/s11357-011-9256-y

Rantanen, T., Volpato, S., Ferrucci, L., Heikkinen, E., Fried, L. P., and Guralnik, J. M. (2003). Handgrip strength and cause-specific and total mortality in older disabled women: exploring the mechanism. *J. Am. Geriatr. Soc.* 51, 636–641. doi: 10.1034/j.1600-0579.2003.00207.x

Razzaque, M. S. (2012). The role of Klotho in energy metabolism. *Nat. Rev. Endocrinol.* 8, 579–587. doi: 10.1038/nrendo.2012.75

Reid, K. F., Naumova, E. N., Carabello, R. J., Phillips, E. M., and Fielding, R. A. (2008). Lower extremity muscle mass predicts functional performance in mobility-limited elders. *J. Nutr. Health Aging* 12, 493–448. doi: 10.1007/BF02982711

Ryall, J. G., Schertzer, J. D., and Lynch, G. S. (2008). Cellular and molecular mechanisms underlying age-related skeletal muscle wasting and weakness. *Biogerontology* 9, 213–228. doi: 10.1007/s10522-008-9131-0

Sandri, M., Coletto, L., Grumati, P., and Bonaldo, P. (2013). Misregulation of autophagy and protein degradation systems in myopathies and muscular dystrophies. *J. Cell Sci.* 126(Pt 23), 5325–5333. doi: 10.1242/jcs.114041

Schefer, V., and Talan, M. I. (1996). Oxygen consumption in adult and AGED C57BL/6J mice during acute treadmill exercise of different intensity. *Exp. Gerontol.* 31, 387–92. doi: 10.1016/0531-5565(95)02032-2

Semba, R. D., Cappola, A. R., Sun, K., Bandinelli, S., Dalal, M., Crasto, C., et al. (2011). Plasma klotho and mortality risk in older community-dwelling adults. *J. Gerontol. A Biol. Sci. Med. Sci.* 66, 794–800. doi: 10.1093/gerona/glr058

Semba, R. D., Cappola, A. R., Sun, K., Bandinelli, S., Dalal, M., Crasto, C., et al. (2012). Relationship of low plasma klotho with poor grip strength in older community-dwelling adults: the InCHIANTI study. *Eur. J. Appl. Physiol.* 112, 1215–1220. doi: 10.1007/s00421-011-2072-3

Semba, R. D., Moghekar, A. R., Hu, J., Sun, K., Turner, R., Ferrucci, L., et al. (2014). Klotho in the cerebrospinal fluid of adults with and without Alzheimer's disease. *Neurosci. Lett.* 558, 37–40. doi: 10.1016/j.neulet.2013.10.058

Shimada, T., Takeshita, Y., Murohara, T., Sasaki, K., Egami, K., Shintani, S., et al. (2004). Angiogenesis and vasculogenesis are impaired in the precocious-aging klotho mouse. *Circulation* 110, 1148–1155. doi: 10.1161/01.CIR.0000139854.74847.99

Sial, S., Coggan, A. R., Carroll, R., Goodwin, J., and Klein, S. (1996). Fat and carbohydrate metabolism during exercise in elderly and young subjects. *Am. J. Physiol.* 271(6 Pt 1), E983–E999.

Simonsick, E. M., Fan, E., and Fleg, J. L. (2006). Estimating cardiorespiratory fitness in well-functioning older adults: treadmill validation of the long distance corridor walk. *J. Am. Geriatr. Soc.* 54, 127–132. doi: 10.1111/j.1532-5415.2005.00530.x

Swain, D. P., and American College of Sports Medicine. (2014). *ACSM's Resource Manual for Guidelines for Exercise Testing and Prescription, 7th Edn.* Philadelphia, PA: Wolters Kluwer Health/Lippincott Williams & Wilkins.

Szulc, P., Beck, T. J., Marchand, F., and Delmas, P. D. (2005). Low skeletal muscle mass is associated with poor structural parameters of bone and impaired balance in elderly men–the MINOS study. *J. Bone Miner Res.* 20, 721–729. doi: 10.1359/JBMR.041230

Tinetti, M. E. (1987). Factors associated with serious injury during falls by ambulatory nursing home residents. *J. Am. Geriatr. Soc.* 35, 644–648.

Verney, J., Kadi, F., Charifi, N., Feasson, L., Saafi, M. A., Castells, J., et al. (2008). Effects of combined lower body endurance and upper body resistance training on the satellite cell pool in elderly subjects. *Muscle Nerve* 38, 1147–1154. doi: 10.1002/mus.21054

Warren, T. Y., Barry, V., Hooker, S. P., Sui, X., Church, T. S., and Blair, S. N. (2010). Sedentary behaviors increase risk of cardiovascular disease mortality in men. *Med. Sci. Sports Exerc.* 42, 879–885. doi: 10.1249/MSS.0b013e3181c3aa7e

Willis, B. C., and Borok, Z. (2007). TGF-beta-induced EMT: mechanisms and implications for fibrotic lung disease. *Am. J. Physiol. Lung Cell. Mol. Physiol.* 293, L525–L534. doi: 10.1152/ajplung.00163.2007

Xiao, N. M., Zhang, Y. M., Zheng, Q., and Gu, J. (2004). Klotho is a serum factor related to human aging. *Chin. Med. J.* 117, 742–747.

Yamamoto, M., Clark, J. D., Pastor, J. V., Gurnani, P., Nandi, A., Kurosu, H., et al. (2005). Regulation of oxidative stress by the anti-aging hormone klotho. *J. Biol. Chem.* 280, 38029–38034. doi: 10.1074/jbc.M509039200

Yamaza, T., Miura, Y., Akiyama, K., Bi, Y., Sonoyama, W., Gronthos, S., et al. (2009). Mesenchymal stem cell-mediated ectopic hematopoiesis alleviates aging-related phenotype in immunocompromised mice. *Blood* 113, 2595–2604. doi: 10.1182/blood-2008-10-182246

Zhang, H., Li, Y., Fan, Y., Wu, J., Zhao, B., Guan, Y., et al. (2008). Klotho is a target gene of PPAR-gamma. *Kidney Int.* 74, 732–739. doi: 10.1038/ki.2008.244

Zhou, L., Li, Y., Zhou, D., Tan, R. J., and Liu, Y. (2013). Loss of Klotho contributes to kidney injury by derepression of Wnt/beta-catenin signaling. *J. Am. Soc. Nephrol.* 24, 771–785. doi: 10.1681/ASN.2012080865

6

Skeletal muscle heat shock protein 70: Diverse functions and therapeutic potential for wasting disorders

Sarah M. Senf*

Department of Physical Therapy, University of Florida, Gainesville, FL, USA

Correspondence:
Sarah M. Senf, Department of Physical Therapy, University of Florida, 1225 Center Drive, HPNP Building Rm. 1142, Gainesville, FL 32610, USA
e-mail: smsenf@ufl.edu

The stress-inducible 70-kDa heat shock protein (HSP70) is a highly conserved protein with diverse intracellular and extracellular functions. In skeletal muscle, HSP70 is rapidly induced in response to both non-damaging and damaging stress stimuli including exercise and acute muscle injuries. This upregulation of HSP70 contributes to the maintenance of muscle fiber integrity and facilitates muscle regeneration and recovery. Conversely, HSP70 expression is decreased during muscle inactivity and aging, and evidence supports the loss of HSP70 as a key mechanism which may drive muscle atrophy, contractile dysfunction and reduced regenerative capacity associated with these conditions. To date, the therapeutic benefit of HSP70 upregulation in skeletal muscle has been established in rodent models of muscle injury, muscle atrophy, modified muscle use, aging, and muscular dystrophy, which highlights HSP70 as a key therapeutic target for the treatment of various conditions which negatively affect skeletal muscle mass and function. This article will review these important findings and provide perspective on the unanswered questions related to HSP70 and skeletal muscle plasticity which require further investigation.

Keywords: heat shock proteins, muscle atrophy, damage, regeneration, dystrophy, sarcopenia, inflammatory response, muscle dysfunction

INTRODUCTION

The 70 kDa heat shock protein (Hsp70/HSPA) family is one of the most evolutionary conserved protein families across both prokaryotic and eukaryotic organisms (Brocchieri et al., 2008). Due to their key roles as molecular chaperones, members of the Hsp70 family are most widely known for their involvement in promoting cellular proteostasis and survival throughout the lifespan and during periods of stress (Morimoto, 1991). However, this important family of proteins possesses several additional functions, including the regulation of various cell signaling pathways involved in cell growth and inflammation (Asea et al., 2000; Nollen and Morimoto, 2002).

In humans, there are at least 13 different genes that encode for distinct Hsp70 proteins, but which share a common domain structure, including *HSPA1A, HSPA1B, HSPA1L, HSPA2, HSPA4, HSPA4L, HSPA5, HSPA6, HSPA7, HSPA8, HSPA9, HSPA12A,* and *HSPA14* (Kampinga et al., 2009). The protein products encoded by these genes are localized to various subcellular compartments, and differ in their pattern of expression across various tissues. Among the most well studied Hsp70 family members are the constitutively expressed 70 kDa heat shock cognate protein (HSC70 or HSC73), encoded by the *HSPA8* gene, and the stress-inducible Hsp70 family members, encoded for by the *HSPA1A* and *HSPA1B* genes and whose protein products differ by only two amino acids. Due to inconsistencies in nomenclature, the proteins produced by these inducible genes are referred to by several different names. HSP70-1/HSP72/HSPA1/HSPA1A each refers to the protein product of *HSPA1A*, while HSP70-2/HSPA1B both refer to the protein product of *HSPA1B*. Moreover, due to the high homology of HSP70-1 and HSP70-2, and the belief that these are fully interchangeable proteins, these proteins are often collectively referred to as simply HSP70, or more commonly in the muscle literature, as HSP72.

In the last decade, the importance of HSP70 in skeletal muscle has gained significant attention, due to its induction in response to various physiological and pathophysiological stimuli, and its speculated role in the muscle adaptations to these stimuli. This article will therefore, review the studies which have provided key experimental evidence surrounding the biological functions of HSP70 in skeletal muscle. More specifically, this article will focus on the studies which have demonstrated its critical role in (1) protecting against muscle damage, (2) promoting muscle regeneration and recovery, and (3) maintaining skeletal muscle mass and integrity. In doing so, the potential of HSP70-targeted therapeutics for the treatment of both skeletal muscle injuries and muscle wasting disorders will be highlighted. Importantly, since the majority of these studies were performed in rodent models, the use of HSP70 in this article will be in reference to the inducible HSP70 proteins encoded by the rodent *Hspa1a* and *Hspa1b* genes.

HSP70 AND SKELETAL MUSCLE DAMAGE AND REGENERATION

HSP70 OVEREXPRESSION

The inducible HSP70 is increased in skeletal muscle following various perturbations such as exercise (Hernando and Manso, 1997; Milne and Noble, 2002; Morton et al., 2009) and muscle injury (Senf et al., 2013), and during the periods of muscle re-growth and regeneration associated with these conditions (Selsby et al., 2007; Senf et al., 2013). In contrast, HSP70 is decreased during prolonged periods of muscle inactivity (Lawler et al., 2006; Chen et al., 2007; Senf et al., 2008) when muscles undergo significant remodeling to reduce myofiber size to match the reduced force demands placed on the muscle. Due to these observations, HSP70 has long been considered to play an important role in regulating skeletal muscle plasticity.

The first definitive evidence that HSP70 regulates skeletal muscle plasticity was demonstrated through the use of muscle-specific Hsp70 transgenic (Tg) mice, and was published by McArdle et al. (2004). In this study, muscles from wild type (WT) mice and Hsp70 Tg mice were damaged through inducing lengthening muscle contractions, and the morphological and functional properties of these muscles subsequently compared. The authors found that 3 days following the lengthening contraction protocol, muscles from Hsp70 Tg mice showed less muscle fiber damage compared to WT, and reduced deficits in muscle specific force. At later time points Hsp70 Tg mice also showed earlier muscle functional recovery than WT. Thus, these findings demonstrate that upregulation of HSP70 is sufficient to protect against muscle damage and enhance muscle functional recovery. In a subsequent study, skeletal muscles from Hsp70 Tg mice were also found to have enhanced morphological recovery following muscle injury induced via cryolesioning (Miyabara et al., 2006). This study similarly linked their findings of enhanced recovery in muscles overexpressing HSP70 to reduced muscle damage in response to the injury stimulus. Markers of muscle satellite cell-activation were also measured in injured muscles, and found to be decreased in Hsp70 Tg mice compared to WT. This finding was not surprising since the extent of satellite cell-mediated repair should match the extent of muscle damage. In a more recent study, muscles from Hsp70 Tg mice also displayed enhanced recovery of fiber cross-sectional area (CSA) and function following a period of disuse muscle atrophy (Miyabara et al., 2012). Thus, these studies together provide considerable evidence that HSP70 upregulation is a feasible countermeasure to protect against muscle damage and enhance the recovery process.

A later study by Moresi et al. (2009) further demonstrated a more specific role of HSP70 in the augmentation of muscle fiber regeneration. In this study, HSP70 was overexpressed specifically in regenerating myofibers via electroporation of an *Hsp70* expression plasmid into muscles 3 days *following* cryolesioning injury. Due to the timing of Hsp70 overexpression in muscles *post-injury*, this therefore, bypassed and eliminated the potential for ectopic HSP70 to interfere with the early damage sequela. When the CSA of regenerating myofibers positive for HSP70 or a control vector were measured and compared in muscles 7 days *post-injury* (4 days following plasmid electroporation), regenerating myofibers positive for HSP70 were significantly larger. Thus, the data from this study provided clear evidence that enhancing HSP70 expression *post-injury* can enhance the muscle regenerative process. This is highly significant from a therapeutic standpoint, since preventative treatments to reduce muscle damage in the event of acute injury are often unrealistic. Thus, HSP70-targeted therapeutics to enhance muscle regeneration and recovery may be particularly relevant to sports-related skeletal muscle strains and contusions, traumatic muscle injures and even spinal cord injury (SCI), since markers of regeneration were recently shown to be elevated in rat skeletal muscle following moderate spinal cord contusion (Jayaraman et al., 2013).

HSP70 KNOCKOUT

Collectively the studies discussed thus, far have provided key experimental evidence that Hsp70 upregulation protects against muscle damage and enhances the recovery process. However, until just recently, it was not clear whether HSP70 is necessary for the regenerative process, and whether a reduction in HSP70 alone is sufficient to enhance muscle damage and interfere with the regenerative process. This question is important in that skeletal muscle expression of HSP70, and the ability to induce its expression, is diminished with age concomitantly with the age-related decline in muscle regenerative capacity and rate of recovery following muscle damage (Vasilaki et al., 2002; McArdle et al., 2004). The study by McArdle et al. (2004) provided important evidence that these two events may be linked, since both adult and aged mice overexpressing HSP70 showed protection against muscle damage and enhanced functional recovery. However, loss of function studies using gene knockdown are also important in confirming this link, through establishing the biological *requirement* of HSP70 for these skeletal muscle processes. Therefore, my colleagues and I recently conducted experiments using mice which lack the inducible HSP70 coded for by *Hspa1a* and *Hspa1b* (*Hsp70*$^{-/-}$ mice). In these experiments muscles from WT and *Hsp70*$^{-/-}$ mice were injured via direct injection with cardiotoxin, which induces widespread muscle fiber necrosis, and is thus, a standardized and reproducible method to study the regenerative process. At various time points following the injury stimulus the extent of muscle inflammation, necrosis, and regeneration were subsequently compared. We found that injured muscles from *Hsp70*$^{-/-}$ mice had a significantly delayed inflammatory response to muscle injury which was followed at later time points by sustained inflammation and muscle fiber necrosis, fibrosis, and reduced CSA of regenerating myofibers (Senf et al., 2013). In addition, injured muscles lacking HSP70 also developed widespread calcifications during the recovery process. These findings therefore, provide strong evidence that HSP70 is necessary for successful muscle regeneration and recovery, and further link the age-related impairments in these critical skeletal muscle processes to deficits in HSP70.

The mechanisms whereby HSP70 regulates muscle regeneration and recovery following injury are still being elucidated. However, in our recent report we uncovered some important mechanistic details. Based on rescue experiments introducing an *Hsp70* plasmid into muscles of *Hsp70*$^{-/-}$ mice either 4 days prior to injury or 4 days post injury, we establish that HSP70 plays an especially critical role within the first 4 days following injury to support the recovery process (Senf et al., 2013). The first several days following muscle injury are dominated by a highly coordinated inflammatory response involving the recruitment of various immune cell populations including neutrophils and macrophages which support muscle regeneration and repair (Tidball and Villalta, 2010). Infiltration of these immune cell populations contribute to muscle healing in various capacities, and their failure to infiltrate in a timely manner can certainly impede the recovery process. One important role is their involvement in the removal of necrotic cellular debris through phagocytosis, which allows viable muscle cells to successfully repopulate damaged areas. Since injured muscles from *Hsp70*$^{-/-}$ mice displayed a significantly impaired ability to recruit these important phagocytic immune cells in a timely manner, we hypothesize that this may have contributed to the persisting muscle inflammation and fiber necrosis seen in these mice at later time points. This notion is supported by the rescue experiments in which reintroduction of HSP70 into muscles of *Hsp70*$^{-/-}$ mice *prior to* cardiotoxin injury (but not post injury) prevented these deficits in muscle recovery.

So exactly how does HSP70 expressed by skeletal muscle fibers contribute to immune cell infiltration in response to injury? One possibility is through the immunostimulatory functions of HSP70 when localized to the extracellular environment. Studies on tissue injury of the heart, liver and skin have in fact demonstrated that HSP70 is released into the extracellular environment following tissue injury and facilitates the activation of pro-inflammatory processes and the recruitment of immune cells to the injury site (Dybdahl et al., 2002, 2005; Kimura et al., 2004; Kovalchin et al., 2006). Thus, a similar mechanism involving extracellular HSP70 may be involved in the inflammatory response to muscle injury. While this concept has previously been suggested by others (Lightfoot et al., 2009; Han et al., 2010), data generated in our recent study were the first to support this notion. In these experiments, recombinant HSP70 protein was directly injected into muscles of *Hsp70*$^{-/-}$ mice at the time of injury to simulate HSP70 release into the extracellular microenvironment. Using this method, we were able to completely restore early immune cell infiltration into injured muscles of *Hsp70*$^{-/-}$ mice, thus, providing a novel link between the inflammatory response to muscle injury and the extracellular functions of HSP70 (Senf et al., 2013). However, our understanding of HSP70 and its involvement in the inflammatory response to muscle injury is still in its infancy. Thus, additional studies are needed to elucidate the precise roles of HSP70 in the initiation of inflammatory processes in damaged muscle, and how this modulates the regenerative process.

As mentioned previously, the CSA of regenerating myofibers in muscles from *Hsp70*$^{-/-}$ mice were significantly smaller than WT (Senf et al., 2013). This indicates that HSP70 is necessary for the normal muscle fiber regeneration, and complements the previous findings of Moresi et al. (2009) which demonstrated that HSP70 overexpression enhances the CSA of regenerating myofibers. Although the mechanisms whereby HSP70 is necessary for myofiber regeneration are currently unclear, markers of satellite cell activation and proliferation in injured muscles from *Hsp70*$^{-/-}$ mice were not significantly compromised. Therefore, HSP70 may be dispensable for these early stages of the myogenic program. In contrast, HSP70 could regulate later stages of the myogenic program which support differentiation and the formation of multinucleated myofibers. This notion is supported by experiments from two separate studies in which introduction of an *Hsp70* plasmid into muscles 3 or 4 days following injury enhanced the CSA and nucleation of regenerating myofibers (Moresi et al., 2009; Senf et al., 2013). However, as mentioned previously, additional studies detailing the effect of HSP70 overexpression and knockdown on each stage of the myogenic program are needed to better understand the role of HSP70 in these important cellular processes. Preferably, these experiments would be performed in both skeletal muscle cells *in vitro* and whole muscle, *in vivo*, to differentiate between the muscle cell autonomous and non-autonomous mechanisms whereby HSP70 regulates the muscle regenerative process following injury.

HSP70 AND MUSCLE WASTING AND DYSFUNCTION

In addition to the roles of HSP70 in facilitating muscle regeneration and recovery following injury, HSP70 also plays an important role in regulating muscle fiber size under baseline conditions and during conditions of muscle atrophy. Indeed, HSP70 is decreased in both adult and aged rats during periods of muscle disuse, and plasmid-mediated restoration of HSP70 expression in muscles during the disuse period significantly inhibits the associated fiber atrophy (Senf et al., 2008; Dodd et al., 2009). These findings were linked to HSP70 negatively regulating the Forkhead BoxO (FoxO) and Nuclear Factor κB (NF-κB) pathways, which are activated during multiple conditions of muscle atrophy and which drive the atrophy phenotype (Cai et al., 2004; Hunter and Kandarian, 2004; Sandri et al., 2004; Judge et al., 2007; Senf et al., 2010; Reed et al., 2012). Thus, reductions in HSP70 during conditions of atrophy may contribute to the atrophy phenotype through weakening the inhibition of these signaling pathways. Evidence that HSP70 is necessary for the maintenance of muscle fiber size and functional integrity is demonstrated by the muscle phenotype of adult *Hsp70*$^{-/-}$ mice, in which muscle fiber CSA and muscle specific force is reduced when compared to controls (Senf et al., 2013). This is further supported by evidence that the age-related decline in muscle specific force is prevented in muscles of aged mice overexpressing HSP70 throughout the lifespan (McArdle et al., 2004). This regulation of skeletal muscle functional integrity by HSP70 may be related to the finding that muscles from Hsp70 Tg mice also displayed enhanced antioxidant capacity (Broome et al., 2006), since oxidative stress may contribute to muscle dysfunction during the aging process. In addition, and perhaps related to this, HSP70 also appears to contribute to the maintenance of skeletal muscle quality during normal physiological conditions, since muscles from *Hsp70*$^{-/-}$ mice also had significant increases in the amount of extracellular tissue (non-muscle fiber tissue) surrounding the already smaller muscle fibers. The mechanisms responsible for the reduced fiber CSA in mice lacking HSP70 throughout the lifespan are not known. However, since induction of intracellular HSP70 represses pathways involved in muscle atrophy and inflammation in skeletal muscle (Chung et al., 2008; Senf et al., 2008), the lack of HSP70 may contribute to increases in these signaling pathways under baseline conditions. Alternatively, deficits in post-natal muscle growth in mice could play a role in this finding, since *Hsp70*$^{-/-}$ mice had

Table 1 | List of studies which have directly manipulated Hsp70 expression to investigate the functions of Hsp70 in regulating skeletal muscle plasticity.

	Condition/model	Skeletal muscle phenotype	References
Hsp70 OVEREXPRESSION			
Hsp70 transgenic mice	10–12 months adult mice	Decreased body and muscle mass	McArdle et al., 2004
	Aging	Preservation of muscle specific force	McArdle et al., 2004
	Muscle damage/eccentric contractions	Decreased muscle damage, improved muscle functional recovery (adult and old mice)	McArdle et al., 2004
	Muscle damage/cryolesioning	Decreased muscle damage, improved morphological recovery	Miyabara et al., 2006
	Modified muscle use/cast-immobilization and recovery	Improved muscle structural and functional recovery	Miyabara et al., 2012
	Muscular dystrophy/crossed with *mdx* mice	Improved muscle morphology and function	Gehrig et al., 2012
Hsp70 plasmid electroporation	Muscle atrophy/cast-immobilization	Attenuation of disuse muscle fiber atrophy (adult and old rats)	Senf et al., 2008; Dodd et al., 2009
	Muscle damage/freeze injury	Increased CSA of regenerating muscle fibers	Moresi et al., 2009
Hsp70 KNOCKDOWN			
Hsp70 knockout mice	12–15 weeks adult mice	Decreased muscle fiber CSA, decreased muscle specific force	Senf et al., 2013
	Muscle damage/direct cardiotoxin injection	Delayed inflammatory response to injury, impaired muscle regeneration and recovery (smaller CSA of regenerating fibers, sustained inflammation, fibrosis and calcium deposition)	Senf et al., 2013
	Modified muscle use/cast-immobilization and recovery	Decreased muscle reloading damage, decreased size of regenerating fibers	Senf et al., 2013

deficits in the growth of regenerating myofibers, and both processes rely upon related cellular mechanisms to support fiber growth. Clearly, numerous unanswered questions still remain surrounding the mechanisms in which HSP70 regulates muscle fiber size and function. Nonetheless, these collective studies confirm that HSP70 is necessary for the maintenance of muscle fiber size and functional integrity, and highlight HSP70 upregulation as a key therapeutic strategy that may be beneficial during various skeletal muscle wasting disorders to maintain muscle mass and function.

One highly significant study surrounding the use of HSP70-targeted therapeutics for genetic muscle wasting disorders was recently published by Gehrig et al. (2012). In this study, the authors demonstrate that upregulation of the inducible HSP70 in mouse skeletal muscle (through either genetic or pharmacological means) ameliorates the dystrophic phenotype. This finding was demonstrated in two models of muscular dystrophy related to the absence of dystrophin, including the mdx model and the more severe dko model in which utrophin is also absent. Importantly, treatment of dystrophic mice with BGP-15, a pharmacological co-inducer of HSP70 that is currently being used in clinical trials, improved the dystrophic pathology of both limb and diaphragm muscles and extended lifespan. Thus, BGP-15 and other pharmacological inducers of HSP70 may be key therapeutic agents for muscular dystrophies. The mechanism whereby HSP70 improved the dystrophy phenotype in this study was linked to its regulation of the sarcoplasmic/endoplasmic reticulum Ca(2+)-ATPase (SERCA) protein, whose activity is compromised in severely dystrophic muscle. The activity of SERCA is critical in removing intracellular calcium, and HSP70 was found to interact with and enhance SERCA activity. Since increased intracellular calcium is a key activator of inflammatory and muscle degenerative pathways, maintenance of SERCA activity was proposed to be a key mechanism for the amelioration of the dystrophic phenotype in muscles overexpressing HSP70. However, since HSP70 also negatively regulates muscle atrophy pathways, enhances regenerative processes and promotes a timely and controlled inflammatory response to muscle damage, the beneficial effects of HSP70 upregulation on the dystrophic pathology could also be related to these additional skeletal muscle functions of HSP70. Regardless of the mechanism, the findings from this study clearly indicate that HSP70-targeted therapeutics have significant potential for the treatment of dystrophic muscle pathologies.

CONCLUSION

In summary, the inducible HSP70 is a critical skeletal muscle protein that positively regulates muscle size and function during health and disease. The studies which directly support this notion are summarized in **Table 1**. While several questions still remain surrounding the mechanisms responsible for this regulation, it is clear that therapeutics targeting HSP70 upregulation have strong potential for success in the treatment of both acquired and genetic muscle wasting disorders and in the treatment of muscle injuries. However, future studies should continue to delineate the cellular mechanisms whereby HSP70 regulates skeletal muscle plasticity. These studies are important not only from a mechanistic standpoint, but from a therapeutic standpoint, since the timing of HSP70 induction, route of administration, and duration of treatment to optimally enhance therapeutic benefits may be revealed from knowledge gained through these studies.

REFERENCES

Asea, A., Kraeft, S. K., Kurt-Jones, E. A., Stevenson, M. A., Chen, L. B., Finberg, R. W., et al. (2000). HSP70 stimulates cytokine production through a CD14-dependant pathway, demonstrating its dual role as a chaperone and cytokine. *Nat. Med.* 6, 435–442. doi: 10.1038/74697

Brocchieri, L., Conway de Macario, E., and Macario, A. J. (2008). hsp70 genes in the human genome: conservation and differentiation patterns predict a wide array of overlapping and specialized functions. *BMC Evol. Biol.* 8:19. doi: 10.1186/1471-2148-8-19

Broome, C. S., Kayani, A. C., Palomero, J., Dillmann, W. H., Mestril, R., Jackson, M. J., et al. (2006). Effect of lifelong overexpression of HSP70 in skeletal muscle on age-related oxidative stress and adaptation after non-damaging contractile activity. *FASEB J.* 20, 1549–1551. doi: 10.1096/fj.05-4935fje

Cai, D., Frantz, J. D., Tawa, N. E. Jr., Melendez, P. A., Oh, B. C., Lidov, H. G., et al. (2004). IKKbeta/NF-kappaB activation causes severe muscle wasting in mice. *Cell* 119, 285–298. doi: 10.1016/j.cell.2004.09.027

Chen, Y. W., Gregory, C. M., Scarborough, M. T., Shi, R., Walter, G. A., and Vandenborne, K. (2007). Transcriptional pathways associated with skeletal muscle disuse atrophy in humans. *Physiol. Genomics* 31, 510–520. doi: 10.1152/physiolgenomics.00115.2006

Chung, J., Nguyen, A. K., Henstridge, D. C., Holmes, A. G., Chan, M. H., Mesa, J. L., et al. (2008). HSP72 protects against obesity-induced insulin resistance. *Proc. Natl. Acad. Sci. U.S.A.* 105, 1739–1744. doi: 10.1073/pnas.0705799105

Dodd, S., Hain, B., and Judge, A. (2009). Hsp70 prevents disuse muscle atrophy in senescent rats. *Biogerontology* 10, 605–611. doi: 10.1007/s10522-008-9203-1

Dybdahl, B., Slordahl, S. A., Waage, A., Kierulf, P., Espevik, T., and Sundan, A. (2005). Myocardial ischaemia and the inflammatory response: release of heat shock protein 70 after myocardial infarction. *Heart* 91, 299–304. doi: 10.1136/hrt.2003.028092

Dybdahl, B., Wahba, A., Lien, E., Flo, T. H., Waage, A., Qureshi, N., et al. (2002). Inflammatory response after open heart surgery: release of heat-shock protein 70 and signaling through toll-like receptor-4. *Circulation* 105, 685–690. doi: 10.1161/hc0602.103617

Gehrig, S. M., Van der Poel, C., Sayer, T. A., Schertzer, J. D., Henstridge, D. C., Church, J. E., et al. (2012). Hsp72 preserves muscle function and slows progression of severe muscular dystrophy. *Nature* 484, 394–398. doi: 10.1038/nature10980

Han, R., Frett, E. M., Levy, J. R., Rader, E. P., Lueck, J. D., Bansal, D., et al. (2010). Genetic ablation of complement C3 attenuates muscle pathology in dysferlin-deficient mice. *J. Clin. Invest.* 120, 4366–4374. doi: 10.1172/JCI42390

Hernando, R., and Manso, R. (1997). Muscle fibre stress in response to exercise: synthesis, accumulation and isoform transitions of 70-kDa heat-shock proteins. *Eur. J. Biochem.* 243, 460–467. doi: 10.1111/j.1432-1033.1997.0460a.x

Hunter, R. B., and Kandarian, S. C. (2004). Disruption of either the Nfkb1 or the Bcl3 gene inhibits skeletal muscle atrophy. *J. Clin. Invest.* 114, 1504–1511. doi: 10.1172/JCI200421696

Jayaraman, A., Liu, M., Ye, F., Walter, G. A., and Vandenborne, K. (2013). Regenerative responses in slow- and fast-twitch muscles following moderate contusion spinal cord injury and locomotor training. *Eur. J. Appl. Physiol.* 113, 191–200. doi: 10.1007/s00421-012-2429-2

Judge, A. R., Koncarevic, A., Hunter, R. B., Liou, H. C., Jackman, R. W., and Kandarian, S. C. (2007). Role for IkappaBalpha, but not c-Rel, in skeletal muscle atrophy. *Am. J. Physiol. Cell Physiol.* 292, C372–C382. doi: 10.1152/ajpcell.00293.2006

Kampinga, H. H., Hageman, J., Vos, M. J., Kubota, H., Tanguay, R. M., Bruford, E. A., et al. (2009). Guidelines for the nomenclature of the human heat shock proteins. *Cell Stress Chaperones* 14, 105–111. doi: 10.1007/s12192-008-0068-7

Kimura, F., Itoh, H., Ambiru, S., Shimizu, H., Togawa, A., Yoshidome, H., et al. (2004). Circulating heat-shock protein 70 is associated with postoperative infection and organ dysfunction after liver resection. *Am. J. Surg.* 187, 777–784. doi: 10.1016/j.amjsurg.2003.08.029

Kovalchin, J. T., Wang, R., Wagh, M. S., Azoulay, J., Sanders, M., and Chandawarkar, R. Y. (2006). *In vivo* delivery of heat shock protein 70 accelerates wound healing by up-regulating macrophage-mediated phagocytosis. *Wound Repair Regen.* 14, 129–137. doi: 10.1111/j.1743-6109.2006.00102.x

Lawler, J. M., Song, W., and Kwak, H. B. (2006). Differential response of heat shock proteins to hindlimb unloading and reloading in the soleus. *Muscle Nerve* 33, 200–207. doi: 10.1002/mus.20454

Lightfoot, A., McArdle, A., and Griffiths, R. D. (2009). Muscle in defense. *Crit. Care Med.* 37, S384–S390. doi: 10.1097/CCM.0b013e3181b6f8a5

McArdle, A., Dillmann, W. H., Mestril, R., Faulkner, J. A., and Jackson, M. J. (2004). Overexpression of HSP70 in mouse skeletal muscle protects against muscle damage and age-related muscle dysfunction. *FASEB J.* 18, 355–357. doi: 10.1096/fj.03-0395fje

Milne, K. J., and Noble, E. G. (2002). Exercise-induced elevation of HSP70 is intensity dependent. *J. Appl. Physiol.* 93, 561–568. doi: 10.1152/japplphysiol.00528.2001

Miyabara, E. H., Martin, J. L., Griffin, T. M., Moriscot, A. S., and Mestril, R. (2006). Overexpression of inducible 70-kDa heat shock protein in mouse attenuates skeletal muscle damage induced by cryolesioning. *Am. J. Physiol. Cell Physiol.* 290, C1128–C1138. doi: 10.1152/ajpcell.00399.2005

Miyabara, E. H., Nascimento, T. L., Rodrigues, D. C., Moriscot, A. S., Davila, W. F., Aitmou, Y., et al. (2012). Overexpression of inducible 70-kDa heat shock protein in mouse improves structural and functional recovery of skeletal muscles from atrophy. *Pflugers Arch.* 463, 733–741. doi: 10.1007/s00424-012-1087-x

Moresi, V., Garcia-Alvarez, G., Pristera, A., Rizzuto, E., Albertini, M. C., Rocchi, M., et al. (2009). Modulation of caspase activity regulates skeletal muscle regeneration and function in response to vasopressin and tumor necrosis factor. *PLoS ONE* 4:e5570. doi: 10.1371/journal.pone.0005570

Morimoto, R. I. (1991). Heat shock: the role of transient inducible responses in cell damage, transformation, and differentiation. *Cancer Cells* 3, 295–301.

Morton, J. P., Kayani, A. C., McArdle, A., and Drust, B. (2009). The exercise-induced stress response of skeletal muscle, with specific emphasis on humans. *Sports Med.* 39, 643–662. doi: 10.2165/00007256-200939080-00003

Nollen, E. A., and Morimoto, R. I. (2002). Chaperoning signaling pathways: molecular chaperones as stress-sensing heat shock proteins. *J. Cell Sci.* 115, 2809–2816.

Reed, S. A., Sandesara, P. B., Senf, S. M., and Judge, A. R. (2012). Inhibition of FoxO transcriptional activity prevents muscle fiber atrophy during cachexia and induces hypertrophy. *FASEB J.* 26, 987–1000. doi: 10.1096/fj.11-189977

Sandri, M., Sandri, C., Gilbert, A., Skurk, C., Calabria, E., Picard, A., et al. (2004). Foxo transcription factors induce the atrophy-related ubiquitin ligase atrogin-1 and cause skeletal muscle atrophy. *Cell* 117, 399–412. doi: 10.1016/S0092-8674(04)00400-3

Selsby, J. T., Rother, S., Tsuda, S., Pracash, O., Quindry, J., and Dodd, S. L. (2007). Intermittent hyperthermia enhances skeletal muscle regrowth and attenuates oxidative damage following reloading. *J. Appl. Physiol.* 102, 1702–1707. doi: 10.1152/japplphysiol.00722.2006

Senf, S. M., Dodd, S. L., and Judge, A. R. (2010). FOXO signaling is required for disuse muscle atrophy and is directly regulated by Hsp70. *Am. J. Physiol. Cell Physiol.* 298, C38–C45. doi: 10.1152/ajpcell.00315.2009

Senf, S. M., Dodd, S. L., McClung, J. M., and Judge, A. R. (2008). Hsp70 overexpression inhibits NF-kappaB and Foxo3a transcriptional activities and prevents skeletal muscle atrophy. *FASEB J.* 22, 3836–3845. doi: 10.1096/fj.08-110163

Senf, S. M., Howard, T. M., Ahn, B., Ferreira, L. F., and Judge, A. R. (2013). Loss of the inducible Hsp70 delays the inflammatory response to skeletal muscle injury and severely impairs muscle regeneration. *PLoS ONE* 8:e62687. doi: 10.1371/journal.pone.0062687

Tidball, J. G., and Villalta, S. A. (2010). Regulatory interactions between muscle and the immune system during muscle regeneration. *Am. J. Physiol. Regul. Integr. Comp. Physiol.* 298, R1173–R1187. doi: 10.1152/ajpregu.00735.2009

7

Emerging gene editing strategies for Duchenne muscular dystrophy targeting stem cells

Carmen Bertoni*

Department of Neurology, David Geffen School of Medicine, University of California Los Angeles, CA, USA

****Correspondence:***
Carmen Bertoni, Department of Neurology, University of California Los Angeles, 710 Westwood Plaza, 4145 RNRC, Los Angeles, CA 90095, USA
e-mail: cbertoni@ucla.edu

The progressive loss of muscle mass characteristic of many muscular dystrophies impairs the efficacy of most of the gene and molecular therapies currently being pursued for the treatment of those disorders. It is becoming increasingly evident that a therapeutic application, to be effective, needs to target not only mature myofibers, but also muscle progenitors cells or muscle stem cells able to form new muscle tissue and to restore myofibers lost as the result of the diseases or during normal homeostasis so as to guarantee effective and lost lasting effects. Correction of the genetic defect using oligodeoxynucleotides (ODNs) or engineered nucleases holds great potential for the treatment of many of the musculoskeletal disorders. The encouraging results obtained by studying *in vitro* systems and model organisms have set the groundwork for what is likely to become an emerging field in the area of molecular and regenerative medicine. Furthermore, the ability to isolate and expand from patients various types of muscle progenitor cells capable of committing to the myogenic lineage provides the opportunity to establish cell lines that can be used for transplantation following *ex vivo* manipulation and expansion. The purpose of this article is to provide a perspective on approaches aimed at correcting the genetic defect using gene editing strategies and currently under development for the treatment of Duchenne muscular dystrophy (DMD), the most sever of the neuromuscular disorders. Emphasis will be placed on describing the potential of using the patient own stem cell as source of transplantation and the challenges that gene editing technologies face in the field of regenerative biology.

Keywords: muscle stem cell, satellite cells, DMD, *mdx*, gene repair, gene correction, ssODN, dystrophin

INTRODUCTION

The discovery of dystrophin as the gene responsible for Duchenne muscular Dystrophy (DMD) has enabled researchers to identify several of the genes linked directly or indirectly to dystrophin and to correlate defects in those genes to many of the different forms of muscular dystrophies (Monaco et al., 1986; Hoffman et al., 1987; Koenig et al., 1987). Despite the diversity in phenotypic and pathological manifestation of various forms of muscular dystrophies identified to date, many display common symptoms. Characteristic is the progressive loss of muscle mass which has been attributed, at least in part, to the inability of muscle stem cells to efficiently regenerate tissue lost as the result of the disease. Great progress has been made toward the identification of therapies for DMD. Potential approaches range from gene augmentation strategies using viral or plasmid vectors aimed at restoring dystrophin expression to upregulation of genes that could be used to overcome the lack of expression of the defected gene. While some of these approaches have sown efficacy, the results obtained to date have also expounded limitations in the clinical applicability of therapeutic applications to DMD. In particular, the progressive loss of expression of the therapeutic gene observed following treatment have clearly indicated that targeting mature myofibers alone is not sufficient to preserve the beneficial effects achieved by the therapeutic approach (Bertoni et al., 2006; Kayali et al., 2010). Critical to the development of effective strategies to treat muscle disorders is the optimization of approaches targeting muscle stem cells and capable of regenerating tissue lost as the result of the disease or as the result of normal muscle turnover.

Muscle stem cells are classically defined as undifferentiated cells characterized by their unique ability to activate in response to specific stimuli and self-renew. Daughter cells originated by the division of stem cells can either retain their stem cell identity or differentiate into a more committed lineage capable of producing new muscle tissue or of fusing with preexisting myofibers to repair damage ones. Among the different types and subtypes of muscle stem cells identified to date, satellite cells (SCs) are probably the most studied. Since their initial identification (Mauro, 1961) studies have clearly demonstrated that SCs are composed by an heterogeneous population of muscle stem cells distinguishable based on their gene expression signatures, their ability to commit into a specific myogenic lineage, their capacity to assume non-myogenic cell-fate and differences in their ability to activate in response to specific queues (Schultz, 1996; Seale et al., 2000; Ono et al., 2010; Bentzinger et al., 2012; Brack and Rando, 2012; Yin et al., 2013). Other types of stem cells capable of assuming a myogenic cell fate and of regenerating muscles have been described. Those include bone marrow stem cells

(Ferrari et al., 1998; Bittner et al., 1999; Gussoni et al., 1999), muscle side population (SP) cells (Gussoni et al., 1999; Asakura et al., 2002; Rivier et al., 2004; Doyle et al., 2011), muscle-derived stem cells (Lee et al., 2000), mesangioblasts (Minasi et al., 2002; Sampaolesi et al., 2003; Galli et al., 2005; Morosetti et al., 2006), pericytes (Dellavalle et al., 2007; Peault et al., 2007), embryonic stem cells (ESCs) (Bhagavati and Xu, 2004; Barberi et al., 2007; Darabi et al., 2009; Filareto et al., 2012) and induced pluripotent stem cells (iPSCs) (Chang et al., 2009; Kazuki et al., 2010; Darabi et al., 2012; Tedesco et al., 2012).

Therapeutic approaches to muscle disorders and targeting stem cells have focused primarily on demonstrating the feasibility of restoring dystrophin expression following transplantation of cells isolated from healthy donors. Proof-of-concept studies have been performed in immunosuppressed *mdx* mice that have been used as models for DMD (Coulton et al., 1988; Sicinski et al., 1989). Some success has been achieved using transplantation of freshly isolated SCs (Collins et al., 2005; Boldrin et al., 2009, 2012) or subpopulations of SCs isolated using fluorescence activate cell sorting (FACS) which have been used primarily to demonstrate the existence of distinguished populations of SCs with regenerative capacity and capable of self-renewing (Cerletti et al., 2008; Sacco et al., 2008; Rocheteau et al., 2012).

Despite the encouraging results obtained to date in the field, issues still remain that may hamper the applicability of cell-mediated regenerative approaches to muscle disorders. Among those, is the need to use heterologous sources for the transplantation procedure and the risk of immune rejection associated with their use. The issue of immune response could be overcome by the use of reprogrammable stem cells capable of differentiate into muscle progenitor cells such as human ESCs human iPSCs (Darabi et al., 2012) or mesoangioblasts (Tedesco et al., 2012) isolated directly from the patient and that have been genetically modified to express dystrophin or other therapeutically relevant genes. Among the technologies currently being investigated for the treatment of DMD, gene editing is perhaps the most exciting as it offers the possibility to correct a genetic defect at the source of the problem, the DNA and can therefore promise to restore a completely functional protein. Critical to the success of gene editing strategies for muscle disorders is to target cells capable of retaining the stem cells properties to ensure that the beneficial effects achieved by the gene correction process is maintained over time. As such, the use of muscle stem cells capable of self-renewing is likely to have advantages over other type of cells, namely due to their ability to actively participate to the regenerative process over prolonged periods of time with virtually little or no loss of regenerative potential.

The use of gene editing in muscle stem cells for therapeutic purposes can be divided into two major applications: strategies aimed at targeting muscle stem cells *ex vivo* that can be used for transplantation purposes and strategies aimed at targeting and correcting stem cells *in situ* following systemic administration of the therapeutic agent into the patient's own stem cells, mainly SCs (**Figure 1**). Both approaches present pros and cons as discussed in more detail below (see Drawbacks and limitations of gene editing mediated by ODNs and endonucleases). Among the hurdles that will need to be overcome before cell-mediated therapies can be brought into the clinic is the need to target a large number of muscles for the therapy to be clinically relevant. Nonetheless, the use of gene editing strategies in muscle stem cells is likely to become a valid therapeutic alternative to gene augmentation therapies. This review will provide an overview of the progress made in the past decade toward the development of gene editing tools for the treatment of DMD and the current state-of-the art of technologies aimed at permanently correct the genetic defect in muscle progenitor cells and stem cells.

OLIGONUCLEOTIDE-MEDIATED GENE CORRECTION

Different areas of investigations have focused on the possibility of using oligodeoxynucleotides (ODNs) as therapeutic vectors. First among those, the success obtained using homologous recombination (HR) technologies, an approach that has been employed extensively to generate animal models to study disease mechanisms (Capecchi, 1989). However, the low frequency of HR and the high frequency of non-homologous integration of such constructs have clearly evidenced serious limitations in the applicability of this approach for the treatment of inherited diseases and have prompted the development of new, safer vectors capable of activating repair mechanisms other than HR and capable of introducing single base pair (bp) alterations at the genomic DNA without the need of integrating into the genome. Gene editing mediated by ODNs generally employs short (less than 100 nucleotides) synthetic DNA or RNA sequences homologous to the region of the genomic DNA targeted for repair. The technology differ substantially from that employing antisense oligonucleotides (AONs), that also uses oligonucleotides, but that act at the messenger RNA (mRNA) level to block and therefore redirect splicing of the mRNA to produce shorter although still functional proteins (Arechavala-Gomeza et al., 2012). Gene editing mediated by ODNs takes advantage of innate repair mechanisms present in the cell and responsible for maintenance of chromosome integrity. The process requires multiple steps which begin with the pairing of the ODN with the region of the genomic DNA targeted for repair, recognition of the mismatch on the targeted base, excision of the mutation, and insertion of the desired base (**Figure 2**).

EVOLUTION OF ODNs FOR GENE EDITING PURPOSES

The initial vectors employed for gene editing strategies consisted of chimeric DNA/RNA ODNs (chODNs) made of 68 residues which were originally given the name of chimeraplasts. The vector contained both RNA and DNA residues complementary to the region of the genomic DNA targeted for repair and flanked by 2′-O-methylated RNA residues which were used to increase resistance to RNase H activity (**Figure 2A**). To increase stability and maintain their secondary structure, ODNs were designed to contain at their 3′ and 5′ ends polythymidine hairpins and a 3′ tag containing a clamp made of guanidine and cytosine residues (**Figure 2A**) (Cole-Strauss et al., 1996; Kren et al., 1999a,b; Bertoni, 2008). These chODNs were designed to pair with both strands of the gene targeted for repair and to activate DNA mismatch repair (MMR) mechanisms though the recognition of the single base mismatch present on the ODN (**Figure 2B**). The activation results in the conversion of the targeted base at the genomic level using the information provided by the chODN. Since their

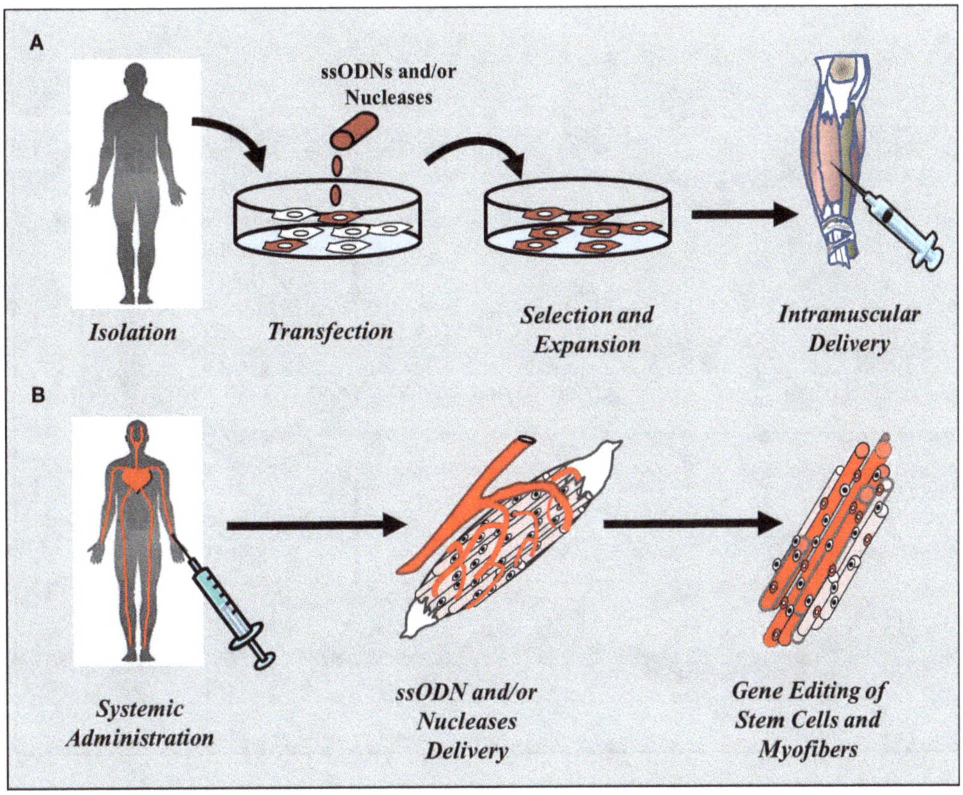

FIGURE 1 | Cell-mediated regenerative approaches to muscle disorders. Gene editing strategies in muscle stem cells are aimed at either correcting the genetic disorder *ex vivo* or at delivery the therapeutic agent *in situ* following systemic administration. **(A)** *Ex vivo* approaches requires harvesting of cells from the patient or healthy donor, reprogramming in cases were the cells being employed are not muscle-derived, editing using the targeting tools, selection of the cells undergone repair and expansion prior to delivery into muscle through local, or systemic administration. **(B)** Delivery of the gene editing tools into muscle typically uses the circulatory system and can employ intraperitoneal, subcutaneous, intra-arterial, or intravenous administration depending on the physico-chemical, and pharmacological properties of the therapeutic agent being employed. The method is much less invasive than direct intramuscular injection and has the potential of targeting a large number of muscles simultaneously.

first application, chODNs have been investigated in their ability to target and induce genomic modifications in a number of different cell types and have been successfully applied in both eukaryotic and prokaryotic cells (Cole-Strauss et al., 1996, 1999; Kren et al., 1998, 1999b; Beetham et al., 1999; Zhu et al., 1999, 2000; Bartlett et al., 2000; Rando et al., 2000; Rice et al., 2000, 2001; Tagalakis et al., 2001; Igoucheva and Yoon, 2002).

The initial studies exploring the feasibility of using chODNs for the treatment of muscular dystrophies were performed in the *mdx* mouse model for DMD (Rando et al., 2000; Bertoni and Rando, 2002; Bertoni et al., 2003). A chODN designed to target and correct the single point mutation present in exon 23 of the dystrophin gene was shown to restore dystrophin expression in both muscle precursor cells in culture (Bertoni and Rando, 2002) as well as *in vivo* following direct intramuscular injection (Rando et al., 2000). Importantly, correction was demonstrated to be stably inherited in dividing cells and to result in restoration of full-length dystrophin expression. When administered intramuscularly at high doses, the chODN was able to distribute into approximately 40% of the SCs present in the muscle (Bertoni and Rando, 2002). Once explanted, SCs that had taken up the chODN targeting the *mdx* mutation, were shown to proliferate and expand *in vitro* to produce myoblasts capable of differentiating and to form myotubes which expressed full-length dystrophin. The level of gene repair detected in those cells remained substantially lower than that achieved in muscle progenitor cells transfected with the targeting chODN in culture demonstrating the presence of intrinsic differences in the ability of SCs to undergo gene repair compared to myoblasts (Bertoni and Rando, 2002). Nonetheless, the results clearly indicated the feasibility of using ODNs to target and correct SCs and demonstrated for the first time the possibility of targeting SCs *in situ* following delivery of ODNs. Studies in the GRMD have confirmed the feasibility of using chODNs to correct defects in the dystrophin gene in larger animals (Bartlett et al., 2000).

A key advancement in vector development was the discovery that ODNs made of single stranded DNA sequences (ssODNs) were as efficient as chODNs in directing the gene correction process (Gamper et al., 2000a,b) rendering this technology widely available to virtually any laboratory interested in exploring its potential application in different prokaryotic and eukaryotic systems and for different applications (Igoucheva et al., 2001, 2008; Dekker et al., 2003, 2006; Nickerson and Colledge, 2003; Pierce et al., 2003; Radecke et al., 2004; Bertoni et al., 2005; Olsen et al.,

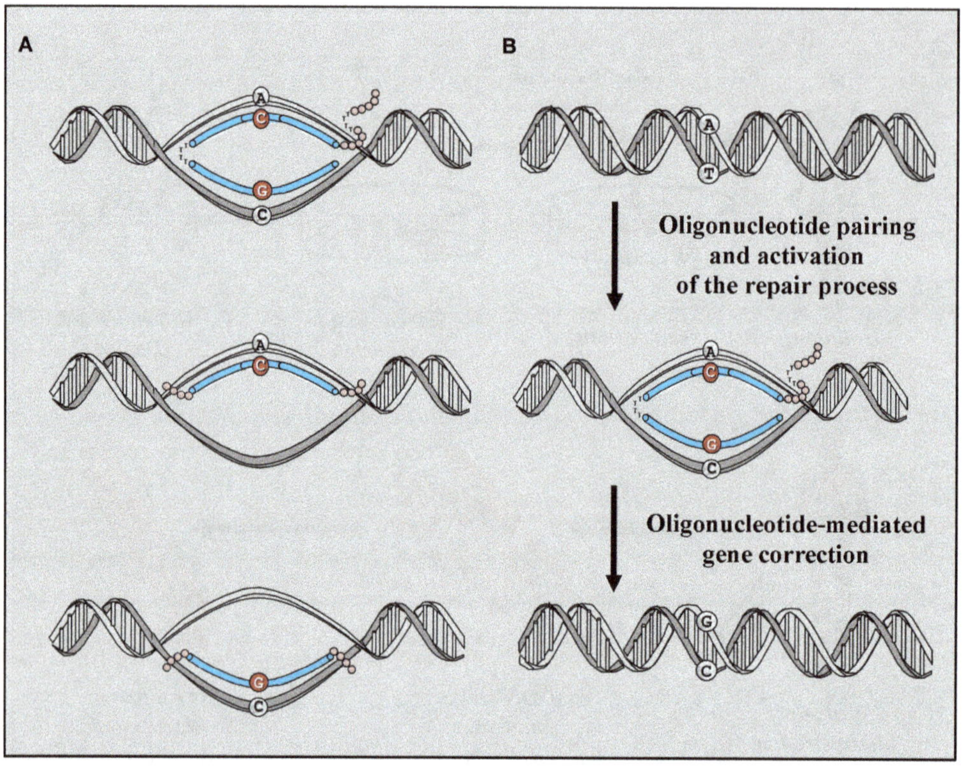

FIGURE 2 | ODN-mediated gene editing. (A) The basic structure of targeting ODNs consists of a stretch of DNA perfectly homologous to the region of the gene that is targeted for correction with the exception of a single base mismatch. A chODN contains a complimentary region composed of 2′-O-methyl RNA interrupted by a pentameric block of DNA bases while ssODNs consist of unmodified DNA bases and can be complimentary to the coding strand or complimentary to the non-coding strand of the gene targeted for correction. Phosphorothioate (PS) bases are added to the each end of the ODNs to increase their stability to endonucleases. **(B)** The correction process is activated by the pairing of ODN with the genomic sequence targeted for repair. Recognition of the mismatch present on the ODNs activates innate repair mechanisms naturally present in the cell nuclei and capable of directing the correction based on the information provided by the ODN template. The process require the presence of protein such as RecA and MSH2 capable of recognizing and correct the mismatch.

2005b; Sorensen et al., 2005; Aarts et al., 2006; Morozov and Wawrousek, 2008; Disterer et al., 2009). ssODN can either be complementary to the leading strand of the genomic loci or complimentary to the lagging strand (**Figure 2A**). In muscle, gene correction mediated by ssODN has been assessed using the *mdx*^{5cv} mouse. In this model, an A-to-T transversion in exon 10 of the dystrophin gene creates a cryptic splice site recognized by the splicing machinery. Thus, the mRNA of the dystrophin gene is aberrantly spliced causing total absence of dystrophin (Im et al., 1996). The use of the *mdx*^{5cv} mouse allows to precisely quantitate frequencies of gene repair achieved at both, the genomic DNA and mRNA levels, making this animal model particularly valuable (Bertoni et al., 2005; Kayali et al., 2010). Results clearly indicated that ssODNs complementary to the coding strand were as effective as chODN in correcting the dystrophin gene defect in *mdx*^{5cv} *in vitro* as well as *in vivo*. A strand bias was observed in the correction abilities of linear DNA ODNs depending on whether the ssODNs were targeting the coding or the non-coding strand of the dystrophin gene, suggesting that transcription may influence the ability of ssODNs to induce the genetic alteration at the chromosome level (Bertoni et al., 2005). Differences in strand bias observed by others seem to confirm the implication of transcription in the processes that take place in gene repair mediated by ssODNs (Igoucheva et al., 2001, 2003; Liu et al., 2001, 2002).

In recent years, studies have focused primarily on identifying new generation of ssODNs that could promote more efficiently the repair process in an effort to increase the frequencies of gene repair to levels that would be considered therapeutically relevant. Some success has been obtained by increasing the stability of the ODNs. The use of ssODNs containing 2′-*O*-methyl RNA residues (Igoucheva et al., 2001; Nickerson and Colledge, 2003), PS linkages (Liu et al., 2002; Olsen et al., 2005b), or Locked Nucleic Acid (LNA) bases (Parekh-Olmedo et al., 2002) at their extremities have been shown to increase targeting frequencies. Several studies have also demonstrated that gene repair can be enhanced by synchronizing the cells in the S phase of the cell cycle or by reducing the rate of replication fork progression (Brachman and Kmiec, 2004; Ferrara and Kmiec, 2004; Ferrara et al., 2004; Olsen et al., 2005a). Promising results have been achieved in muscle using ssODNs made of peptide nucleic acids (PNAs) bases (Kayali et al., 2010). PNAs are DNA mimics capable of forming stable duplex structures with Watson-Crick complementary DNA or RNA with a higher binding affinity than that of DNA/DNA or DNA/RNA duplexes made of unmodified bases (Nielsen, 2005). In general, ssODNs stretching from 12 to 18 nucleotides are sufficient to allow strong duplex formation with their complementary DNA or RNA sequences and to distinguish single base mutations. Kayali et al demonstrated that ssODNs made of PNA (PNA-ssODNs) containing the appropriate mismatch were capable of targeting and correcting the *mdx*^{5cv} mutation in the dystrophin gene more efficiently than ssODNs made of unmodified bases (Kayali et al., 2010). Expression of full-length dystrophin was sustained for up to four months after injection although correction was shown to decrease over time as the result of normal muscle turnover (Kayali et al., 2010). These results were particularly important to the field fo gene editing for DMD because provided the first evidence of how correction of the genetic defect in mature myofibers alone is not sufficient to guarantee long lasting effects and paved the way for subsequent studies aimed at studying the feasibility of targeting and correcting SCs and their therapeutic relevance for the treatment of DMD.

MECHANISMS OF ACTION OF ODN-MEDIATED GENE REPAIR

It is believed that chODNs and ssODNs act through similar mechanisms and that the repair process involves multiple steps (Gamper et al., 2000a,b; Igoucheva et al., 2004). The first steps requires the annealing of the ODN to the region of the genomic DNA targeted for repair (Liu et al., 2003; Jensen et al., 2011; Papaioannou et al., 2012). Pairing leads to the formation of a heteroduplex between the ssODN and the double-stranded target site (**Figure 2B**) (Bertoni, 2005, 2008; Engstrom et al., 2009). Msh2, a member of the family of proteins involved in the MMR mechanism has been shown to inhibit the repair process, potentially by preventing recombination between the ODN and the targeted genomic sequence, a phenomenon known as heteroduplex rejection (Dekker et al., 2003; Pierce et al., 2003; Aarts et al., 2006; Maguire and Kmiec, 2007; Igoucheva et al., 2008; Papaioannou et al., 2009). Furthermore, a two- to three-fold increase in frequencies of gene repair has been reported recently in primary cultures isolated from *mdx*^{5cv} muscle transfected with targeting ssODNs in conjunction with a siRNA designed to transiently downregulate Msh2 expression supporting the implication of the MMR as one of the mechanisms that controls ssODN-mediated gene repair in muscle cells (Maguire et al., 2009). Interestingly, the authors also failed to detect an effect when Msh2 was downregulated in purified myoblasts maintained in culture for prolonged period of time suggesting that the MMR may not be the only mechanism involved in the correction process in myoblasts and that culturing conditions of these cells may influence the repair process.

The second phase implicated in the correction process mediated by ODNs, involves the activation of the repair process. Some studies have implicated the HR pathway through homology-directed repair (HDR) and non-homologous end-joining (NHEJ) mechanisms as one of the mechanisms responsible for the correction induced at the genomic level through evidences that demonstrate that a portion of the ODN becomes integral part of the genomic DNA (Radecke et al., 2006; Aarts and te Riele, 2010). However, it is evident that mechanisms other than HR may be involved in the process catalyzed by ODNs. Among those, the nucleotide excision repair (NER) pathway appear to play a role and it was demonstrated that two of the proteins involved in this repair pathway, XPG and ERCC4, are required to facilitate ssODN-mediated gene repair, whereas components in the NHEJ pathway was found to inhibit the correction process (Igoucheva et al., 2006).

Recent studies aimed at improving the specificity and efficacy of ssODNs in directing single base alterations at the genomic level have also evidenced the possibility of recruiting repair mechanisms other than HR and NER (Bertoni et al., 2009). The approach involves the use of ssODNs containing methyl-CpG sequences and capable of activating the base excision repair (BER) mechanism through the recruitment of the methyl-CpG binding domain protein 4 (MBD4) also known as MED1. MBD4 is thought to be responsible for maintaining genome integrity by recognizing G:T or G:U mismatches at m^{5}CpG sites on double-stranded DNA (Bellacosa et al., 1999; Hendrich et al., 1999). *In vitro* studies have demonstrated that MBD4 can efficiently recognize and hydrolyze G:T or G:U mismatches at hemi-methylated m^{5}CpG sites as well as G:T and G:U mismatches in non-methylated CpG sequences (Hendrich et al., 1999). The introduction of the DNA mismatch is recognized by DNA glycosylases which excise the damaged base from the genomic DNA creating an apurinic/apyrimidinic site (AP site). The DNA strand is subsequently processed by specific endonucleases and ligases to direct the addition of a new cytosine at the AP site and to complete the repair process using the ssODNs as template (Bertoni et al., 2009). This new generation of ssODNs was shown to efficiently correct a single point mutation introduced in a GFP reporter system which was stably transfected in myoblasts. The drawback of using methyl-CpG-modified ssODNs is represented by the sequence specificity of the mutations that can be targeted by this approach which limits its broad applications in all genetic defects (Bertoni et al., 2003, 2009).

THERAPIES FOR DMD USING ODNs TARGETING STEM CELLS

The feasibility of using ssODNs to correct gene defects in SCs and restore full-length dystrophin expression has recently been demonstrated by Nick-Ahd et al. In the study, the authors isolated SCs from the *mdx*^{5cv} mouse and transfected PNA-ssODNs targeting the *mdx*^{5cv} mutation prior to engraftment into immunocompromised *mdx*/nude mice (Nik-Ahd and Bertoni, 2014). Clusters of dystrophin-positive fibers were clearly detected immediately following transplantation and expression of dystrophin, resulting from the contribution of donor-derived SCs that had undergone gene repair, were shown to increase over time. The work represent the first evidence of the feasibility of inducing *ex vivo* gene repair of SCs without compromising the ability of isolated cells to self-renew following transplantation (Nik-Ahd and Bertoni, 2014).

More recently, gene editing strategies mediated by ssODNs has been extended to iPSCs isolated from human skin fibroblasts of two patients affected by type I spinal muscular atrophy (SMA). SMA is an autosomal recessive genetic disorder caused by a genetic defect in the survival motor neuron 1 (*SMN1*) gene, which encodes SMN. Loss of SMN protein is thought to be responsible for the progressive loss of motor neurons which is paralleled by the progressive muscle wasting characteristic of SMA patients (Brzustowicz et al., 1990; Lefebvre et al., 1995; Coovert et al., 1997). Corti et al used a 75 bp ssODN was used to target and redirect splicing of the *SMN2* gene, a gene paralogous to *SMN1* and to induce expression of a protein similar to SMN1. This strategy has previously been shown to partially rescue motor neuron loss in animal models and is considered a valuable approach to treat the disease in patients (Lefebvre et al., 1997; Le et al., 2005). Correction mediated by ssODNs targeting the *SMN2* gene was achieved in approximately 4% of the transfected cells suggesting frequencies of gene repair similar to those observed in muscle culture and demonstrating that iPSCs are equally amenable to gene repair than myoblasts and SCs (Bertoni et al., 2005, 2009; Maguire et al., 2009; Kayali et al., 2010; Nik-Ahd and Bertoni, 2014). Importantly, when transplanted into the spinal cords of 1-day-old SMA mice, donor-derived motor neuron engrafted in the anterior spinal cords of transplanted mice and ameliorated defects in neuromuscular function in SMA mice (Corti et al., 2012). These results are particularly encouraging as they represent the first evidence of how gene editing mediated by ssODNs could have a clinical applicability to disorders other than DMD demonstrating that the field of gene repair is slowly but steadily growing toward the development of clinical applications for the treatment of different neuromuscular disorders.

NUCLEASE-MEDIATED GENE EDITING

During the past 10 years, the field of gene editing has witnessed a tremendous growth in the number of laboratories interested in developing corrections strategies using engineered nucleases. These nucleases are artificial restriction enzymes that can be designed to target virtually any site in the genome. Their use has enabled routine reprogramming of prokaryotic and eukaryotic systems for a variety of applications ranging from site-directed mutagenesis of bacterial systems, generation of animal models to study diseases, or simply proof-of-concept studies to demonstrate the specificity of a biological system. The ability of nucleases to recognize specific sequences in the genome and introduce a cleavage at specific sites has been known for almost two decades, but this technology has boomed only recently. This rapid growth is in part due to the crescent interest of commercial sources in developing new products that could be brought to the market and in part to the recognition of public and government sources of the potential that this application could have in basic and translational biology. More recently, nucleases have moved into preclinical and clinical applications for numerous diseases and three phase I and phase II clinical trials are on their way in Human Immunodeficiency Virus (HIV) patients (Tang, 2013a,b; Tebas and Stein, 2013).

There are three major families of engineered nucleases being employed in gene editing approaches: zinc finger nucleases (ZFNs), transcription activator-like effector nucleases (TALENs), and engineered meganuclease (MNs) (**Figure 3**). A fourth family termed clustered regularly interspaced short palindromic repeats (CRISPR) has been recently developed as an additional approach to alter genomic sequences at the DNA level (Pauwels et al., 2013). Despite its early stages of development, the use of CRISPR has already proven to be a valid alternative to ZFNs, TALENs, and MNs (Jinek et al., 2012, 2013; Chang et al., 2013; Cong et al., 2013; DiCarlo et al., 2013; Mali et al., 2013; Wang et al., 2013), but its potential for the treatment of neuromuscular disorders has yet to be explored.

The mechanisms of action of nucleases are common to all system and rely on their ability to create a double-strand break (DSB) which is either repaired by NHEJ, or, in the presence of a donor DNA, can be repaired by HR (**Figure 4**). Several hurdles still need to be overcome before this approach can have a wide-spread use in the context of clinical applications to genetic disorders. Among those, is the limited level of gene editing frequencies achieved in cells, the relative difficulty and time consuming process required to assemble the nucleases *in vitro*, the need to use viral or plasmid vectors to ensure high levels of expression of nucleases in the nucleus required to achieve an effect and the risk of off-target mutations that have been associated with their use (as described in more detail below). Nonetheless, the results reported to date have clearly proven the validity of using engineered nucleases for therapeutic purposes.

ZFNs, TALENS, AND MNs

ZFNs are engineered restriction enzymes obtained by fusing a zinc finger DNA-binding domain to a DNA-cleavage domain originated from the *Fok*I restriction endonuclease (**Figure 3A**). Each zinc finger domain interacts with 3 bps of DNA and can be engineered to target unique sequences within complex genomes (Bibikova et al., 2003). The DNA-binding domains of individual ZFNs typically contain between three and six individual zinc finger repeats allowing the recognition of sequences of the genome comprised between 9 and 18 bps respectively. Introduction of the DSB is mediated by the dimer formed by the association of two *Fok*I domains. As a result, two ZFNs need to be expressed and bound to opposite strands of the targeted genomic DNA for the cleavage to occur (**Figure 3A**). Furthermore, each *Fok*I domain needs to be separated by 5–7 bp to allow proper formation of the *Fok*I dimer. To date, ZFNs have been successfully employed to target drosophila (Bibikova et al., 2002, 2003; Beumer et al., 2006, 2008, 2013; Bozas et al., 2009), plants (Shukla et al., 2009; Tovkach et al., 2009; Townsend et al., 2009; Marton et al., 2010; Osakabe et al., 2010; Zhang et al., 2010; Curtin et al., 2011; Qi et al., 2013), *Caenorhabditis elegans* (Morton et al., 2006; Wood et al., 2011), zebrafish (Doyon et al., 2008; Meng et al., 2008; Foley et al., 2009a,b; McCammon and Amacher, 2010; Sander et al., 2011b; Zhu et al., 2011), rat and mouse (Mani et al., 2005; Carbery et al., 2010; Mashimo et al., 2010; Meyer et al., 2010; Cui et al., 2011; Osiak et al., 2011; Chou et al., 2012; Hermann et al., 2012; Bhakta et al., 2013; Shen et al., 2013) and human cells (Alwin et al., 2005; Urnov et al., 2005; Lombardo et al., 2007; Miller et al., 2007; Perez et al., 2008; Hockemeyer et al., 2009; Zou et al., 2009; Holt et al., 2010; Lei et al., 2011; Dreyer and Cathomen, 2012; Handel et al., 2012; Wang et al., 2012).

One of the major drawbacks that has restricted the wide use of ZFNs in the research and clinical settings is the limited availability of DNA-binding domains targeting all trinucleotide combinations and required to guarantee specificity of the ZFN to its target (Desjarlais and Berg, 1992; Pabo et al., 2001), the high cost of purchasing engineered zinc-finger units available in proprietary

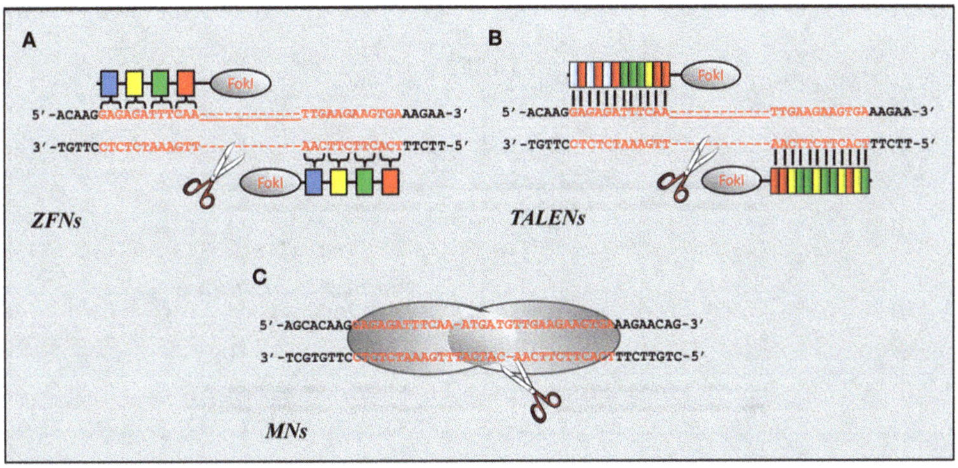

FIGURE 3 | Nucleases currently used as gene editing tools for muscle disorders. (A) Schematic representation of a ZFN dimer bound to its target. Each ZFN contains the cleavage domain of *FokI* linked to a series of zinc fingers each designed to specifically recognize trinucleotide sequences (colored boxes) flanking the cleavage site. **(B)** Schematic representation of a TALEN dimer. Like ZFNs each TALEN contains the catalytic domain of the *FokI* endonuclease flanked by modules responsible for the recognition of the sequence targeted for repair. Unlike ZFNs, however, each modular repeat binds to a specific bp. Each color represents a module for each of the four nucleotide bases. **(C)** Schematic representation of a LAGLIDADG homing endonuclease (LHE) bound to a DNA target through its catalytic motif. Sequence specificity toward most DNA targets is usually achieved through the association or fusion of protein domains from different enzymes to generate chimeric MNs.

archives (Pearson, 2008) and, even when DNA-binding domains can be obtained from publically available libraries, the difficulty encountered to assemble and select the ZFNs specific to the desired sequence (Isalan et al., 1997). These limitations have been largely overcome by the introduction of a second generation of engineered nucleases that display similar binding affinity for their target, but higher specificity and relative ease in assembly. TALENs are artificial restriction enzymes generated by fusing a TAL effector DNA binding domain to a DNA cleavage domain (**Figure 3B**). The DNA-binding domain is generally composed of repeats ranging in number from 33 to 35 amino acids with the exception of the 12th and 13th amino acids which vary for each of the four nucleotides that compose the DNA (Boch et al., 2009; Moscou and Bogdanove, 2009; Mahfouz et al., 2011). Therefore, assembly of the TALEN requires the simple combination of the four possible DNA-binding domains in the order specified by the sequence of the genomic DNA targeted for repair. Similarly to ZFNs, a recognition sequence of 14–20 bp is sufficient to confer specify toward the target site of the genomic DNA, while a separation of 12–19 bp between *Fok*I domains appears to be ideal to guarantee efficient dimerization of the catalytic domain of the nuclease. The relative ease by which these nuclease can be assembled and the much lower cost of producing or purchasing custom vectors expressing a specific nuclease has enable gene editing mediated by TALENs to boom in a relatively short period of time (Cermak et al., 2011; Mahfouz and Li, 2011; Mahfouz et al., 2011; Sander et al., 2011a; Tesson et al., 2011; Wood et al., 2011; Carlson et al., 2012; Li et al., 2012; Liu et al., 2012; Moore et al., 2012; Tong et al., 2012).

A third class of nucleases has also been implemented as potential gene editing tools (**Figure 3C**). MNs (also known as homing endonucleases) have been developed based on studies that were originally conducted in yeast and that identified mobile elements in the genome (HO and I-SceI) encoded by the mitochondrial genome and responsible for triggering recombination events (Orr-Weaver et al., 1981; Kostriken et al., 1983; Jacquier and Dujon, 1985; Nickoloff et al., 1986; Colleaux et al., 1988). MNs recognize DNA sequences of 12–40 bp in length and are classified in five families based on key sequence and structure motifs. Among those, the LAGLIDADG family is the largest and best characterized one, and the one currently being used for designing MNs (Epinat et al., 2013). The initial studies employed a neomycin resistance reporter gene that was used to demonstrate the feasibility of targeting NIH3T3 and mouse ESCs (Rouet et al., 1994; Smih et al., 1995). Since then, MNs have been successfully applied to induce mutagenesis, recombination or gene targeting in bacteria (Cox et al., 2007; Flannagan et al., 2008), plants (Siebert and Puchta, 2002; Puchta and Fauser, 2013) and mammalian cells (Thermes et al., 2002; Epinat et al., 2003, 2013; Grosse et al., 2011; Izmiryan et al., 2011; Munoz et al., 2011; Menoret et al., 2013). Extensive work conducted on better understanding the mechanisms of action and the amino acid structure of different members of the LAGLIDADG family has enable the construction of chimeric MNs with improved activity and targetability (Seligman et al., 2002; Arnould et al., 2006; Rosen et al., 2006; Smith et al., 2006). Nonetheless, the still limited numbers of sequences that can be targeted combined with the inability of précising direct the recombination of heterodimers necessary to induce target specificity mediated by chimeric MNs (Arnould et al., 2006) has limited its applicability to a large number of genetic disorders.

APPLICATION OF ENGINEERED NUCLEASE FOR THE TREATMENT OF MUSCLE DISORDERS

The use of engineered nucleases to precisely direct genomic alterations in specific genes known to cause muscle disorders

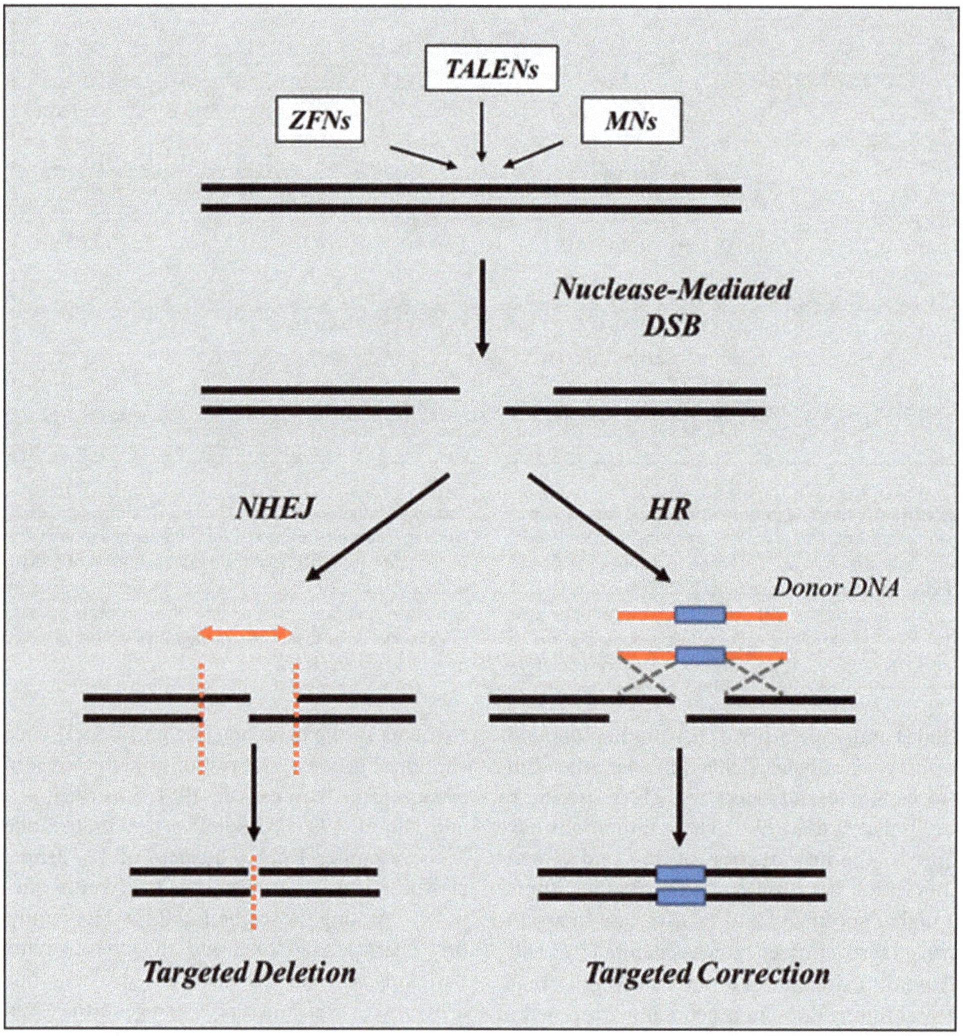

FIGURE 4 | Gene editing using nucleases. Upon introduction into the cell and following recognition of the region of the genomic DNA targeted for repair, the binding domains of the nucleases associate and generate a DSB which triggers the activation of specific repair mechanisms. In the absence of donor DNA sequences, the break is repaired by the NHEJ repair pathway by cleaving non-compatible overhang sequences and by joining the ends of the cleaved sequences (targeted deletion). This usually results in deletions of one or more bases (indels). Depending on the type of mutation targeted for repair, these deletions can lead to either, the inactivation of the gene or to the expression of in-frame transcripts encoding for shorter, although still functional proteins. Introduction of single base alterations can only occur in the presence of a donor DNA containing the desired sequence (targeted correction). The process is directed by the HR pathway and requires the exchange of DNA sequences from the donor DNA to the genomic DNA targeted for repair.

has so far been limited to proof-of-concept studies and have focused primarily on determining their applicability for the treatment of DMD (Chapdelaine et al., 2010; Rousseau et al., 2011; Benabdallah et al., 2013; Ousterout et al., 2013). MNs and ZFNs have been used to test the feasibility of activating the NHEJ repair mechanism and of restoring the normal reading frame of a dog microdystrophin gene containing a frame-shift mutation (Chapdelaine et al., 2010; Rousseau et al., 2011). The ability of MNs to induce indels in the dystrophin locus has also been demonstrated through studies aimed at determining the effect of chromatin accessibility on genome editing mediated by MNs (Daboussi et al., 2012). In this study, Daboussi et al designed 37 MNs capable of cleaving different genomic targets. Among those, 5 MNs were shown to efficiently target intronic regions of the dystrophin gene. Although the study was not designed to assess the feasibility of using MNs to restore dystrophin expression, it clearly demonstrated that the dystrophin locus is amenable to gene editing mediated by MNs paving the way for further work aimed at developing effective gene repair strategies to DMD using MNs.

Nuclease-mediated editing of dystrophin gene defects has been recently demonstrated in human cells. TALENs have been tested in primary dermal fibroblasts isolated from a DMD patient harboring a deletion of exons 46–50 (Δ46–50) and have been used to induce targeted deletions of exon 51 to restore the coding reading frame of the dystrophin gene (Ousterout et al., 2013). Clonal analysis identified a clone with an NHEJ event expected to correct the dystrophin reading frame. When transdifferentiated into myoblasts following ectopic expression of MyoD, cells generated from the clone were shown to form myotubes expressing a dystrophin protein of a molecular weight identical to that predicted as a result of the expression of an in frame transcript lacking exon 46 through 50 of the dystrophin mRNA. The robustness of the approach was further confirmed in immortalized myoblast cells lines isolated from two DMD patients with a deletion of exons 48–50 (Δ48–50) also treatable by the same pair of TALENs used to correct the Δ46–50 fibroblasts. In addition to confirm the ability of nucleases of targeting the human DMD gene, these studies have also established the feasibility of using TALEN-mediated NHEJ to target and correct dystrophin gene defects caused by large deletions further extending the applicability of the approach to the majority of the mutations causing DMD.

DRAWBACKS AND LIMITATIONS OF GENE EDITING MEDIATED BY ODNs AND ENDONUCLEASES

As any technology currently being tested and optimized for the treatment of genetic disorders, limitations do exist that may ultimately preclude the use of ODNs or engineered nucleases from entering the clinic for the treatment of DMD. In the case of ODNs, perhaps the major drawback is the low efficiency of the correction process achieved to date. While the use of specific modifications inserted on the oligonucleotides to stabilize the structure of ssODNs (Kayali et al., 2010) or those used to recruit specific repair mechanisms (Bertoni et al., 2009) have proven to significantly increase the gene correction frequencies achieved in muscle *in vitro* and *in vivo*, the frequencies obtained remain low. Other factors are likely to influence the clinical applicability of ODNs including the possibility to induce mutations at regions of the genome different from that targeted for repair, a phenomenon that has not been studied in detail. Additional parameters such as possible toxicity of the ODNs once introduced into patients will also have to be examined.

One of the limiting factors that preclude the use of engineered nucleases, particularly for clinical applications, is represented by the inability to efficiently control the level of expression of the nucleases once delivered to the cell and by the fact that certain endonucleases such as ZFNs and TALENs require the formation of dimers to be active which implies the use of at least two vectors to efficiently express each endonuclease. To date, delivery of endonuclease into the cells has employed, for the most part, the use of plasmid vectors. Although this method of delivery result in efficient expression of the vectors sustained only for a short period of time, potentially the time needed for the nucleases to induce the desired genomic alteration, the level of expression achieved cannot be easily controlled and the efficiency of delivery is limited particularly when targeting stem cells or muscle progenitor cells. An alternative approach is to use lentiviral vectors which have been shown to efficiently transduce stem cells and to be able to achieve high levels of transgene expression. Although effective, these vectors are known to randomly integrate into the genome and therefore they can potentially be mutagenic. This problem has been recently addressed through extensive studies aimed at better characterizing the sequences encoded by the lentiviral vector that direct the recombination process and has led to the development of a new generation of lentiviral vectors unable of integrating (Cornu and Cathomen, 2007; Lombardo et al., 2007). Although safer, these vectors can only achieve limited levels of expression into cells which have been associated with significant lower levels of gene correction frequencies. Promising results have been obtained using adenoviral vectors (Perez et al., 2008; Holkers et al., 2013) and adeno-associated virus vectors which have been shown to drive efficient expression of the nucleases into cells (Porteus et al., 2003; Gellhaus et al., 2010; Metzger et al., 2011). Nonetheless, these vectors still require systems to control their expression once introduced into the cell.

An alternative to the use of viral vectors is the introduction into the cell of mRNA encoding for the nuclease (Geurts et al., 2010; Meyer et al., 2010; Zou et al., 2011) or purified nuclease proteins (Gaj et al., 2012). This method, however, has shown only limited efficacy and is associated with higher costs of production and purification of the endonucleases at the doses required to achieve significant effects.

A major concern that limits the use of endonuclease particularly in the context of therapeutic applications, is the potential off-target effects that have been associated with their use. These effects appear to be related, for the most part, to the lack of binding specificity of the DNA-binding domain toward its recognition sequence (Bibikova et al., 2002; Olsen et al., 2009). As such, cleavage of regions other than those targeted for repair may result in the generation of indels that, once repaired through NHEJ events, could lead to the inactivation of genes. If the inactivation occurs in genes responsible for muscle stem cells maintenance or necessary for the proper function of muscle progenitor cells poses serious safety concerns. Future applications of gene editing targeting and employing stem cells for therapeutic purposes will have to be further refined and issues of toxicity as well as possible side effects will have to be evaluated in detail so as to guarantee safe and long lasting effects.

FUTURE OF GENE EDITING STRATEGIES IN MUSCLE STEM CELLS

Several parameters need to be considered and optimized before we can reach the stage of designing clinical trials using gene editing approaches that specifically target muscle stem cells. First among all, is the efficacy of the approach being used and the benefits that can be achieved by the different systems being employed. Approaches aimed at correcting stem cells *ex vivo* have clear advantages over systems that target stem cells *in situ* (**Figure 1**). First, delivery of ODNs or nucleases in cells maintained in culture it is easier to accomplish as it can rely on both chemical as well as physical methods of delivery. For instance, the use of chemical-based reagents such as Lipofectamine™ 2000, Fugene® HD and other of transfection reagents currently in the market, as well as electroporation devices such as Amaxa Nucleofector™ and Neon® Electroporation System have proven to be effective in delivering naked DNA, including ssODNs as well as plasmids encoding nucleases into muscle progenitor cells, SCs, and ESCs (Bertoni and Rando, 2002; Bertoni et al., 2003, 2005; Dekker et al., 2003, 2006; Pierce et al., 2003; Aarts et al., 2006; Flagler et al., 2008; Kayali et al., 2010; Corti et al., 2012; Fontes and Lakshmipathy, 2013). Additionally, viral vectors can be used to express nucleases in cases where chemical and electroporation methods pose a challenge. Another advantage of targeting and correcting stem cells *ex vivo*, is represented by the fact that cells that have undergone repair can be selected, expanded in culture and characterized to ensure that they are safe to use in patients. Importantly, cells to be transplanted into muscle can undergo quality checks to ensure they are devoided of off-target mutations introduced by the ODN or the nuclease in region of the genome other than that targeted for repair. Great progress has been made toward the development of technologies capable of sequencing the entire genome or of studying changes in gene expression at a single cell level. These technologies are likely to become integral part of study design for future clinical trials and will be instrumental to the progress of gene editing technologies toward a safe and effective approach to treat muscle disorders. Finally, clones obtained following selection and expansion can potentially be stored over prolonged periods of times, virtually the lifetime of the patient, and could serve as a reservoir of cells to be used in the event that repeated administrations are required.

The major drawback of *ex vivo* approaches is represented by the difficulty encountered in delivering stem cells into skeletal muscles and the need to target a large number of muscles for the therapeutic approach to be clinically relevant. So far, most of the studies aimed at determining the efficacy of the genetically modified cells to restore muscle function have focused on delivering the cells intramuscularly. Although perfectly suitable for applications aimed at studying the efficacy of the cells being introduced into tissues to engraft and to regenerate muscle, this approach is not applicable in a clinical setting due to the number of injections that would be required to achieve functional effects in patients. Clinical applications to muscle disorders are likely to rely on the use of procedures capable of deliver genetically modified cells systemically. Intravenous or intrarterial injections have been successfully used to deliver Sca-1^{+}CD34^{+} (Torrente et al., 2001) and CD133^{+} (Torrente et al., 2004) muscle derived stem cells, mesoangioblasts (Sampaolesi et al., 2006), and pericytes (Dellavalle et al., 2007), but appear to have limited applicability with other cell types. Factors that can promote migration, survival, and engraftment of cells following administration are likely to have important implications for the success of cell-mediated regenerative approaches for the treatment of neuromuscular diseases. Some success has already been achieved following pretreatment of mesoangioblasts with stromal-derived factor-1 (SDF-1) and tumor necrosis factor-α (TNF-α) prior to administration of mesoangioblasts into dystrophic mice (Galvez et al., 2006) and, more recently using inhibitors of junctional adhesion molecule-A (JAM-A) expression, a small immunoglobulin that is located at endothelial and epithelial cell junctions (Giannotta et al., 2014).

Direct delivery of ODNs or nucleases into skeletal muscles may represent a valuable alternative to transplantation of genetically modified cells. In general, this approach will only be able to target endogenous muscle stem cells that are actively participating to the regeneration process such as SCs. Furthermore, it would be applicable only to patients that are at an early stage during the disease process before the reservoir of cells capable of regenerating muscles is exhausted or before their regenerative capacity is compromised as a result of the continue activation typical of muscles that undergo repeated rounds of degeneration and regeneration. Several methods of delivery are currently being optimized and tested for their ability to distribute ODNs and nucleases into different organs and tissues following systemic administration. In the case of ODN-based therapies some success has been achieved using trans-activator of transcription (Tat) protein of the HIV (Frankel and Pabo, 1988; Green and Loewenstein, 1988; Green et al., 1989; Brooks et al., 2005; Bechara and Sagan, 2013). More recently, efforts have been directed toward the identification of short peptide sequences that could be linked to ODNs and used to enhance their uptake through mechanisms of endocytosis and/or direct translocation across the plasma membrane (Joliot et al., 1991; Bechara and Sagan, 2013; Betts and Wood, 2013; Moulton, 2013; Regberg et al., 2013). Some success has been achieved using ODNs tagged to cell penetrating peptides (CPPs) which have been shown to successfully target and distribute ODNs into myofibers following systemic administration (Lescop et al., 2005; Moulton et al., 2007; Ivanova et al., 2008; Wu et al., 2008; Yin et al., 2008; Betts and Wood, 2013). Moreover, the use of CPPs has been implemented in gene editing technologies aimed at enhancing delivery of engineered nucleases with promising results further highlighting the potential of using peptide as carriers to enhance delivery (Nain et al., 2010; Puria et al., 2012; Chen et al., 2013). However, most of the studies thus far have been focused on targeting myofibers and little is known on the ability of CPPs to penetrate SCs or other types of muscle stem cells following systemic delivery.

The main drawback of directly delivering systemically ODNs or nucleases into muscles is represented by the inability to control the repair process once the therapeutic agent reaches it targeted stem cell. As a result, issues of toxicity, off-target effects, and low frequencies of gene repair may limit the beneficial effects achieved. Studies aimed at further refine the efficacy and specificity of the repair process mediated by ODNs or nucleases is likely to have important implications for the success of gene editing approaches.

Independently from the approach used to correct the genetic defect and whether restoration of the missing protein is achieved through delivery of genetically modified cells *ex vivo* or systemic administration of gene editing tools *in situ*, other factors may hamper the efficacy and stability of the repair process. Considerations should be given to possible immune response toward the protein being restored as the result of the therapeutic application. Preconditioning of patients using immunosuppressive reagent as well as administration of chemotherapeutic drugs that are toxic to proliferating cells may be necessary to ensure efficient cell engraftment and rapid clonogenic growth of the transplanted cells.

SUMMARY AND CONCLUSIONS

The past decade or so has seen an exponential growth in the development of therapeutic applications for muscle disorders specifically designed to target stem cells. Clinical trials are currently undergoing to test the feasibility and efficacy of restoring dystrophin expression in skeletal muscles of DMD patients following systemic administration of mesoangioblasts highlighting the fact that the field is rapidly advancing toward clinical applications for this disease. Approaches aimed at using the patient own stem cells as source for the transplantation procedures has clear advantages over those using heterologous sources of stem cells. As such, it is likely that gene editing approaches will become integral part of future applications to treat muscle disorders using genetically modified cells.

Additional parameters will have to be taken into account and defined before these approaches can enter into the clinic. For instance, gene editing strategies targeting stem cells *ex vivo* will require to refine culturing techniques to ensure that, once explanted, muscle stem cells can be efficiently propagated *in vitro* while maintaining maximal regenerative potential. Furthermore, a better understanding of the mechanisms that regulate stem-cell properties will help redefine and select a specific population of cells that is safe to use in patients without compromising the beneficial effects that can be achieved using the approach. Along the same line, the development of new delivery systems or vectors capable of targeting muscle stem cells *in situ* will be a key to the optimization of gene editing strategies. Ultimately, a key component of preclinical and clinical studies will remain the efficacy and safety of the approach being employed. The trials currently under way for muscle disorders as well as other genetic diseases and the clinical trials that are planned to start within the next few years will be instrumental in determining the key parameters necessary to achieve sustained effects in patients and to ensure the safety and efficacy of the approach being employed. Despite the early stages of gene editing approaches aimed at targeting and correcting stem cells for the treatment of muscle disorders, the results obtained to date are encouraging. Collaborations among different laboratories interested in pursuing these technologies for the treatment of inherited genetic disease affecting muscle could result in advancing gene editing strategies more rapidly and more efficiently into the clinic.

ACKNOWLEDGMENTS

This work was supported by a grant from the Muscular Dystrophy Association (MDA) USA (277016).

REFERENCES

Aarts, M., Dekker, M., de Vries, S., van der Wal, A., and te Riele, H. (2006). Generation of a mouse mutant by oligonucleotide-mediated gene modification in ES cells. *Nucleic Acids Res.* 34, e147. doi: 10.1093/nar/gkl896

Aarts, M., and te Riele, H. (2010). Subtle gene modification in mouse ES cells: evidence for incorporation of unmodified oligonucleotides without induction of DNA damage. *Nucleic Acids Res.* 38, 6956–6967. doi: 10.1093/nar/gkq589

Alwin, S., Gere, M. B., Guhl, E., Effertz, K., Barbas, C. F. 3rd., Segal, D. J., et al. (2005). Custom zinc-finger nucleases for use in human cells. *Mol. Ther.* 12, 610–617. doi: 10.1016/j.ymthe.2005.06.094

Arechavala-Gomeza, V., Anthony, K., Morgan, J., and Muntoni, F. (2012). Antisense oligonucleotide-mediated exon skipping for Duchenne muscular dystrophy: progress and challenges. *Curr. Gene Ther.* 12, 152–160. doi: 10.2174/156652312800840621

Arnould, S., Chames, P., Perez, C., Lacroix, E., Duclert, A., Epinat, J. C., et al. (2006). Engineering of large numbers of highly specific homing endonucleases that induce recombination on novel DNA targets. *J. Mol. Biol.* 355, 443–458. doi: 10.1016/j.jmb.2005.10.065

Asakura, A., Seale, P., Girgis-Gabardo, A., and Rudnicki, M. A. (2002). Myogenic specification of side population cells in skeletal muscle. *J. Cell Biol.* 159, 123–134. doi: 10.1083/jcb.200202092

Barberi, T., Bradbury, M., Dincer, Z., Panagiotakos, G., Socci, N. D., and Studer, L. (2007). Derivation of engraftable skeletal myoblasts from human embryonic stem cells. *Nat. Med.* 13, 642–648. doi: 10.1038/nm1533

Bartlett, R. J., Stockinger, S., Denis, M. M., Bartlett, W. T., Inverardi, L., Le, T. T., et al. (2000). *In vivo* targeted repair of a point mutation in the canine dystrophin gene by a chimeric RNA/DNA oligonucleotide. *Nat. Biotechnol.* 18, 615–622. doi: 10.1038/76448

Bechara, C., and Sagan, S. (2013). Cell-penetrating peptides: 20 years later, where do we stand? *FEBS Lett.* 587, 1693–1702. doi: 10.1016/j.febslet.2013.04.031

Beetham, P. R., Kipp, P. B., Sawycky, X. L., Arntzen, C. J., and May, G. D. (1999). A tool for functional plant genomics: chimeric RNA/DNA oligonucleotides cause *in vivo* gene-specific mutations. *Proc. Natl. Acad. Sci. U.S.A.* 96, 8774–8778. doi: 10.1073/pnas.96.15.8774

Bellacosa, A., Cicchillitti, L., Schepis, F., Riccio, A., Yeung, A. T., Matsumoto, Y., et al. (1999). MED1, a novel human methyl-CpG-binding endonuclease, interacts with DNA mismatch repair protein MLH1. *Proc. Natl. Acad. Sci. U.S.A.* 96, 3969–3974. doi: 10.1073/pnas.96.7.3969

Benabdallah, B. F., Duval, A., Rousseau, J., Chapdelaine, P., Holmes, M. C., Haddad, E., et al. (2013). Targeted gene addition of microdystrophin in mice skeletal muscle via human myoblast transplantation. *Mol. Ther. Nucleic Acids* 2, e68. doi: 10.1038/mtna.2012.55

Bentzinger, C. F., Wang, Y. X., and Rudnicki, M. A. (2012). Building muscle: molecular regulation of myogenesis. *Cold Spring Harb. Perspect. Biol.* 4:a008342. doi: 10.1101/cshperspect.a008342

Bertoni, C. (2005). Oligonucleotide-mediated gene editing for neuromuscular disorders. *Acta Myol.* 24, 194–201.

Bertoni, C. (2008). Clinical approaches in the treatment of Duchenne muscular dystrophy (DMD) using oligonucleotides. *Front. Biosci.* 13, 517–527. doi: 10.2741/2697

Bertoni, C., Jarrahian, S., Wheeler, T. M., Li, Y., Olivares, E. C., Calos, M. P., et al. (2006). Enhancement of plasmid-mediated gene therapy for muscular dystrophy by directed plasmid integration. *Proc. Natl. Acad. Sci. U.S.A.* 103, 419–424. doi: 10.1073/pnas.0504505102

Bertoni, C., Lau, C., and Rando, T. A. (2003). Restoration of dystrophin expression in mdx muscle cells by chimeraplast-mediated exon skipping. *Hum. Mol. Genet.* 12, 1087–1099. doi: 10.1093/hmg/ddg133

Bertoni, C., Morris, G. E., and Rando, T. A. (2005). Strand bias in oligonucleotide-mediated dystrophin gene editing. *Hum. Mol. Genet.* 14, 221–233. doi: 10.1093/hmg/ddi020

Bertoni, C., and Rando, T. A. (2002). Dystrophin gene repair in mdx muscle precursor cells *in vitro* and *in vivo* mediated by RNA-DNA chimeric oligonucleotides. *Hum. Gene Ther.* 13, 707–718. doi: 10.1089/104303402317322276

Bertoni, C., Rustagi, A., and Rando, T. A. (2009). Enhanced gene repair mediated by methyl-CpG-modified single-stranded oligonucleotides. *Nucleic Acids Res.* 37, 7468–7482. doi: 10.1093/nar/gkp757

Betts, C. A., and Wood, M. J. (2013). Cell penetrating peptide delivery of splice directing oligonucleotides as a treatment for Duchenne muscular dystrophy. *Curr. Pharm. Des.* 19, 2948–2962. doi: 10.2174/1381612811319160009

Beumer, K., Bhattacharyya, G., Bibikova, M., Trautman, J. K., and Carroll, D. (2006). Efficient gene targeting in Drosophila with zinc-finger nucleases. *Genetics* 172, 2391–2403. doi: 10.1534/genetics.105.052829

Beumer, K. J., Trautman, J. K., Bozas, A., Liu, J..L., Rutter, J., Gall, J. G., et al. (2008). Efficient gene targeting in Drosophila by direct embryo injection with zinc-finger nucleases. *Proc. Natl. Acad. Sci. U.S.A.* 105, 19821–19826. doi: 10.1073/pnas.0810475105

Beumer, K. J., Trautman, J. K., Mukherjee, K., and Carroll, D. (2013). Donor DNA utilization during gene targeting with zinc-finger nucleases. *G3 (Bethesda.)* 3, 657–664. doi: 10.1534/g3.112.005439

Bhagavati, S., and Xu, W. (2004). Isolation and enrichment of skeletal muscle progenitor cells from mouse bone marrow. *Biochem. Biophys. Res. Commun.* 318, 119–124. doi: 10.1016/j.bbrc.2004.03.192

Bhakta, M. S., Henry, I. M., Ousterout, D. G., Das, K. T., Lockwood, S. H., Meckler, J. F., et al. (2013). Highly active zinc-finger nucleases by extended modular assembly. *Genome Res.* 23, 530–538. doi: 10.1101/gr.143693.112

Bibikova, M., Beumer, K., Trautman, J. K., and Carroll, D. (2003). Enhancing gene targeting with designed zinc finger nucleases. *Science* 300, 764. doi: 10.1126/science.1079512

Bibikova, M., Golic, M., Golic, K. G., and Carroll, D. (2002). Targeted chromosomal cleavage and mutagenesis in Drosophila using zinc-finger nucleases. *Genetics* 161, 1169–1175.

Bittner, R. E., Schofer, C., Weipoltshammer, K., Ivanova, S., Streubel, B., Hauser, E., et al. (1999). Recruitment of bone-marrow-derived cells by skeletal and cardiac muscle in adult dystrophic mdx mice. *Anat. Embryol. (Berl)* 199, 391–396. doi: 10.1007/s004290050237

Boch, J., Scholze, H., Schornack, S., Landgraf, A., Hahn, S., Kay, S., et al. (2009). Breaking the code of DNA binding specificity of TAL-type III effectors. *Science* 326, 1509–1512. doi: 10.1126/science.1178811

Boldrin, L., Neal, A., Zammit, P. S., Muntoni, F., and Morgan, J. E. (2012). Donor satellite cell engraftment is significantly augmented when the host niche is preserved and endogenous satellite cells are incapacitated. *Stem Cells* 30, 1971–1984. doi: 10.1002/stem.1158

Boldrin, L., Zammit, P., Muntoni, F., and Morgan, J. (2009). The mature adult dystrophic mouse muscle environment does not impede efficient engrafted satellite cell regeneration and self-renewal. *Stem Cells* 27, 2478–2487. doi: 10.1002/stem.162

Bozas, A., Beumer, K. J., Trautman, J. K., and Carroll, D. (2009). Genetic analysis of zinc-finger nuclease-induced gene targeting in Drosophila. *Genetics* 182, 641–651. doi: 10.1534/genetics.109.101329

Brachman, E. E., and Kmiec, E. B. (2004). DNA replication and transcription direct a DNA strand bias in the process of targeted gene repair in mammalian cells. *J. Cell Sci.* 117, 3867–3874. doi: 10.1242/jcs.01250

Brack, A. S., and Rando, T. A. (2012). Tissue-specific stem cells: lessons from the skeletal muscle satellite cell. *Cell Stem Cell* 10, 504–514. doi: 10.1016/j.stem.2012.04.001

Brooks, H., Lebleu, B., and Vives, E. (2005). Tat peptide-mediated cellular delivery: back to basics. *Adv. Drug Deliv. Rev.* 57, 559–577. doi: 10.1016/j.addr.2004.12.001

Brzustowicz, L. M., Lehner, T., Castilla, L. H., Penchaszadeh, G. K., Wilhelmsen, K. C., Daniels, R., et al. (1990). Genetic mapping of chronic childhood-onset spinal muscular atrophy to chromosome 5q11.2-13.3. *Nature* 344, 540–541. doi: 10.1038/344540a0

Capecchi, M. R. (1989). Altering the genome by homologous recombination. *Science* 244, 1288–1292. doi: 10.1126/science.2660260

Carbery, I. D., Ji, D., Harrington, A., Brown, V., Weinstein, E. J., Liaw, L., et al. (2010). Targeted genome modification in mice using zinc-finger nucleases. *Genetics* 186, 451–459. doi: 10.1534/genetics.110.117002

Carlson, D. F., Tan, W., Lillico, S. G., Stverakova, D., Proudfoot, C., Christian, M., et al. (2012). Efficient TALEN-mediated gene knockout in livestock. *Proc. Natl. Acad. Sci. U.S.A.* 109, 17382–17387. doi: 10.1073/pnas.1211446109

Cerletti, M., Jurga, S., Witczak, C. A., Hirshman, M. F., Shadrach, J. L., Goodyear, L. J., et al. (2008). Highly efficient, functional engraftment of skeletal muscle stem cells in dystrophic muscles. *Cell* 134, 37–47. doi: 10.1016/j.cell.2008.05.049

Cermak, T., Doyle, E. L., Christian, M., Wang, L., Zhang, Y., Schmidt, C., et al. (2011). Efficient design and assembly of custom TALEN and other TAL effector-based constructs for DNA targeting. *Nucleic Acids Res.* 39, e82. doi: 10.1093/nar/gkr218

Chang, H., Yoshimoto, M., Umeda, K., Iwasa, T., Mizuno, Y., Fukada, S., et al. (2009). Generation of transplantable, functional satellite-like cells from mouse embryonic stem cells. *FASEB J.* 23, 1907–1919. doi: 10.1096/fj.08-123661

Chang, N., Sun, C., Gao, L., Zhu, D., Xu, X., Zhu, X., et al. (2013). Genome editing with RNA-guided Cas9 nuclease in zebrafish embryos. *Cell Res.* 23, 465–472. doi: 10.1038/cr.2013.45

Chapdelaine, P., Pichavant, C., Rousseau, J., Paques, F., and Tremblay, J. P. (2010). Meganucleases can restore the reading frame of a mutated dystrophin. *Gene Ther.* 17, 846–858. doi: 10.1038/gt.2010.26

Chen, Z., Jaafar, L., Agyekum, D. G., Xiao, H., Wade, M. F., Kumaran, R. I., et al. (2013). Receptor-mediated delivery of engineered nucleases for genome modification. *Nucleic Acids Res.* 41, e182. doi: 10.1093/nar/gkt710

Chou, S. T., Leng, Q., and Mixson, A. J. (2012). Zinc finger nucleases: tailor-made for gene therapy. *Drugs Future* 37, 183–196.

Cole-Strauss, A., Gamper, H., Holloman, W. K., Munoz, M., Cheng, N., and Kmiec, E. B. (1999). Targeted gene repair directed by the chimeric RNA/DNA oligonucleotide in a mammalian cell-free extract. *Nucleic Acids Res.* 27, 1323–1330. doi: 10.1093/nar/27.5.1323

Cole-Strauss, A., Yoon, K., Xiang, Y., Byrne, B. C., Rice, M. C., Gryn, J., et al. (1996). Correction of the mutation responsible for sickle cell anemia by an RNA-DNA oligonucleotide. *Science* 273, 1386–1389. doi: 10.1126/science.273.5280.1386

Colleaux, L., D'Auriol, L., Galibert, F., and Dujon, B. (1988). Recognition and cleavage site of the intron-encoded omega transposase. *Proc. Natl. Acad. Sci. U.S.A.* 85, 6022–6026. doi: 10.1073/pnas.85.16.6022

Collins, C. A., Olsen, I., Zammit, P. S., Heslop, L., Petrie, A., Partridge, T. A., et al. (2005). Stem cell function, self-renewal, and behavioral heterogeneity of cells from the adult muscle satellite cell niche. *Cell.* 122, 289–301. doi: 10.1016/j.cell.2005.05.010

Cong, L., Ran, F. A., Cox, D., Lin, S., Barretto, R., Habib, N., et al. (2013). Multiplex genome engineering using CRISPR/Cas systems. *Science* 339, 819–823. doi: 10.1126/science.1231143

Coovert, D. D., Le, T. T., McAndrew, P. E., Strasswimmer, J., Crawford, T. O., Mendell, J. R., et al. (1997). The survival motor neuron protein in spinal muscular atrophy. *Hum. Mol. Genet.* 6, 1205–1214. doi: 10.1093/hmg/6.8.1205

Cornu, T. I., and Cathomen, T. (2007). Targeted genome modifications using integrase-deficient lentiviral vectors. *Mol. Ther.* 15, 2107–2113. doi: 10.1038/sj.mt.6300345

Corti, S., Nizzardo, M., Simone, C., Falcone, M., Nardini, M., Ronchi, D., et al. (2012). Genetic correction of human induced pluripotent stem cells from patients with spinal muscular atrophy. *Sci. Transl. Med.* 4, 165ra162. doi: 10.1126/scitranslmed.3004108

Coulton, G. R., Morgan, J. E., Partridge, T. A., and Sloper, J. C. (1988). The mdx mouse skeletal muscle myopathy: I. A histological, morphometric and biochemical investigation. *Neuropathol. Appl. Neurobiol.* 14, 53–70. doi: 10.1111/j.1365-2990.1988.tb00866.x

Cox, M. M., Layton, S. L., Jiang, T., Cole, K., Hargis, B. M., Berghman, L. R., et al. (2007). Scarless and site-directed mutagenesis in *Salmonella enteritidis* chromosome. *BMC Biotechnol.* 7:59. doi: 10.1186/1472-6750-7-59

Cui, X., Ji, D., Fisher, D. A., Wu, Y., Briner, D. M., and Weinstein, E. J. (2011). Targeted integration in rat and mouse embryos with zinc-finger nucleases. *Nat. Biotechnol.* 29, 64–67. doi: 10.1038/nbt.1731

Curtin, S. J., Zhang, F., Sander, J. D., Haun, W. J., Starker, C., Baltes, N. J., et al. (2011). Targeted mutagenesis of duplicated genes in soybean with zinc-finger nucleases. *Plant Physiol.* 156, 466–473. doi: 10.1104/pp.111.172981

Daboussi, F., Zaslavskiy, M., Poirot, L., Loperfido, M., Gouble, A., Guyot, V., et al. (2012). Chromosomal context and epigenetic mechanisms control the efficacy of genome editing by rare-cutting designer endonucleases. *Nucleic Acids Res.* 40, 6367–6379. doi: 10.1093/nar/gks268

Darabi, R., Arpke, R. W., Irion, S., Dimos, J. T., Grskovic, M., Kyba, M., et al. (2012). Human ES- and iPS-derived myogenic progenitors restore DYSTROPHIN and improve contractility upon transplantation in dystrophic mice. *Cell Stem Cell* 10, 610–619. doi: 10.1016/j.stem.2012.02.015

Darabi, R., Baik, J., Clee, M., Kyba, M., Tupler, R., and Perlingeiro, R. C. (2009). Engraftment of embryonic stem cell-derived myogenic progenitors in a dominant model of muscular dystrophy. *Exp. Neurol.* 220, 212–216. doi: 10.1016/j.expneurol.2009.08.002

Dekker, M., Brouwers, C., Aarts, M., van der Torre, J., de Vries, S., van de Vrugt, H., et al. (2006). Effective oligonucleotide-mediated gene disruption in ES cells lacking the mismatch repair protein MSH3. *Gene Ther.* 13, 686–694. doi: 10.1038/sj.gt.3302689

Dekker, M., Brouwers, C., and te Riele, H. (2003). Targeted gene modification in mismatch-repair-deficient embryonic stem cells by single-stranded DNA oligonucleotides. *Nucleic Acids Res.* 31:e27. doi: 10.1093/nar/gng027

Dellavalle, A., Sampaolesi, M., Tonlorenzi, R., Tagliafico, E., Sacchetti, B., Perani, L., et al. (2007). Pericytes of human skeletal muscle are myogenic precursors distinct from satellite cells. *Nat. Cell Biol.* 9, 255–267. doi: 10.1038/ncb1542

Desjarlais, J. R., and Berg, J. M. (1992). Toward rules relating zinc finger protein sequences and DNA binding site preferences. *Proc. Natl. Acad. Sci. U.S.A.* 89, 7345–7349. doi: 10.1073/pnas.89.16.7345

DiCarlo, J. E., Norville, J. E., Mali, P., Rios, X., Aach, J., and Church, G. M. (2013). Genome engineering in *Saccharomyces cerevisiae* using CRISPR-Cas systems. *Nucleic Acids Res.* 41, 4336–4343. doi: 10.1093/nar/gkt135

Disterer, P., Simons, J. P., and Owen, J. S. (2009). Validation of oligonucleotide-mediated gene editing. *Gene Ther.* 16, 824–826. doi: 10.1038/gt.2009.32

Doyle, M. J., Zhou, S., Tanaka, K. K., Pisconti, A., Farina, N. H., Sorrentino, B. P., et al. (2011). Abcg2 labels multiple cell types in skeletal muscle and participates in muscle regeneration. *J. Cell Biol.* 195, 147–163. doi: 10.1083/jcb.201103159

Doyon, Y., McCammon, J. M., Miller, J. C., Faraji, F., Ngo, C., Katibah, G. E., et al. (2008). Heritable targeted gene disruption in zebrafish using designed zinc-finger nucleases. *Nat. Biotechnol.* 26, 702–708. doi: 10.1038/nbt1409

Dreyer, A. K., and Cathomen, T. (2012). Zinc-finger nucleases-based genome engineering to generate isogenic human cell lines. *Methods Mol. Biol.* 813, 145–156. doi: 10.1007/978-1-61779-412-4_8

Engstrom, J. U., Suzuki, T., and Kmiec, E. B. (2009). Regulation of targeted gene repair by intrinsic cellular processes. *Bioessays* 31, 159–168. doi: 10.1002/bies.200800119

Epinat, J. C., Arnould, S., Chames, P., Rochaix, P., Desfontaines, D., Puzin, C., et al. (2003). A novel engineered meganuclease induces homologous recombination in yeast and mammalian cells. *Nucleic Acids Res.* 31, 2952–2962. doi: 10.1093/nar/gkg375

Epinat, J., Silva, G., Pâques, F., Smith, J., and Duchateau, P. (2013). "Engineered meganucleases for genome engineering purposes," in *Site-Directed Insertion of Transgenes*, eds S. Renault and P. Duchateau (Dordrecht; Heidelberg; New York, NY; London: Springer), 147–185.

Ferrara, L., and Kmiec, E. B. (2004). Camptothecin enhances the frequency of oligonucleotide-directed gene repair in mammalian cells by inducing DNA damage and activating homologous recombination. *Nucleic Acids Res.* 32, 5239–5248. doi: 10.1093/nar/gkh822

Ferrara, L., Parekh-Olmedo, H., and Kmiec, E. B. (2004). Enhanced oligonucleotide-directed gene targeting in mammalian cells following treatment with DNA damaging agents. *Exp. Cell Res.* 300, 170–179. doi: 10.1016/j.yexcr.2004.06.021

Ferrari, G., Cusella-De, A. G., Coletta, M., Paolucci, E., Stornaiuolo, A., Cossu, G., et al. (1998). Muscle regeneration by bone marrow-derived myogenic progenitors. *Science.* 279, 1528–1530. doi: 10.1126/science.279.5356.1528

Filareto, A., Darabi, R., and Perlingeiro, R. C. (2012). Engraftment of ES-derived myogenic progenitors in a severe mouse model of muscular dystrophy. *J. Stem Cell Res. Ther.* 10:S10-001. doi: 10.4172/2157-7633.S10-001

Flagler, K., Alexeev, V., Pierce, E. A., and Igoucheva, O. (2008). Site-specific gene modification by oligodeoxynucleotides in mouse bone marrow-derived mesenchymal stem cells. *Gene Ther.* 15, 1035–1048. doi: 10.1038/gt.2008.31

Flannagan, R. S., Linn, T., and Valvano, M. A. (2008). A system for the construction of targeted unmarked gene deletions in the genus Burkholderia. *Environ. Microbiol.* 10, 1652–1660. doi: 10.1111/j.1462-2920.2008.01576.x

Foley, J. E., Maeder, M. L., Pearlberg, J., Joung, J. K., Peterson, R. T., and Yeh, J. R. (2009a). Targeted mutagenesis in zebrafish using customized zinc-finger nucleases. *Nat. Protoc.* 4, 1855–1867. doi: 10.1038/nprot.2009.209

Foley, J. E., Yeh, J. R., Maeder, M. L., Reyon, D., Sander, J. D., Peterson, R. T., et al. (2009b). Rapid mutation of endogenous zebrafish genes using zinc finger nucleases made by Oligomerized Pool ENgineering (OPEN). *PLoS ONE* 4:e4348. doi: 10.1371/journal.pone.0004348

Fontes, A., and Lakshmipathy, U. (2013). Advances in genetic modification of pluripotent stem cells. *Biotechnol. Adv.* 31, 994–1001. doi: 10.1016/j.biotechadv.2013.07.003

Frankel, A. D., and Pabo, C. O. (1988). Cellular uptake of the tat protein from human immunodeficiency virus. *Cell* 55, 1189–1193. doi: 10.1016/0092-8674(88)90263-2

Gaj, T., Guo, J., Kato, Y., Sirk, S. J., and Barbas, C. F. 3rd (2012). Targeted gene knockout by direct delivery of zinc-finger nuclease proteins. *Nat. Methods* 9, 805–807. doi: 10.1038/nmeth.2030

Galli, D., Innocenzi, A., Staszewsky, L., Zanetta, L., Sampaolesi, M., Bai, A., et al. (2005). Mesoangioblasts, vessel-associated multipotent stem cells, repair the infarcted heart by multiple cellular mechanisms: a comparison with bone marrow progenitors, fibroblasts, and endothelial cells. *Arterioscler. Thromb. Vasc. Biol.* 25, 692–697. doi: 10.1161/01.ATV.0000156402.52029.ce

Galvez, B. G., Sampaolesi, M., Brunelli, S., Covarello, D., Gavina, M., Rossi, B., et al. (2006). Complete repair of dystrophic skeletal muscle by mesoangioblasts with enhanced migration ability. *J. Cell Biol.* 174, 231–243. doi: 10.1083/jcb.200512085

Gamper, H. B. Jr., Cole-Strauss, A., Metz, R., Parekh, H., Kumar, R., and Kmiec, E. B. (2000a). A plausible mechanism for gene correction by chimeric oligonucleotides. *Biochemistry* 39, 5808–5816. doi: 10.1021/bi9921891

Gamper, H. B., Parekh, H., Rice, M. C., Bruner, M., Youkey, H., and Kmiec, E. B. (2000b). The DNA strand of chimeric RNA/DNA oligonucleotides can direct gene repair/conversion activity in mammalian and plant cell-free extracts 69. *Nucleic Acids Res.* 28, 4332–4339. doi: 10.1093/nar/28.21.4332

Gellhaus, K., Cornu, T. I., Heilbronn, R., and Cathomen, T. (2010). Fate of recombinant adeno-associated viral vector genomes during DNA double-strand break-induced gene targeting in human cells. *Hum. Gene Ther.* 21, 543–553. doi: 10.1089/hum.2009.167

Geurts, A. M., Cost, G. J., Remy, S., Cui, X., Tesson, L., Usal, C., et al. (2010). Generation of gene-specific mutated rats using zinc-finger nucleases. *Methods Mol. Biol.* 597, 211–225. doi: 10.1007/978-1-60327-389-3_15

Giannotta, M., Benedetti, S., Tedesco, F. S., Corada, M., Trani, M., D'Antuono, R., et al. (2014). Targeting endothelial junctional adhesion molecule-A/ EPAC/ Rap-1 axis as a novel strategy to increase stem cell engraftment in dystrophic muscles. *EMBO Mol. Med.* 6, 239–258. doi: 10.1002/emmm.201302520

Green, M., Ishino, M., and Loewenstein, P. M. (1989). Mutational analysis of HIV-1 Tat minimal domain peptides: identification of trans-dominant mutants that suppress HIV-LTR-driven gene expression. *Cell* 58, 215–223. doi: 10.1016/0092-8674(89)90417-0

Green, M., and Loewenstein, P. M. (1988). Autonomous functional domains of chemically synthesized human immunodeficiency virus tat trans-activator protein. *Cell* 55, 1179–1188. doi: 10.1016/0092-8674(88)90262-0

Grosse, S., Huot, N., Mahiet, C., Arnould, S., Barradeau, S., Clerre, D. L., et al. (2011). Meganuclease-mediated inhibition of HSV1 infection in cultured cells. *Mol. Ther.* 19, 694–702. doi: 10.1038/mt.2010.302

Gussoni, E., Soneoka, Y., Strickland, C. D., Buzney, E. A., Khan, M. K., Flint, A. F., et al. (1999). Dystrophin expression in the mdx mouse restored by stem cell transplantation. *Nature* 401, 390–394. doi: 10.1038/43919

Handel, E. M., Gellhaus, K., Khan, K., Bednarski, C., Cornu, T. I., Muller-Lerch, F., et al. (2012). Versatile and efficient genome editing in human cells by combining zinc-finger nucleases with adeno-associated viral vectors. *Hum. Gene Ther.* 23, 321–329. doi: 10.1089/hum.2011.140

Hendrich, B., Hardeland, U., Ng, H. H., Jiricny, J., and Bird, A. (1999). The thymine glycosylase MBD4 can bind to the product of deamination at methylated CpG sites. *Nature* 401, 301–304. doi: 10.1038/45843

Hermann, M., Maeder, M. L., Rector, K., Ruiz, J., Becher, B., Burki, K., et al. (2012). Evaluation of OPEN zinc finger nucleases for direct gene targeting of the ROSA26 locus in mouse embryos. *PLoS ONE* 7:e41796. doi: 10.1371/journal.pone.0041796

Hockemeyer, D., Soldner, F., Beard, C., Gao, Q., Mitalipova, M., DeKelver, R. C., et al. (2009). Efficient targeting of expressed and silent genes in human ESCs and iPSCs using zinc-finger nucleases. *Nat. Biotechnol.* 27, 851–857. doi: 10.1038/nbt.1562

Hoffman, E. P., Brown, R. H. Jr., and Kunkel, L. M. (1987). Dystrophin: the protein product of the Duchenne muscular dystrophy locus. *Cell.* 51, 919–928. doi: 10.1016/0092-8674(87)90579-4

Holkers, M., Maggio, I., Liu, J., Janssen, J. M., Miselli, F., Mussolino, C., et al. (2013). Differential integrity of TALE nuclease genes following adenoviral and lentiviral vector gene transfer into human cells. *Nucleic Acids Res.* 41, e63. doi: 10.1093/nar/gks1446

Holt, N., Wang, J., Kim, K., Friedman, G., Wang, X., Taupin, V., et al. (2010). Human hematopoietic stem/progenitor cells modified by zinc-finger nucleases targeted to CCR5 control HIV-1 *in vivo*. *Nat. Biotechnol.* 28, 839–847. doi: 10.1038/nbt.1663

Igoucheva, O., Alexeev, V., Anni, H., and Rubin, E. (2008). Oligonucleotide-mediated gene targeting in human hepatocytes: implications of mismatch repair. *Oligonucleotides* 18, 111–122. doi: 10.1089/oli.2008.0120

Igoucheva, O., Alexeev, V., Pryce, M., and Yoon, K. (2003). Transcription affects formation and processing of intermediates in oligonucleotide-mediated gene alteration. *Nucleic Acids Res.* 31, 2659–2670. doi: 10.1093/nar/gkg360

Igoucheva, O., Alexeev, V., Scharer, O., and Yoon, K. (2006). Involvement of ERCC1/XPF and XPG in oligodeoxynucleotide-directed gene modification. *Oligonucleotides* 16, 94–104. doi: 10.1089/oli.2006.16.94

Igoucheva, O., Alexeev, V., and Yoon, K. (2001). Targeted gene correction by small single-stranded oligonucleotides in mammalian cells. *Gene Ther.* 8, 391–399. doi: 10.1038/sj.gt.3301414

Igoucheva, O., Alexeev, V., and Yoon, K. (2004). Mechanism of gene repair open for discussion. *Oligonucleotides* 14, 311–321. doi: 10.1089/oli.2004.14.311

Igoucheva, O. A., and Yoon, K. (2002). Gene correction frequency by chimeric RNA-DNA oligonucleotide using nuclear extracts. *Methods Mol. Med.* 69, 95–107.

Im, W. B., Phelps, S. F., Copen, E. H., Adams, E. G., Slightom, J. L., and Chamberlain, J. S. (1996). Differential expression of dystrophin isoforms in strains of mdx mice with different mutations. *Hum. Mol. Genet.* 5, 1149–1153. doi: 10.1093/hmg/5.8.1149

Isalan, M., Choo, Y., and Klug, A. (1997). Synergy between adjacent zinc fingers in sequence-specific DNA recognition. *Proc. Natl. Acad. Sci. U.S.A.* 94, 5617–5621. doi: 10.1073/pnas.94.11.5617

Ivanova, G. D., Arzumanov, A., Abes, R., Yin, H., Wood, M. J., Lebleu, B., et al. (2008). Improved cell-penetrating peptide-PNA conjugates for splicing redirection in HeLa cells and exon skipping in mdx mouse muscle. *Nucleic Acids Res.* 36, 6418–6428. doi: 10.1093/nar/gkn671

Izmiryan, A., Basmaciogullari, S., Henry, A., Paques, F., and Danos, O. (2011). Efficient gene targeting mediated by a lentiviral vector-associated meganuclease. *Nucleic Acids Res.* 39, 7610–7619. doi: 10.1093/nar/gkr524

Jacquier, A., and Dujon, B. (1985). An intron-encoded protein is active in a gene conversion process that spreads an intron into a mitochondrial gene. *Cell* 41, 383–394. doi: 10.1016/S0092-8674(85)80011-8

Jensen, N. M., Dalsgaard, T., Jakobsen, M., Nielsen, R. R., Sorensen, C. B., Bolund, L., et al. (2011). An update on targeted gene repair in mammalian cells: methods and mechanisms. *J. Biomed. Sci.* 18:10. doi: 10.1186/1423-0127-18-10

Jinek, M., Chylinski, K., Fonfara, I., Hauer, M., Doudna, J. A., and Charpentier, E. (2012). A programmable dual-RNA-guided DNA endonuclease in adaptive bacterial immunity. *Science* 337, 816–821. doi: 10.1126/science.1225829

Jinek, M., East, A., Cheng, A., Lin, S., Ma, E., and Doudna, J. (2013). RNA-programmed genome editing in human cells. *Elife* 2:e00471. doi: 10.7554/eLife.00471

Joliot, A., Pernelle, C., Deagostini-Bazin, H., and Prochiantz, A. (1991). Antennapedia homeobox peptide regulates neural morphogenesis. *Proc. Natl. Acad. Sci. U.S.A.* 88, 1864–1868. doi: 10.1073/pnas.88.5.1864

Kayali, R., Bury, F., Ballard, M., and Bertoni, C. (2010). Site directed gene repair of the dystrophin gene mediated by PNA-ssODNs. *Hum. Mol. Genet.* 19, 3266–3281. doi: 10.1093/hmg/ddq235

Kazuki, Y., Hiratsuka, M., Takiguchi, M., Osaki, M., Kajitani, N., Hoshiya, H., et al. (2010). Complete genetic correction of ips cells from Duchenne muscular dystrophy. *Mol. Ther.* 18, 386–393. doi: 10.1038/mt.2009.274

Koenig, M., Hoffman, E. P., Bertelson, C. J., Monaco, A. P., Feener, C., and Kunkel, L. M. (1987). Complete cloning of the Duchenne muscular dystrophy (DMD) cDNA and preliminary genomic organization of the DMD gene in normal and affected individuals. *Cell* 50, 509–517. doi: 10.1016/0092-8674(87)90504-6

Kostriken, R., Strathern, J. N., Klar, A. J., Hicks, J. B., and Heffron, F. (1983). A site-specific endonuclease essential for mating-type switching in *Saccharomyces cerevisiae*. *Cell* 35, 167–174. doi: 10.1016/0092-8674(83)90219-2

Kren, B. T., Bandyopadhyay, P., and Steer, C. J. (1998). *In vivo* site-directed mutagenesis of the factor IX gene by chimeric RNA/DNA oligonucleotides. *Nat. Med.* 4, 285–290. doi: 10.1038/nm0398-285

Kren, B. T., Metz, R., Kumar, R., and Steer, C. J. (1999a). Gene repair using chimeric RNA/DNA oligonucleotides. *Semin. Liver Dis.* 19, 93–104. doi: 10.1055/s-2007-1007101

Kren, B. T., Parashar, B., Bandyopadhyay, P., Chowdhury, N. R., Chowdhury, J. R., and Steer, C. J. (1999b). Correction of the UDP-glucuronosyltransferase gene defect in the gunn rat model of crigler-najjar syndrome type I with a chimeric oligonucleotide. *Proc. Natl. Acad. Sci. U.S.A.* 96, 10349–10354. doi: 10.1073/pnas.96.18.10349

Lee, J. Y., Qu-Petersen, Z., Cao, B., Kimura, S., Jankowski, R., Cummins, J., et al. (2000). Clonal isolation of muscle-derived cells capable of enhancing muscle regeneration and bone healing. *J. Cell Biol.* 150, 1085–1100. doi: 10.1083/jcb.150.5.1085

Lefebvre, S., Burglen, L., Reboullet, S., Clermont, O., Burlet, P., Viollet, L., et al. (1995). Identification and characterization of a spinal muscular atrophy-determining gene. *Cell* 80, 155–165. doi: 10.1016/0092-8674(95)90460-3

Lefebvre, S., Burlet, P., Liu, Q., Bertrandy, S., Clermont, O., Munnich, A., et al. (1997). Correlation between severity and SMN protein level in spinal muscular atrophy. *Nat. Genet.* 16, 265–269. doi: 10.1038/ng0797-265

Lei, Y., Lee, C. L., Joo, K. I., Zarzar, J., Liu, Y., Dai, B., et al. (2011). Gene editing of human embryonic stem cells via an engineered baculoviral vector carrying zinc-finger nucleases. *Mol. Ther.* 19, 942–950. doi: 10.1038/mt.2011.12

Lescop, C., Herzner, H., Siendt, H., Bolliger, R., Hennebohle, M., Weyermann, P., et al. (2005). Novel cell-penetrating alpha-keto-amide calpain inhibitors as potential treatment for muscular dystrophy. *Bioorg. Med. Chem. Lett.* 15, 5176–5181. doi: 10.1016/j.bmcl.2005.08.064

Le, T. T., Pham, L. T., Butchbach, M. E., Zhang, H. L., Monani, U. R., Coovert, D. D., et al. (2005). SMNDelta7, the major product of the centromeric survival motor neuron (SMN2) gene, extends survival in mice with spinal muscular atrophy and associates with full-length SMN. *Hum. Mol. Genet.* 14, 845–857. doi: 10.1093/hmg/ddi078

Li, T., Liu, B., Spalding, M. H., Weeks, D. P., and Yang, B. (2012). High-efficiency TALEN-based gene editing produces disease-resistant rice. *Nat. Biotechnol.* 30, 390–392. doi: 10.1038/nbt.2199

Liu, J., Li, C., Yu, Z., Huang, P., Wu, H., Wei, C., et al. (2012). Efficient and specific modifications of the Drosophila genome by means of an easy TALEN strategy. *J. Genet. Genomics* 39, 209–215. doi: 10.1016/j.jgg.2012.04.003

Liu, L., Parekh-Olmedo, H., and Kmiec, E. B. (2003). The development and regulation of gene repair. *Nat. Rev. Genet.* 4, 679–689. doi: 10.1038/nrg1156

Liu, L., Rice, M. C., Drury, M., Cheng, S., Gamper, H., and Kmiec, E. B. (2002). Strand bias in targeted gene repair is influenced by transcriptional activity. *Mol. Cell. Biol.* 22, 3852–3863. doi: 10.1128/MCB.22.11.3852-3863.2002

Liu, L., Rice, M. C., and Kmiec, E. B. (2001). *In vivo* gene repair of point and frameshift mutations directed by chimeric RNA/DNA oligonucleotides and modified single-stranded oligonucleotides. *Nucleic Acids Res.* 29, 4238–4250. doi: 10.1093/nar/29.20.4238

Lombardo, A., Genovese, P., Beausejour, C. M., Colleoni, S., Lee, Y. L., Kim, K. A., et al. (2007). Gene editing in human stem cells using zinc finger nucleases and integrase-defective lentiviral vector delivery. *Nat. Biotechnol.* 25, 1298–1306. doi: 10.1038/nbt1353

Maguire, K. K., and Kmiec, E. B. (2007). Multiple roles for MSH2 in the repair of a deletion mutation directed by modified single-stranded oligonucleotides. *Gene* 386, 107–114. doi: 10.1016/j.gene.2006.08.014

Maguire, K., Suzuki, T., DiMatteo, D., Parekh-Olmedo, H., and Kmiec, E. (2009). Genetic correction of splice site mutation in purified and enriched myoblasts isolated from mdx5cv mice. *BMC Mol. Biol.* 10:15. doi: 10.1186/1471-2199-10-15

Mahfouz, M. M., and Li, L. (2011). TALE nucleases and next generation GM crops. *GM Crops* 2, 99–103. doi: 10.4161/gmcr.2.2.17254

Mahfouz, M. M., Li, L., Shamimuzzaman, M., Wibowo, A., Fang, X., and Zhu, J. K. (2011). De novo-engineered transcription activator-like effector (TALE) hybrid nuclease with novel DNA binding specificity creates double-strand breaks. *Proc. Natl. Acad. Sci. U.S.A.* 108, 2623–2628. doi: 10.1073/pnas.1019533108

Mali, P., Yang, L., Esvelt, K. M., Aach, J., Guell, M., DiCarlo, J. E., et al. (2013). RNA-guided human genome engineering via Cas9. *Science* 339, 823–826. doi: 10.1126/science.1232033

Mani, M., Kandavelou, K., Dy, F. J., Durai, S., and Chandrasegaran,S. (2005). Design, engineering, and characterization of zinc finger nucleases. *Biochem. Biophys. Res. Commun.* 335, 447–457. doi: 10.1016/j.bbrc.2005.07.089

Marton, I., Zuker, A., Shklarman, E., Zeevi, V., Tovkach, A., Roffe, S., et al. (2010). Nontransgenic genome modification in plant cells. *Plant Physiol.* 154, 1079–1087. doi: 10.1104/pp.110.164806

Mashimo, T., Takizawa, A., Voigt, B., Yoshimi, K., Hiai, H., and Kuramoto, T. (2010). Generation of knockout rats with X-linked severe combined immunodeficiency (X-SCID) using zinc-finger nucleases. *PLoS ONE* 5:e8870. doi: 10.1371/journal.pone.0008870

Mauro, A. (1961). Satellite cell of skeletal muscle fibers. *J. Biophys. Biochem. Cytol.* 9, 493–495. doi: 10.1083/jcb.9.2.493

McCammon, J. M., and Amacher, S. L. (2010). Using zinc finger nucleases for efficient and heritable gene disruption in zebrafish. *Methods Mol. Biol.* 649, 281–298. doi: 10.1007/978-1-60761-753-2_18

Meng, X., Noyes, M. B., Zhu, L. J., Lawson, N. D., and Wolfe, S. A. (2008). Targeted gene inactivation in zebrafish using engineered zinc-finger nucleases. *Nat. Biotechnol.* 26, 695–701. doi: 10.1038/nbt1398

Menoret, S., Fontaniere, S., Jantz, D., Tesson, L., Thinard, R., Remy, S., et al. (2013). Generation of Rag1-knockout immunodeficient rats and mice using engineered meganucleases. *FASEB J.* 27, 703–711. doi: 10.1096/fj.12-219907

Metzger, M. J., McConnell-Smith, A., Stoddard, B. L., and Miller, A. D. (2011). Single-strand nicks induce homologous recombination with less toxicity than double-strand breaks using an AAV vector template. *Nucleic Acids Res.* 39, 926–935. doi: 10.1093/nar/gkq826

Meyer, M., de Angelis, M. H., Wurst, W., and Kuhn, R. (2010). Gene targeting by homologous recombination in mouse zygotes mediated by zinc-finger nucleases. *Proc. Natl. Acad. Sci. U.S.A.* 107, 15022–15026. doi: 10.1073/pnas.1009424107

Miller, J. C., Holmes, M. C., Wang, J., Guschin, D. Y., Lee, Y. L., Rupniewski, I., et al. (2007). An improved zinc-finger nuclease architecture for highly specific genome editing. *Nat. Biotechnol.* 25, 778–785. doi: 10.1038/nbt1319

Minasi, M. G., Riminucci, M., De, A. L., Borello, U., Berarducci, B., Innocenzi, A., et al. (2002). The meso-angioblast: a multipotent, self-renewing cell that originates from the dorsal aorta and differentiates into most mesodermal tissues. *Development* 129, 2773–2783.

Monaco, A. P., Neve, R. L., Colletti-Feener, C., Bertelson, C. J., Kurnit, D. M., and Kunkel, L. M. (1986). Isolation of candidate cDNAs for portions of the Duchenne muscular dystrophy gene. *Nature* 323, 646–650. doi: 10.1038/323646a0

Moore, F. E., Reyon, D., Sander, J. D., Martinez, S. A., Blackburn, J. S., Khayter, C., et al. (2012). Improved somatic mutagenesis in zebrafish using transcription activator-like effector nucleases (TALENs). *PLoS ONE* 7:e37877. doi: 10.1371/journal.pone.0037877

Morosetti, R., Mirabella, M., Gliubizzi, C., Broccolini, A., De, A. L., Tagliafico, E., et al. (2006). MyoD expression restores defective myogenic differentiation of human mesoangioblasts from inclusion-body myositis muscle. *Proc. Natl. Acad. Sci. U.S.A.* 103, 16995–17000. doi: 10.1073/pnas.0603386103

Morozov, V., and Wawrousek, E. F. (2008). Single-strand DNA-mediated targeted mutagenesis of genomic DNA in early mouse embryos is stimulated by Rad51/54 and by Ku70/86 inhibition. *Gene Ther.* 15, 468–472. doi: 10.1038/sj.gt.3303088

Morton, J., Davis, M. W., Jorgensen, E. M., and Carroll, D. (2006). Induction and repair of zinc-finger nuclease-targeted double-strand breaks in *Caenorhabditis elegans* somatic cells. *Proc. Natl. Acad. Sci. U.S.A* 103, 16370–16375. doi: 10.1073/pnas.0605633103

Moscou, M. J., and Bogdanove, A. J. (2009). A simple cipher governs DNA recognition by TAL effectors. *Science* 326, 1501. doi: 10.1126/science.1178817

Moulton, H. M. (2013). *In vivo* delivery of morpholino oligos by cell-penetrating peptides. *Curr. Pharm. Des.* 19, 2963–2969. doi: 10.2174/1381612811319160010

Moulton, H. M., Fletcher, S., Neuman, B. W., McClorey, G., Stein, D. A., Abes, S., et al. (2007). Cell-penetrating peptide-morpholino conjugates alter pre-mRNA splicing of DMD (Duchenne muscular dystrophy) and inhibit murine coronavirus replication *in vivo*. *Biochem. Soc. Trans.* 35, 826–828. doi: 10.1042/BST0350826

Munoz, I. G., Prieto, J., Subramanian, S., Coloma, J., Redondo, P., Villate, M., et al. (2011). Molecular basis of engineered meganuclease targeting of the endogenous human RAG1 locus. *Nucleic Acids Res.* 39, 729–743. doi: 10.1093/nar/gkq801

Nain, V., Sahi, S., and Verma, A. (2010). CPP-ZFN: a potential DNA-targeting anti-malarial drug. *Malar. J.* 9, 258. doi: 10.1186/1475-2875-9-258

Nickerson, H. D., and Colledge, W. H. (2003). A comparison of gene repair strategies in cell culture using a lacZ reporter system. *Gene Ther.* 10, 1584–1591. doi: 10.1038/sj.gt.3302049

Nickoloff, J. A., Chen, E. Y., and Heffron, F. (1986). A 24-base-pair DNA sequence from the MAT locus stimulates intergenic recombination in yeast. *Proc. Natl. Acad. Sci. U.S.A.* 83, 7831–7835. doi: 10.1073/pnas.83.20.7831

Nielsen, P. E. (2005). Gene targeting using peptide nucleic acid. *Methods Mol. Biol.* 288, 343–358.

Nik-Ahd, F., and Bertoni, C. (2014). *Ex vivo* gene editing of the dystrophin gene in muscle stem cells using peptide nucleic acid single stranded oligodeoxynucleotides (PNA-SsODNs) induces stable expression of dystrophin in a mouse model for Duchenne muscular dystrophy. *Stem Cells*. doi: 10.1002/stem.1668

Olsen, P. A., Randol, M., and Krauss, S. (2005a). Implications of cell cycle progression on functional sequence correction by short single-stranded DNA oligonucleotides. *Gene Ther.* 12, 546–551. doi: 10.1038/sj.gt.3302454

Olsen, P. A., Randol, M., Luna, L., Brown, T., and Krauss, S. (2005b). Genomic sequence correction by single-stranded DNA oligonucleotides: role of DNA synthesis and chemical modifications of the oligonucleotide ends. *J. Gene Med.* 7, 1534–1544. doi: 10.1002/jgm.804

Olsen, P. A., Solhaug, A., Booth, J. A., Gelazauskaite, M., and Krauss, S. (2009). Cellular responses to targeted genomic sequence modification using single-stranded oligonucleotides and zinc-finger nucleases. *DNA Repair (Amst)* 8, 298–308. doi: 10.1016/j.dnarep.2008.11.011

Ono, Y., Boldrin, L., Knopp, P., Morgan, J. E., and Zammit, P. S. (2010). Muscle satellite cells are a functionally heterogeneous population in both somite-derived and branchiomeric muscles. *Dev. Biol.* 337, 29–41. doi: 10.1016/j.ydbio.2009.10.005

Orr-Weaver, T. L., Szostak, J. W., and Rothstein, R. J. (1981). Yeast transformation: a model system for the study of recombination. *Proc. Natl. Acad. Sci. U.S.A.* 78, 6354–6358. doi: 10.1073/pnas.78.10.6354

Osakabe, K., Osakabe, Y., and Toki, S. (2010). Site-directed mutagenesis in Arabidopsis using custom-designed zinc finger nucleases. *Proc. Natl. Acad. Sci. U.S.A.* 107, 12034–12039. doi: 10.1073/pnas.1000234107

Osiak, A., Radecke, F., Guhl, E., Radecke, S., Dannemann, N., Lutge, F., et al. (2011). Selection-independent generation of gene knockout mouse embryonic stem cells using zinc-finger nucleases. *PLoS ONE* 6:e28911. doi: 10.1371/journal.pone.0028911

Ousterout, D. G., Perez-Pinera, P., Thakore, P. I., Kabadi, A. M., Brown, M. T., Qin, X., et al. (2013). Reading frame correction by targeted genome editing restores dystrophin expression in cells from Duchenne muscular dystrophy patients. *Mol. Ther.* 21, 1718–1726. doi: 10.1038/mt.2013.111

Pabo, C. O., Peisach, E., and Grant, R. A. (2001). Design and selection of novel Cys2His2 zinc finger proteins. *Annu. Rev. Biochem.* 70, 313–340. doi: 10.1146/annurev.biochem.70.1.313

Papaioannou, I., Disterer, P., and Owen, J. S. (2009). Use of internally nuclease-protected single-strand DNA oligonucleotides and silencing of the mismatch repair protein, MSH2, enhances the replication of corrected cells following gene editing. *J. Gene Med.* 11, 267–274. doi: 10.1002/jgm.1296

Papaioannou, I., Simons, J. P., and Owen, J. S. (2012). Oligonucleotide-directed gene-editing technology: mechanisms and future prospects. *Expert Opin. Biol Ther.* 12, 329–342. doi: 10.1517/14712598.2012.660522

Parekh-Olmedo, H., Drury, M., and Kmiec, E. B. (2002). Targeted Nucleotide exchange in Saccharomyces cerevisiae directed by short oligonucleotides containing locked nucleic acids. *Chem. Biol.* 9, 1073–1084. doi: 10.1016/S1074-5521(02)00236-3

Pauwels, K., Podevin, N., Breyer, D., Carroll, D., and Herman, P. (2013). Engineering nucleases for gene targeting: safety and regulatory considerations. *N. Biotechnol.* 31, 18–27. doi: 10.1016/j.nbt.2013.07.001

Pearson, H. (2008). Protein engineering: the fate of fingers. *Nature* 455, 160–164. doi: 10.1038/455160a

Peault, B., Rudnicki, M., Torrente, Y., Cossu, G., Tremblay, J. P., Partridge, T., et al. (2007). Stem and progenitor cells in skeletal muscle development, maintenance, and therapy. *Mol. Ther.* 15, 867–877. doi: 10.1038/mt.sj.6300145

Perez, E. E., Wang, J., Miller, J. C., Jouvenot, Y., Kim, K. A., Liu, O., et al. (2008). Establishment of HIV-1 resistance in CD4+ T cells by genome editing using zinc-finger nucleases. *Nat. Biotechnol.* 26, 808–816. doi: 10.1038/nbt1410

Pierce, E. A., Liu, Q., Igoucheva, O., Omarrudin, R., Ma, H., Diamond, S. L., et al. (2003). Oligonucleotide-directed single-base DNA alterations in mouse embryonic stem cells. *Gene Ther.* 10, 24–33. doi: 10.1038/sj.gt.3301857

Porteus, M. H., Cathomen, T., Weitzman, M. D., and Baltimore, D. (2003). Efficient gene targeting mediated by adeno-associated virus and DNA double-strand breaks. *Mol. Cell. Biol.* 23, 3558–3565. doi: 10.1128/MCB.23.10.3558-3565.2003

Puchta, H., and Fauser, F. (2013). Synthetic nucleases for genome engineering in plants: prospects for a bright future. *Plant J.* doi: 10.1111/tpj.12338. [Epub ahead of print].

Puria, R., Sahi, S., and Nain, V. (2012). HER2+ breast cancer therapy: by CPP-ZFN mediated targeting of mTOR? *Technol. Cancer Res. Treat.* 11, 175–180. doi: 10.7785/tcrt.2012.500247

Qi, Y., Zhang, Y., Zhang, F., Baller, J. A., Cleland, S. C., Ryu, Y., et al. (2013). Increasing frequencies of site-specific mutagenesis and gene targeting in Arabidopsis by manipulating DNA repair pathways. *Genome Res.* 23, 547–554. doi: 10.1101/gr.145557.112

Radecke, F., Radecke, S., and Schwarz, K. (2004). Unmodified oligodeoxynucleotides require single-strandedness to induce targeted repair of a chromosomal EGFP gene. *J. Gene Med.* 6, 1257–1271. doi: 10.1002/jgm.613

Radecke, S., Radecke, F., Peter, I., and Schwarz, K. (2006). Physical incorporation of a single-stranded oligodeoxynucleotide during targeted repair of a human chromosomal locus. *J. Gene Med.* 8, 217–228. doi: 10.1002/jgm.828

Rando, T. A., Disatnik, M. H., and Zhou, L. Z. (2000). Rescue of dystrophin expression in mdx mouse muscle by RNA/DNA oligonucleotides. *Proc. Natl. Acad. Sci. U.S.A.* 97, 5363–5368. doi: 10.1073/pnas.97.10.5363

Regberg, J., Eriksson, J. N., and Langel, U. (2013). Cell-penetrating peptides: from cell cultures to *in vivo* applications. *Front. Biosci. (Elite Ed.)* 5, 509–516. doi: 10.2741/E632

Rice, M. C., Bruner, M., Czymmek, K., and Kmiec, E. B. (2001). *In vitro* and *in vivo* nucleotide exchange directed by chimeric RNA/DNA oligonucleotides in Saccharomyces cerevisae 66. *Mol. Microbiol.* 40, 857–868. doi: 10.1046/j.1365-2958.2001.02407.x

Rice, M. C., May, G. D., Kipp, P. B., Parekh, H., and Kmiec, E. B. (2000). Genetic repair of mutations in plant cell-free extracts directed by specific chimeric oligonucleotides 70. *Plant Physiol.* 123, 427–438. doi: 10.1104/pp.123.2.427

Rivier, F., Alkan, O., Flint, A. F., Muskiewicz, K., Allen, P. D., Leboulch, P., et al. (2004). Role of bone marrow cell trafficking in replenishing skeletal muscle SP and MP cell populations. *J. Cell Sci.* 117, 1979–1988. doi: 10.1242/jcs.01051

Rocheteau, P., Gayraud-Morel, B., Siegl-Cachedenier, I., Blasco, M. A., and Tajbakhsh, S. (2012). A subpopulation of adult skeletal muscle stem cells retains all template DNA strands after cell division. *Cell* 148, 112–125. doi: 10.1016/j.cell.2011.11.049

Rosen, L. E., Morrison, H. A., Masri, S., Brown, M. J., Springstubb, B., Sussman, D., et al. (2006). Homing endonuclease I-CreI derivatives with novel DNA target specificities. *Nucleic Acids Res.* 34, 4791–4800. doi: 10.1093/nar/gkl645

Rouet, P., Smih, F., and Jasin, M. (1994). Introduction of double-strand breaks into the genome of mouse cells by expression of a rare-cutting endonuclease. *Mol. Cell. Biol* 14, 8096–8106.

Rousseau, J., Chapdelaine, P., Boisvert, S., Almeida, L. P., Corbeil, J., Montpetit, A., et al. (2011). Endonucleases: tools to correct the dystrophin gene. *J. Gene Med.* 13, 522–537. doi: 10.1002/jgm.1611

Sacco, A., Doyonnas, R., Kraft, P., Vitorovic, S., and Blau, H. M. (2008). Self-renewal and expansion of single transplanted muscle stem cells. *Nature* 456, 502–506. doi: 10.1038/nature07384

Sampaolesi, M., Blot, S., D'Antona, G., Granger, N., Tonlorenzi, R., Innocenzi, A., et al. (2006). Mesoangioblast stem cells ameliorate muscle function in dystrophic dogs. *Nature* 444, 574–579. doi: 10.1038/nature05282

Sampaolesi, M., Torrente, Y., Innocenzi, A., Tonlorenzi, R., D'Antona, G., Pellegrino, M. A., et al. (2003). Cell therapy of alpha-sarcoglycan null dystrophic mice through intra-arterial delivery of mesoangioblasts. *Science* 301, 487–492. doi: 10.1126/science.1082254

Sander, J. D., Cade, L., Khayter, C., Reyon, D., Peterson, R. T., Joung, J. K., et al. (2011a). Targeted gene disruption in somatic zebrafish cells using engineered TALENs. *Nat. Biotechnol.* 29, 697–698. doi: 10.1038/nbt.1934

Sander, J. D., Yeh, J. R., Peterson, R. T., and Joung, J. K. (2011b). Engineering zinc finger nucleases for targeted mutagenesis of zebrafish. *Methods Cell Biol.* 104, 51–58. doi: 10.1016/B978-0-12-374814-0.00003-3

Schultz, E. (1996). Satellite cell proliferative compartments in growing skeletal muscles. *Dev. Biol.* 175, 84–94. doi: 10.1006/dbio.1996.0097

Seale, P., Sabourin, L. A., Girgis-Gabardo, A., Mansouri, A., Gruss, P., and Rudnicki, M. A. (2000). Pax7 is required for the specification of myogenic satellite cells. *Cell* 102, 777–786. doi: 10.1016/S0092-8674(00)00066-0

Seligman, L. M., Chisholm, K. M., Chevalier, B. S., Chadsey, M. S., Edwards, S. T., Savage, J. H., et al. (2002). Mutations altering the cleavage specificity of a homing endonuclease. *Nucleic Acids Res.* 30, 3870–3879. doi: 10.1093/nar/gkf495

Shen, B., Zhang, X., Du, Y., Wang, J., Gong, J., Zhang, X., et al. (2013). Efficient knockin mouse generation by ssDNA oligonucleotides and zinc-finger nuclease assisted homologous recombination in zygotes. *PLoS ONE* 8:e77696. doi: 10.1371/journal.pone.0077696

Shukla, V. K., Doyon, Y., Miller, J. C., DeKelver, R. C., Moehle, E. A., Worden, S. E., et al. (2009). Precise genome modification in the crop species Zea mays using zinc-finger nucleases. *Nature* 459, 437–441. doi: 10.1038/nature07992

Sicinski, P., Geng, Y., Ryder-Cook, A. S., Barnard, E. A., Darlison, M. G., and Barnard, P. J. (1989). The molecular basis of muscular dystrophy in the mdx mouse: a point mutation. *Science* 244, 1578–1580. doi: 10.1126/science.2662404

Siebert, R., and Puchta, H. (2002). Efficient repair of genomic double-strand breaks by homologous recombination between directly repeated sequences in the plant genome. *Plant Cell* 14, 1121–1131. doi: 10.1105/tpc.001727

Smih, F., Rouet, P., Romanienko, P. J., and Jasin, M. (1995). Double-strand breaks at the target locus stimulate gene targeting in embryonic stem cells. *Nucleic Acids Res.* 23, 5012–5019. doi: 10.1093/nar/23.24.5012

Smith, J., Grizot, S., Arnould, S., Duclert, A., Epinat, J. C., Chames, P., et al. (2006). A combinatorial approach to create artificial homing endonucleases cleaving chosen sequences. *Nucleic Acids Res.* 34, e149. doi: 10.1093/nar/gkl720

Sorensen, C. B., Krogsdam, A. M., Andersen, M. S., Kristiansen, K., Bolund, L., and Jensen,T. G. (2005). Site-specific strand bias in gene correction using single-stranded oligonucleotides. *J. Mol. Med. (Berl.)* 83, 39–49. doi: 10.1007/s00109-004-0592-6

Tagalakis, A. D., Graham, I. R., Riddell, D. R., Dickson, J. G., and Owen, J. S. (2001). Gene correction of the apolipoprotein (Apo) E2 phenotype to wild-type ApoE3 by in situ chimeraplasty. *J. Biol. Chem.* 276, 13226–13230. doi: 10.1074/jbc.C000883200

Tang, W. (2013a). *Phase 1 Dose Escalation Study of Autologous T-cells Genetically Modified at the CCR5 Gene by Zinc Finger Nucleases in HIV-Infected Patients.* Available online at: http://clinicaltrials.gov/ct2/show/NCT01044654

Tang, W. (2013b). *Study of Autologous T-cells Genetically Modified at the CCR5 Gene by Zinc Finger Nucleases in HIV-Infected Subjects.* Available online at: http://clinicaltrials.gov/ct2/show/record/NCT01252641

Tebas, T., and Stein, D. (2013). *Autologous T-cells Genetically Modified at the CCR5 Gene by Zinc Finger Nucleases SB-728 for HIV (zinc-finger).* http://clinicaltrials.gov/ct2/show/NCT00842634

Tedesco, F. S., Gerli, M. F., Perani, L., Benedetti, S., Ungaro, F., Cassano, M., et al. (2012). Transplantation of genetically corrected human iPSC-derived progenitors in mice with limb-girdle muscular dystrophy. *Sci. Transl. Med.* 4, 140ra89. doi: 10.1126/scitranslmed.3003541

Tesson, L., Usal, C., Menoret, S., Leung, E., Niles, B. J., Remy, S., et al. (2011). Knockout rats generated by embryo microinjection of TALENs. *Nat. Biotechnol.* 29, 695–696. doi: 10.1038/nbt.1940

Thermes, V., Grabher, C., Ristoratore, F., Bourrat, F., Choulika, A., Wittbrodt, J., et al. (2002). I-SceI meganuclease mediates highly efficient transgenesis in fish. *Mech. Dev.* 118, 91–98. doi: 10.1016/S0925-4773(02)00218-6

Tong, C., Huang, G., Ashton, C., Wu, H., Yan, H., and Ying, Q. L. (2012). Rapid and cost-effective gene targeting in rat embryonic stem cells by TALENs. *J. Genet. Genomics* 39, 275–280. doi: 10.1016/j.jgg.2012.04.004

Torrente, Y., Belicchi, M., Sampaolesi, M., Pisati, F., Meregalli, M., D'Antona, G., et al. (2004). Human circulating AC133(+) stem cells restore dystrophin expression and ameliorate function in dystrophic skeletal muscle. *J. Clin. Invest* 114, 182–195. doi: 10.1172/JCI20325

Torrente, Y., Tremblay, J. P., Pisati, F., Belicchi, M., Rossi, B., Sironi, M., et al. (2001). Intraarterial injection of muscle-derived CD34(+)Sca-1(+) stem cells restores dystrophin in mdx mice. *J. Cell Biol.* 152, 335–348. doi: 10.1083/jcb.152.2.335

Tovkach, A., Zeevi, V., and Tzfira, T. (2009). A toolbox and procedural notes for characterizing novel zinc finger nucleases for genome editing in plant cells. *Plant J.* 57, 747–757. doi: 10.1111/j.1365-313X.2008.03718.x

Townsend, J. A., Wright, D. A., Winfrey, R. J., Fu, F., Maeder, M. L., Joung, J. K., et al. (2009). High-frequency modification of plant genes using engineered zinc-finger nucleases. *Nature* 459, 442–445. doi: 10.1038/nature07845

Urnov, F. D., Miller, J. C., Lee, Y. L., Beausejour, C. M., Rock, J. M., Augustus, S., et al. (2005). Highly efficient endogenous human gene correction using designed zinc-finger nucleases. *Nature* 435, 646–651. doi: 10.1038/nature03556

Wang, H., Yang, H., Shivalila, C. S., Dawlaty, M. M., Cheng, A. W., Zhang, F., et al. (2013). One-step generation of mice carrying mutations in multiple genes by CRISPR/Cas-mediated genome engineering. *Cell* 153, 910–918. doi: 10.1016/j.cell.2013.04.025

Wang, J., Friedman, G., Doyon, Y., Wang, N. S., Li, C. J., Miller, J. C., et al. (2012). Targeted gene addition to a predetermined site in the human genome using a ZFN-based nicking enzyme. *Genome Res.* 22, 1316–1326. doi: 10.1101/gr.122879.111

Wood, A. J., Lo, T. W., Zeitler, B., Pickle, C. S., Ralston, E. J., Lee, A. H., et al. (2011). Targeted genome editing across species using ZFNs and TALENs. *Science* 333, 307. doi: 10.1126/science.1207773

Wu, B., Moulton, H. M., Iversen, P. L., Jiang, J., Li, J., Li, J., et al. (2008). Effective rescue of dystrophin improves cardiac function in dystrophin-deficient mice by a modified morpholino oligomer. *Proc. Natl. Acad. Sci U.S.A.* 105, 14814–14819. doi: 10.1073/pnas.0805676105

Yin, H., Moulton, H. M., Seow, Y., Boyd, C., Boutilier, J., Iverson, P., et al. (2008). Cell-penetrating peptide-conjugated antisense oligonucleotides restore systemic muscle and cardiac dystrophin expression and function. *Hum. Mol. Genet.* 17, 3909–3918. doi: 10.1093/hmg/ddn293

Yin, H., Price, F., and Rudnicki, M. A. (2013). Satellite cells and the muscle stem cell niche. *Physiol. Rev.* 93, 23–67. doi: 10.1152/physrev.00043.2011

Zhang, F., Maeder, M. L., Unger-Wallace, E., Hoshaw, J. P., Reyon, D., Christian, M., et al. (2010). High frequency targeted mutagenesis in Arabidopsis thaliana using zinc finger nucleases. *Proc. Natl. Acad. Sci. U.S.A.* 107, 12028–12033. doi: 10.1073/pnas.0914991107

Zhu, C., Smith, T., McNulty, J., Rayla, A. L., Lakshmanan, A., Siekmann, A. F., et al. (2011). Evaluation and application of modularly assembled zinc-finger nucleases in zebrafish. *Development* 138, 4555–4564. doi: 10.1242/dev.066779

Zhu, T., Mettenburg, K., Peterson, D. J., Tagliani, L., and Baszczynski, C. L. (2000). Engineering herbicide-resistant maize using chimeric RNA/DNA oligonucleotides. *Nat. Biotechnol.* 18, 555–558. doi: 10.1038/75435

Zhu, T., Peterson, D. J., Tagliani, L., St Clair, G., Baszczynski, C. L., and Bowen, B. (1999). Targeted manipulation of maize genes *in vivo* using chimeric RNA/DNA oligonucleotides. *Proc. Natl. Acad. Sci. U.S.A.* 96, 8768–8773. doi: 10.1073/pnas.96.15.8768

Zou, J., Maeder, M. L., Mali, P., Pruett-Miller, S. M., Thibodeau-Beganny, S., Chou, B. K., et al. (2009). Gene targeting of a disease-related gene in human induced pluripotent stem and embryonic stem cells. *Cell Stem Cell* 5, 97–110. doi: 10.1016/j.stem.2009.05.023

Zou, J., Sweeney, C. L., Chou, B. K., Choi, U., Pan, J., Wang, H., et al. (2011). Oxidase-deficient neutrophils from X-linked chronic granulomatous disease iPS cells: functional correction by zinc finger nuclease-mediated safe harbor targeting. *Blood* 117, 5561–5572. doi: 10.1182/blood-2010-12-328161

8

Structural alterations of skeletal muscle in COPD

Sunita Mathur[1], Dina Brooks[1] and Celso R. F. Carvalho[2]*

[1] Department of Physical Therapy, University of Toronto, Toronto, ON, Canada
[2] Department of Physical Therapy, University of São Paulo, São Paulo, Brazil

***Correspondence:**
Celso R. F. Carvalho, Department of Physical Therapy, University of São Paulo, Av Dr Arnaldo 455 room 1210, São Paulo, Brazil
e-mail: cscarval@usp.br

Background: Chronic obstructive pulmonary disease (COPD) is a respiratory disease associated with a systemic inflammatory response. Peripheral muscle dysfunction has been well characterized in individuals with COPD and results from a complex interaction between systemic and local factors.

Objective: In this narrative review, we will describe muscle wasting in people with COPD, the associated structural changes, muscle regenerative capacity and possible mechanisms for muscle wasting. We will also discuss how structural changes relate to impaired muscle function and mobility in people with COPD.

Key Observations: Approximately 30–40% of individuals with COPD experience muscle mass depletion. Furthermore, muscle atrophy is a predictor of physical function and mortality in this population. Associated structural changes include a decreased proportion and size of type-I fibers, reduced oxidative capacity and mitochondrial density mainly in the quadriceps. Observations related to impaired muscle regenerative capacity in individuals with COPD include a lower proportion of central nuclei in the presence or absence of muscle atrophy and decreased maximal telomere length, which has been correlated with reduced muscle cross-sectional area. Potential mechanisms for muscle wasting in COPD may include excessive production of reactive oxygen species (ROS), altered amino acid metabolism and lower expression of peroxisome proliferator-activated receptors-gamma-coactivator 1-alpha mRNA. Despite a moderate relationship between muscle atrophy and function, impairments in oxidative metabolism only seems weakly related to muscle function.

Conclusion: This review article demonstrates the cellular modifications in the peripheral muscle of people with COPD and describes the evidence of its relationship to muscle function. Future research will focus on rehabilitation strategies to improve muscle wasting and maximize function.

Keywords: COPD, skeletal muscle, deconditioning, muscle fiber types, mytochondria, protein balance

INTRODUCTION

Chronic obstructive pulmonary disease (COPD) is the fourth leading cause of death worldwide and presents a major burden of disease in middle and high-income countries (World Health Organization, 2008). COPD is primarily a disease of the respiratory system and is diagnosed based on abnormal lung function evaluated by spirometry (low forced expiratory volume); and symptoms such as dyspnea, chronic cough and/or sputum production (Vestbo et al., 2013). However, impairments in lung function and breathing only explain one aspect of the disability experienced by individuals with COPD. There are several secondary consequences of COPD and skeletal muscle dysfunction poses a key limitation in these patients. In fact, muscle mass has been shown to be an independent predictor of mortality from lung function in people with COPD (Marquis et al., 2002; Schols et al., 2005). Muscle size and muscle strength are also associated with important clinical outcomes such as reduced quality of life (Mostert et al., 2000), greater healthcare resource utilization (Decramer et al., 1996) and exercise intolerance in this population (Hamilton et al., 1995; Gosselink et al., 1996).

The concept that skeletal muscle dysfunction could be an important limitation to exercise capacity in people with COPD was first described by Killian et al. (1992) in a study where the symptoms limiting peak exercise capacity were systematically assessed using ratings of perceived exertion. Approximately 40% of people with COPD had an early termination of exercise due to symptoms of leg fatigue which were greater than their rating of shortness of breath at the end of a progressive exercise test; and in another 30% of patients, ratings of leg fatigue and dyspnea were equal. These findings led to further investigations of skeletal muscle dysfunction in people with COPD including examinations of muscle fiber typing (Jobin et al., 1998; Whittom et al., 1998), mitochondrial enzyme concentrations (Maltais et al., 2000), muscle metabolism (Kutsuzawa et al., 1995), functional deficits in muscle strength (Gosselink et al., 2000) and endurance (Serres et al., 1998) and the relationship between muscle function and peak exercise capacity (Hamilton et al., 1995; Gosselink et al., 1996). The early literature on skeletal muscle dysfunction in COPD was summarized in a comprehensive review by the American Thoracic Society and European

Respiratory Society (ATS/ERS, 1999). The body of literature on skeletal muscle dysfunction has continued to explode and recent studies suggest that about one third of patients with COPD exhibit quadriceps muscle weakness (Seymour et al., 2010) and that muscle weakness and muscle atrophy are observed not only in moderate to severe disease but also earlier in the course of the disease (Seymour et al., 2010; Shrikrishna et al., 2012; Kelly et al., 2013).

Several factors are thought to contribute to the development of skeletal muscle dysfunction in people with COPD. Low physical inactivity or the effects of chronic deconditioning is likely a major factor contributing to muscle dysfunction in patients with COPD, who tend to be sedentary (Pitta et al., 2005; Watz et al., 2009). Although a causal link between inactivity and muscle dysfunction is difficult to establish in COPD, low physical activity has been associated with quadriceps muscle wasting even in people with mild airflow obstruction (Shrikrishna et al., 2012). Typically, muscle disuse atrophy has a pattern of inducing greater lower limb atrophy and weakness compared to upper limb (de Boer et al., 2008; Pisot et al., 2008). This pattern has also been observed in people with COPD where hadgrip strength tends to be better preserved than lower limb strength (Gosselink et al., 2000; Heijdra et al., 2003). Furthermore, studies examining muscle strength during and after an acute exacerbation of COPD, demonstrate that muscle weakness is apparent as early as the third day of the exacerbation (Spruit et al., 2003) and further decreased by about 5% after 5 days of hospitalization. The result of this study also showed that handgrip force also declined during the hospitalization initially, but did not decline further with longer hospitalization as it did for quadriceps force (Spruit et al., 2003).These finding suggests that muscle disuse is an important factor contributing to weakness in people with COPD.

Other factors that are associated with skeletal muscle dysfunction include the use of oral corticosteroid medications that causes "steroid-induced myopathy" in COPD (Decramer et al., 1996); low circulation testosterone (Van Vliet et al., 2005); hypoxemia (Koechlin et al., 2005), nutritional depletion (Engelen et al., 1994), oxidative stress (Couillard et al., 2003) and systemic inflammation (Spruit et al., 2003). Exposure to tobacco smoke, the main cause of COPD, is also recognized to contribute to muscle dysfunction even prior to the development of lung disease. In an observational study of over a 1000 healthy young adults (21–36 years old), an inverse relationship between smoking tobacco and knee extensor muscle strength was reported (Kok et al., 2012). Furthermore, this study demonstrated that 100 g of tobacco a week resulted in a reduction of 3% in muscle strength in men and 5% in women and this association existed independently of lifestyle physical fitness and body fat percentage (Kok et al., 2012). In addition, an inverse relationship between smoking tobacco and increased fatigability (Wüst et al., 2008) and muscle fiber atrophy (Montes de Oca et al., 2008) has also been described in non-COPD smokers. These results clearly demonstrate that smoking has an adverse effect of muscle function even in healthy subjects without COPD diagnosis. The combination of these factors likely leads to the complex set of adaptations that is observed in the peripheral muscles of people with COPD.

The purpose of this narrative review is to describe structural changes in skeletal muscle of people with COPD and describe the main mechanisms hypothesized to contribute to muscle atrophy. The relationship between skeletal muscle dysfunction to physical function and mobility will also be discussed.

STRUCTURAL CHANGES IN THE SKELETAL MUSCLE

SKELETAL MUSCLE ATROPHY IN COPD

Approximately 30–40% of people with COPD experience muscle atrophy (Schols et al., 1993; Engelen et al., 1994; Vermeeren et al., 2006) and a proportion of these patients may present normal body mass since the amount of fat mass is relatively maintained (Engelen et al., 1999; Eid et al., 2001; Vermeeren et al., 2006). Loss of muscle mass has been observed at the whole body level using D-XA and bioelectrical impedance measures, at the level of individual muscles using computed tomography (Bernard et al., 1998), magnetic resonance imaging (Mathur et al., 2007, 2008) and ultrasound (Seymour et al., 2010), as well as from muscle biopsy studies (Whittom et al., 1998; Gosker et al., 2002a,b). In an early study by Marquis et al. (2002), it was found that mid-thigh cross-sectional area measured using CT was a stronger predictor of mortality than lung function (FEV_1) in a large cohort of patients with moderate to severe COPD. Similarly Schols et al. (2005) found that fat-free mass but not fat mass was an independent predictor of survival.

Muscle atrophy has important consequences for mobility, as muscle strength and power are closely related with muscle size. Furthermore, the loss of muscle mass and quality have been shown to have important multi-system consequences in other chronic disease conditions. For example in diabetes, muscle atrophy and fat infiltration is associated with poor glucose tolerance (Goodpaster et al., 2003) and may also be related to the immunologic status of an individual (Jo et al., 2012). These multi-system issues require further attention in the COPD population. The mechanism of muscle atrophy and how it may be accelerated in people with COPD is a growing area of investigation.

MUSCLE FIBER TYPE

The first study evaluating peripheral muscle fiber types in people with COPD was performed by Hughes et al. (1983) using biopsy analyses from the quadriceps of patients with moderate COPD. While they did not observe any change in fiber type proportions, they observed a significant atrophy in the type II fibers that was associated with weight loss. Since then, several studies have quantified changes in proportion and size in skeletal muscle fiber types of the lower limb of COPD and they have mainly focused in the vastus lateralis (VL) muscle. Jakobsson et al. (1990) showed a reduced percentage of type I fibers in the quadriceps, which was confirmed by the findings of Whittom et al. (1998). Another study in patients with COPD reported fiber-type analysis by quantifying myosin heavy-chain (MHC) and myosin light-chain (MLC) isoforms and observed a significantly greater proportion of MHC-2B in the VL compared with control subjects (Satta et al., 1997). They also observed that the pattern of distribution of MLC isoforms was shifted toward fast isoforms in COPD patients. A meta-analysis established a pathological proportion of slow to fast fiber types in people with COPD patients aged 60–70 years old. The authors evaluated eight studies with 84 patients and determined that, compared with reference values, a proportion of type I fibers less than 27% and of type IIX fibers greater than 29% in the VL could be defined as pathological (Gosker et al., 2007b). Gosker et al. suggested that COPD patients present a reduction in the type I fibers that is strongly associated with the severity of the disease.

Although the precise causes for such changes is not fully understood, it has been suggested that multiple factors such as hypoxemia and long-term disuse are related to the higher proportion of type II fibers. Hildebrand et al. (1991) reported that the high proportion of type II fibers was positively correlated with hypoxemia suggesting this may be a factor underlying muscle fiber differentiation in COPD (Hildebrand et al., 1991). It also appears that these changes are more profound in the lower limb muscles since no changes have been observed in the proportion of type I fibers of the biceps brachii muscle of people with severe COPD and matched control subjects (Sato et al., 1997); which suggests that disuse may play a role in fiber type changes in COPD.

METABOLIC ENZYMES

There is substantial evidence to suggest a decrease in the activity of key oxidative enzymes in peripheral muscles of COPD patients, such as citrate synthase and succinate dehydrogenase. Muscle biopsy from the VL muscle in people with severe COPD have demonstrated lower oxidative enzyme activity compared with healthy subjects; however, no significant difference was observed in the activity of the glycolytic enzyme between COPD and controls (Jakobsson et al., 1995; Maltais et al., 1996). Other studies have found increased activity of glycolytic enzymes such as phosphofructokinase (Whittom et al., 1998). It has been also suggested that hypoxemia contributes to these metabolic alterations in people with COPD; however, no reversal in the activities of any enzyme was observed even after long-term oxygen therapy (Jakobsson et al., 1995). Interestingly, muscle cytochrome oxidase activity is inversely related to arterial oxygen levels (PaO_2) in COPD patients what suggests a compensatory response to reduced O_2 availability to augment ATP production (Wagner, 2006).

MUSCLE CAPILLARITY

The oxidative metabolism in skeletal muscle is dependent on mitochondrial volume, density and activity and on muscle blood supply, therefore alterations in the muscle capillary network or mitochondria can lead to decreased exercise tolerance in COPD. A study by Simard et al. (1996) reported that the number of capillaries per surface area in the VL of patients with COPD was 53% lower than in age-matched normal subjects. Similarly, Jobin et al. (1998) observed a lower number of capillaries per square millimeter and lower ratio of capillaries per fiber ratio in COPD patients compared with controls. However, when normalized for fiber cross-sectional area, the number of capillary contacts per fiber were similar between patients with COPD and control subjects. A possible explanation for the reduced number of capillaries could be hypoxemia; however, patients from Jobin's study did not present with marked hypoxemia either at rest or during exercise. Only recently, Eliason et al. (2010) provided evidence of a disturbed muscle-to-capillary interface in COPD patients and a positive correlation between the degree of muscle capillarization, airflow obstruction and exercise capacity. The authors also showed that muscle capillarization decreased with the severity of the disease. Hypoxemia may be a possible explanation for the reduced vascularization. This hypothesis is strengthened by findings that COPD patients present an overexpression of the von Hippel-Lindau tumor suppression protein (Jatta et al., 2009) that lead to an adverse effect on tissue capillarization and impair the transduction of hypoxic-angiogenetic transcription factors such as vascular endothelial growth factor (Kondo and Kaelin, 2001).

MITOCHONDRIA DYSFUNCTION

Although cardiac output and ventilatory limitation have been observed during exercise in COPD patients (Cuttica et al., 2011), there is a noteworthy observation that the oxidative capacity of peripheral skeletal muscle is significant and remains reduced even following lung transplantation (Lands et al., 1999). Several studies have suggested that mitochondrial dysfunction exists in people with COPD. At least three changes in mitochondria have been suggested: an impairment in density and biogenesis, increased oxidative stress and apoptosis (Meyer et al., 2013). Gosker et al. (2007a) reported a reduction in the mitochondrial area along with reduced proportion of type I fibers suggesting that the reduction in the number of mitochondria might be related to changes slow type fibers. The role of oxidative stress in mitochondrial dysfunction was observed by Puente-Maestu et al. (2012) and recently reviewed by Kirkham and Barnes (2013). The highest sources of reactive oxygen species (ROS) are the alveolar macrophages and activated neutrophils from the circulation that release superoxide radicals and hydrogen peroxide. ROS are chemically reactive molecules containing oxygen, and include oxygen ions and peroxides. These are natural byproducts of normal oxygen metabolism and have important roles in cell signaling and homeostasis. In addition, mitochondrial respiration can also generate ROS due to the constant exposure to sources of inflammatory responses to bacterial and viral infections within the lungs. For instance, airway epithelial cells exposed to lipid soluble components from the tobacco induce the production of mitochondria-derived ROS (van der Toorn et al., 2009). Mitochondrial dysfunction has also been described in the airway epithelium of chronic cigarette smokers. Hoffmann and coworkers evaluated changes in mitochondrial morphology and expression of markers for mitochondrial capacity in the human bronchial epithelial cell line from ex-smokers with COPD (GOLD stage IV) and compared with age-matched smoking and never-smoking controls. Their results demonstrated that long-term cigarette smoking induces robust and persistent changes in mitochondrial structure and function in human bronchial epithelial cells, including increased fragmentation, branching, density of the matrix and reduced numbers of cristae. Interestingly, they also showed that most of these changes persisted upon smoking cessation. The authors speculated that an attenuated antioxidant response with elevated ROS in COPD may lead to an increased oxidant burden, possibly contributing to the observed mitochondrial defects in bronchial epithelial cells from COPD patients (Hoffmann et al., 2013). Hara and colleagues compared mitochondrial morphology in lung tissues from smokers without COPD and from COPD patients (Hara et al., 2013). Analyzing the electron microscopic of lung tissues, they demonstrated that mitochondria in bronchial epithelial cells tended to be fragmented in COPD but not in smokers without COPD, suggesting the fission process dominancy of mitochondrial dynamics in COPD pathogenesis. Tobacco smoke can also affect mitochondrial function in skeletal muscle. There is evidence that carbon monoxide has a direct inhibitory effect *in vitro* on cytochrome *c* oxidase (an enzyme related to the ATP synthesis in the mitochondria) activity in the human VL (Alonso et al., 2003); as well as its classical effect of oxygen depletion (Young and Caughey, 1990). Tobacco smoke may also act on muscle mitochondria through an increased expression of tumor necrosis factor-α (Tang et al., 2010).

MECHANISMS OF MUSCLE ATROPHY IN COPD

There are several interactive mechanisms that may contribute to the underlying development of muscle wasting in people with COPD. For a thorough review of the pathways leading to muscle atrophy, the reader to referred to the review by Langen et al. (2013). We present a brief overview of the major mechanisms that have been studied to date in the section below.

REGULATION OF MYONUCLEAR TURNOVER

Muscle apoptosis was hypothesized to be one factor underlying the development of muscle atrophy in COPD, however there are limited data in this area. Agusti et al. (2002) found that TUNEL positive nuclei were higher in people with COPD who had a low BMI; and there was an inverse relationship between TUNEL and BMI. However, specific measures of muscle size were not included in this study. Barreiro et al. (2011) found a relationship between muscle mass and apoptotic nuclei in people with severe COPD but no difference in caspase-3 between the COPD patients and healthy controls. Lastly, Gosker et al. (2003) found no evidence of active caspase-3 in muscle fibers of people with COPD and TUNEL-positive fibers were similar between people with COPD and healthy controls. However, the authors did report changes in the muscle fibers indicative of impaired muscle regenerative capacity such as the presence of fibrosis and adipocyte replacement in the muscle tissue.

There are some data to suggest that muscle regenerative capacity may be impaired in people with COPD. Theriault et al. (2012) described significantly shorter telomere lengths in people with COPD with low mid-thigh cross-sectional area. Also, people with COPD who had relatively preserved muscle mass had a significantly higher proportion of central nuclei, indicating past muscle regeneration. Although these results were based on a limited sample of 16 patients with COPD, they provide some evidence for exhausted muscle regenerative capacity in people with COPD who present with low muscle mass. Other markers of muscle regeneration such as Myf5, MyoD and myogenin have been shown to be similar between COPD patients and controls (Plant et al., 2010); whereas other studies have found a difference in these factors between COPD patients and controls; and between cachetic and non-cachetic patients with COPD (Vogiatzis et al., 2010; Fermoselle et al., 2012). Myostatin, an inhibitor of muscle growth, has been shown to be higher in COPD patients compared with controls (Man et al., 2010; Plant et al., 2010; Ju and Chen, 2012).

REGULATION OF PROTEIN BALANCE

Muscle mass is regulated through a balance of protein synthesis and degradation. In COPD, it is not clear whether protein synthesis is downregulated, protein degradation is upregulated or whether muscle mass depletion is a result of both processes. One of the proteolytic systems which has been studied in COPD is the ubiquitin-protease system. There is evidence for increased activation of this system in people with COPD, which may contribute to muscle wasting (Fermoselle et al., 2012; Lemire et al., 2012). People with COPD who exhibit muscle atrophy also have increased levels of atrogin-1 and MuRF-1 (muscle ring finger 1), both of which regulators of muscle atrophy (Plant et al., 2010; Lemire et al., 2012) as well as regulators FOXO-1 and FOXO-3 (Doucet et al., 2007; Debigare et al., 2010). The autophagy-lysosome pathway has also been hypothesized to be a factor in protein degrading leading to muscle wasting in people with COPD (Hussain and Sandri, 2013). A recent study found evidence for autophagy in the VL and tibialis anterior muscles of people with COPD (Guo et al., 2013). The number of autophagosomes was also inversely correlated with FEV_1; and the degree of lipidation of the LCB3 protein was associated with low thigh muscle cross-sectional area. Further studies are needed to understand the contributions of the ubiquitin-proteasome pathway and autophagy-lysosome pathway in muscle wasting in COPD.

In terms of protein synthesis, the IGF-1-Akt pathway has been studied in people with COPD, however the results are conflicting. Circulating levels of IGF-1 have been shown to be similar between people with COPD and controls across disease severities (Piehl-Aulin et al., 2009) and in cachetic vs. non-cachetic patients with COPD (Debigare et al., 2003). However, during periods of acute exacerbation, IGF-1 levels have been shown to be decreased (Crul et al., 2007). The discrepancy in findings may be due to heterogeneous patient samples and stability of the disease; periods of acute exacerbation for example, are known to result in muscle atrophy.

CLINICAL RELEVANCE OF MUSCLE ATROPHY IN COPD

Reduced exercise capacity, poor quality of life, difficulty with activities of daily living and recurrent acute exacerbation are not simply the consequence of pulmonary impairment, but also impacted by peripheral muscle dysfunction.

Although a causal relationship has not been established, significant association have been observed between measures of muscle function, lung function and exercise performance. Lower quadriceps strength is correlated with lower FEV_1 (Bernard et al., 1998). In addition, lower extremity muscle strength is significantly correlated with the 6-min walking distance, incremental shuttle walk performance, maximal oxygen update and symptoms on incremental exercise test but not endurance shuttle walking test performance (Hamilton et al., 1995; Gosselink et al., 1996; Saey et al., 2003; Steiner et al., 2005). More specifically, reduced fat free mass is correlated with decreased walking distance and maximal oxygen uptake (Schols et al., 1991; Baarends et al., 1997).

Reduced limb muscle strength also contributes to increased dyspnea, poor quality of life and health status (Shoup et al., 1997; Mostert et al., 2000); whereas improvement in muscle strength result in better in quality of life (Simpson et al., 1992). Furthermore, quadriceps wasting is independently associated with lower levels of physical activity in early COPD disease (Shrikrishna et al., 2012). In addition, there is a tendency for patients with muscle wasting to have higher depression scores than those without wasting (Chavannes et al., 2005; Al-shair et al., 2009) although the direction of the relationship is not known. On one hand, depression could result in altered appetite and decrease physical activity contributing to muscle wasting. On the other, muscle wasting could impact the ability to perform activities of daily living as well as community integration and therefore lead to depression and isolation.

Although lower extremity strength has received most of the attention, upper extremity strength is also compromised in individuals with COPD. The force-generating capacity of upper limb muscles are reduced in patients with COPD compared to healthy control (Gosselink et al., 2000). Specifically, arm elevation affects lung volume and respiratory muscles resulting in reduction in force-generating capacity (Janaudis-Ferreira et al., 2009). The reduction in upper extremity muscle strength in COPD contributes to difficulties in performing arm activities.

Finally, there is increasing evidence of impaired postural control in patients with COPD (Butcher et al., 2004; Beauchamp et al., 2009; Roig et al., 2009). Although the underlying mechanisms for reduced postural control among individuals with COPD remain unclear, many hypotheses have been proposed, including decreased levels of physical activity, peripheral muscle weakness and altered trunk muscle mechanics among others (Butcher et al., 2004; Beauchamp et al., 2009; Roig et al., 2009). Thus, skeletal muscle dysfunction may play an important role in the balance impairment in individuals with COPD.

Impaired exercise capacity and peripheral muscle dysfunction contribute to increased mortality and reduced health status, even when accounting for age and lung function status (Marquis et al., 2002; Schols et al., 2005). Specifically, mid-thigh muscle cross sectional area, an index of muscle mass has a strong impact on mortality in individuals with FEV1 of less than 50% (Schols et al., 2005). Although lower body mass index is a predictor of mortality in individuals with COPD, loss of muscle has more implications for survival than loss in other compartments (Schols et al., 2005). Decramer et al. (1997) also found that lower quadriceps muscle force was more strongly associated with higher utilization of health care resources compared to pulmonary function and exercise capacity.

CONCLUSION

Despite COPD being primarily a respiratory disease, these individuals present with important secondary dysfunction in their peripheral muscles characterized by muscle atrophy alterations in muscle fiber type, fiber composition as well as reduction in oxidative enzymatic activity, capillarity and mitochondrial dysfunction. These muscle changes have important clinical consequences such as impaired exercise tolerance, low physical activity and quality of life in people with COPD.

REFERENCES

Agusti, A. G., Sauleda, J., Miralles, C., Gomez, C., Togores, B., Sala, E., et al. (2002). Skeletal muscle apoptosis and weight loss in chronic obstructive pulmonary disease. *Am. J. Respir. Crit. Care Med.* 166, 485–489. doi: 10.1164/rccm.2108013

Alonso, J. R., Cardellach, F., Lopez, S., Casademont, J., and Miro, O. (2003). Carbon monoxide specifically inhibits cytochrome c oxidase of human mitochondrial respiratory chain. *Pharmacol. Toxicol.* 93, 142–146. doi: 10.1034/j.1600-0773.2003.930306.x

Al-shair, K., Dockry, R., Mallia-Milanes, B., Kolsum, U., Singh, D., and Vestbo, J. (2009). Depression and its relationship with poor exercise capacity, BODE index and muscle wasting in COPD. *Respir. Med.* 103, 1572–1579. doi: 10.1016/j.rmed.2008.11.021

ATS/ERS. (1999). Skeletal muscle dysfunction in chronic obstructive pulmonary disease. A statement of the American Thoracic Society and European Respiratory Society. *Am. J. Respir. Crit. Care Med.* 159, S1–S40.

Baarends, E. M., Schols, A. M., Mostert, R., and Wouters, E. F. (1997). Peak exercise response in relation to tissue depletion in patients with chronic obstructive pulmonary disease. *Eur. Respir. J.* 10, 2807–2813. doi: 10.1183/09031936.97.10122807

Barreiro, E., Ferrer, D., Sanchez, F., Minguella, J., Marin-Corral, J., Martinez-Llorens, J., et al. (2011). Inflammatory cells and apoptosis in respiratory and limb muscles of patients with COPD. *J. Appl. Physiol.* 111, 808–817. doi: 10.1152/japplphysiol.01017.2010

Beauchamp, M. K., Hill, K., Goldstein, R. S., Janaudis-Ferreira, T., and Brooks, D. (2009). Impairments in balance discriminate fallers from non-fallers in COPD. *Respir. Med.* 103, 1885–1891. doi: 10.1016/j.rmed.2009.06.008

Bernard, S., LeBlanc, P., Whittom, F., Carrier, G., Jobin, J., Belleau, R., et al. (1998). Peripheral muscle weakness in patients with chronic obstructive pulmonary disease. *Am. J. Respir. Crit. Care Med.* 158, 629–634. doi: 10.1164/ajrccm.158.2.9711023

Butcher, S. J., Meshke, J. M., and Sheppard, M. S. (2004). Reductions in functional balance, coordination, and mobility measures among patients with stable chronic obstructive pulmonary disease. *J. Cardiopulm. Rehabil.* 24:274e80. doi: 10.1097/00008483-200407000-00013

Chavannes, N. H., Huibers, M. J., Schermer, T. R., Hendriks, A., van Weel, C., Wouters, E. F., et al. (2005). Associations of depressive symptoms with gender, body mass index and dyspnea in primary care COPD patients. *Fam. Pract.* 22, 604–607. doi: 10.1093/fampra/cmi056

Couillard, A., Maltais, F., Saey, D., Debigare, R., Michaud, A., Koechlin, C., et al. (2003). Exercise-induced quadriceps oxidative stress and peripheral muscle dysfunction in patients with chronic obstructive pulmonary disease. *Am. J. Respir. Crit. Care Med.* 167, 1664–1669. doi: 10.1164/rccm.200209-1028OC

Crul, T., Spruit, M. A., Gayan-Ramirez, G., Quarck, R., Gosselink, R., Troosters, T., et al. (2007). Markers of inflammation and disuse in vastus lateralis of chronic obstructive pulmonary disease patients. *Eur. J. Clin. Invest.* 37, 897–904. doi: 10.1111/j.1365-2362.2007.01867.x

Cuttica, M. J., Shah, S. J., Rosenberg, S. R., Orr, R., Beussink, L., Dematte, J. E., et al. (2011). Right heart structural changes are independently associated with exercise capacity in non-severe COPD. *PLoS ONE* 6:e29069. doi: 10.1371/journal.pone.0029069

Debigare, R., Cote, C. H., and Maltais, F. (2010). Ubiquitination and proteolysis in limb and respiratory muscles of patients with chronic obstructive pulmonary disease. *Proc. Am. Thorac. Soc.* 7, 84–90. doi: 10.1513/pats.200906-051JS

Debigare, R., Marquis, K., Cote, C. H., Tremblay, R. R., Michaud, A., LeBlanc, P., et al. (2003). Catabolic/anabolic balance and muscle wasting in patients with COPD. *Chest* 124, 83–89. doi: 10.1378/chest.124.1.83

de Boer, M. D., Seynnes, O. R., di Prampero, P. E., Pisot, R., Mekjaviæ, I. B., Biolo, G., et al. (2008). Effect of 5 weeks horizontal bed rest on human muscle thickness and architecture of weight bearing and non-weight bearing muscles. *Eur. J. Appl. Physiol.* 104, 401–407. doi: 10.1007/s00421-008-0703-0

Decramer, M., de Bock, V., and Dom, R. (1996). Functional and histologic picture of steroid-induced myopathy in chronic obstructive pulmonary disease. *Am. J. Respir. Crit. Care Med.* 153, 1958–1964. doi: 10.1164/ajrccm.153.6.8665061

Decramer, M., Gosselink, R., Troosters, T., Verschueren, M., and Evers, G. (1997). Muscle weakness is related to utilization of health care resources in COPD patients. *Eur. Respir. J.* 10, 417–423. doi: 10.1183/09031936.97.10020417

Doucet, M., Russell, A. P., Leger, B., Debigare, R., Joanisse, D. R., Caron, M. A., et al. (2007). Muscle atrophy and hypertrophy signaling in patients with chronic obstructive pulmonary disease. *Am. J. Respir. Crit. Care Med.* 176, 261–269. doi: 10.1164/rccm.200605-704OC

Eid, A. A., Ionescu, A. A., Nixon, L. S., Lewis-Jenkins, V., Matthews, S. B., Griffiths, T. L., et al. (2001). Inflammatory response and body composition in chronic obstructive pulmonary disease. *Am. J. Respir. Crit. Care Med.* 164, 1414–1418. doi: 10.1164/ajrccm.164.8.2008109

Eliason, G., Abdel-Halim, S. M., Piehl-Aulin, K., and Kadim, F. (2010). Alterations in the muscle-to-capillary interface in patients with different degrees of chronic obstructive pulmonary disease. *Respir. Res.* 11, 97–104. doi: 10.1186/1465-9921-11-97

Engelen, M. P., Schols, A. M., Baken, W. C., Wesseling, G. J., and Wouters, E. F. (1994). Nutritional depletion in relation to respiratory and peripheral skeletal muscle function in out-patients with COPD. *Eur. Respir. J.* 7, 1793–1797. doi: 10.1183/09031936.94.07101793

Engelen, M. P., Schols, A. M., Lamers, R. J., and Wouters, E. F. (1999). Different patterns of chronic tissue wasting among patients with chronic obstructive pulmonary disease. *Clin. Nutr.* 18, 275–280. doi: 10.1016/S0261-5614(98)80024-1

Fermoselle, C., Rabinovich, R., Ausin, P., Puig-Vilanova, E., Coronell, C., Sanchez, F., et al. (2012). Does oxidative stress modulate limb muscle atrophy in severe COPD patients? *Eur. Respir. J.* 40, 851–862. doi: 10.1183/09031936.00137211

Goodpaster, B. H., Krishnaswami, S., Resnick, H., Kelley, D. E., Haggerty, C., Harris, T. B., et al. (2003). Association between regional adipose tissue distribution and both type 2 diabetes and impaired glucose tolerance in elderly men and women. *Diabetes Care* 26, 372–379. doi: 10.2337/diacare.26.2.372

Gosker, H. R., Engelen, M. P., van Mameren, H., van Dijk, P. J., van der Vusse, G. J., Wouters, E. F., et al. (2002a). Muscle fiber type IIX atrophy is involved in the loss of fat-free mass in chronic obstructive pulmonary disease. *Am. J. Clin. Nutr.* 76, 113–119.

Gosker, H. R., Hesselink, M. K., Duimel, H., Ward, K. A., and Schols, A. M. (2007a). Reduced mitochondrial density in the vastus lateralis muscle of patients with COPD. *Eur. Respir. J.* 30, 73–79. doi: 10.1183/09031936.00146906

Gosker, H. R., Kubat, B., Schaart, G., van der Vusse, G. J., Wouters, E. F., and Schols, A. M. (2003). Myopathological features in skeletal muscle of patients with chronic obstructive pulmonary disease. *Eur. Respir. J.* 22, 280–285. doi: 10.1183/09031936.03.00012803

Gosker, H. R., van Mameren, H., van Dijk, P. J., Engelen, M. P., van der Vusse, G. J., Wouters, E. F., et al. (2002b). Skeletal muscle fibre-type shifting and metabolic profile in patients with chronic obstructive pulmonary disease. *Eur. Respir. J.* 19, 617–625. doi: 10.1183/09031936.02.00762001

Gosker, H. R., Zeegers, M. P., Wouter, E. F., and Schols, A. M. (2007b). Muscle fiber type shifting in the vastus lateralis of patients with COPD is associated with disease severity: a systematic review and meta-analysis. *Thorax* 62, 944–949. doi: 10.1136/thx.2007.078980

Gosselink, R., Troosters, T., and Decramer, M. (1996). Peripheral muscle weakness contributes to exercise limitation in COPD. *Am. J. Respir. Crit. Care Med.* 153, 976–980. doi: 10.1164/ajrccm.153.3.8630582

Gosselink, R., Troosters, T., and Decramer, M. (2000). Distribution of muscle weakness in patients with stable chronic obstructive pulmonary disease. *J. Cardiopulm. Rehabil.* 20, 353–360. doi: 10.1097/00008483-200011000-00004

Guo, Y., Gosker, H. R., Schols, A. M., Kapchinsky, S., Bourbeau, J., Sandri, M., et al. (2013). Autophagy in locomotor muscles of patients with chronic obstructive pulmonary disease. *Am. J. Respir. Crit. Care Med.* 188, 1313–1320. doi: 10.1164/rccm.201304-0732OC

Hamilton, A. L., Killian, K. J., Summers, E., and Jones, N. L. (1995). Muscle strength, symptom intensity, and exercise capacity in patients with cardiorespiratory disorders. *Am. J. Respir. Crit. Care Med.* 152, 2021–2031. doi: 10.1164/ajrccm.152.6.8520771

Hara, H., Araya, J., Ito, S., Kobayashi, K., Takasaka, N., Yoshii, Y., et al. (2013). Mitochondrial fragmentation in cigarette smoke-induced bronchial epithelial cell senescence. *Am. J. Physiol. Lung Cell. Mol. Physiol.* 305, L737–L746. doi: 10.1152/ajplung.00146.2013

Heijdra, Y. F., Pinto-Plata, V., Frants, R., Rassulo, J., Kenney, L., and Celli, B. R. (2003). Muscle strength and exercise kinetics in COPD patients with a normal fat-free mass index are comparable to control subjects. *Chest* 124, 75–82. doi: 10.1378/chest.124.1.75

Hildebrand, I. L., Sylvén, C., Esbjörnsson, M., Hellström, K., and Jansson, E. (1991). Does chronic hypoxaemia induce transformations of fibre types? *Acta Physiol. Scand.* 141, 435–439. doi: 10.1111/j.1748-1716.1991.tb09102.x

Hoffmann, R. F., Zarrintan, S., Brandenburg, S. M., Kol, A., de Bruin, H. G., Jafari, S., et al. (2013). Prolonged cigarette smoke exposure alters mitochondrial structure and function in airway epithelial cells. *Respir. Res.* 14, 97–109. doi: 10.1186/1465-9921-14-97

Hughes, R. L., Katz, H., Sahgal, V., Campbell, J. A., Hartz, R., and Shields, T. W. (1983). Fiber size and energy metabolites in five separate muscles from patients with chronic obstructive lung diseases. *Respiration* 44, 321–328. doi: 10.1159/000194564

Hussain, S. N., and Sandri, M. (2013). Role of autophagy in COPD skeletal muscle dysfunction. *J. Appl. Physiol.* 114, 1273–1281. doi: 10.1152/japplphysiol.00893.2012

Jakobsson, P., Jorfeldt, L., and Burndin, A. (1990). Skeletal muscle metabolites and fibre types in patients with advanced chronic obstructive pulmonary disease (COPD), with and without chronic respiratory failure. *Eur. Respir. J.* 3, 192–196.

Jakobsson, P. L., Jordfelt, L., and Henriksson, J. (1995). Metabolic enzyme activity in the quadriceps femoris muscle in patients with severe chronic obstructive pulmonary disease. *Am. J. Respir. Crit. Care Med.* 151, 374–377. doi: 10.1164/ajrccm.151.2.7842194

Janaudis-Ferreira, T., Hill, K., Goldstein, R., Wadell, K., and Brooks, D. (2009). Arm exercise training in patients with chronic obstructive pulmonary disease: a systematic review. *J. Cardiopulm. Rehabil. Prev.* 29, 277–283. doi: 10.1097/HCR.0b013e3181b4c8d0

Jatta, K., Eliason, G., Portela-Gomes, G. M., Grimelius, L. P., Caro, O., Nilholm, L., et al. (2009). Overexpression of von Hippel- Lindau (VHL) in skeletal muscles of patients with chronic obstructive pulmonary disease (COPD). *J. Clin. Pathol.* 62, 70–76. doi: 10.1136/jcp.2008.057190

Jo, E., Lee, S. R., Park, B. S., and Kim, J. S. (2012). Potential mechanisms underlying the role of chronic inflammation in age-related muscle wasting. *Aging Clin. Exp. Res.* 24, 412–422. doi: 10.3275/8464

Jobin, J., Maltais, F., Doyon, J. F., LeBlanc, P., Simard, P. M., Simard, A. A., et al. (1998). Chronic obstructive pulmonary disease: capillarity and fiber-type characteristics of skeletal muscle. *J. Cardiopulm. Rehabil.* 18, 432–437. doi: 10.1097/00008483-199811000-00005

Ju, C. R., and Chen, R. C. (2012). Serum myostatin levels and skeletal muscle wasting in chronic obstructive pulmonary disease. *Respir. Med.* 106, 102–108. doi: 10.1016/j.rmed.2011.07.016

Kelly, J. L., Elkin, S. L., Fluxman, J., Polkey, M. I., Soljak, M. A., and Hopkinson, N. S. (2013). Breathlessness and skeletal muscle weakness in patients undergoing lung health screening in primary care. *COPD* 10, 40–54. doi: 10.3109/15412555.2012.727923

Killian, K. J., Leblanc, P., Martin, D. H., Summers, E., Jones, N. L., and Campbell, E. J. (1992). Exercise capacity and ventilatory, circulatory, and symptom limitation in patients with chronic airflow limitation. *Am. Rev. Respir. Dis.* 146, 935–940. doi: 10.1164/ajrccm/146.4.935

Kirkham, P. A., and Barnes, P. J. (2013). Oxidative stress in COPD. *Chest* 144, 266–273. doi: 10.1378/chest.12-2664

Koechlin, C., Maltais, F., Saey, D., Michaud, A., LeBlanc, P., Hayot, M., et al. (2005). Hypoxaemia enhances peripheral muscle oxidative stress in chronic obstructive pulmonary disease. *Thorax* 60, 834–841. doi: 10.1136/thx.2004.037531

Kok, M. O., Hoekstra, T., and Twisk, J. W. (2012). The longitudinal relationship between smoking and muscle strength in healthy adults. *Eur. Addict. Res.* 18, 70–75. doi: 10.1159/000333600

Kondo, K., and Kaelin, W. G. (2001). The von Hippel-Lindau tumor suppressor gene. *Exp. Cell Res.* 264, 117–125. doi: 10.1006/excr.2000.5139

Kutsuzawa, T., Shioya, S., Kurita, D., Haida, M., Ohta, Y., and Yamabayashi, H. (1995). Muscle energy metabolism and nutritional status in patients with chronic obstructive pulmonary disease. A 31P magnetic resonance study. *Am. J. Respir. Crit. Care Med.* 152, 647–652. doi: 10.1164/ajrccm.152.2.7633721

Lands, L. C., Smountas, A. A., Mesiano, G., Brosseau, L., Shennib, H., Charbonneau, M.et al. (1999). Maximal exercise capacity and peripheral skeletal muscle function following lung transplantation. *J. Heart Lung Transplant.* 18, 113–120. doi: 10.1016/S1053-2498(98)00027-8

Langen, R. C., Gosker, H. R., Remels, A. H., and Schols, A. M. (2013). Triggers and mechanisms of skeletal muscle wasting in chronic obstructive pulmonary disease. *Int. J. Biochem. Cell Biol.* 45, 2245–2256. doi: 10.1016/j.biocel.2013.06.015

Lemire, B. B., Debigarr, R., Dube, A., Theriault, M. E., Cote, C. H., and Maltais, F. (2012). MAPK signaling in the quadriceps of patients with chronic obstructive pulmonary disease. *J. Appl. Physiol.* 113, 159–166. doi: 10.1152/japplphysiol.01518.2011

Maltais, F., LeBlanc, P., Whittom, F., Simard, C., Marquis, K., Belanger, M., et al. (2000). Oxidative enzyme activities of the vastus lateralis muscle and the functional status in patients with COPD. *Thorax* 55, 848–853. doi: 10.1136/thorax.55.10.848

Maltais, F., Simard, A. A., Simard, C., Jobin, J., Desgagnés, P., and Le- Blanc, P. (1996). Oxidative capacity of the skeletal muscle and lactic acid kinetics during exercise in normal subjects and in patients with COPD. *Am. J. Respir. Crit. Care Med.* 153, 288–293. doi: 10.1164/ajrccm.153.1.8542131

Man, W. D., Natanek, S. A., Riddoch-Contreras, J., Lewis, A., Marsh, G. S., Kemp, P. R., et al. (2010). Quadriceps myostatin expression in COPD. *Eur. Respir. J.* 36, 686–688. doi: 10.1183/09031936.00032510

Marquis, K., Debigare, R., Lacasse, Y., LeBlanc, P., Jobin, J., Carrier, G., et al. (2002). Midthigh muscle cross-sectional area is a better predictor of mortality than body mass index in patients with chronic obstructive pulmonary disease. *Am. J. Respir. Crit. Care Med.* 166, 809–813. doi: 10.1164/rccm.2107031

Mathur, S., MacIntyre, D. L., Forster, B. B., Road, J. D., Levy, R. D., and Reid, W. D. (2007). Preservation of eccentric torque of the knee extensors and flexors in patients with COPD. *J. Cardiopulm. Rehabil. Prev.* 27, 411–416. doi: 10.1097/01.HCR.0000300271.45881.99

Mathur, S., Takai, K. P., Macintyre, D. L., and Reid, D. (2008). Estimation of thigh muscle mass with magnetic resonance imaging in older adults and people with chronic obstructive pulmonary disease. *Phys. Ther.* 88, 219–230. doi: 10.2522/ptj.20070052

Meyer, A., Zoll, J., Charles, A. L., Chraloux, A., Blay, F., Diemunsch, P., et al. (2013). Skeletal muscle mithochondrial dysfunction during chronic obstructive pulmonary disease: central actor and therapeutic target. *Exp. Physiol.* 98, 1063–1078. doi: 10.1113/expphysiol.2012.069468

Montes de Oca, M., Loeb, E., Torres, S. H., De Sanctis, J., Hernandez, N., and Tálamo, C. (2008). Peripheral muscle alterations in non-COPD smokers. *Chest* 133, 13–18. doi: 10.1378/chest.07-1592

Mostert, R., Goris, A., Weling-Scheepers, C., Wouters, E. F., and Schols, A. M. (2000). Tissue depletion and health related quality of life in patients with chronic obstructive pulmonary disease. *Respir. Med.* 94, 859–867. doi: 10.1053/rmed.2000.0829

Piehl-Aulin, K., Jones, I., Lindvall, B., Magnuson, A., and Abdel-Halim, S. M. (2009). Increased serum inflammatory markers in the absence of clinical and skeletal muscle inflammation in patients with chronic obstructive pulmonary disease. *Respiration* 78, 191–196. doi: 10.1159/000207793

Pisot, R., Narici, M. V., Simunic, B., De Boer, M., Seynnes, O., Jurdana, M., et al. (2008). Whole muscle contractile parameters and thickness loss during 35-day bed rest. *Eur. J. Appl. Physiol.* 104, 409–414. doi: 10.1007/s00421-008-0698-6

Pitta, F., Troosters, T., Spruit, M. A., Probst, V. S., Decramer, M., and Gosselink, R. (2005). Characteristics of physical activities in daily life in chronic obstructive pulmonary disease. *Am. J. Respir. Crit. Care Med.* 171, 972–977. doi: 10.1164/rccm.200407-855OC

Plant, P. J., Brooks, D., Faughnan, M., Bayley, T., Bain, J., Singer, L., et al. (2010). Cellular markers of muscle atrophy in chronic obstructive pulmonary disease. *Am. J. Respir. Cell Mol. Biol.* 42, 461–471. doi: 10.1165/rcmb.2008-0382OC

Puente-Maestu, L., Tejedor, A., Lázaro, A., de Miguel, J., Alvarez-Sala, L., González-Aragoneses, F., et al. (2012). Site of mitochondrial ROS production in skeletal muscle of COPD and its relationship with exercise oxidative stress. *Am. J. Respir. Cell Mol. Biol.* 47, 358–362. doi: 10.1165/rcmb.2011-0382OC

Roig, M., Eng, J. J., Road, J. D., and Reid, W. D. (2009). Falls in patients with chronic obstructive pulmonary disease: a call for further research. *Respir. Med.* 103, 1257–1269. doi: 10.1016/j.rmed.2009.03.022

Saey, D., Debigare, R., LeBlanc, P., Mador, M. J., Cote, C. H., Jobin, J., et al. (2003). Contractile leg fatigue after cycle exercise: a factor limiting exercise in patients with chronic obstructive pulmonary disease. *Am. J. Respir. Crit. Care Med.* 168, 425–430. doi: 10.1164/rccm.200208-856OC

Sato, Y., Asoh, T., Honda, Y., Fujimatsu, Y., Higuchi, I., and Oizumi, K. (1997). Morphologic and histochemical evaluation of muscle in patients with chornic pulmonary emphysema manifesting generalized emaciation. *Eur. Neurol.* 37, 116–121.

Satta, A., Migliori, G. B., Spanevello, A., Neri, M., Bottinelli, R., Canepari, M., et al. (1997). Fibre types in skeletal muscles of chronic obstructive pulmonary disease patients related to respiratory function and exercise tolerance. *Eur. Respir. J.* 10, 2853–2860. doi: 10.1183/09031936.97.10122853

Schols, A. M., Broekhuizen, R., Weling-Scheepers, C. A., and Wouters, E. F. (2005). Body composition and mortality in chronic obstructive pulmonary disease. *Am. J. Clin. Nutr.* 82, 53–59. doi: 10.1016/j.rmedu.2005.09.028

Schols, A. M., Fredrix, E. W., Soeters, P. B., Westerterp, K. R., and Wouters, E. F. (1991). Resting energy expenditure in patients with chronic obstructive pulmonary disease. *Am. J. Clin. Nutr.* 54, 983–987.

Schols, A. M., Soeters, P. B., Dingemans, A. M., Mostert, R., Frantzen, P. J., and Wouters, E. F. (1993). Prevalence and characteristics of nutritional depletion in patients with stable COPD eligible for pulmonary rehabilitation. *Am. Rev. Respir. Dis.* 147, 1151–1156. doi: 10.1164/ajrccm/147.5.1151

Serres, I., Gautier, V., Varray, A., and Prefaut, C. (1998). Impaired skeletal muscle endurance related to physical inactivity and altered lung function in COPD patients. *Chest* 113, 900–905. doi: 10.1378/chest.113.4.900

Seymour, J. M., Spruit, M. A., Hopkinson, N. S., Natanek, S. A., Man, W. D., Jackson, A., et al. (2010). The prevalence of quadriceps weakness in COPD and the relationship with disease severity. *Eur. Respir. J.* 36, 81–88. doi: 10.1183/09031936.00104909

Shoup, R., Dalsky, G., Warner, S., Davies, M., Connors, M., Khan, M., et al. (1997). Body composition and health-related quality of life in patients with obstructive airways disease. *Eur. Respir. J.* 10, 1576–1580. doi: 10.1183/09031936.97.10071576

Shrikrishna, D., Patel, M., Tanner, R. J., Seymour, J. M., Connolly, B. A., Puthucheary, Z. A., et al. (2012). Quadriceps wasting and physical inactivity in patients with COPD. *Eur. Respir. J.* 40, 1115–1122. doi: 10.1183/09031936.00170111

Simard, C. F., Maltais, P., Leblanc, P., Simard, M., and Jobin, J. (1996). Mitochondrial and capillarity changes in vastus lateralis muscle of COPD patients: electron microscopy study. *Med. Sci. Sports Exerc.* 28, S95. doi: 10.1097/00005768-199605001-00564

Simpson, K., Killian, K., McCartney, N., Stubbing, D. G., and Jones, N. L. (1992). Randomised controlled trial of weightlifting exercise in patients with chronic airflow limitation. *Thorax* 47, 70–75. doi: 10.1136/thx.47.2.70

Spruit, M. A., Gosselink, R., Troosters, T., Kasran, A., Gayan-Ramirez, G., Bogaerts, P., et al. (2003). Muscle force during an acute exacerbation in hospitalised patients with COPD and its relationship with CXCL8 and IGF-I. *Thorax* 58, 752–756. doi: 10.1136/thorax.58.9.752

Steiner, M. C., Singh, S. J., and Morgan, M. D. (2005). The contribution of peripheral muscle function to shuttle walking performance in patients with chronic obstructive pulmonary disease. *J. Cardiopulm. Rehabil.* 25, 43–49. doi: 10.1097/00008483-200501000-00010

Tang, K., Wagner, P. D., and Breen, E. C. (2010). TNF-α-mediated reduction in PGC-1α may impair skeletal muscle function after cigarette smoke exposure. *J. Cell. Physiol.* 222, 320–327. doi: 10.1002/jcp.21955

Theriault, M. E., Pare, M. E., Maltais, F., and Debigare, R. (2012). Satellite cells senescence in limb muscle of severe patients with COPD. *PLoS ONE.* 7:e39124. doi: 10.1371/journal.pone.0039124

van der Toorn, M., Rezayat, D., Kauffman, H. F., Bakker, S. J., Gans, R. O., Koëter, G. H., et al. (2009). Lipidsoluble components in cigarette smoke induce mitochondrial production of reactive oxygen species in lung epithelial cells. *Am. J. Physiol. Lung Cell. Mol. Physiol.* 297, L109–L114. doi: 10.1152/ajplung.90461.2008

Van Vliet, M., Spruit, M. A., Verleden, G., Kasran, A., Van Herck, E., Pitta, F., et al. (2005). Hypogonadism, quadriceps weakness, and exercise intolerance in chronic obstructive pulmonary disease. *Am. J. Respir. Crit. Care Med.* 172, 1105–1111. doi: 10.1164/rccm.200501-114OC

Vermeeren, M. A., Creutzberg, E. C., Schols, A. M., Postma, D. S., Pieters, W. R., Roldaan, A. C., et al. (2006). COSMIC Study Group. Prevalence of nutritional depletion in a large out-patient population of patients with COPD. *Respir. Med.* 100, 1349–1355. doi: 10.1016/j.rmed.2005.11.023

Vestbo, J., Hurd, S. S., Agustí, A. G., Jones, P. W., Vogelmeier, C., Anzueto, A., et al. (2013). Global strategy for the diagnosis, management, and prevention of chronic obstructive pulmonary disease: GOLD executive summary. *Am. J. Respir. Crit. Care Med.* 187, 347–365. doi: 10.1164/rccm.201204-0596PP

Vogiatzis, I., Simoes, D. C., Stratakos, G., Kourepini, E., Terzis, G., Manta, P., et al. (2010). Effect of pulmonary rehabilitation on muscle remodelling in cachectic patients with COPD. *Eur. Respir. J.* 36, 301–310. doi: 10.1183/09031936.00112909

Wagner, P. D. (2006). Skeletal muscles in chronic obstructive pulmonary disease: deconditioning, or myopathy? *Respirology* 11, 681–686. doi: 10.1111/j.1440-1843.2006.00939.x

Watz, H., Waschki, B., Meyer, T., and Magnussen, H. (2009). Physical activity in patients with COPD. *Eur. Respir. J.* 33, 262–272. doi: 10.1183/09031936.00024608

Whittom, F., Jobin, J., Simard, P. M., Leblanc, P., Simard, C., Bernard, S., et al. (1998). Histochemical and morphological characteristics of the vastus lateralis muscle in patients with chronic obstructive pulmonary disease. *Med. Sci. Sports Exerc.* 30, 1467–1474. doi: 10.1097/00005768-199810000-00001

World Health Organization. (2008). *Global Burden of Disease: 2004 Update*. Geneva: WHO Press.

Wüst, R. C., Morse, C. I., de Haan, A., Rittweger, J., Jones, D. A., and Degens, H. (2008). Skeletal muscle properties and fatigue resistance in relation to smoking history. *Eur. J. Appl. Physiol.* 104, 103–110. doi: 10.1007/s00421-008-0792-9

Young, L. J., and Caughey, W. S. (1990). Pathobiochemistry of CO poisoning. *FEBS Lett.* 272, 1–6. doi: 10.1016/0014-5793(90)80436-M

9

Advancements in stem cells treatment of skeletal muscle wasting

Mirella Meregalli†, Andrea Farini†, Clementina Sitzia and Yvan Torrente*

Stem Cell Laboratory, Dipartimento di Fisiopatologia Medico-Chirurgica e dei Trapianti, Centro Dino Ferrari, Fondazione IRCCS Ca' Granda Ospedale Maggiore Policlinico, Università degli Studi di Milano, Milano, Italy

Correspondence:
Yvan Torrente, Stem Cell Laboratory, Dipartimento di Fisiopatologia Medico-Chirurgica e dei Trapianti, Fondazione IRCCS Ca' Granda Ospedale Maggiore Policlinico, Università degli Studi di Milano, Via F. Sforza 35, 20122 Milan, Italy e-mail: yvan.torrente@unimi.it

† These authors have contributed equally to this work.

Muscular dystrophies (MDs) are a heterogeneous group of inherited disorders, in which progressive muscle wasting and weakness is often associated with exhaustion of muscle regeneration potential. Although physiological properties of skeletal muscle tissue are now well known, no treatments are effective for these diseases. Muscle regeneration was attempted by means transplantation of myogenic cells (from myoblast to embryonic stem cells) and also by interfering with the malignant processes that originate in pathological tissues, such as uncontrolled fibrosis and inflammation. Taking into account the advances in the isolation of new subpopulation of stem cells and in the creation of artificial stem cell niches, we discuss how these emerging technologies offer great promises for therapeutic approaches to muscle diseases and muscle wasting associated with aging.

Keywords: muscle wasting, stem cell niche, fibrosis, inflammation, myogenic stem cell

INTRODUCTION

Skeletal muscle is a highly complex system formed by thousands of contractile units called muscle fibers. Each muscle fiber is limited by a plasma membrane called sarcolemma and by a basal lamina, that are surrounded by an extra cellular matrix constituted of connective tissue (Buckingham et al., 2003). Muscle remodeling occurs throughout the entire life although at different rate considering the developmental stages. Starting from embryo until childhood, protein synthesis is upregulated and satellite cells (SCs) actively develop new muscle fibers while in adults cellular turnover is strongly reduced (Schiaffino et al., 2007). In response to exogenous stimuli or to biological factors such as age or nutrition, the muscle increases its size, the amount of contractile proteins and consequently force production. The regulation of muscle cell size is a tightly regulated phenomena, and it is a balance between muscle proliferation and degradation of preexisting proteins. Uncontrolled events, often associated with diseases, lead to hypertrophy or atrophy, respectively (Sandri, 2008). The complex hierarchy of events that triggers muscle remodeling is often unbalanced in muscular diseases. For instance, Duchenne muscular dystrophy (DMD), the most frequent among all the dystrophies, is characterized by a rapid atrophy in youth, muscular wasting and inability to walk in adolescence and premature death for cardiorespiratory failure by the age of 30. As the genetic nature of these pathologies leads to uncontrolled fiber degeneration, different treatments were proven to delay the progression of the diseases. The main goal was to retard the atrophy and replace diseased muscle with new healthy and functional muscle fibers by using myogenic stem cells (Brunelli and Rovere-Querini, 2008). Unfortunately, the use of stem cell in regenerative medicine is limited by the poor engraftment and persistence of transplanted cells and the risk of neoplastic formation (Suuronen et al., 2008; Kuraitis et al., 2012). Due to these findings, other aspects were deeply investigated to increase the survival of injected stem cells into pathological muscle. Modulation of the inflammatory reaction is a key step for stem cell transplantation (Smythe et al., 2000): myeloid cells (Suzuki et al., 1999; Mcnally et al., 2000), macrophages (Wehling et al., 2001; Villalta et al., 2009), neutrophils (Hodgetts et al., 2006) and eosinophils (Cai et al., 2000) actively contribute to development of pathogenesis in several myophaties but only macrophages and sometimes eosinophils play a role in muscle regeneration (Tidball and Villalta, 2010). Pathological conditions modify the microenvironment of stem cells (the so-called niche) preventing the activation of resident stem cells and reducing the success of exogenous cell therapies. Tissue engineering technologies may create a novel *in vitro* niche allowing the maintenance and propagation of SCs and enhancing their muscular potential.

In this review, we will describe the efforts that are necessary to design a successful therapeutic approach for muscular diseases, relating to find a functional stem cell population, to identify feasible matrix/polymer to engineer stem cells' niche and to modulate secondary—but relevant—effects of impaired muscle regeneration, as fibrosis and inflammation.

MYOGENIC STEM CELLS

EMBRYONIC STEM CELLS (ESCs)

Introduction to ESCs

Embryonic stem cells (ESCs) are pluripotent cells derived from the early embryo that are characterized by the ability to proliferate over prolonged periods of culture remaining undifferentiated and maintaining a stable karyotype (Amit and Itskovitz-Eldor, 2002; Carpenter et al., 2003; Hoffman and Carpenter, 2005). ESCs differentiate into cells forming all 3 embryonic germ layers, and are characterized by self-renewal, immortality, and pluripotency (Strulovici et al., 2007). As ESCs possess the potential to differentiate into all normal tissues, the ability to derive and maintain these cells in culture opened the possibility to have an unlimited supply of differentiated cells to replace pathological tissues (Moon et al., 2006; Skottman et al., 2006).

Markers of ESCs

Cell origins are often defined by one or more cell-surface markers and intracellular epitopes unique to that particular cell type. hESCs are maintained in culture on feeder layers of heterologous cells and then differentiated into specific cell lineages (Takahashi and Yamanaka, 2006; Conrad et al., 2008). Stage-specific embryonic antigen citation(SSEA) markers are used to distinguish early stages of cell development and to denote pluripotency: hESCs express SSEA-3 and -4 during pluripotency and only SSEA-1 upon differentiation (Andrews et al., 1996; Thomson and Marshall, 1998; Thomson et al., 1998; Reubinoff et al., 2001). Nanog is a NK-2-type homeodomain gene encoding for a transcription factor that is critically involved in the self-renewal of stem cells. In 2005, Lin's group demonstrated that the tumor suppressor p53 binds to the promoter of Nanog, stimulating p53 (Lin et al., 2005). Octamer-binding transcription factor 4 (Oct-4) down-regulation is observed in differentiating cells (Rosner et al., 1990). It was suggested that only Oct-4 was necessary for the maintenance of pluripotency, but its expression level governed three cell fates once differentiation occurs. Similarly, Xu et al. published that the catalytic component of telomerase, telomerase reverse transcriptase (hTERT), was expressed in undifferentiated cells and down-regulated upon differentiation (Xu et al., 2001).

Limits of ESCs

Although the attentions that received, scientific and medical issues need to be addressed before hESCs can be considered safe for clinical applications (Leist et al., 2008). The American federal government severely restricted access and use of hESCs in 2001 but they were largely overturned by the Obama administration. Many organizations and countries have already banned reproductive cloning of human beings. As this procedure can be used to generate stem cells for therapeutic purposes, in countries where this type of cloning is legal, such as Australia and the United Kingdom, the created embryos must be destroyed within 14 days. Guidelines in using ESCs were proposed by the International Society of Stem Cell Research citation (http://www.isscr.org/guidelines/index.htm).

Myogenic potential of ESCs

Several lineages (blood, cardiac muscle and endothelial cells) were obtained by *in vitro* differentiation of ESCs, however for skeletal muscle several drawbacks arose, especially for the difficulty to identify a temporal expression of myogenic regulatory factors (Rohwedel et al., 1994). This way, in 2005 Bhagavati et al. co-cultured ESCs derived from normal mice with a preparation from mouse muscle enriched for myogenic stem and precursor cells. They transplanted ESCs into dystrophic mdx mice but unfortunately newly-formed muscle was occasionally seen (Bhagavati and Xu, 2005). Similarly, Barberi et al. described a stroma-free induction system to derive mesenchymal precursors and skeletal myoblast from hESCs. Following *in vitro* maturation, these cells were injected into tibialis anterior of immunodeficient scid mice and it was observed a long-term myoblast engraftment and the lack of teratomas (Barberi et al., 2007). As it was suggested that the lack of myogenic differentiation of ESCs was due to the impairment of myogenic signals in the mesoderm (Darabi et al., 2008a), Darabi et al. transiently expressed paired box 3 (Pax3) and paired box 7 (Pax7) during early mesoderm development and obtained several early embryonic skeletal myogenic progenitors (Darabi et al., 2008b, 2011). These cells were also implanted into mdx mice and gave rise to large numbers of skeletal muscle fibers and SCs, so that muscle force was ameliorated (Darabi et al., 2009, 2011). More recently, Sakurai et al. described that the elimination of bone morphogenetic protein 4 (BMP4) from serum-free ESC cultures together with the implementation of lithium chloride (LiCl) allowed the differentiation of these cells to myogenic progenitors cells. hESCs-derived progenitors showed a notable capacity of differentiation into skeletal muscle cells (Sakurai et al., 2009).

INDUCED PLURIPOTENT STEM CELLS (iPSCs)

Generation of iPSCs

Recent advances in the understanding of ESC biology included the identification of several master regulators of ESC pluripotency and differentiation (Takahashi and Yamanaka, 2006). Intensive study of ESC growth conditions has not yet produced a complete picture of the unique transcriptional and epigenetic state that is responsible for pluripotency and self-renewal in ESCs. Yamanaka's group identified four factors (Oct3/4, Klf4, Sox2, and c-myc) whose expression is sufficient to produce cells similar to ESCs, called induced pluripotent stem cells (iPSCs). The same factors were used to reprogram human fibroblasts to an ESC-like pluripotent state.

The new era of iPSCs

Now that embryonic tissue is no longer required to make a pluripotent cell, investigators have the ability to create tissue-based models of human disease based on cells derived from individual patients (Dimos et al., 2008; Park et al., 2008; Ebert et al., 2009; Soldner et al., 2009). Accordingly, iPSCs were efficiently used in murine models of sickle cells anemia and Parkinson's disease. Even if these cells were showed to be suitable for cell therapy, it has to be yet demonstrated the possibility to generate human iPSCs without introduction of DNA into the genome (to avoid oncogenic potential of undifferentiated iPSCs following the unsafe reintroduction of these genes), to ameliorate the efficiency of manipulation of human iPSCs and the capacity to obtain any desired cell types.

iPSCs and human disease

Since the work of Yamanaka was published, reprogramming of cells provided a realistic way not only to obtain lines from patients with incurable pathologies to investigate disease mechanisms and drug screening but to generate sufficient numbers of patient-specific pluripotent stem cells (Egawa et al., 2012). The generation of patient-specific iPSCs has the advantage of avoiding many of the ethical concerns associated with the use of embryonic or foetal material, and have no risk of immune rejection. Many cell types like motor neurons (Dimos et al., 2008), hepatocytes (Song et al., 2009), pancreatic insulin producing cells (Zhang et al., 2006), hematopoietic cells (Hanna et al., 2007), retinal cells (Carr et al., 2009), cardiomyocyte (Zwi et al., 2009) and mesenchymal stem cells (Lian et al., 2010), have been successfully derived from human iPSCs. Nelson et al. reported the use of iPSCs for myocardial repair in animal models of acute myocardial infarction (Nelson et al., 2009) while Ye used iPSCs in different hematological disorders (Ye et al., 2009).

Myogenic potential of iPSCs

As described above, to be used for clinical applications, iPSCs need to be generated in large amount in safety; this way, protocols to isolate and characterize these cells were largely improved. Mizuno et al. identified iPS-derived satellite-like cells by means the expression of the SM/C-2.6 antibody (Mizuno et al., 2010) while Darabi purified PDGFαR+Flk−1− murine iPS cells that expressed the myogenic factor Pax7 (Darabi et al., 2008a, 2011). In fact, the group of Perlingeiro recently isolated large quantity of Pax7+ human iPSCs (and ESCs) that, transplanted into dystrophic mice, engrafted well producing high amount of dystrophin and replenishing the satellite cell compartment (Darabi et al., 2012). Similarly, the expression of MyoD and Myf5 allowed the purification of myogenic iPS cells (Iacovino et al., 2011; Goudenege et al., 2012). Filareto et al. successfully obtained iPSCs from fibroblast of dystrophin/utrophin double knockout mice and engineered them with the micro-dystrophin gene. Injected into dystrophic mice, these cells engrafted well and improved muscle strength (Filareto et al., 2013). In parallel, Tedesco et al. generated mesoangioblast/mesenchymal-like cells from iPSCs of healthy and dystrophic patients: these cells were also modified to express constitutively the MyoD gene. Transplanted into model mice of LGMD-2A, iPSCs cells ameliorated their dystrophic phenotype (Tedesco et al., 2012).

SATELLITE CELLS (SCs)

SCs are small progenitor cells originating from somites that lie between the basement membrane and sarcolemma of individual muscle fibers (Shi and Garry, 2006; Sambasivan and Tajbakhsh, 2007). SCs are normally present in healthy adult mammalian muscle as quiescent cells and are characterized by the expression of Pax7, that is fundamental for their maintenance and self-renewal, and by the absence of Myogenic differentiation 1 (MyoD) and myogenin, that conversely are necessary for myogenic differentiation. Once activated in response to specific stimuli such as oxidative stress, SCs up-regulate the expression of Myf5 to start their proliferation so that they differentiate into new myofibers, driven by specific factors such as MyoD, myogenin and myosin heavy chain (Whalen et al., 1990). Since the work of Montarras and colleagues (Montarras et al., 2005), different techniques for SCs isolation were assessed. Sacco et al. derived SCs from transplantation of one intact myofiber and demonstrated that once transplanted into dystrophic mice, SCs proliferated and contributed to form new muscle fibers (Sacco et al., 2008). Cerletti et al. isolated the skeletal muscle precursors (SMPs): injected into animal models, these SC-like cells restored dystrophin expression and, more importantly, were positioned into the SC niche, where they regulated the subsequent rounds of injury and repair (Cerletti et al., 2008). Similarly, the muscle side-population cells (mSP) isolated by Tanaka et al. engrafted into host SC niche, giving rise both to SCs and myonuclear population (Tanaka et al., 2009).

Autologous transplantation of genetically corrected SCs into patients suffering from muscular diseases could be our ideal approach (Price et al., 2007): unfortunately, it was demonstrated that the growth of SCs *in vitro* significantly reduced their *in vivo* myogenic potential, rendering their transplantation an inefficient technique (Tremblay et al., 1993; Mendell et al., 1995; Gussoni et al., 1997). To overcome these problems, several studies investigated the SC niches, as described in detail in section Satellite cells niche.

MUSCLE-DERIVED STEM CELLS (MDSCs)

Besides SCs, muscle-derived stem cells (MDSCs) were isolated within the muscle, with the capacity of self-renewal and mesodermal differentiation. Sarig et al. identified a subpopulation of MyoD+ stem cells that formed muscle fibers but also osteogenic and adipogenic cells (Sarig et al., 2006). Tamaki et al. purified a subpopulation of CD34-CD45- cells that proliferated into myogenic, vasculogenic and neural cell lineages (Tamaki et al., 2007). Sca−1+CD34+ stem cells purified from murine muscle differentiated into myogenic and multimyeloid lineages *in vitro* and regenerated muscle *in vivo* (Torrente et al., 2001). Alessandri et al. showed that muscle-derived stem cells positive for desmin and vimentin differentiated *in vitro* into skeletal muscle fibers and neurons (Alessandri et al., 2004). Notably, Rouger et al. identified early myogenic progenitors that originated from SC niche, the MuStem cells; transplanted into Golden retriever muscular dystrophy (GRMD) dogs, these cells allowed the re-expression of dystrophin (Rouger et al., 2011).

MESENCHYMAL STEM CELLS (MSCs)

Mesenchymal stem cells (MSCs) are clonogenic and adherent cells, isolated from adult and foetal bone marrow and from other tissues and organs (Alhadlaq and Mao, 2004; Le Blanc and Pittenger, 2005; Beyer Nardi and Da Silva Meirelles, 2006): they are able to differentiate into several lineages (Zheng et al., 2007; Nesti et al., 2008). As MSCs were identified into muscle tissue biopsies, it was suggested that skeletal muscle could be an important source of MSCs for therapeutic interventions (Jackson et al., 2010). Transplanted into DMD patients, MSCs fused with host fibers and enhanced the activity of endogenous stem cells through the secretion of trophic factors (Ichim et al., 2010). Interestingly, De Bari et al. described the *in vitro* myogenic potential of MSCs isolated from adult human synovial membrane (De Bari et al., 2001). Following injection into dystrophic mice, these cells formed new myofibers, re-expressed the dystrophin and contributed to SCs replenishment (De Bari et al., 2003). Gang et al. showed that MSCs from umbilical cord blood differentiated into skeletal muscle, expressing late myogenic markers as MyoD (Gang et al., 2004). Riordan et al. described that hematopoietic precursors present in the bone marrow were protected from inflammatory damage by MSCs (Riordan et al., 2007) while Nemeth et al. demonstrated that MSCs can modulate the activity of macrophages and consequently inhibit inflammatory processes (Nemeth et al., 2009). The capacity of MSCs to modulate inflammation could be an important feature in the perspective of cell therapy in dystrophic patients as inflammation is a prominent component of the disease (as reviewed in detail in section Inflammation and repair mechanisms in skeletal muscle). Following these evidences, MSCs injection were proven to reduce inflammation in animal models for several human diseases, such as autoimmune arthritis and diabetes (Fiorina et al., 2009; Madec et al., 2009), multiple sclerosis (Constantin et al., 2009; Rafei et al., 2009a), lupus (Zhou et al., 2008), rheumatoid arthritis (Song et al., 2010) and autoimmune encephalomyelitis (Rafei et al., 2009b). Although all these encouraging results, several problems need to be solved. First of all, more efforts are needed to elucidate the origin of MSCs; moreover, protocols for isolation of the cells and their expansion *in vivo* have to be standardized.

MUSCLE-DERIVED CD133+ STEM CELLS

Torrente et al. isolated stem cells from human normal and DMD biopsies expressing the glycoprotein CD133. CD133+ stem cells co-expressed CD34, CD45, and kinase insert domain receptor (KDR) and differentiated into muscle (Torrente et al., 2007). Moreover, Negroni et al. found that muscle-derived CD133+ stem cells co-expressed the satellite cell marker CD56 and eventually formed myosin heavy chain (MyHC)+ multinucleated myotubes (Negroni et al., 2009). As Phase I clinic trial demonstrated that infusion of these cells was safe and feasible (Torrente et al., 2007), muscle-derived dystrophic CD133+ stem cells were engineered to express a shorter but still functional dystrophin. Transplanted into dystrophic mice, CD133+ stem cells allowed the expression of dystrophin and the formation of new myofibers, improving murine muscular force. Interestingly, some of injected CD133+ stem cells were identified beneath the basal lamina, in SC-like position, thus expressing M-Cadherin (Benchaouir et al., 2007).

MESOANGIOBLASTS

Physically associated with the embryonic dorsal aorta in avian and mammalian species, mesoangioblasts are multipotent progenitors of mesodermal tissues, expressing α-smooth muscle actin (SMA) and retaining myogenic capacity (Tagliafico et al., 2004). Cossu et al. engineered these cells with human microdystrophin and demonstrated that they improved muscle function after injection into GRMDs (Sampaolesi et al., 2006; Cossu and Sampaolesi, 2007). In order to ameliorate their ability of migration, mesoangioblasts were exposed to Stromal cell-derived factor (SDF)-1 and tumor necrosis factor (TNF)-α so that, following transplantation into α-sarcoglycan KO mice, the large majority of α-sarcoglycan-expressing myofibers was reconstituted (Galvez et al., 2006). Similarly, Tedesco et al. transduced mdx-derived mesoangioblasts with a vector carrying the entire human dystrophin genetic locus. Injected into scid/mdx mice, these cells formed several muscle fibers expressing dystrophin and replenished the SC compartments (Tedesco et al., 2011). More recently, Cossu's group obtained mesoangioblasts from iPSCs of LGMD-2D patients that rescued the expression of α-sarcoglycans in dystrophic mice (Tedesco et al., 2012). According to these evidences, mesoangioblasts seemed to be feasible to treat MDs and they are currently being utilized in a phase I/II clinical trial (EudraCT no. 2011-000176-33).

ARTIFICIAL STEM CELL NICHE

SATELLITE CELLS NICHE

SCs behavior is influenced by factors that are secreted by myofibers. SDF-1 can bind to receptor CXCR4 on the surface of SC activating a migratory response (Sherwood et al., 2004; Ratajczak et al., 2006) while M-cadherin enhance the adhesion of SC to myofibers allowing their fusion (Irintchev et al., 1994). Interestingly, SCs can regulate their own quiescence and self-renewal according to the expression of ligands for the Notch receptor family (Conboy and Rando, 2002; Conboy et al., 2003; Kuang et al., 2007). Like other stem cells, SCs can proliferate in a asymmetric manner, giving rise to one stem cell and one differentiated cell; and in a symmetric manner, originating two daughter cells retaining full stem cell potential (Morrison and Kimble, 2006). Asymmetric self-renewal is preferred in quiescient conditions while the other is typical in case of injury or disease. Each tissue-specific stem cell is located inside anatomically-defined microenvironment, called niche, surrounded by extracellular matrix (ECM) composed of a network of fibrillar proteins, growth factors, chemokines, cytokines and proteins that are present on the surface of neighboring cells. According to the interactions with these components, the cell choose self-renewal or a pathway of differentiation, following specific stimuli (Lutolf and Hubbell, 2005; Cosgrove et al., 2009). SCs reside in the niches that are positioned in a compartment between the myofiber plasma membrane and the basal lamina that surrounds the myofiber so that in the apical part of the niche they receive the signals from the myofibers while on their basal surface they are influenced by basal lamina signals (Collins et al., 2005; Kuang et al., 2008). SCs express several molecules to interact with the basal lamina and all its components (collagen, laminin, fibronectin) (Burkin and Kaufman, 1999). Conversely, the proteoglycan components of the basal lamina bind growth factors secreted by SCs such as basic Fibroblast Growth Factors (bFGF), and Insulin-like growth factor 1 (IGF-1) that regulate SC survival and proliferation (Golding et al., 2007; Le Grand et al., 2009). Other factors derived from cells that are not proximal to the niches or from the systemic circulation can influence SCs, such as myostatin, and wingless-type MMTV integration site family, member 3a (Wnt3a) (Mccroskery et al., 2003; Brack and Rando, 2007). These extrinsic factors play a fundamental role in aging, when the regenerative capacity of skeletal muscle declines (Grounds, 1987): for example, increased levels of circulating Wnt3a allowed the activation of β-catenin pathway in SCs, so that muscle regeneration is reduced and fibrosis is enhanced (Brack et al., 2008). The incredible complexity of niche regulation is the reason why, after removal from their *in vivo* localization,

SCs—and other adult stem cells—rapidly lost their myogenic ability (Dykstra et al., 2006) so that they cannot be used in clinical trials (Farini et al., 2009). As Kuang and collaborators suggested, the balance among the signals deriving from the various components of the niche is necessary to maintain the myogenic potential of the SCs (Kuang et al., 2008).

Recent studies have focused on imitate the regulatory machinery of the *in vivo* SC niche, as a powerful tool to control stem cell function. Three dimensional (3-D) matrices are the model system that mimics the *in vivo* microenvironment, allowing the investigation of these physiologic events (Cukierman et al., 2001; Abbott, 2003). They can derive from cells or tissues while others can be composed of ECM proteins. Natural ECMs can be formed by various protein fibrils and fibers interwoven within a hydrated network of glycosaminoglycan chains, providing a structural scaffold. Fibrils, pores, elastin and collagen can be present and alter the biophysical properties of ECMs. Moreover, artificial synthetic materials were produced with similar structure. Polyethylene glycol (PEG)-based hydrogels were used for the maintenance of SCs *in vitro* (Lutolf and Hubbell, 2005) while, recently, Kloxin and colleagues developed PEG hydrogels that controlled matrix stiffness without toxicity to cells (Kloxin et al., 2009). As these matrices were able to alter biophysical properties in a non-invasive manner, they were used to investigate the progression of biophysical changes associated with muscle fibrosis or disease (Engler et al., 2004). Moreover, Lutolf et al. demonstrated that PEG hydrogels were suitable for single-stem cell clonal assays and resistant to non-specific cell adhesion mediated by protein adsorption (Lutolf et al., 2009a). However, further studies are necessary to define exactly all the components that constitute the microenvironment of the SCs and the molecular steps that regulate the transition between SCs quiescence and proliferation.

TEM CELL FATE *IN VITRO*

In vitro stem-cell colture is carried out on flat coated with different substrates like collagen or laminin, on feeder-cell layers and within hydrogels synthetized from ECM components (for example collagen or Matrigel). Most frequently culture of stem cells was performed on rigid polystyrene tissue-culture plastic exposing cells to soluble factors in liquid media (Lutolf et al., 2009b).

These culture conditions are far from resemble the *in vivo* condition, where cells live in close proximity to each other and in contact with the ECM. Recently, 3D niche are still being explored and should be considered. Blau's group are studying the two-dimensional (2D) biomaterial culture systems deconstructing the niche and identifying and assessing the effects of individual niche components on stem-cell fate (Lutolf et al., 2009b). Normally, the effects of cell–cell interactions are studied by co-culturing; this strategy makes it difficult to discriminate the role of particular molecules.

In vivo, secreted growth factors and cytokines are mostly tethered to ECM components like proteoglycans. At the same time, receptor ligands are presented to stem cells surface and to nearby support cells. In both cases, molecule immobilization probably has the critical role of increasing protein stability, promoting persistent signaling and inducing receptor clustering (Irvine et al., 2002). A covalent binding of fibroblast growth factor 2 (FGF2) to a synthetic polymer stabilized the growth factor and increased its potency 100-fold relative to FGF2 in solution. Similarly, the epidermal growth factor (EGF) covalently tethered to a biomaterial scaffold, was shown to be more effective than its soluble counterpart in inducing mesenchymal stem cells differentiation and preventing Fas-ligand-induced death (Fan et al., 2007). Natural and synthetic matrices can be used to create cell-culture substrates with known elastic modulus providing diffusion of soluble molecules to the basal surface and the apical one, and can be used to test the relevance of homeostatic and disease related matrix stiffness to stem-cell behavior. Soluble factors in culture media used in combination with the tissue-culture matrix affect cell fate. Human MSCs expressed genes consistent with differentiation into distinct tissue-specific cell types when exposed to polyacrylamide gels with a range of stiffness typical of brain, muscle and bone (Engler et al., 2006). The effects of the physical properties of culture substrate on stem-cell fate are fully appreciated, culture platforms based on soft biomaterials are likely to replace, rigid, tissue-culture plastic. Within the niche, cells dialog with the surrounding ECM during development and in adulthood (Folkman and Moscona, 1978). Although some of these effects are probably due to alterations in the adhesive interactions and crosstalk between the ECM and the cell as they work to define each other, there is ample evidence suggesting that physical control of cell shape alone can act as a potent regulator of cell signaling and fate determination (Wozniak and Chen, 2009).

STEM CELL FATE *IN VIVO*

Biomaterials technologies offer great opportunities to control the stem cell fate *in vivo*, especially in case of tissue damage. Two main modes of application have been proposed: one in which biomaterials are used as carriers for introducing stem cells into damaged, diseased or aged tissue, and one in which biomaterials are used to augment endogenous stem-cell function (Lutolf et al., 2009b). In regenerative medicine, stem cell transplantation has some limitations: survival and engraftment of transplanted stem cells and the disrupted biological environment characterized by abundant cell and tissue necrosis. Biomaterials have to be designed to act as carriers for local delivery of stem cells, supporting cells or molecular niche cues. Biomaterials may improve the effect of stem cell transplantation; they may be used as multifunctional stem-cell microenvironments. They have to increase the delivering and enhancing the viability of the cells, to function as support in order to increase the numbers of the cells and stimulate the function of endogenous stem cells. Moreover, biomaterials can deliver diffusible cytokines in order to promote the mobilization of endogenous cells involved in repair, to enhance survival and to stimulate self-renewal and expansion of the transplanted cells. Materials would enhance tissue regeneration, tissue function and overcome the adverse effects of disease or ageing (Conboy et al., 2005; Adams et al., 2007). Therefore, they could permit local and specific delivery of bioactive niche components able to inhibit and stimulate molecules and drugs that have to increase the number and the functions of transplanted stem cells. In order to obtain these benefits *in vivo*, materials have to be achieved by forming a scaffold that deliver biomolecules near the stem-cell niche or by targeted delivery of soluble microparticles or as carriers of such bioactive niche components (Adams et al., 2007). Recently, Rothenfluh et al. isolated polymer nanoparticles, sufficiently small to enter the matrix of the targeted tissues; then, they modified them with a biomolecular ligand for matrix binding. This way, the modified the matrix into a source of nanoparticles (Gu et al., 2008; Rothenfluh et al., 2008). Similarly, Gu and co-workers modified existing nanoparticles so that they were used for differential delivery and controlled release of drugs (Gu et al., 2008). Biomaterials aim is not only to create materials to control spatially and temporally the components of the niche but also to study microenvironmental regulation of stem cell proliferation and fate (Conboy et al., 2005). Artificial niches could incorporate appropriate "homing" signals that would attract endogenous stem cells and localize them by means of known cell—cell or cell—matrix adhesive interactions. Biomaterial research is focused on create artificial niche where cells could to be exposed to tethered signals that control stem-cell function and expansion by self-renewal division.

MUSCLE PATHOPHYSIOLOGY

MUSCLE FIBROSIS

Following injury, a cascade of events starts to repair damaged tissues. First of all, inflammatory cells phagocyte the cell debris and secrete growth factors and cytokines that allow the proliferation of other cell types in the site of injury, as described in details below (see section Inflammation and repair mechanisms in skeletal muscle). Then, SCs start to proliferate and differentiate, a process which ultimately ends with the formation of new muscle fibers. Unfortunately, in muscular pathologies, the deficiency of structural proteins leads to continuous cycles of myofiber degeneration and regeneration, so that the damaged muscle fibers cannot be replaced by new fibers, causing myofiber degeneration, inflammation and fibrosis (Grounds et al., 2005; Serrano and Munoz-Canoves, 2010). In particular, the inflammatory cells eliminate the basement membranes of necrotic fibers that cannot be used to build the new fibers: this condition leads to abnormal muscle fiber arrangement in dystrophic muscles. Due to the chronic persistence of inflammatory cells, dystrophic muscles are characterized by higher concentration of growth factors and cytokines, that induce the massive proliferation and activation of fibroblasts. Their activity causes the accumulation of fibrotic elements that are responsible for uncontrolled events such as remodeling of the basal lamina and formation of collagenous tissues (Serrano and Munoz-Canoves, 2010). Normally, the events of muscle regeneration are tightly controlled by the interplay among different molecules. Insulin-like growth factor (IGF) is a key element in controlling tissue activity: it binds to cell surface receptors and to IGF-binding proteins, exerting a fundamental role in modulating myofibroblast and SCs proliferation. The matrix metallo-proteases (MMPs) have the function to degrade the ECM and to recruit inflammatory and myogenic cells in the site of injury while Sca-1 inhibits myoblast proliferation, preserving the progenitor cells (Serrano and Munoz-Canoves, 2010). Transforming growth factor (TGF)-β is highly expressed in regenerating muscle and it is a key regulator of fibrosis' development (Zhou et al., 2006); often, it functions in synergy with connective tissue growth factor (CTGF), inducing fibrosis and promoting dedifferentiation of myoblasts (Vial et al., 2008). CTGF binds to IGF-binding proteins and it is associated with fibrotic remodeling.

In the case of MDs, especially in DMD, membranes lacking the members of the dystroglycan complex are vulnerable to mechanical and oxidative stress. Due to myofiber breakdown, myofibroblasts remained activated: these phenomena are associated with altered production of ECM components and the accumulation of these molecules that lead to muscle cell necrosis and fibrosis (Klingler et al., 2012). Fibrosis development was considered a progressive and irreversible pathologic phenomenon, but recent advances in knowledge of its development steps render this pathological feature amenable for clinical treatments. A better understanding of the factors that participate in fibrosis may help identify pharmacological targets capable of attenuating the progression of untreatable muscular diseases.

MUSCULAR HYPERTROPHY AND ATROPHY: TWO OPPOSITES OF THE SAME PHENOMENON

Skeletal muscle is the most abundant tissue in mammals and muscle remodeling occurs throughout the entire life. A fine regulated pathway determines the balance between new protein accumulation and degradation of pre-existing ones (Sandri, 2008). Different stimuli, originated by functional overload or aging, can modulate this pathway causing a shift in this balance toward one side. Besides of physiological conditions, this pathway is influenced by lots of inherited and acquired disorders such as MDs, cancer cachexia and commons drugs as glucocorticoids (Cassano et al., 2009). Among signals that can produce hypertrophy, IGF1 pathway is one of the best characterized. IGF-1Ec is expressed in response to mechanical stimuli and cellular damage and promotes both proliferation and differentiation of satellite cells, while in adult myofibers it increases DNA content per myofiber and can influence myosin phenotype (Bamman et al., 2001). The binding of IGF-1 to its receptor IGF1R, triggers the activation of several kinases including phosphatidylinositol-3-kinase (PI3K), the consequent production of PIP3 recruits protein kinase B (AKT). AKT plays a central role in muscle remodeling: it acts by either activating positive signal (mTor) or blocking negative pathway (Myostatin, apoptotic cascade, GSK3β). A trophy results from degradation of both myofiber number and protein contents, through calpain system, lysosomal and the ubiquitin-proteasoma pathways (Voisin et al., 1996; Lecker et al., 1999). Two genes were found up-regulated in atrophy models: muscle-specific ubiquitin ligase atrogin-1 (MAFbx) and muscle RING-finger protein-1 (MURF1); further studies showed that they were ubiquitin-ligase expressed only in skeletal and cardiac muscle (Bodine et al., 2001). Another important factor is nuclear factor kappa-light-chain-enhancer of activated B cells (NF-kB) which is involved in inflammatory pathway leading to TNF-α and INF-γ expression and it can induce the degradation of MyoD. Moreover, knock out of myostatin, a member of the TGF-β family, can lead to an enormous enlargement of skeletal muscle mass (Mcpherron et al., 1997). Myostatin is in fact the most important negative regulatory element of fiber synthesis and it is strictly regulated during myogenesis thanks to the presence of E-boxes, MEF2 and GRE binding sites (Spiller et al., 2002). In particular, myostatin is synthesized as a precursor, that is processed by furin proteases to generate a dimer composed by an N-terminal pro-peptide, bound to biologically active C-terminal fragment. When the pro-peptide is cleaved, myostatin is activated and interact with several proteins, such as follistatin. Interestingly, mice without the expression of this protein have a reduced body mass (Matzuk et al., 1995) while follistatin forced expression leads to muscular hyper-growth (Nakatani et al., 2008). To test whether lack of myostatin could ameliorate the symptoms of muscular diseases, Whittemore et al. demonstrated that in wild type mice the blocking of the protein increased muscle mass (Whittemore et al., 2003) while Bogdanovich et al. showed that this condition in mdx mice improved myofibers size and muscular force (Bogdanovich et al., 2002). According to these studies, Wagner et al. described a phase I/II clinical trial of MYO-029 (a neutralizing antibody to myostatin) in dystrophic patients. This trial did not demonstrate any improvement in muscle strength, but no side effects were assessed, except for hypersensitivity skin reactions. This trial was originally designed to test safety so that a bigger cohort of patient or different choice of samples are required to detect arrest of disease progression or minimal improvements in strength. Furthermore, results could be explained by the fact that the patients were selected at late stage of the disease when the regenerative response is exhausted and the myostatin substrate was eliminated (Wagner et al., 2008). Similar studies were conducted also with animal models of other muscular diseases but opposite results were obtained (Li et al., 2005; Ohsawa et al., 2006). Further works demonstrated that myostatin not only downregulates the expression of several myogenic genes (Amthor et al., 2002; Mcfarlane et al., 2008) but efficiently inhibits the proliferation of muscle progenitor cells (Thomas et al., 2000). The complexity of mechanism involving muscle growth and regeneration is further increased by the discovery of microRNA. Recently, skeletal muscle specific microRNAs able to interact with master regulatory genes in muscle development were found (O'rourke et al., 2007). As an example, miRNA206 can influence satellite cells behavior by modulating Pax3 and MET transforming gene (cMet) (Clop et al., 2006; Mccarthy et al., 2007).

INFLAMMATION AND REPAIR MECHANISMS IN SKELETAL MUSCLE

Injuries affecting skeletal muscle determine the activation of the immune system and activate a cascade of events that are required to clean cellular debris and to allow the replacement of lost fibers with new ones. Furthermore, immune cells promote regeneration through the release of growth factors (Brunelli and Rovere-Querini, 2008). After acute muscular damage neutrophils rapidly appear, followed by phagocytic macrophages which continue to increase in numbers until about 2 days post-injury. A second population of macrophages develops at about 4 days post-injury and it is characterized by a non-phagocytic phenotype (Tidball and Villalta, 2010). In parallel, myogenic precursors start to proliferate and differentiate by recapitulating developmental steps. Firstly, response to injury is mediated by Th1 cytokines (INFγ and TNFα) which trigger the activation of classic M1 pro-inflammatory macrophages (Gordon and Taylor, 2005). At a second stage, a population of M2 anti-inflammatory macrophages is predominant thanks to Th2 cytokines stimulation, such as interleukin (IL)−4, −10, −13. This phenotype-switch is required to stop inflammation and to permit the differentiation and fusion of satellite cells. This process is strictly regulated and several signals are known to be involved (Fadok et al., 2001; Arnold et al., 2007) but further studies are needed to better understand each phase. In MDs, skeletal muscles are subjected to chronic injuries that maintain a continue activation of the immune system. In fact, inflammatory infiltrates consisting of both macrophages and lymphocytes are present and elevated serum cytokines levels are detectable. Furthermore, a partial adaptive response to treatment with corticosteroid supports a role for the immune system in exacerbating muscular wasting (Backman and Henriksson, 1995). Progressive MDs like DMD are characterized by an initial phase that recapitulates the event observed in acute injury and repair. A second phase is dominated by chronic inflammation which triggers fibrosis deposition and atrophy. In fact in adult mdx mice a transition from M2a macrophages to M2c macrophages occurs in an attempt to control M1 cytolitic macrophages and to promote muscle regeneration through the release of IL-10 and IL-4 (Gordon, 2003; Horsley et al., 2003). M2 macrophages may also partecipate in activation of cytotoxic T-cells (which promote muscle damage through perforin-mediate process) and promote muscle fibrosis through arginase metabolism of arginine (Villalta et al., 2009; Tidball and Villalta, 2010).

The importance of modulating immune system cells was proven in different animal model of MDs, for example depletion of macrophages from mdx mice resulted in reduced muscle membrane lysis (Petrof et al., 1993). Furthermore, non-steroidal anti-inflammatory drug (NSAID) treatment was effective both in ameliorating muscle morphology and reducing macrophage infiltration (Serra et al., 2012) and anti-oxidant drugs (N-acetylcysteine) in mdx mice reduced necrosis by regulating TNF-α level (De Senzi Moraes Pinto et al., 2013). Recently an important role for acquired immunity in DMD pathogenesis has been pointed out by (Mendell et al., 1995; Hemmati et al., 2003; Flanigan et al., 2013) opening new perspectives in treatment of MDs.

CONCLUSIONS

Skeletal muscle emerged as a promising tissue source for stem and progenitor cells that can be used in a variety of therapeutic applications. Skeletal muscle constitutes around one third of body weight in a healthy subjects (Gates et al., 2008). Muscle has an high capacity to repair itself after injury; this characteristic suggests that it serves as a reservoir for cells that participate in tissue regeneration processes (Usas and Huard, 2007). Several works described the ability of different muscle-derived stem cell populations to differentiate into multiple cell types, including osteoblasts, adipocytes, chondrocytes, myoblasts and endothelial cells. In addition, these cells showed regenerative, anti-inflammatory and anti-apoptotic properties. Each of these cell types is characterized primarily on the basis of their *in vitro* characteristics after they have been isolated from the body. *In vivo* they exhibited the capacity to migrate through different tissues where they are exposed to different extracellular and environmental signals. While rudimentary models were developed to describe the *in vivo* relationship among these stem cell populations, substantial additional studies are needed to refine and verify these relationships.

New approaches using organisms genetically modified and transgenic mouse models proposed the importance of the microenvironment—like the niche and the extrinsic factors—to be a key component in stem cell regulation. Particularly, significant progress has been made in understanding how satellite cells can act as tissue-specific adult stem cells in skeletal muscle. In the same time, many studies investigated the satellite cell properties in term of efficacy after *in vivo* transplantation using novel approaches such as non-invasive bioluminescence imaging. These tools provided information for assessing not only satellite cell function but, in general, stem cell function. Investigations on the molecular nature of stem cell niche signals on *in vivo* models and short-term cultures of isolated myofibers, are now on-going. Bioengineering offers significant tools for the development of strategies to mimic biochemical and biophysical features of the *in vivo* niche microenvironment (Lutolf et al., 2009b). We hope that the synthesis of biomaterials, micro-fabrication technology and stem cell biology will provide systems potentially innovative to better understand how stem cell fate is controlled. The analysis of the niche and the dynamic responses of stem cells to well-defined artificial microenvironments, might give us the possibility to understand the role of specific niche components and niche architecture in regulating fundamental cellular mechanisms such as cellular division, self-renewal, and differentiation *in vitro* and *in vivo*. Development of biomaterials able to re-create an *in vitro* SCs niche could give rise to novel insights into understanding the molecular cues, critical for the *in vitro* maintenance and expansion of muscle stem cells. Above all, these *in vitro* systems can well lead to the generation of adequate numbers of stem cells and the ability to control their differentiation in order to maximize their utility, not only as cell-based therapeutics for tissue regeneration and replacement, but also as the control of inflammation after muscle damage (Cosgrove et al., 2009). In conclusion, all these considerations will be important not only to better characterize satellite cell biology and therapeutic approaches to treat muscle diseases and aging-related muscle wasting, but also to give necessary information for the study of adult tissue-specific stem cells.

AUTHOR CONTRIBUTIONS

Mirella Meregalli and Yvan Torrente designed the approach, Andrea Farini and Clementina Sitzia wrote the manuscript.

ACKNOWLEDGMENTS

This work was supported by Associazione La Nostra Famiglia Fondo DMD Gli Amici di Emanuele, Associazione Amici del Centro Dino Ferrari, Ministry of Health (RF-2009-1547384).

REFERENCES

Abbott, A. (2003). Cell culture: biology's new dimension. *Nature* 424, 870–872. doi: 10.1038/424870a

Adams, G. B., Martin, R. P., Alley, I. R., Chabner, K. T., Cohen, K. S., Calvi, L. M., et al. (2007). Therapeutic targeting of a stem cell niche. *Nat. Biotechnol.* 25, 238–243. doi: 10.1038/nbt1281

Alessandri, G., Pagano, S., Bez, A., Benetti, A., Pozzi, S., Iannolo, G., et al. (2004). Isolation and culture of human muscle-derived stem cells able to differentiate into myogenic and neurogenic cell lineages. *Lancet* 364, 1872–1883. doi: 10.1016/S0140-6736(04)17443-6

Alhadlaq, A., and Mao, J. J. (2004). Mesenchymal stem cells: isolation and therapeutics. *Stem Cells Dev.* 13, 436–448. doi: 10.1089/scd.2004.13.436

Amit, M., and Itskovitz-Eldor, J. (2002). Derivation and spontaneous differentiation of human embryonic stem cells. *J. Anat.* 200, 225–232. doi: 10.1046/j.1469-7580.2002.00032.x

Amthor, H., Huang, R., Mckinnell, I., Christ, B., Kambadur, R., Sharma, M., et al. (2002). The regulation and action of myostatin as a negative regulator of muscle development during avian embryogenesis. *Dev. Biol.* 251, 241–257. doi: 10.1006/dbio.2002.0812

Andrews, P. W., Casper, J., Damjanov, I., Duggan-Keen, M., Giwercman, A., Hata, J., et al. (1996). Comparative analysis of cell surface antigens expressed by cell lines derived from human germ cell tumours. *Int. J. Cancer* 66, 806–816. doi: 10.1002/(SICI)1097-0215(19960611)66:6<806::AID-IJC17>3.0.CO;2-0

Arnold, L., Henry, A., Poron, F., Baba-Amer, Y., Van Rooijen, N., Plonquet, A., et al. (2007). Inflammatory monocytes recruited after skeletal muscle injury switch into antiinflammatory macrophages to support myogenesis. *J. Exp. Med.* 204, 1057–1069. doi: 10.1084/jem.20070075

Backman, E., and Henriksson, K. G. (1995). Low-dose prednisolone treatment in Duchenne and Becker muscular dystrophy. *Neuromuscul. Disord.* 5, 233–241. doi: 10.1016/0960-8966(94)00048-E

Bamman, M. M., Shipp, J. R., Jiang, J., Gower, B. A., Hunter, G. R., Goodman, A. Jr., et al. (2001). Mechanical load increases muscle IGF-I and androgen receptor mRNA concentrations in humans. *Am. J. Physiol. Endocrinol. Metab.* 280, E383–E390.

Barberi, T., Bradbury, M., Dincer, Z., Panagiotakos, G., Socci, N. D., and Studer, L. (2007). Derivation of engraftable skeletal myoblasts from human embryonic stem cells. *Nat. Med.* 13, 642–648. doi: 10.1038/nm1533

Benchaouir, R., Meregalli, M., Farini, A., D'antona, G., Belicchi, M., Goyenvalle, A., et al. (2007). Restoration of human dystrophin following transplantation of exon-skipping-engineered DMD patient stem cells into dystrophic mice. *Cell Stem Cell* 1, 646–657. doi: 10.1016/j.stem.2007.09.016

Beyer Nardi, N., and Da Silva Meirelles, L. (2006). Mesenchymal stem cells: isolation, *in vitro* expansion and characterization. *Handb. Exp. Pharmacol.* 174, 249–282. doi: 10.1007/978-3-540-77855-4_11

Bhagavati, S., and Xu, W. (2005). Generation of skeletal muscle from transplanted embryonic stem cells in dystrophic mice. *Biochem. Biophys. Res. Commun.* 333, 644–649. doi: 10.1016/j.bbrc.2005.05.135

Bodine, S. C., Latres, E., Baumhueter, S., Lai, V. K., Nunez, L., Clarke, B. A., et al. (2001). Identification of ubiquitin ligases required for skeletal muscle atrophy. *Science* 294, 1704–1708. doi: 10.1126/science.1065874

Bogdanovich, S., Krag, T. O., Barton, E. R., Morris, L. D., Whittemore, L. A., Ahima, R. S., et al. (2002). Functional improvement of dystrophic muscle by myostatin blockade. *Nature* 420, 418–421. doi: 10.1038/nature01154

Brack, A. S., Conboy, I. M., Conboy, M. J., Shen, J., and Rando, T. A. (2008). A temporal switch from notch to Wnt signaling in muscle stem cells is necessary for normal adult myogenesis. *Cell Stem Cell* 2, 50–59. doi: 10.1016/j.stem.2007.10.006

Brack, A. S., and Rando, T. A. (2007). Intrinsic changes and extrinsic influences of myogenic stem cell function during aging. *Stem Cell Rev.* 3, 226–237. doi: 10.1007/s12015-007-9000-2

Brunelli, S., and Rovere-Querini, P. (2008). The immune system and the repair of skeletal muscle. *Pharmacol. Res.* 58, 117–121. doi: 10.1016/j.phrs.2008.06.008

Buckingham, M., Bajard, L., Chang, T., Daubas, P., Hadchouel, J., Meilhac, S., et al. (2003). The formation of skeletal muscle: from somite to limb. *J. Anat.* 202, 59–68. doi: 10.1046/j.1469-7580.2003.00139.x

Burkin, D. J., and Kaufman, S. J. (1999). The alpha7beta1 integrin in muscle development and disease. *Cell Tissue Res.* 296, 183–190. doi: 10.1007/s004410051279

Cai, B., Spencer, M. J., Nakamura, G., Tseng-Ong, L., and Tidball, J. G. (2000). Eosinophilia of dystrophin-deficient muscle is promoted by perforin-mediated cytotoxicity by T cell effectors. *Am. J. Pathol.* 156, 1789–1796. doi: 10.1016/S0002-9440(10)65050-X

Carpenter, M. K., Rosler, E., and Rao, M. S. (2003). Characterization and differentiation of human embryonic stem cells. *Cloning Stem Cells* 5, 79–88. doi: 10.1089/153623003321512193

Carr, A. J., Vugler, A. A., Hikita, S. T., Lawrence, J. M., Gias, C., Chen, L. L., et al. (2009). Protective effects of human iPS-derived retinal pigment epithelium cell transplantation in the retinal dystrophic rat. *PLoS ONE* 4:e8152. doi: 10.1371/journal.pone.0008152

Cassano, M., Quattrocelli, M., Crippa, S., Perini, I., Ronzoni, F., and Sampaolesi, M. (2009). Cellular mechanisms and local progenitor activation to regulate skeletal muscle mass. *J. Muscle Res. Cell Motil.* 30, 243–253. doi: 10.1007/s10974-010-9204-y

Cerletti, M., Jurga, S., Witczak, C. A., Hirshman, M. F., Shadrach, J. L., Goodyear, L. J., et al. (2008). Highly efficient, functional engraftment of skeletal muscle stem cells in dystrophic muscles. *Cell* 134, 37–47. doi: 10.1016/j.cell.2008.05.049

Clop, A., Marcq, F., Takeda, H., Pirottin, D., Tordoir, X., Bibe, B., et al. (2006). A mutation creating a potential illegitimate microRNA target site in the myostatin gene affects muscularity in sheep. *Nat. Genet.* 38, 813–818. doi: 10.1038/ng1810

Collins, C. A., Olsen, I., Zammit, P. S., Heslop, L., Petrie, A., Partridge, T. A., et al. (2005). Stem cell function, self-renewal, and behavioral heterogeneity of cells from the adult muscle satellite cell niche. *Cell* 122, 289–301. doi: 10.1016/j.cell.2005.05.010

Conboy, I. M., Conboy, M. J., Smythe, G. M., and Rando, T. A. (2003). Notch-mediated restoration of regenerative potential to aged muscle. *Science* 302, 1575–1577. doi: 10.1126/science.1087573

Conboy, I. M., Conboy, M. J., Wagers, A. J., Girma, E. R., Weissman, I. L., and Rando, T. A. (2005). Rejuvenation of aged progenitor cells by exposure to a young systemic environment. *Nature* 433, 760–764. doi: 10.1038/nature03260

Conboy, I. M., and Rando, T. A. (2002). The regulation of Notch signaling controls satellite cell activation and cell fate determination in postnatal myogenesis. *Dev. Cell* 3, 397–409. doi: 10.1016/S1534-5807(02)00254-X

Conrad, S., Renninger, M., Hennenlotter, J., Wiesner, T., Just, L., Bonin, M., et al. (2008). Generation of pluripotent stem cells from adult human testis. *Nature* 456, 344–349. doi: 10.1038/nature07404

Constantin, G., Marconi, S., Rossi, B., Angiari, S., Calderan, L., Anghileri, E., et al. (2009). Adipose-derived mesenchymal stem cells ameliorate chronic experimental autoimmune encephalomyelitis. *Stem Cells* 27, 2624–2635. doi: 10.1002/stem.194

Cosgrove, B. D., Sacco, A., Gilbert, P. M., and Blau, H. M. (2009). A home away from home: challenges and opportunities in engineering *in vitro* muscle satellite cell niches. *Differentiation* 78, 185–194. doi: 10.1016/j.diff.2009.08.004

Cossu, G., and Sampaolesi, M. (2007). New therapies for Duchenne muscular dystrophy: challenges, prospects and clinical trials. *Trends Mol. Med.* 13, 520–526. doi: 10.1016/j.molmed.2007.10.003

Cukierman, E., Pankov, R., Stevens, D. R., and Yamada, K. M. (2001). Taking cell-matrix adhesions to the third dimension. *Science* 294, 1708–1712. doi: 10.1126/science.1064829

Darabi, R., Arpke, R. W., Irion, S., Dimos, J. T., Grskovic, M., Kyba, M., et al. (2012). Human ES- and iPS-derived myogenic progenitors restore DYSTROPHIN and improve contractility upon transplantation in dystrophic mice. *Cell Stem Cell* 10, 610–619. doi: 10.1016/j.stem.2012.02.015

Darabi, R., Baik, J., Clee, M., Kyba, M., Tupler, R., and Perlingeiro, R. C. (2009). Engraftment of embryonic stem cell-derived myogenic progenitors in a dominant model of muscular dystrophy. *Exp. Neurol.* 220, 212–216. doi: 10.1016/j.expneurol.2009.08.002

Darabi, R., Gehlbach, K., Bachoo, R. M., Kamath, S., Osawa, M., Kamm, K. E., et al. (2008a). Functional skeletal muscle regeneration from differentiating embryonic stem cells. *Nat. Med.* 14, 134–143. doi: 10.1038/nm1705

Darabi, R., Santos, F. N., and Perlingeiro, R. C. (2008b). The therapeutic potential of embryonic and adult stem cells for skeletal muscle regeneration. *Stem Cell Rev.* 4, 217–225. doi: 10.1007/s12015-008-9023-3

Darabi, R., Santos, F. N., Filareto, A., Pan, W., Koene, R., Rudnicki, M. A., et al. (2011). Assessment of the myogenic stem cell compartment following transplantation of Pax3/Pax7-induced embryonic stem cell-derived progenitors. *Stem Cells* 29, 777–790. doi: 10.1002/stem.625

De Bari, C., Dell'accio, F., Tylzanowski, P., and Luyten, F. P. (2001). Multipotent mesenchymal stem cells from adult human synovial membrane. *Arthritis Rheum.* 44, 1928–1942. doi: 10.1002/1529-0131(200108)44:8<1928::AID-ART331>3.0.CO;2-P

De Bari, C., Dell'accio, F., Vandenabeele, F., Vermeesch, J. R., Raymackers, J. M., and Luyten, F. P. (2003). Skeletal muscle repair by adult human mesenchymal stem cells from synovial membrane. *J. Cell Biol.* 160, 909–918. doi: 10.1083/jcb.200212064

De Senzi Moraes Pinto, R., Ferretti, R., Moraes, L. H., Neto, H. S., Marques, M. J., and Minatel, E. (2013). N-acetylcysteine treatment reduces TNF-alpha levels and myonecrosis in diaphragm muscle of mdx mice. *Clin. Nutr.* 32, 472–475. doi: 10.1016/j.clnu.2012.06.001

Dimos, J. T., Rodolfa, K. T., Niakan, K. K., Weisenthal, L. M., Mitsumoto, H., Chung, W., et al. (2008). Induced pluripotent stem cells generated from patients with ALS can be differentiated into motor neurons. *Science* 321, 1218–1221. doi: 10.1126/science.1158799

Dykstra, B., Ramunas, J., Kent, D., Mccaffrey, L., Szumsky, E., Kelly, L., et al. (2006). High-resolution video monitoring of hematopoietic stem cells cultured in single-cell arrays identifies new features of self-renewal. *Proc. Natl. Acad. Sci. U.S.A.* 103, 8185–8190. doi: 10.1073/pnas.0602548103

Ebert, A. D., Yu, J., Rose, F. F. Jr., Mattis, V. B., Lorson, C. L., Thomson, J. A., et al. (2009). Induced pluripotent stem cells from a spinal muscular atrophy patient. *Nature* 457, 277–280. doi: 10.1038/nature07677

Egawa, N., Kitaoka, S., Tsukita, K., Naitoh, M., Takahashi, K., Yamamoto, T., et al. (2012). Drug screening for ALS using patient-specific induced pluripotent stem cells. *Sci. Transl. Med.* 4, 145ra104. doi: 10.1126/scitranslmed.3004052

Engler, A. J., Griffin, M. A., Sen, S., Bonnemann, C. G., Sweeney, H. L., and Discher, D. E. (2004). Myotubes differentiate optimally on substrates with tissue-like stiffness: pathological implications for soft or stiff microenvironments. *J. Cell Biol.* 166, 877–887. doi: 10.1083/jcb.200405004

Engler, A. J., Sen, S., Sweeney, H. L., and Discher, D. E. (2006). Matrix elasticity directs stem cell lineage specification. *Cell* 126, 677–689. doi: 10.1016/j.cell.2006.06.044

Fadok, V. A., Bratton, D. L., Guthrie, L., and Henson, P. M. (2001). Differential effects of apoptotic versus lysed cells on macrophage production of cytokines: role of proteases. *J. Immunol.* 166, 6847–6854.

Fan, V. H., Tamama, K., Au, A., Littrell, R., Richardson, L. B., Wright, J. W., et al. (2007). Tethered epidermal growth factor provides a survival advantage to mesenchymal stem cells. *Stem Cells* 25, 1241–1251. doi: 10.1634/stemcells.2006-0320

Farini, A., Razini, P., Erratico, S., Torrente, Y., and Meregalli, M. (2009). Cell based therapy for Duchenne muscular dystrophy. *J. Cell Physiol.* 221, 526–534. doi: 10.1002/jcp.21895

Filareto, A., Parker, S., Darabi, R., Borges, L., Iacovino, M., Schaaf, T., et al. (2013). An *ex vivo* gene therapy approach to treat muscular dystrophy using inducible pluripotent stem cells. *Nat Commun* 4, 1549. doi: 10.1038/ncomms2550

Fiorina, P., Jurewicz, M., Augello, A., Vergani, A., Dada, S., La Rosa, S., et al. (2009). Immunomodulatory function of bone marrow-derived mesenchymal stem cells in experimental autoimmune type 1 diabetes. *J. Immunol.* 183, 993–1004. doi: 10.4049/jimmunol.0900803

Flanigan, K. M., Campbell, K., Viollet, L., Wang, W., Gomez, A. M., Walker, C. M., et al. (2013). Anti-dystrophin T cell responses in Duchenne muscular dystrophy: prevalence and a glucocorticoid treatment effect. *Hum. Gene Ther.* 24, 797–806. doi: 10.1089/hum.2013.092

Folkman, J., and Moscona, A. (1978). Role of cell shape in growth control. *Nature* 273, 345–349. doi: 10.1038/273345a0

Galvez, B. G., Sampaolesi, M., Brunelli, S., Covarello, D., Gavina, M., Rossi, B., et al. (2006). Complete repair of dystrophic skeletal muscle by mesoangioblasts with enhanced migration ability. *J. Cell Biol.* 174, 231–243. doi: 10.1083/jcb.200512085

Gang, E. J., Jeong, J. A., Hong, S. H., Hwang, S. H., Kim, S. W., Yang, I. H., et al. (2004). Skeletal myogenic differentiation of mesenchymal stem cells isolated from human umbilical cord blood. *Stem Cells* 22, 617–624. doi: 10.1634/stemcells.22-4-617

Gates, C. B., Karthikeyan, T., Fu, F., and Huard, J. (2008). Regenerative medicine for the musculoskeletal system based on muscle-derived stem cells. *J. Am. Acad. Orthop. Surg.* 16, 68–76.

Golding, J. P., Calderbank, E., Partridge, T. A., and Beauchamp, J. R. (2007). Skeletal muscle stem cells express anti-apoptotic ErbB receptors during activation from quiescence. *Exp. Cell. Res.* 313, 341–356. doi: 10.1016/j.yexcr.2006.10.019

Gordon, S. (2003). Alternative activation of macrophages. *Nat. Rev. Immunol.* 3, 23–35. doi: 10.1038/nri978

Gordon, S., and Taylor, P. R. (2005). Monocyte and macrophage heterogeneity. *Nat. Rev. Immunol.* 5, 953–964. doi: 10.1038/nri1733

Goudenege, S., Lebel, C., Huot, N. B., Dufour, C., Fujii, I., Gekas, J., et al. (2012). Myoblasts derived from normal hESCs and dystrophic hiPSCs efficiently fuse with existing muscle fibers following transplantation. *Mol. Ther.* 20, 2153–2167. doi: 10.1038/mt.2012.188

Grounds, M. D. (1987). Phagocytosis of necrotic muscle in muscle isografts is influenced by the strain, age, and sex of host mice. *J. Pathol.* 153, 71–82. doi: 10.1002/path.1711530110

Grounds, M. D., Sorokin, L., and White, J. (2005). Strength at the extracellular matrix-muscle interface. *Scand J Med Sci Sports* 15, 381–391. doi: 10.1111/j.1600-0838.2005.00467.x

Gu, F., Zhang, L., Teply, B. A., Mann, N., Wang, A., Radovic-Moreno, A. F., et al. (2008). Precise engineering of targeted nanoparticles by using self-assembled biointegrated block copolymers. *Proc. Natl. Acad. Sci. U.S.A.* 105, 2586–2591. doi: 10.1073/pnas.0711714105

Gussoni, E., Blau, H. M., and Kunkel, L. M. (1997). The fate of individual myoblasts after transplantation into muscles of DMD patients. *Nat. Med.* 3, 970–977. doi: 10.1038/nm0997-970

Hanna, J., Wernig, M., Markoulaki, S., Sun, C. W., Meissner, A., Cassady, J. P., et al. (2007). Treatment of sickle cell anemia mouse model with iPS cells generated from autologous skin. *Science* 318, 1920–1923. doi: 10.1126/science.1152092

Hemmati, H. D., Nakano, I., Lazareff, J. A., Masterman-Smith, M., Geschwind, D. H., Bronner-Fraser, M., et al. (2003). Cancerous stem cells can arise from pediatric brain tumors. *Proc. Natl. Acad. Sci. U.S.A.* 100, 15178–15183. doi: 10.1073/pnas.2036535100

Hodgetts, S., Radley, H., Davies, M., and Grounds, M. D. (2006). Reduced necrosis of dystrophic muscle by depletion of host neutrophils, or blocking TNFalpha function with Etanercept in mdx mice. *Neuromuscul. Disord.* 16, 591–602. doi: 10.1016/j.nmd.2006.06.011

Hoffman, L. M., and Carpenter, M. K. (2005). Characterization and culture of human embryonic stem cells. *Nat. Biotechnol.* 23, 699–708. doi: 10.1038/nbt1102

Horsley, V., Jansen, K. M., Mills, S. T., and Pavlath, G. K. (2003). IL-4 acts as a myoblast recruitment factor during mammalian muscle growth. *Cell* 113, 483–494. doi: 10.1016/S0092-8674(03)00319-2

Iacovino, M., Bosnakovski, D., Fey, H., Rux, D., Bajwa, G., Mahen, E., et al. (2011). Inducible cassette exchange: a rapid and efficient system enabling conditional gene expression in embryonic stem and primary cells. *Stem Cells* 29, 1580–1588. doi: 10.1002/stem.715

Ichim, T. E., Alexandrescu, D. T., Solano, F., Lara, F., Campion Rde, N., Paris, E., et al. (2010). Mesenchymal stem cells as anti-inflammatories: implications for treatment of Duchenne muscular dystrophy. *Cell Immunol.* 260, 75–82. doi: 10.1016/j.cellimm.2009.10.006

Irintchev, A., Zeschnigk, M., Starzinski-Powitz, A., and Wernig, A. (1994). Expression pattern of M-cadherin in normal, denervated, and regenerating mouse muscles. *Dev. Dyn.* 199, 326–337. doi: 10.1002/aja.10019 90407

Irvine, D. J., Hue, K. A., Mayes, A. M., and Griffith, L. G. (2002). Simulations of cell-surface integrin binding to nanoscale-clustered adhesion ligands. *Biophys. J.* 82, 120–132. doi: 10.1016/S0006-3495(02)75379-4

Jackson, W. M., Nesti, L. J., and Tuan, R. S. (2010). Potential therapeutic applications of muscle-derived mesenchymal stem and progenitor cells. *Expert Opin. Biol. Ther.* 10, 505–517. doi: 10.1517/14712591003610606

Klingler, W., Jurkat-Rott, K., Lehmann-Horn, F., and Schleip, R. (2012). The role of fibrosis in Duchenne muscular dystrophy. *Acta Myol.* 31, 184–195.

Kloxin, A. M., Kasko, A. M., Salinas, C. N., and Anseth, K. S. (2009). Photodegradable hydrogels for dynamic tuning of physical and chemical properties. *Science* 324, 59–63. doi: 10.1126/science.1169494

Kuang, S., Gillespie, M. A., and Rudnicki, M. A. (2008). Niche regulation of muscle satellite cell self-renewal and differentiation. *Cell Stem Cell* 2, 22–31. doi: 10.1016/j.stem.2007.12.012

Kuang, S., Kuroda, K., Le Grand, F., and Rudnicki, M. A. (2007). Asymmetric self-renewal and commitment of satellite stem cells in muscle. *Cell* 129, 999–1010. doi: 10.1016/j.cell.2007.03.044

Kuraitis, D., Giordano, C., Ruel, M., Musaro, A., and Suuronen, E. J. (2012). Exploiting extracellular matrix-stem cell interactions: a review of natural materials for therapeutic muscle regeneration. *Biomaterials* 33, 428–443. doi: 10.1016/j.biomaterials.2011.09.078

Le Blanc, K., and Pittenger, M. (2005). Mesenchymal stem cells: progress toward promise. *Cytotherapy* 7, 36–45. doi: 10.1080/14653240510018118

Lecker, S. H., Solomon, V., Price, S. R., Kwon, Y. T., Mitch, W. E., and Goldberg, A. L. (1999). Ubiquitin conjugation by the N-end rule pathway and mRNAs for its components increase in muscles of diabetic rats. *J. Clin. Invest.* 104, 1411–1420. doi: 10.1172/JCI7300

Le Grand, F., Jones, A. E., Seale, V., Scime, A., and Rudnicki, M. A. (2009). Wnt7a activates the planar cell polarity pathway to drive the symmetric expansion of satellite stem cells. *Cell Stem Cell* 4, 535–547. doi: 10.1016/j.stem.2009.03.013

Leist, M., Bremer, S., Brundin, P., Hescheler, J., Kirkeby, A., Krause, K. H., et al. (2008). The biological and ethical basis of the use of human embryonic stem cells for *in vitro* test systems or cell therapy. *ALTEX* 25, 163–190.

Li, Z. F., Shelton, G. D., and Engvall, E. (2005). Elimination of myostatin does not combat muscular dystrophy in dy mice but increases postnatal lethality. *Am J Pathol* 166, 491–497. doi: 10.1016/S0002-9440(10)62271-7

Lian, Q., Zhang, Y., Zhang, J., Zhang, H. K., Wu, X., Zhang, Y., et al. (2010). Functional mesenchymal stem cells derived from human induced pluripotent stem cells attenuate limb ischemia in mice. *Circulation* 121, 1113–1123. doi: 10.1161/CIRCULATIONAHA.109.898312

Lin, T., Chao, C., Saito, S., Mazur, S. J., Murphy, M. E., Appella, E., et al. (2005). p53 induces differentiation of mouse embryonic stem cells by suppressing Nanog expression. *Nat. Cell Biol.* 7, 165–171. doi: 10.1038/ncb1211

Lutolf, M. P., Doyonnas, R., Havenstrite, K., Koleckar, K., and Blau, H. M. (2009a). Perturbation of single hematopoietic stem cell fates in artificial niches. *Integr. Biol. (Camb.)* 1, 59–69. doi: 10.1039/b815718a

Lutolf, M. P., Gilbert, P. M., and Blau, H. M. (2009b). Designing materials to direct stem-cell fate. *Nature* 462, 433–441. doi: 10.1038/nature08602

Lutolf, M. P., and Hubbell, J. A. (2005). Synthetic biomaterials as instructive extracellular microenvironments for morphogenesis in tissue engineering. *Nat. Biotechnol.* 23, 47–55. doi: 10.1038/nbt1055

Madec, A. M., Mallone, R., Afonso, G., Abou Mrad, E., Mesnier, A., Eljaafari, A., et al. (2009). Mesenchymal stem cells protect NOD mice from diabetes by inducing regulatory T cells. *Diabetologia* 52, 1391–1399. doi: 10.1007/s00125-009-1374-z

Matzuk, M. M., Lu, N., Vogel, H., Sellheyer, K., Roop, D. R., and Bradley, A. (1995). Multiple defects and perinatal death in mice deficient in follistatin. *Nature* 374, 360–363. doi: 10.1038/374360a0

Mccarthy, J. J., Esser, K. A., and Andrade, F. H. (2007). MicroRNA-206 is overexpressed in the diaphragm but not the hindlimb muscle of mdx mouse. *Am. J. Physiol. Cell Physiol.* 293, C451–C457. doi: 10.1152/ajpcell.00077.2007

Mccroskery, S., Thomas, M., Maxwell, L., Sharma, M., and Kambadur, R. (2003). Myostatin negatively regulates satellite cell activation and self-renewal. *J. Cell Biol.* 162, 1135–1147. doi: 10.1083/jcb.200207056

Mcfarlane, C., Hennebry, A., Thomas, M., Plummer, E., Ling, N., Sharma, M., et al. (2008). Myostatin signals through Pax7 to regulate satellite cell self-renewal. *Exp. Cell Res.* 314, 317–329. doi: 10.1016/j.yexcr.2007.09.012

Mcnally, E. M., Ly, C. T., Rosenmann, H., Mitrani Rosenbaum, S., Jiang, W., Anderson, L. V., et al. (2000). Splicing mutation in dysferlin produces limb-girdle muscular dystrophy with inflammation. *Am. J. Med. Genet.* 91, 305–312. doi: 10.1002/(SICI)1096-8628(20000410)91:4%3C305::AID-AJMG12%3E3.0.CO;2-S

Mcpherron, A. C., Lawler, A. M., and Lee, S. J. (1997). Regulation of skeletal muscle mass in mice by a new TGF-beta superfamily member. *Nature* 387, 83–90. doi: 10.1038/387083a0

Mendell, J. R., Kissel, J. T., Amato, A. A., King, W., Signore, L., Prior, T. W., et al. (1995). Myoblast transfer in the treatment of Duchenne's muscular dystrophy. *N. Engl. J. Med.* 333, 832–838. doi: 10.1056/NEJM199509283331303

Mizuno, Y., Chang, H., Umeda, K., Niwa, A., Iwasa, T., Awaya, T., et al. (2010). Generation of skeletal muscle stem/progenitor cells from murine induced pluripotent stem cells. *FASEB J.* 24, 2245–2253. doi: 10.1096/fj.09-137174

Montarras, D., Morgan, J., Collins, C., Relaix, F., Zaffran, S., Cumano, A., et al. (2005). Direct isolation of satellite cells for skeletal muscle regeneration. *Science* 309, 2064–2067. doi: 10.1126/science.1114758

Moon, S. Y., Park, Y. B., Kim, D. S., Oh, S. K., and Kim, D. W. (2006). Generation, culture, and differentiation of human embryonic stem cells for therapeutic applications. *Mol. Ther.* 13, 5–14. doi: 10.1016/j.ymthe.2005.09.008

Morrison, S. J., and Kimble, J. (2006). Asymmetric and symmetric stem-cell divisions in development and cancer. *Nature* 441, 1068–1074. doi: 10.1038/nature04956

Nakatani, M., Takehara, Y., Sugino, H., Matsumoto, M., Hashimoto, O., Hasegawa, Y., et al. (2008). Transgenic expression of a myostatin inhibitor derived from follistatin increases skeletal muscle mass and ameliorates dystrophic pathology in mdx mice. *FASEB J.* 22, 477–487. doi: 10.1096/fj.07-8673com

Negroni, E., Riederer, I., Chaouch, S., Belicchi, M., Razini, P., Di Santo, J., et al. (2009). *In vivo* myogenic potential of human CD133+ muscle-derived stem cells: a quantitative study. *Mol. Ther.* 17, 1771–1778. doi: 10.1038/mt.2009.167

Nelson, T. J., Martinez-Fernandez, A., Yamada, S., Perez-Terzic, C., Ikeda, Y., and Terzic, A. (2009). Repair of acute myocardial infarction by human stemness factors induced pluripotent stem cells. *Circulation* 120, 408–416. doi: 10.1161/CIRCULATIONAHA.109.865154

Nemeth, K., Leelahavanichkul, A., Yuen, P. S., Mayer, B., Parmelee, A., Doi, K., et al. (2009). Bone marrow stromal cells attenuate sepsis via prostaglandin E(2)-dependent reprogramming of host macrophages to increase their interleukin-10 production. *Nat. Med.* 15, 42–49. doi: 10.1038/nm.1905

Nesti, L. J., Jackson, W. M., Shanti, R. M., Koehler, S. M., Aragon, A. B., Bailey, J. R., et al. (2008). Differentiation potential of multipotent progenitor cells derived from war-traumatized muscle tissue. *J. Bone Joint Surg. Am.* 90, 2390–2398. doi: 10.2106/JBJS.H.00049

Ohsawa, Y., Hagiwara, H., Nakatani, M., Yasue, A., Moriyama, K., Murakami, T., et al. (2006). Muscular atrophy of caveolin-3-deficient mice is rescued by myostatin inhibition. *J. Clin. Invest.* 116, 2924–2934. doi: 10.1172/JCI28520

O'rourke, J. R., Georges, S. A., Seay, H. R., Tapscott, S. J., Mcmanus, M. T., Goldhamer, D. J., et al. (2007). Essential role for Dicer during skeletal muscle development. *Dev. Biol.* 311, 359–368. doi: 10.1016/j.ydbio.2007.08.032

Park, I. H., Zhao, R., West, J. A., Yabuuchi, A., Huo, H., Ince, T. A., et al. (2008). Reprogramming of human somatic cells to pluripotency with defined factors. *Nature* 451, 141–146. doi: 10.1038/nature06534

Petrof, B. J., Shrager, J. B., Stedman, H. H., Kelly, A. M., and Sweeney, H. L. (1993). Dystrophin protects the sarcolemma from stresses developed during muscle contraction. *Proc. Natl. Acad. Sci. U.S.A.* 90, 3710–3714. doi: 10.1073/pnas.90.8.3710

Price, F. D., Kuroda, K., and Rudnicki, M. A. (2007). Stem cell based therapies to treat muscular dystrophy. *Biochim. Biophys. Acta* 1772, 272–283. doi: 10.1016/j.bbadis.2006.08.011

Rafei, M., Birman, E., Forner, K., and Galipeau, J. (2009a). Allogeneic mesenchymal stem cells for treatment of experimental autoimmune encephalomyelitis. *Mol. Ther.* 17, 1799–1803. doi: 10.1038/mt.2009.157

Rafei, M., Campeau, P. M., Aguilar-Mahecha, A., Buchanan, M., Williams, P., Birman, E., et al. (2009b). Mesenchymal stromal cells ameliorate experimental autoimmune encephalomyelitis by inhibiting CD4 Th17 T cells in a CC chemokine ligand 2-dependent manner. *J. Immunol.* 182, 5994–6002. doi: 10.4049/jimmunol.0803962

Ratajczak, J., Miekus, K., Kucia, M., Zhang, J., Reca, R., Dvorak, P., et al. (2006). Embryonic stem cell-derived microvesicles reprogram hematopoietic progenitors: evidence for horizontal transfer of mRNA and protein delivery. *Leukemia* 20, 847–856. doi: 10.1038/sj.leu.2404132

Reubinoff, B. E., Itsykson, P., Turetsky, T., Pera, M. F., Reinhartz, E., Itzik, A., et al. (2001). Neural progenitors from human embryonic stem cells. *Nat. Biotechnol.* 19, 1134–1140. doi: 10.1038/nbt1201-1134

Riordan, N. H., Chan, K., Marleau, A. M., and Ichim, T. E. (2007). Cord blood in regenerative medicine: do we need immune suppression? *J. Transl. Med.* 5, 8. doi: 10.1186/1479-5876-5-8

Rohwedel, J., Maltsev, V., Bober, E., Arnold, H. H., Hescheler, J., and Wobus, A. M. (1994). Muscle cell differentiation of embryonic stem cells reflects myogenesis *in vivo*: developmentally regulated expression of myogenic determination genes and functional expression of ionic currents. *Dev. Biol.* 164, 87–101. doi: 10.1006/dbio.1994.1182

Rosner, M. H., Vigano, M. A., Ozato, K., Timmons, P. M., Poirier, F., Rigby, P. W., et al. (1990). A POU-domain transcription factor in early stem cells and germ cells of the mammalian embryo. *Nature* 345, 686–692. doi: 10.1038/345686a0

Rothenfluh, D. A., Bermudez, H., O'neil, C. P., and Hubbell, J. A. (2008). Biofunctional polymer nanoparticles for intra-articular targeting and retention in cartilage. *Nat. Mater.* 7, 248–254. doi: 10.1038/nmat2116

Rouger, K., Larcher, T., Dubreil, L., Deschamps, J. Y., Le Guiner, C., Jouvion, G., et al. (2011). Systemic delivery of allogenic muscle stem cells induces long-term muscle repair and clinical efficacy in duchenne muscular dystrophy dogs. *Am. J. Pathol.* 179, 2501–2518. doi: 10.1016/j.ajpath.2011.07.022

Sacco, A., Doyonnas, R., Kraft, P., Vitorovic, S., and Blau, H. M. (2008). Self-renewal and expansion of single transplanted muscle stem cells. *Nature* 456, 502–506. doi: 10.1038/nature07384

Sakurai, H., Inami, Y., Tamamura, Y., Yoshikai, T., Sehara-Fujisawa, A., and Isobe, K. (2009). Bidirectional induction toward paraxial mesodermal derivatives from mouse ES cells in chemically defined medium. *Stem Cell Res.* 3, 157–169. doi: 10.1016/j.scr.2009.08.002

Sambasivan, R., and Tajbakhsh, S. (2007). Skeletal muscle stem cell birth and properties. *Semin. Cell Dev. Biol.* 18, 870–882. doi: 10.1016/j.semcdb.2007.09.013

Sampaolesi, M., Blot, S., D'antona, G., Granger, N., Tonlorenzi, R., Innocenzi, A., et al. (2006). Mesoangioblast stem cells ameliorate muscle function in dystrophic dogs. *Nature* 444, 574–579. doi: 10.1038/nature05282

Sandri, M. (2008). Signaling in muscle atrophy and hypertrophy. *Physiology (Bethesda)* 23, 160–170. doi: 10.1152/physiol.00041.2007

Sarig, R., Baruchi, Z., Fuchs, O., Nudel, U., and Yaffe, D. (2006). Regeneration and transdifferentiation potential of muscle-derived stem cells propagated as myospheres. *Stem Cells* 24, 1769–1778. doi: 10.1634/stemcells.2005-0547

Schiaffino, S., Sandri, M., and Murgia, M. (2007). Activity-dependent signaling pathways controlling muscle diversity and plasticity. *Physiology (Bethesda)* 22, 269–278. doi: 10.1152/physiol.00009.2007

Serra, F., Quarta, M., Canato, M., Toniolo, L., De Arcangelis, V., Trotta, A., et al. (2012). Inflammation in muscular dystrophy and the beneficial effects of non-steroidal anti-inflammatory drugs. *Muscle Nerve* 46, 773–784. doi: 10.1002/mus.23432

Serrano, A. L., and Munoz-Canoves, P. (2010). Regulation and dysregulation of fibrosis in skeletal muscle. *Exp. Cell Res.* 316, 3050–3058. doi: 10.1016/j.yexcr.2010.05.035

Sherwood, R. I., Christensen, J. L., Conboy, I. M., Conboy, M. J., Rando, T. A., Weissman, I. L., et al. (2004). Isolation of adult mouse myogenic progenitors: functional heterogeneity of cells within and engrafting skeletal muscle. *Cell* 119, 543–554. doi: 10.1016/j.cell.2004.10.021

Shi, X., and Garry, D. J. (2006). Muscle stem cells in development, regeneration, and disease. *Genes Dev.* 20, 1692–1708. doi: 10.1101/gad.1419406

Skottman, H., Dilber, M. S., and Hovatta, O. (2006). The derivation of clinical-grade human embryonic stem cell lines. *FEBS Lett.* 580, 2875–2878. doi: 10.1016/j.febslet.2006.03.083

Smythe, G. M., Fan, Y., and Grounds, M. D. (2000). Enhanced migration and fusion of donor myoblasts in dystrophic and normal host muscle. *Muscle Nerve* 23, 560–574. doi: 10.1002/(SICI)1097-4598(200004)23:4%3C560::AID-MUS16%3E3.3.CO;2-7

Soldner, F., Hockemeyer, D., Beard, C., Gao, Q., Bell, G. W., Cook, E. G., et al. (2009). Parkinson's disease patient-derived induced pluripotent stem cells free of viral reprogramming factors. *Cell* 136, 964–977. doi: 10.1016/j.cell.2009.02.013

Song, H. Y., Lee, M. J., Kim, M. Y., Kim, K. H., Lee, I. H., Shin, S. H., et al. (2010). Lysophosphatidic acid mediates migration of human mesenchymal stem cells stimulated by synovial fluid of patients with rheumatoid arthritis. *Biochim. Biophys. Acta* 1801, 23–30. doi: 10.1016/j.bbalip.2009.08.011

Song, Z., Cai, J., Liu, Y., Zhao, D., Yong, J., Duo, S., et al. (2009). Efficient generation of hepatocyte-like cells from human induced pluripotent stem cells. *Cell Res.* 19, 1233–1242. doi: 10.1038/cr.2009.107

Spiller, M. P., Kambadur, R., Jeanplong, F., Thomas, M., Martyn, J. K., Bass, J. J., et al. (2002). The myostatin gene is a downstream target gene of basic helix-loop-helix transcription factor MyoD. *Mol. Cell Biol.* 22, 7066–7082. doi: 10.1128/MCB.22.20.7066-7082.2002

Strulovici, Y., Leopold, P. L., O'connor, T. P., Pergolizzi, R. G., and Crystal, R. G. (2007). Human embryonic stem cells and gene therapy. *Mol. Ther.* 15, 850–866.

Suuronen, E. J., Kuraitis, D., and Ruel, M. (2008). Improving cell engraftment with tissue engineering. *Semin. Thorac. Cardiovasc. Surg.* 20, 110–114. doi: 10.1053/j.semtcvs.2008.03.005

Suzuki, K., Totsuka, M., Nakaji, S., Yamada, M., Kudoh, S., Liu, Q., et al. (1999). Endurance exercise causes interaction among stress hormones, cytokines, neutrophil dynamics, and muscle damage. *J. Appl. Physiol.* 87, 1360–1367.

Tagliafico, E., Brunelli, S., Bergamaschi, A., De Angelis, L., Scardigli, R., Galli, D., et al. (2004). TGFbeta/BMP activate the smooth muscle/bone differentiation programs in mesoangioblasts. *J. Cell Sci.* 117, 4377–4388. doi: 10.1242/jcs.01291

Takahashi, K., and Yamanaka, S. (2006). Induction of pluripotent stem cells from mouse embryonic and adult fibroblast cultures by defined factors. *Cell* 126, 663–676. doi: 10.1016/j.cell.2006.07.024

Tamaki, T., Okada, Y., Uchiyama, Y., Tono, K., Masuda, M., Wada, M., et al. (2007). Clonal multipotency of skeletal muscle-derived stem cells between mesodermal and ectodermal lineage. *Stem Cells* 25, 2283–2290. doi: 10.1634/stemcells.2006-0746

Tanaka, K. K., Hall, J. K., Troy, A. A., Cornelison, D. D., Majka, S. M., and Olwin, B. B. (2009). Syndecan-4-expressing muscle progenitor cells in the SP engraft as satellite cells during muscle regeneration. *Cell Stem Cell* 4, 217–225. doi: 10.1016/j.stem.2009.01.016

Tedesco, F. S., Gerli, M. F., Perani, L., Benedetti, S., Ungaro, F., Cassano, M., et al. (2012). Transplantation of genetically corrected human iPSC-derived progenitors in mice with limb-girdle muscular dystrophy. *Sci. Transl. Med.* 4, 140ra189. doi: 10.1126/scitranslmed.3003541

Tedesco, F. S., Hoshiya, H., D'antona, G., Gerli, M. F., Messina, G., Antonini, S., et al. (2011). Stem cell-mediated transfer of a human artificial chromosome ameliorates muscular dystrophy. *Sci. Transl. Med.* 3, 96ra78. doi: 10.1126/scitranslmed.3002342

Thomas, M., Langley, B., Berry, C., Sharma, M., Kirk, S., Bass, J., et al. (2000). Myostatin, a negative regulator of muscle growth, functions by inhibiting myoblast proliferation. *J. Biol. Chem.* 275, 40235–40243. doi: 10.1074/jbc.M004356200

Thomson, J. A., Itskovitz-Eldor, J., Shapiro, S. S., Waknitz, M. A., Swiergiel, J. J., Marshall, V. S., and Jones, J. M. (1998). Embryonic stem cell lines derived from human blastocysts. *Science* 282, 1145–1147. doi: 10.1126/science.282.5391.1145

Thomson, J. A., and Marshall, V. S. (1998). Primate embryonic stem cells. *Curr. Top Dev. Biol.* 38, 133–165. doi: 10.1016/S0070-2153(08)60246-X

Tidball, J. G., and Villalta, S. A. (2010). Regulatory interactions between muscle and the immune system during muscle regeneration. *Am. J. Physiol. Regul. Integr. Comp. Physiol.* 298, R1173–R1187. doi: 10.1152/ajpregu.00735.2009

Torrente, Y., Belicchi, M., Marchesi, C., Dantona, G., Cogiamanian, F., Pisati, F., et al. (2007). Autologous transplantation of muscle-derived CD133+ stem cells in Duchenne muscle patients. *Cell Transplant.* 16, 563–577. doi: 10.3727/000000007783465064

Torrente, Y., Tremblay, J. P., Pisati, F., Belicchi, M., Rossi, B., Sironi, M., et al. (2001). Intraarterial injection of muscle-derived CD34(+)Sca-1(+) stem cells restores dystrophin in mdx mice. *J. Cell Biol.* 152, 335–348. doi: 10.1083/jcb.152.2.335

Tremblay, J. P., Malouin, F., Roy, R., Huard, J., Bouchard, J. P., Satoh, A., et al. (1993). Results of a triple blind clinical study of myoblast transplantations without immunosuppressive treatment in young boys with Duchenne muscular dystrophy. *Cell Transplant.* 2, 99–112.

Usas, A., and Huard, J. (2007). Muscle-derived stem cells for tissue engineering and regenerative therapy. *Biomaterials* 28, 5401–5406. doi: 10.1016/j.biomaterials.2007.09.008

Vial, C., Zuniga, L. M., Cabello-Verrugio, C., Canon, P., Fadic, R., and Brandan, E. (2008). Skeletal muscle cells express the profibrotic cytokine connective tissue growth factor (CTGF/CCN2), which induces their dedifferentiation. *J. Cell. Physiol.* 215, 410–421. doi: 10.1002/jcp.21324

Villalta, S. A., Nguyen, H. X., Deng, B., Gotoh, T., and Tidball, J. G. (2009). Shifts in macrophage phenotypes and macrophage competition for arginine metabolism affect the severity of muscle pathology in muscular dystrophy. *Hum. Mol. Genet.* 18, 482–496. doi: 10.1093/hmg/ddn376

Voisin, L., Gray, K., Flowers, K. M., Kimball, S. R., Jefferson, L. S., and Vary, T. C. (1996). Altered expression of eukaryotic initiation factor 2B in skeletal muscle during sepsis. *Am. J. Physiol.* 270, E43–E50.

Wagner, K. R., Fleckenstein, J. L., Amato, A. A., Barohn, R. J., Bushby, K., Escolar, D. M., et al. (2008). A phase I/IItrial of MYO-029 in adult subjects with muscular dystrophy. *Ann. Neurol.* 63, 561–571. doi: 10.1002/ana.21338

Wehling, M., Spencer, M. J., and Tidball, J. G. (2001). A nitric oxide synthase transgene ameliorates muscular dystrophy in mdx mice. *J. Cell Biol.* 155, 123–131. doi: 10.1083/jcb.200105110

Whalen, R. G., Harris, J. B., Butler-Browne, G. S., and Sesodia, S. (1990). Expression of myosin isoforms during notexin-induced regeneration of rat soleus muscles. *Dev. Biol.* 141, 24–40. doi: 10.1016/0012-1606(90)90099-5

Whittemore, L. A., Song, K., Li, X., Aghajanian, J., Davies, M., Girgenrath, S., et al. (2003). Inhibition of myostatin in adult mice increases skeletal muscle mass and strength. *Biochem. Biophys. Res. Commun.* 300, 965–971. doi: 10.1016/S0006-291X(02)02953-4

Wozniak, M. A., and Chen, C. S. (2009). Mechanotransduction in development: a growing role for contractility. *Nat. Rev. Mol. Cell Biol.* 10, 34–43. doi: 10.1038/nrm2592

Xu, C., Inokuma, M. S., Denham, J., Golds, K., Kundu, P., Gold, J. D., and Carpenter, M. K. (2001). Feeder-free growth of undifferentiated human embryonic stem cells. *Nat. Biotechnol.* 19, 971–974. doi: 10.1038/nbt 1001-971

Ye, L., Chang, J. C., Lin, C., Sun, X., Yu, J., and Kan, Y. W. (2009). Induced pluripotent stem cells offer new approach to therapy in thalassemia and sickle cell anemia and option in prenatal diagnosis in genetic diseases. *Proc. Natl. Acad. Sci. U.S.A.* 106, 9826–9830. doi: 10.1073/pnas.0904689106

Zhang, X., Stojkovic, P., Przyborski, S., Cooke, M., Armstrong, L., Lako, M., et al. (2006). Derivation of human embryonic stem cells from developing and arrested embryos. *Stem Cells* 24, 2669–2676. doi: 10.1634/stemcells.2006-0377

Zheng, B., Cao, B., Crisan, M., Sun, B., Li, G., Logar, A., et al. (2007). Prospective identification of myogenic endothelial cells in human skeletal muscle. *Nat. Biotechnol.* 25, 1025–1034. doi: 10.1038/nbt1334

Zhou, K., Zhang, H., Jin, O., Feng, X., Yao, G., Hou, Y., et al. (2008). Transplantation of human bone marrow mesenchymal stem cell ameliorates the autoimmune pathogenesis in MRL/lpr mice. *Cell. Mol. Immunol.* 5, 417–424. doi: 10.1038/cmi.2008.52

Zhou, L., Porter, J. D., Cheng, G., Gong, B., Hatala, D. A., Merriam, A. P., et al. (2006). Temporal and spatial mRNA expression patterns of TGF-beta1, 2, 3 and TbetaRI, II, III in skeletal muscles of mdx mice. *Neuromuscul. Disord.* 16, 32–38. doi: 10.1016/j.nmd.2005.09.009

Zwi, L., Caspi, O., Arbel, G., Huber, I., Gepstein, A., Park, I. H., et al. (2009). Cardiomyocyte differentiation of human induced pluripotent stem cells. *Circulation* 120, 1513–1523. doi: 10.1161/CIRCULATIONAHA.109.868885

10

Skeletal muscle wasting with disuse atrophy is multi-dimensional: The response and interaction of myonuclei, satellite cells and signaling pathways

Naomi E. Brooks[1]* and Kathryn H. Myburgh[2]

[1] *Health and Exercise Science Research Group, School of Sport, University of Stirling, Stirling, UK*
[2] *Muscle Research Group, Department of Physiological Sciences, Stellenbosch University, Stellenbosch, South Africa*

****Correspondence:***
Naomi E. Brooks, Health and Exercise Science Research Group, School of Sport, University of Stirling, Stirling FK9 4LA, UK
e-mail: n.e.brooks@stir.ac.uk

Maintenance of skeletal muscle is essential for health and survival. There are marked losses of skeletal muscle mass as well as strength and physiological function under conditions of low mechanical load, such as space flight, as well as ground based models such as bed rest, immobilization, disuse, and various animal models. Disuse atrophy is caused by mechanical unloading of muscle and this leads to reduced muscle mass without fiber attrition. Skeletal muscle stem cells (satellite cells) and myonuclei are integrally involved in skeletal muscle responses to environmental changes that induce atrophy. Myonuclear domain size is influenced differently in fast and slow twitch muscle, but also by different models of muscle wasting, a factor that is not yet understood. Although the myonuclear domain is 3-dimensional this is rarely considered. Apoptosis as a mechanism for myonuclear loss with atrophy is controversial, whereas cell death of satellite cells has not been considered. Molecular signals such as myostatin/SMAD pathway, MAFbx, and MuRF1 E3 ligases of the ubiquitin proteasome pathway and IGF1-AKT-mTOR pathway are 3 distinctly different contributors to skeletal muscle protein adaptation to disuse. Molecular signaling pathways activated in muscle fibers by disuse are rarely considered within satellite cells themselves despite similar exposure to unloading or low mechanical load. These molecular pathways interact with each other during atrophy and also when various interventions are applied that could alleviate atrophy. Re-applying mechanical load is an obvious method to restore muscle mass, however how nutrient supplementation (e.g., amino acids) may further enhance recovery (or reduce atrophy despite unloading or ageing) is currently of great interest. Satellite cells are particularly responsive to myostatin and to growth factors. Recently, the hibernating squirrel has been identified as an innovative model to study resistance to atrophy.

Keywords: skeletal muscle atrophy, muscle cell signaling, myostatin, MuRF1, MAFbx, IGF1-AKT-mTOR, unloading, resistance exercise

INTRODUCTION

Skeletal muscle plays a significant role in quality of life and is essential for health and survival. It is highly organized at the micro- and macroscopic level and plays a major role in mobility of the human body. Skeletal muscle accounts for ~40% of body mass, permits precise movements and is highly adaptive. The characteristic of plasticity allows skeletal muscle to change and adapt depending on the stimuli placed upon it. Increases in mechanical load and increasing workload will stimulate muscle hypertrophy, while removal of mechanical load will lead to muscle atrophy as an appropriate adaptation to hypogravity (Goldberg et al., 1975).

Skeletal muscle has the uncanny ability to alter its phenotype depending on the mechanical load placed upon it. Disuse is an expansive label for the low mechanical load or mechanical unloading of muscle; with the most severe example being that of lack of gravity in spaceflight. The ground-based model, bed rest, simulates spaceflight. Physiological changes during bed rest include 6–24% reduction in muscle mass and strength (Narici and de Boer, 2011) and other disuse associated changes in skeletal muscle (Brooks et al., 2008).

Morphological changes with atrophy include a decreased cross-sectional area of muscle fibers, concomitant reduced whole muscle volume and mass, but no decrease in number of fibers (Nicks et al., 1989). This is different to age-related muscle fiber atrophy which is accompanied by a reduction in number of muscle fibers (Lexell et al., 1988). The process of muscle atrophy is highly regulated and results in reduced protein content, reduced force production, increased fatigability and decreased insulin sensitivity (Fauteck and Kandarian, 1995; Harrison et al., 2003), decreased capillary density of both fiber types and disruption of the 3-dimensional architecture of skeletal muscle (Hikida et al., 1997). Skeletal muscle also undergoes a shift in contractile capacity of the fibers toward fast glycolytic phenotypes (Fauteck and Kandarian, 1995; Fitts et al., 2000). For example, the soleus muscle which is predominantly composed of slow twitch fibers is a postural muscle and highly susceptible to disuse and fiber type switching (Booth and Baldwin, 1996).

Disease-induced atrophy (cachexia) is seen in disease states such as cancer, AIDS, renal failure, congestive heart failure, chronic obstructive pulmonary disease (COPD) and burns. In addition to disuse atrophy, cachexia involves an intricate cytokine and inflammatory response inducing signaling cascades and gene transcription. This review will focus on disuse atrophy and selected growth factor-related signaling. Human models of disuse, such as immobilization and sedentary lifestyle (inactivity) include decreased mechanical loading. Immobilization can occur as a result of various injuries, mostly not of skeletal muscle so the influence on skeletal muscle is considered a side effect. Immobilization can also be used as a model to investigate disuse and load reduction on skeletal muscle as a research intervention. Unilateral lower limb suspension involves suspension of one limb while the other is used for movement assisted by crutches. This model resulted in 5–10% reduction in CSA of Quadriceps muscle after 4 weeks (for more detailed review about ULLS, the reader is referred to Hackney and Ploutz-Snyder, 2012). Immobilization (cast or leg brace) in humans can lead to ~12% decrease in leg mass (for more detailed review about immobilization, the reader is referred to Marimuthu et al., 2011).

Skeletal muscle unloading in rodents is best modeled by hindlimb suspension (HS; Morey-Holton and Globus, 2002), which also leads to significant skeletal muscle atrophy particularly in postural, slow-twitch muscles, such as the soleus muscle (Templeton et al., 1984; Fitts et al., 1986; Riley et al., 1987). The HS model involves the animal being suspended by the tail which prevents the back legs from bearing any weight whilst the animals support their weight on the front legs. The front legs do not take on the entire weight of the animal since some of the loading is compensated for by the pulley and wire system that allows the animal to still move freely in the cage. For a recent extensive review on disuse atrophy and unloading models, the reader is directed to Baldwin et al. (2013). Of particular interest are the alterations in MHC and fiber shifting away from slow-oxidative fiber type toward fast glycolytic fiber type in the soleus muscle with HS (Templeton et al., 1984; Elder and McComas, 1987; Riley et al., 1987; Tsika et al., 1987). This observation is consistent regardless of the duration of unloading in different studies. Because of the location of the MHC genes this suggests that the basal gene expression by the myonuclei is altered. Thus a concept not frequently considered arises: constitutive gene expression is altered once the adaptive phase is complete. To understand the role of the myonuclear response to atrophy it is important to investigate myonuclei as entities in their own right. The fact that a muscle fiber is multinucleated and large adds to the complexity of the myonuclear responses. On the other hand the muscle precurser cells (satellite cells; SCs) are mononuclear and typically quiescent, hence their response to disuse may not be similar to those of the myonuclei.

There is a plethora of research which has been carried out in human subjects with differing methods and timescales of atrophy-inducing stimulation. Two recent studies from van Loon's laboratory demonstrate that after 5 days cast immobilization (Dirks et al., 2014) and 14 days cast immobilization (Wall et al., 2013) there are significant losses in muscle strength and size. Five days of immobilization led to 3.5% reduction in quadriceps CSA and 9% muscle strength (Dirks et al., 2014). In young males, there was a 8% decrease in muscle cross-sectional area and a 23% reduction in quadriceps strength after 14 days immobilization (Wall et al., 2013). In addition, data from the Kjaer laboratory also report decreases in fiber size (10; 20%) and strength (13; 20%) after 4 and 14 days, respectively (Suetta et al., 2012, 2013). The decrease in whole muscle strength is also reflected in reduced specific force of single muscle fibers (Hvid et al., 2013). Bed rest studies of longer duration (e.g., 28 days) consistently show reduced muscle strength and size (Hikida et al., 1989; LeBlanc et al., 1992; Edgerton et al., 1995; Ferrando et al., 1996; Bloomfield, 1997; Brooks et al., 2008). In skeletal muscle from individuals who were 9 years post-spinal cord injury, there was considerable atrophy compared to controls and 90% of the fibers were type II fibers (Verdijk et al., 2012).

Skeletal muscle is a key tissue in maintaining functional ability and contributing to health status. The aim of this review is to highlight the important and integrative role of SCs and myonuclei in skeletal muscle homeostasis with the focus particularly on atrophy. Understanding the role of myonuclei and SCs both in load-bearing and a variety of disuse conditions may lead to therapies to combat deleterious alterations in skeletal muscle that are specifically targeted to these progenitor cells. Since both SCs and myonuclei respond to environmental changes, the involvement of SCs in skeletal muscle health as well as for skeletal muscle therapies should be further investigated.

MYONUCLEI AND MYONUCLEAR DOMAIN

Despite being post-mitotic and unable to divide and replicate, myonuclei remain essential for skeletal muscle homeostasis, maintenance and adaptive responses. Therefore analysis of myonuclei may shed light on mechanisms responsible for muscle fiber loss or on responses to interventions to fight physical disability such as that seen with ageing and disease (Malatesta and Meola, 2010).

The theory of myonuclear domain suggests that each skeletal muscle nucleus governs an area of surrounding cytoplasm (Hall and Ralston, 1989) and produces enough protein to support the limited area of cytoplasmic and structural proteins within the local "domain" (Pavlath et al., 1989). Research has consistently reported that in situations of positive change in fiber size, i.e., with muscle growth, hypertrophy or overload, there are increases in myonuclear number as the fiber increases in size (Allen et al., 1995; McCall et al., 1998; Roy et al., 1999a; Adams et al., 2002; Petrella et al., 2006; VanderMeer et al., 2011). However, a somewhat flexible myonuclear domain size is likely especially during e.g., the early phase of an adaptive response (Kadi et al., 2004), either increase or decrease in fiber size or change in metabolic status.

Myonuclear domain size is different between fast and slow fiber types (Burleigh, 1977). Slow muscle fibers have higher rates of protein turnover (Booth and Thomason, 1991) and higher oxidative capacity has been associated with a higher level of protein synthesis (Roy et al., 1999b). In general, slow fibers have larger numbers of myonuclei (Edgerton and Roy, 1991) which leads to a smaller calculated myonuclear domain size (Tseng et al., 1994; Allen et al., 1995; Hikida et al., 1997; Brooks et al.,

2009). Fast muscle fibers have lower oxidative capacity, relatively lower numbers of myonuclei and larger myonuclear domain sizes (Burleigh, 1977; Tseng et al., 1994). However, it is well known that fast twitch fiber sub-types have widely varying oxidative capacity and multiple hybrid isoforms (Kohn et al., 2007). It has also been reported that there is a positive correlation between myonuclear number and fiber size in young mice and this relationship is lost during adulthood (Bruusgaard et al., 2006). More research needs to be done to unravel the fiber type/oxidative capacity and age and myonuclear domain relationship.

MYONUCLEAR DOMAIN AND DISUSE ATROPHY

While the myonuclear domain theory is well substantiated for the increase and incorporation of myonuclei with muscle hypertrophy (see above), the response of the myonuclear number and myonuclear domain size with atrophy is less conclusive. Despite less being known about the influence of disuse on myonuclei, the alterations in muscle morphology, biochemistry and physiology suggest that the myonuclei are influencing features of change within the muscle as well as being influenced by these alterations. Furthermore, atrophy from disuse occurs rapidly and its development is not simply the reverse of skeletal muscle hypertrophy. Myonuclear loss may follow a different timescale, occurring at a slower pace than the loss in muscle fiber size (VanderMeer et al., 2011). This may further complicate our understanding of change vs. no change of myonuclear domain size in response to an intervention. It is therefore important to distinguish between the adaptive phase and the new steady state when considering the muscle response to unloading.

Based on the myonuclear domain theory and the response to muscle growth, it could perhaps be inferred that with muscle atrophy there would be an accompanying loss of myonuclei resulting in maintenance of the myonuclear domain size (Siu and Alway, 2009). This inference relies on acceptance of the myonuclear domain theory that hypothesizes that each myonucleus can control only a certain domain for protein synthesis and general "maintenance." Although this hypothesis was based on solid observational data, the mechanisms controlling the removal of nuclei under conditions that cell death (myofiber necrosis) is absent, is far from understood. Nonetheless, decreased myonuclear numbers are noted in muscles undergoing a variety of atrophy-inducing experimental conditions in humans and animals such as spinal cord isolation and transection, microgravity, hind limb suspension and chronic denervation (Darr and Schultz, 1989; Schmalbruch et al., 1991; Allen et al., 1995, 1996, 1997b, 1999; Day et al., 1995; Rodrigues Ade and Schmalbruch, 1995; Hikida et al., 1997). However, there have also been recent reports to suggest that atrophy with HS does not lead to loss of myonuclei (Bruusgaard et al., 2012).

Myonuclei can be removed by a number of different processes, mainly apoptosis or autophagy. Apoptosis is a tightly regulated process of highly coordinated "programmed cell death." The process of apoptosis is a vital mechanism to allow normal development, tissue turnover and immunological function (Thompson, 1995) and to maintain tissue homeostasis throughout the lifespan. Apoptosis as a means of cell death is easy to conceptualize for mononuclear cells or cells with low nuclear number. However, in a multi-dimensional, multinucleated cell, how and why are particular nuclei targeted and not adjacent nuclei? There appears to be a fiber type-specific response of myonuclear loss, with a greater decrease in myonuclear number in Type I (Zhong et al., 2005) fibers that respond to unloading with more severe atrophy. In contrast excess glucocorticoid production such as that with cachexia results in fast glycolytic fibers being more affected (recently reviewed by Schakman et al., 2013). This further highlights the specificity and complexity inherent in regulation of disuse atrophy and by extension the control of myonuclear domain.

Regardless of the unknown mechanisms initiating myonuclear loss, elimination of myonuclei by nuclear apoptosis remains a rational idea to explain myonuclear domain size consistency in the face of atrophy, reviewed by Siu and Alway (2009). Allen et al. (1997a) published the first research demonstrating that the myonuclei lost with atrophy (HS) were eliminated by "programmed nuclear death," apoptosis. Myonuclear apoptosis has been identified with muscle disuse/unloading/wasting and can be measured with the terminal deoxynucleotidyl transferase-mediated deoxyuridine triphosphate nick end-labeling (TUNEL) or by DNA fragmentation in gel electrophoresis (Allen et al., 1997a; Dupont-Versteegden et al., 1999, 2006; Smith et al., 2000; Leeuwenburgh et al., 2005). For example, after 16 days of HS, rat soleus muscle had reduced number of myonuclei and the size of the myonuclei were increased after HS but the DNA content did not differ (Wang et al., 2006). However, recent advances in techniques for measuring apoptosis, particularly the ability to measure *in vivo* and to differentiate between nuclear loss inside and outside the muscle cell have permitted more accurate assessment of apoptosis in the muscle. In a number of recent publications, small increases in TUNEL+ nuclei have been reported but the location of these nuclei was outside the sarcolemma and thus they have been identified as stroma cells (Bruusgaard et al., 2012; Suetta et al., 2012).

In light of the above discussion, the concept of muscle atrophy coinciding with loss of myonuclei to maintain myonuclear domain size is not conclusive. Nutritional restriction has been reported to reduce muscle fiber size but not myonuclear number thus decreasing the myonuclear domain size (Winick and Noble, 1966; Pitts, 1986). Some studies have found no loss of myonuclei or myonuclear apoptosis with situations of atrophy (Wada et al., 2002; Gundersen and Bruusgaard, 2008). As highlighted in an excellent review on myonuclear domains and muscle atrophy (Gundersen and Bruusgaard, 2008), a lot of the research findings noting myonuclear loss are based on cross-sectional histological assessment of myonuclei at a specific time point. Bruusgaard and Gundersen (2008) conducted an elegant study measuring *in vivo* time lapse of single fibers and found that after 4 weeks of denervation there was a 50% decrease in size of muscle fiber and no change in myonuclear number. Other studies using single fiber analysis have also found no change in myonuclear number in rodent muscle (Wada et al., 2002; Aravamudan et al., 2006).

The method used to measure myonuclei and myonuclear domain size is also important to consider for careful interpretation. Cell culture techniques provide a means for easy myonuclear analysis after intervention. However, the number of myonuclei available for analysis is high and the proportion of myonuclei for a given volume of myotube is more prominent than in whole muscle where the contractile protein content overwhelms the internal content of the fiber. The timing of the myonuclear sampling is also important when determining whether apoptosis actually occurs and it is difficult to maintain myotubes in culture for long periods. Myotubes in culture are also often not subjected to contractile forces and the relevance to disuse atrophy might be questioned, although this does not preclude the investigation of atrophy induced by other methods.

Loading of muscle prior to the induction of atrophy may also influence the acute responses, especially to unloading. Siu et al. (2005) reported that in recently hypertrophied muscle (with increase in myonuclei) myonuclei undergo apoptosis during disuse. Bruusgaard et al. (2010) investigated this further by investigating the concept of "muscle memory" by overloading EDL muscle of mice and rats to stimulate hypertrophy. The EDL muscle was then denervated to induce muscle atrophy. In contrast to Siu et al.'s work, this model of overload led to myonuclear accretion with hypertrophy, and the new myonuclei persisted even with atrophy after denervation (Bruusgaard et al., 2010). This maintenance of myonuclei in the animals with overload and denervation was not seen in the animals who underwent only denervation. The authors suggest that previous hypertrophy bouts may protect skeletal muscle against myonuclear loss with atrophy. This may be of benefit for individuals who will undergo bouts of enforced disuse such as that seen with immobilization and/or bed rest following elective surgical procedures.

It is also important to highlight that the various experimental models used to investigate disuse atrophy differ substantially and hence have varying degrees of physiological application. Although animal models may seem too different from human models, it is of extreme importance for development in the area that both human and animal models are included in the research, whilst still keeping in mind that these choices may differ in the extent that the intervention can be applied. The most typical models of disuse atrophy are: denervation or hindlimb suspension in rodents; immobilization or bed rest in humans. Previously, the techniques used for analysis included histology, immunohistochemistry, gene expression and protein content, but *in vivo* assessment, single fiber assessment, myonuclear assessment, myonuclear domain size estimations were typically lacking in most studies. Further, the timing of muscle or myotube sampling will influence the response recorded. As discussed in this review, this is particularly evident when assessing the SC count in humans after short immobilization bouts, longer bed rest and/or longer disuse seen with spinal cord injury (Brooks et al., 2010; Verdijk et al., 2012; Snijders et al., 2014). The muscle chosen for analysis i.e., slow twitch soleus muscle, or fast twitch EDL muscle, or mixed muscle from humans, are key factors in unraveling the complex but enticing role of myonuclei in skeletal muscle atrophic situations. Recent human research has highlighted sex differences in skeletal muscle response to immobilization (Yasuda et al., 2005) which should also be taken into consideration. Finally, new methods should be developed or taken up by more researchers, for example the 3-dimensional analysis of myonuclear domain size and muscle volume measurements.

A fundamental question related to myonuclei, myonuclear domain and the response to atrophic situations is the involvement of skeletal muscle stem cells (SCs) in the maintenance of muscle mass, and the response to muscle loss.

SATELLITE CELLS

Myonuclei in skeletal muscle are post-mitotic and cannot replicate. Therefore, any increase in myonuclear number such as required for growth and repair is a result of SC fusion, although also to a very minor extent other stem- or stem cell-like cells (Boppart et al., 2013). The quantity of SCs differs between muscles, fiber types, developmental stages and species. In general, there are more SCs in type I fibers than type II fibers; the number of SC number does not change from birth to adulthood despite increases in fiber size (Verdijk et al., 2013). However, this is age, species and muscle specific (Gibson and Schultz, 1982; Mackey et al., 2009; Verdijk et al., 2013). SCs are responsive to various environmental influences, including disuse.

SCs have distinctive morphological features, including large nuclear-to-cytoplasmic ratio, few organelles, small nuclei and condensed interphase chromatin clearly visible using electron microscopy (Mauro, 1961). While the gold standard measurement of SCs is with electron-microscopy, SCs can also be identified with light microscopy and immunohistochemical labeling of factors expressed by the SCs (for further details on transcription factors and other markers expressed by SCs see the recent review by Yin et al., 2013). While SCs express these markers, labeling with some of these will also identify other cells. Where this is the case, the marker should not be used alone to identify SCs but rather in combination with another or several other known markers that (i) label the SCs but not the alternate cell; (ii) label the alternate cell but not the SCs; or (iii) label adjacent structures such as the sarcolemma or basal lamina. The choices for labeling with immunohistochemistry should be carefully considered, particularly when one is assessing SCs after an unusual intervention such as disuse that may affect SCs and myonuclei substantially.

Under normal situations SCs remain quiescent (Bischoff, 1990). Upon activation in response to stimuli present during injury or growth, SCs enter the cell cycle (Bischoff, 1990). When activated, SCs proliferate and express myogenic regulatory factors (MRFs), MyoD and Myf5 (Yablonka-Reuveni and Rivera, 1994; Zammit et al., 2002). After proliferation, most cells maintain MyoD but downregulate Pax7 and commit to differentiation via activation of myogenin. Other myoblasts maintain Pax7 but down-regulate MyoD and withdraw from the cell cycle regaining markers that characterize quiescence (Nagata et al., 2006; Day et al., 2007). All SCs undergo a stage of co-expressing Pax7 and MyoD before the decision to self-renew or differentiate is made. SCs have the ability to undergo both asymmetric as well as symmetric divisions (Kuang et al., 2007) either producing identical progeny or different progeny (Kuang et al., 2007).

Over recent years, a number of key publications have demonstrated that SCs are not all the same (Zammit, 2008; Biressi and Rando, 2010; Scharner and Zammit, 2011) and variations exist even between SCs in the same muscle (Ono et al., 2012). It is thought that the surrounding area (niche) of the SC plays a role in the fate and adaptive responsiveness of the SC (Kuang et al.,

2007). Therefore, the environment that influences muscle fibers and myonuclei will also have an effect on SCs. The role of SCs in skeletal muscle atrophy and recovery is less well characterized than their role in growth and injury repair. However, any reduction in the ability of SCs to respond to injury and trauma during atrophy or upon reloading will be a further detrimental episode for the muscle (Chargé and Rudnicki, 2004).

Although this review is focused on muscle atrophy, it is important to highlight that recent research has questioned the absolute requirement of SCs for muscle hypertrophy. Skeletal muscle can respond to hypertrophy stimulation even in animals without SCs. In adult Pax7-DTA mice, which have greater than 90% of SCs removed, the muscle can respond to an overload stimulus (McCarthy et al., 2011). These muscles without SC have a blunted response to regeneration, but are still able to hypertrophy (McCarthy et al., 2011). A number of studies in animals have reported skeletal muscle hypertrophy without SC activation or incorporation of myonuclei (Amthor et al., 2009; Blaauw et al., 2009; Raffaello et al., 2010; Lee et al., 2012; Wang and McPherron, 2012). These studies demonstrate that hypertrophy can occur independently of both SC proliferation as well as myonuclear accretion. This highlights the ability of rodent skeletal muscle to respond to overexpression induced hypertrophy (i.e., AKT overexpression—Blaauw et al., 2009), myostatin knock-out induced hypertrophy (Amthor et al., 2009), hypertrophy with overexpression of JunB in cell culture (Raffaello et al., 2010). Further, hypertrophy induced by myostatin inhibition in adult mice preceded incorporation of myonuclei (Wang and McPherron, 2012). This is also reported in animals which are transgenically modified to inhibit syndecan4 or Pax7, there is a hypertrophy response to hypertrophy stimulated by myostatin blockade, even without SC proliferation and fusion (Lee et al., 2012).

SATELLITE CELLS AND DISUSE ATROPHY

Early studies indicated that atrophic conditions lead to increases in the number of apoptotic myonuclei both inside and outside myofibers (Allen et al., 1997a; Vescovo et al., 1998). However, more recent studies indicate no change in myonuclear numbers with atrophy, and loss of SCs with atrophy is not a consistent finding. For example, in recent human studies of 14 days immobilization (Snijders et al., 2014), 28 days bed rest (Brooks et al., 2010) there appears to be no change in SC number, but Suetta et al. (Suetta et al., 2013) report an increase in SCs after 14 days immobilization. In contrast, in a recently published paper reporting SC numbers in states of severe disuse atrophy, spinal cord injury, individuals had significantly lower SC numbers in both type I and type II fibers (Verdijk et al., 2012). Thus, the severity of disuse induced atrophy and the duration of the condition must be considered when interpreting the existing literature.

Whether or not some SCs are lost during atrophy, it is still an open question how and why function (e.g., mitotic ability) of remaining SCs are is altered during atrophy and if so, whether their functionality is can be restored with reloading. In studies investigating alterations in SC content and proliferative ability, the age and growth stage of the animals is important. To investigate the role of SCs and the effect which atrophy has on their function, using young animals whose growth has not stabilized can shed light on factors not investigated in other models. For example, the SC may be more responsive during growth and this may alter their response to the atrophy-inducing intervention (see Darr and Schultz, 1989). SC response to potential interventions to reduce atrophy may also be different when comparing the growing, the adult or aged animal, thus interpretation and application should be done with care. Mechanical unloading appears to reduce the number of SCs (Darr and Schultz, 1989; Mozdziak et al., 1998; Matsuba et al., 2009). This may be due to apoptosis of SCs as well as myonuclei in situations of atrophy (Jejurikar et al., 2002; Jejurikar and Kuzon, 2003; Ferreira et al., 2006). Wang et al. (2006) investigated the mechanisms underlying the SC response to HS, particularly the distribution of SCs and the level of mechanical load applied to the muscle. Their results suggest that the regulation of SCs is dependent on the mechanical loading and the location of the SC along the muscle fiber. Unloading resulted in a significant decrease in SC number, particularly at the central region of the muscle fibers (Wang et al., 2006).

In contrast, Darr and Schultz (1989) showed that the alterations in myonuclear and SC population were dependent on the time course of HS. They investigated 30 days of HS in rat muscle, particularly fast-twitch extensor digitorum longus (EDL) and slow-twitch soleus muscle. After 3 days of HS, the authors report a reduction in SC number and halting of mitotic activity in both soleus and EDL muscle. Between 3 and 10 days of HS the SCs began dividing and there was an increase throughout the remainder of the HS. In addition to the increase in dividing cells, the EDL muscle also appeared to have a compensation response with 4x increase in active SCs in EDL myofibers. Although this study found that the earlier response was reduced SC number and mitotic activity, Ferreira et al. (2006) reported an intense peak of proliferating activity in SCs after 6 h of HS (SC duplication) followed by an increase in myonuclei at 12 h of HS (Ferreira et al., 2006). During this time there also appeared to be apoptosis (Ferreira et al., 2006). Investigating the morphometric and ultrastructural properties of SCs in rat soleus during immobilization, Kujawa et al. (2005) found caveolae on the SCs and a decrease in SC activity. Clearly, the SC response to atrophy is biologically complicated. Interestingly, in a human study, when specifically labeled with Pax7 and TUNEL+, there were no apoptotically marked SCs after 14 days of immobilization (Suetta et al., 2012).

In a seminal set of experiments, Mitchell and Pavlath examined the properties of muscle precursor cells (MPCs include both SCs and other stem-like cells between myofibers, fat and in blood vessels) after 14 days of HS in mice (Mitchell and Pavlath, 2004) and subsequent recovery. HS led to decreased number of MPCs and these MPCs taken from atrophied muscle cells could not proliferate and differentiate *in vitro* into normal myonucleated myotubes. Recovery appeared to lead to reversal of the dysfunctional properties highlighting that these changes are transient, lasting only until normal weight bearing activities are resumed. This would seem to imply that SC reactivation is integral to recovery. However, in young animals Jackson et al. (2012) concluded that SCs are not required for muscle growth following atrophy since restoration of myonuclear domain size with reloading after HS was independent of SCs.

Mozdziak et al. (2001) investigated the interaction between injury and HS, specifically the myofiber size, SC mitotic activity and DNA unit size after resumption of normal activities in soleus muscles of rats. They found muscle injury combined with inactivity (HS) caused long-term reduction in muscle size compared with injury in weight bearing animals. After HS the SCs responded to compensate for the muscle injury but this was not enough to return myonuclear numbers to levels similar to that of the animals who had not undergone HS (Mozdziak et al., 2001). The authors speculated that the HS caused a disruption in "DNA expression unit size" (such as seen in Mozdziak et al., 2000) and combined with the reduction in SC mitotic activity results in a reduced size of soleus muscle even after 9 weeks of reloading. This interpretation indicates that the myonuclear domain size is not necessarily primarily responsive to changes in muscle size, but may itself have an active influence on muscle size.

Interestingly, while the number of SCs does not appear to change in human muscle with short-term disuse (28 days or less), it should be highlighted that alterations in MRFs have been documented. During 14 days of immobilization, Snijders et al. (2014) report myogenin mRNA expression doubled. Further, after 28 days bed rest and essential AA supplementation without exercise, MyoD transcripts were elevated after 28 days and remained elevated after recovery (Brooks et al., 2010). Thus, SCs are not quiescent when the environment is changing and there may be a myogenic response occurring despite muscle proteolysis.

Investigations into treatments to reduce atrophic response during HS have found that application of low-frequency electrical stimulation (LFES) partially rescues the loss of SCs and lessens the reduction in muscle cross-sectional area (Zhang et al., 2010); rescues SCs and maintains their viability for muscle regeneration (Guo et al., 2012) and reduces loss of myonuclear domain size (Zhang et al., 2010). Zhang et al. (2010) applied LFES during HS in a rat model and investigated SC response in soleus and EDL muscles. The authors reported evidence of a reduced capacity for SC activation, proliferation and differentiation in soleus muscle after 28 days HS, findings that were partially attenuated by LFES. Interestingly, there was no atrophy in the EDL muscle and no alteration in myonuclear domain size in the EDL muscle (Zhang et al., 2010).

In summary, the balance of data indicates that in animals SC numbers decrease while in human studies SC numbers remain similar or even increase unless the atrophic environment is particularly severe. Furthermore it seems the regenerative capacity, and indeed the myogenic regulation of the remaining SC is maintained. Atrophy occurs under many conditions and unraveling how SCs respond in the various conditions will need to include better examination of the niche environments in which the SCs reside and not only the quantitative responses. The response of SCs to disuse atrophy is further complicated by the time course of exposure to the condition and therefore research should be including a broader timescale without sacrificing investigation of the rapid early responses. Investigation of early responses should include cell signaling events within SC and not only muscle tissue itself. Extensive research has been done on the molecular pathways which influence atrophy (see below) and some evidence exists that SC are also influenced significantly by these pathways.

MOLECULAR SIGNALING PATHWAYS

The molecular mechanisms underpinning muscle atrophy with disuse remain to be fully elucidated. The next section aims to describe 3 of the key molecular pathways which are linked to skeletal muscle atrophy: Atrogin-1/MAFbx and MuRF1; the IGF-1-AKT-mTOR pathway; and the Myostatin Pathway. Existing authoritative review articles will be highlighted. Further, we aim to discuss how these pathways are related to SCs and myonuclear responses to atrophy.

UBIQUITIN PROTEASOME PATHWAY (MAFbx/MuRF1) AND DISUSE ATROPHY

The ATP-dependent ubiquitin proteasome pathway is the primary degradation pathway of skeletal muscle in response to inactivity and disuse. The ubiquitin-proteasome pathway is involved in breakdown of short-lived proteins or long-lived myofibrillar proteins in skeletal muscle. Three distinct components are required for muscle breakdown using the ubiquitin proteasome pathway. E1 ligases which activate ubiquitin, E2 ligases that are responsible for transferring the activated ubiquitin to the protein molecule that is then targeted for degradation and the E3 ligases which regulate the actual transfer of ubiquitin to the protein. Two important skeletal muscle specific ubiquitin E3 ligases are Muscle-specific RING Finger protein1 (MuRF1) and Muscle Atrophy F-box (MAFbx/atrogin-1).

MAFbx and MuRF1 are both primarily expressed in skeletal muscle and are upregulated in several models of disuse (Bodine et al., 2001). MAFbx and MuRF1 were first identified following profiling in mouse atrophy after fasting and immobilization in a profound set of experiments published by both Bodine et al. (2001) and Gomes et al. (2001). In knock-out models, animals which cannot make MAFbx or MuRF1 proteins appear to be similar to the wild-type animals with phenotypically similar muscle and normal body weight (Bodine et al., 2001). However, MAFbx knockout mice had a reduced loss of muscle mass (56% sparing) after 7 and 14 days (Bodine et al., 2001). MuRF1 knockout mice had a 36% sparing of muscle compared to wild-type mice 14 days after denervation.

Both MAFbx and MuRF1 appear to be early markers of disuse atrophy. MAFbx and MuRF1 mRNA levels are rapidly increased in numerous models of atrophy and are thought to contribute to the initiation of the atrophy process (Foletta et al., 2011). They are increased after spaceflight in rodents (Allen et al., 2009), after 3 days of ULLS in humans (Gustafsson et al., 2010); and after immobilization (Jones et al., 2004; Abadi et al., 2009). MAFbx and MuRF1 are regulated by the family of Forkhead box O (FOXO) transcription factors (Stitt et al., 2004). FOXO is a family of transcription factors that are involved in metabolism, apoptosis and cell cycle progression (Carlsson and Mahlapuu, 2002). When FOXO transcription factors are dephosphorylated they enter the nucleus and act to suppress growth and promote apoptosis (Ramaswamy et al., 2002). AKT (also called protein kinase B or PKB) phosphorylates FOXO transcription factors on multiple sites leading to their exclusion from the nucleus. Under normal physiological conditions, AKT thus inhibits the transcriptional functions of FOXO and FOXO is unable to suppress growth or upregulate atrophy and myonuclei are maintained.

IGF-1-PI3K-AKT-mTOR AND DISUSE ATROPHY

Extensive literature supports the role of the IGF-1-PI3K-AKT-mTOR pathway in regulation of skeletal muscle hypertrophy (for example see reviews Glass, 2003; Schiaffino et al., 2013). Activation of this pathway leads to increases in translation initiation factors ultimately leading to increased protein synthesis: IGF1 activates Phosphatidylinositol 3 kinase (PI3K), which phosphorylates phosphatidylinositol-4,5-bisphosphate to phosphatidylinositol-3,4,5-trisphosphate in the membrane; this creates a binding site for AKT; activation of AKT phosphorylates and activates mammalian target of rapamycin (mTOR) kinase; mTOR increases protein synthesis by phosphorylation and activation of p70S6kinase and eukaryotic translation initiation factor 4E binding protein 1, both of which are involved in translation and protein synthesis. The activation of AKT appears to be a crucial determinant of the cellular signaling processes and appears to sit at the transition point between atrophy and hypertrophy (again, see Glass, 2003; Schiaffino et al., 2013 for review).

With situations of disuse, AKT is not activated and this contributes to muscle atrophy via FOXO (Sandri et al., 2004). Animals with overexpression of FOXO have reduced muscle mass and this appears to be related to increases in MAFbx and MuRF1 (see above). Increased FOXO transcript levels in rodents were reported after spaceflight (Allen et al., 2009) and decreased phosphorylation of AKT levels were reported after 10 days HS (Sugiura et al., 2005). Alterations in the IGF1-AKT-mTOR pathway are linked directly to alterations in the ubiquitin proteasome ligases, MAFbx and MuRF1 (Kandarian and Jackman, 2006). Activation of the IGF-1 pathway is significant in reducing FOXO translocation. Inhibition of the IGF-1 pathway caused FOXO translocation to the nucleus, promoted growth suppression and stimulated proteolysis (Stitt et al., 2004). In humans, after 5 days of immobilization without intervention, transcript levels of MAFbx and MuRF1 were increased (Dirks et al., 2014). However, no increases in FOXO were noted after 4 or 14 days of immobilization (Suetta et al., 2012).

Relocation of FOXO to the nucleus also activates genes involved in cell death and cell cycle inhibition (Stitt et al., 2004) and may therefore potentially affect SC proliferation. IGF-1 is known to act directly on SCs. IGF-1 leads to SC proliferation and its absence is associated with lower proliferation capacity. Therefore, interventions that focus on the IGF-1/mTOR pathway will also induce activation of the support-system for addition of myonuclei. IGF-1 acts both intracellularly and extracellularly to induce both proliferation and differentiation of SCs (Bischoff, 1986; Adams and Haddad, 1996; Adams, 1998; Cameron-Smith, 2002; Mourkioti and Rosenthal, 2005) and different isoforms of IGF-1 may be responsible for these (see Review for further reading of the IGF-1 and skeletal muscle regeneration and hypertrophy: Philippou et al., 2007). mTOR has been described as the master regulator of cellular processes and has been linked to differentiation in C2C12 myobalsts (Erbay et al., 2003; Han et al., 2008). While its role in myogenic differentiation has not been conclusively clarified, mTOR is thought to play a role in regulating MyoD stability (Sun et al., 2010). Further clarification of the interaction of mTOR, as well as other key components of the pathway, with SC function remain to be elucidated.

MYOSTATIN AND DISUSE ATROPHY

Myostatin (growth-differentiation factor 8, GDF8) is a member of the transforming growth factor (TGF)β superfamily and a negative regulator of muscle mass. Myostatin appears to be primarily found in muscle tissue (McPherron et al., 1997). It has been widely reported that either natural mutations or scientific knock-out animals without myostatin gene have hypertrophied muscles such as the "double muscled" cattle (Grobet et al., 1997; Kambadur et al., 1997; McPherron and Lee, 1997) and the significant hypertrophy in a child (Schuelke et al., 2004). Myostatin knockout mice were larger in size than wild-type littermates and had over 200% greater muscle mass (McPherron et al., 1997). When myostatin gene expression is blocked experimentally, there are 13–30% increases in skeletal muscle hypertrophy (Whittemore et al., 2003).

The relationship between myostatin and atrophy is less concrete. Overexpression of myostatin appears to lead to muscle atrophy in transgenic mice (Reisz-Porszasz et al., 2003). Increased levels of myostatin mRNA and protein levels are seen as early as 1 day after HS (Carlson et al., 1999), after sciatic nerve resection (Shao et al., 2007) and after 11 days of spaceflight in mice (Allen et al., 2009) and in humans after chronic disuse (Reardon et al., 2001). Serum myostatin levels were increased by 12% after 25 days of head down bed rest (Zachwieja et al., 1999) while myostatin transcript and protein levels were both increased after 3 days of ULLS (Gustafsson et al., 2010). Increased myostatin transcript levels have been report after 5 days (Dirks et al., 2014) while after 14 days of immobilization the same group report decreased protein levels of myostatin (Snijders et al., 2014).

Myostatin appears to inhibit muscle growth through inhibiting the AKT-mTOR pathway (less protein synthesis), upregulating the ubiquitin proteasomal pathway via FOXO (more protein breakdown) (McFarlane et al., 2006) and reducing SC differentiation (Langley et al., 2002; Zimmers et al., 2002). Myostatin activates withdrawal from the cell cycle in mammalian myoblasts and stimulates quiescence rather than differentiation or apoptosis (McFarlane et al., 2008) by inhibiting MyoD activity (Langley et al., 2002; McCroskery et al., 2003; Amthor et al., 2006; Manceau et al., 2008).

Promoting quiescence is not the only influence that myostatin has on SCs. It also seems to play a role in regulating SC self-renewal in cell culture (McFarlane et al., 2008). Excess myostatin inhibited Pax-7 expression, whereas inactivation of myostatin (by genetic inactivation or functional antagonism of myostatin) resulted in increased Pax7 expression (McFarlane et al., 2008). Increased myostatin protein levels have been linked with dysfunctional SCs in aging human muscle (McKay et al., 2012). While the intricate response of skeletal muscle to ageing is outside the scope of this review, this evidence suggests that increased myostatin levels seen with atrophy may contribute to the reduced proliferative ability of SCs and the reduction in the pool of parent SCs.

Myostatin activates the SMAD pathway and SMAD3 null mice had significant atrophy combined with increased levels of MuRF1 and decreased SC function (Ge et al., 2011). This response was initiated by increased myostatin levels in the SMAD3 null mice, and the response was abolished when myostatin was inactivated in these mice (Ge et al., 2011). SMAD3 may contribute to self-renewal of SCs. Myostatin also acts via other SMAD pathways and cell signaling downstream of myostatin interacts with the IGF-1 pathway.

Follistatin is a natural inhibitor of myostatin. Animals with overexpression of follistatin have increased muscle mass (Lee and McPherron, 2001; Haidet et al., 2008), and the muscles are larger than with myostatin knock-out alone (Lee, 2007). Overexpression of follistatin appears to result in increased SC activation as well as increased protein synthesis (Gilson et al., 2009). In this study, increased fiber size was accompanied by increases in myonuclear number (Gilson et al., 2009). The further study of the role of follistatin as a therapeutic aid in maintenance of muscle mass despite atrophy-stimulating conditions is certainly warranted.

SCs have the ability to differentiate across lineages including adipogenic and myogenic lineages. In situations of disuse, there are increased levels of intramuscular adipose tissue (IMAT). The increase in adipose may be due to the reduction of regenerative capacity of SCs (Chargé and Rudnicki, 2004) which may contribute to an abnormal shift toward the adipogenic lineage such as that seen in ageing skeletal muscle (Kirkland et al., 2002). SCs from obese animals produce myotubes that have impaired insulin sensitivity. In SCs cultured from obese animals there is an increased number progressing to the adipogenic lineage rather than the myogenic lineage which suggests that metabolic conditions lead to an increased proportion of SCs entering the adipogenic pathway which may contribute to the greater fat deposit in skeletal muscle (Scarda et al., 2010). It is thought that myostatin may be one of the key regulators of SCs and may play a role in determining the fate of SCs to adipogenic lineage or myogenic lineage (Deng et al., 2012).

In summary, despite atrophy occurring in the multinucleated muscle fibers, SCs are also influenced by the molecular pathways activated during the atrophy process. The alterations in both number and mitotic ability of SCs with atrophy are mediated, at least in part through increased myostatin. The influence of myostatin (and follistatin) on the potential of both SCs and pluripotent stem cells to differentiate into different lineages, is of extreme significance for skeletal muscle health as well as for prospects of clinical medicine and therapies aimed at maintaining and positively influencing skeletal muscle.

RESTORATION OF SKELETAL MUSCLE AFTER DISUSE ATROPHY

Reapplying mechanical load appears to be the most effective method to restore muscle mass, and increase myonuclear number, SC number and regenerative capacity.

Resistance exercise increases muscle mass and by increasing the load placed on the muscle which activates the PI3-AKT-mTOR pathway and increases protein synthesis. As little as one bout of resistance exercise in healthy individuals has been reported to increase IGF1 gene expression (Chesley et al., 1992). In young individuals, resistance exercise leads to increased protein synthesis after 2–4 h (Phillips et al., 1997) and this increase is maintained for 24–48 h in untrained individuals (Phillips et al., 1997).

In models of disuse, such as bed rest and immobilization, resistance exercise alone has been reported to reduce, but not completely alleviate muscle loss. Resistance exercise during 14 days of single leg immobilization in humans was sufficient to preserve quadriceps muscle mass (Oates et al., 2010) and during bed rest exercise alone reduces loss in muscle mass (Ferrando et al., 1997). As mentioned earlier, SCs appear to be activated and used with increases in mass from resistance exercise. In an interesting model to attempt to alleviate muscle loss with immobilization, during 5 days of HS, animals undertook resistance exercise with one leg (a combination of concentric, eccentric and isometric contractions) and the other leg remained as control. The leg which exercised during the HS maintained muscle mass and myofibril content (Adams et al., 2007). The stimulus was sufficient to increase gene expression of IGF1, myogenin and decrease myostatin. Further, increased p70S6K was reported. Thus, combination resistance exercise was sufficient to counter the initial alterations of disuse-induced muscle atrophy in mice (Adams et al., 2007).

Another form of atrophy prevention is electrical stimulation and stretching. However, these interventions did not reduce atrophy after 7 days following denervation in rats (Russo et al., 2010). This intervention reduced gene expression of MyoD, MAFbx, and MuRF1 levels whilst Myostatin gene expression was maintained, but there was no reduction in atrophy (Russo et al., 2010). Neuromuscular electrical stimulation has shown promising results in 5 days of immobilization in humans (Dirks et al., 2014). Applying electrical stimulation during 5 days of immobilization prevented the muscle loss and prevented the increase in myostatin, MAFbx and MuRF1 transcript levels (Dirks et al., 2014).

Protein synthesis and degradation are influenced by nutrient intake and intake of proteins and amino acids stimulate muscle protein synthesis and inhibits protein breakdown (Rennie et al., 1982). In particular, leucine, an essential amino acid, is a powerful stimulator of protein synthesis. Carbohydrate and protein are known to stimulate protein synthesis and can positively influence IGF1-mTOR-AKT pathway to stimulate protein synthesis and prevent upregulation of FOXO, MuRF1, and MAFbx; therefore nutritional intake could be a countermeasure in reducing muscle mass loss with disuse, particularly in situations where exercise is not feasible (such as hospitalized bed rest). Essential AA have consistently been shown to influence protein synthesis and alleviate some, but not all, of the loss of skeletal muscle experienced with bed rest (Paddon-Jones et al., 2004) but not to the same extent as exercise. However, with immobilization, amino acid supplementation does not appear to reduce loss of muscle mass (Stein and Blanc, 2011). An "anabolic resistance" was observed in healthy young individuals after immobilization (Glover et al., 2008) where there was decrease in muscle size and protein synthesis was 68% greater in the non-immobilized leg compared to the immobilized leg. There was also a reduced phosphorylation of AKT and p70S6K (Glover et al., 2008). Amino acid supplementation with immobilization improved protein synthesis but did not completely alleviate alterations with immobilization (Glover et al., 2008). Twenty-eight days of immobilization with protein and amino acid supplementation (28 g protein) did not prevent increases in myostatin, MuRF1 or MAFbx compared with immobilization alone (Bunn et al., 2011). In addition, after 14 days of immobilization there was a 31% decrease in post-prandial protein synthesis rate after consuming 20 g protein (Wall et al., 2013) demonstrating that the concept of anabolic resistance to protein ingestion occurs prior to 28 days. Studies assessing the influence of amino acid supplementation on SC and myonuclear response are an essential part of the keys to understanding the role of SCs and influence of exercise and nutrition.

Amino acid supplementation alone does not appear to reduce muscle atrophy, however combined with resistance exercise they provide an effective countermeasure. Some, but not complete, preservation of muscle mass and strength was reported after 28 days of bed rest with resistance exercise combined with amino acid supplementation (Brooks et al., 2008). Interestingly, the myogenic response was more pronounced in those who did not exercise during bed rest (receiving only the AA supplement) who had greater atrophy than those who exercised (Brooks et al., 2010). Myostatin transcript levels were increased significantly in the group who did not exercise compared with those who did. There was no difference in SC numbers after 28 days of bed rest or recovery indicating that the stimulus was not sufficient to increase and sustain SCs (Brooks et al., 2010). One can speculate that gravity combined with resistance exercise is needed to stimulate SC response.

Overexpression of IGF-1 did not protect mice against muscle loss with cast immobilization. After 1 week of reambulation after immobilization, mice with IGF-1 overexpression had enhanced muscle regeneration including increased muscle size, central myonuclei and Pax7+ cells (Stevens-Lapsley et al., 2010).

During rehabilitation exercise after disuse in humans, myostatin levels were supressed and sustained at lower levels throughout rehabilitation (Jones et al., 2004; Hittel et al., 2010). The reduced myostatin levels during rehabilitation exercise may act, at least in part, by releasing the inhibition on SCs and promoting muscle recovery via SCs (as discussed earlier) as well as increased AKT levels and activity (Morissette et al., 2009; Trendelenburg et al., 2009). These interventions are key to recovery from disuse atrophy and rehabilitation to functional status.

An excellent natural model to study resistance to atrophy is hibernation. Small mammals undergo long periods of reduced activity and hypocaloric intake. Hibernating animals are protected against muscle loss—despite inactivity and anorexia (for review, see Storey and Storey, 2007). Compared to the response of non-hibernating animals, such as humans and rodents, hibernating animals appear to be resistant to atrophy with disuse (Rourke et al., 2004a,b). Larger hibernating animals also appear to avoid protein loss and maintain functional capacity of skeletal muscle (Harlow et al., 2001; Lohuis et al., 2007). Hibernating animals have elevated MAFbx levels but this is not associated with atrophy (Rourke et al., 2004b). Myostatin protein levels are not increased during early hibernation and torpor, but increase during early arousal prior to resuming normal body temperature (Brooks et al., 2011).

In general, mammals lack the ability to prevent significant atrophy with disuse or disease. Hibernating grounds squirrels provide a natural model to study mechanism of resistance to atrophy in conditions of disuse and hypocaloric intake. The response of SCs and myonuclei could prove to be extremely insightful as to the natural response of muscle to resisting atrophy. By understanding the natural response to maintain myonuclear and SC function as well as with muscle atrophy will provide insight into the factors influencing atrophy and reduced function with disuse, normally an atrophy-inducing state.

SUMMARY

Since their first discovery in the 1960s, SCs have rightly played a prominent role in skeletal muscle research. Both SCs and myonuclei respond to the environmental changes which occur with disuse atrophy. The full role which they play to establish a new homeostatic environment for the muscle fiber, and/or the surrounding niche area, and the influence that the environment has on them, remains to be elucidated. The alterations in skeletal muscle with disuse atrophy such as myostatin and IGF1-AKT-mTOR appear to influence SCs as well as muscle mass. Despite no change in SC numbers with short duration human studies (<30 days), the SCs are not quiescent when their environment is changing but rather they are responding to the alterations in the niche area. This review brings together the current knowledge of myonuclear and SC response to disuse atrophy and highlights the complexity of the response in animals and humans.

REFERENCES

Abadi, A., Glover, E. I., Isfort, R. J., Raha, S., Safdar, A., Yasuda, N., et al. (2009). Limb immobilization induces a coordinate down-regulation of mitochondrial and other metabolic pathways in men and women. *PLoS ONE* 4:e6518. doi: 10.1371/journal.pone.0006518

Adams, G. R. (1998). Role of insulin-like growth factor-I in the regulation of skeletal muscle adaptation to increased loading. *Exerc. Sport. Sci. Rev.* 26, 31–60. doi: 10.1249/00003677-199800260-00004

Adams, G. R., Caiozzo, V. J., Haddad, F., and Baldwin, K. M. (2002). Cellular and molecular responses to increased skeletal muscle loading after irradiation. *Am. J. Physiol. Cell Physiol.* 283, C1182–C1195. doi: 10.1152/ajpcell.00173.2002

Adams, G. R., and Haddad, F. (1996). The relationships among IGF-1, DNA content, and protein accumulation during skeletal muscle hypertrophy. *J. Appl. Physiol.* 81, 2509–2516.

Adams, G. R., Haddad, F., Bodell, P. W., Tran, P. D., and Baldwin, K. M. (2007). Combined isometric, concentric, and eccentric resistance exercise prevents unloading-induced muscle atrophy in rats. *J. Appl. Physiol.* 103, 1644–1654. doi: 10.1152/japplphysiol.00669.2007

Allen, D. L., Bandstra, E. R., Harrison, B. C., Thorng, S., Stodieck, L. S., Kostenuik, P. J., et al. (2009). Effects of spaceflight on murine skeletal muscle gene expression. *J. Appl. Physiol.* 106, 582–595. doi: 10.1152/japplphysiol.90780.2008

Allen, D. L., Linderman, J. K., Roy, R. R., Bigbee, A. J., Grindeland, R. E., Mukku, V., et al. (1997a). Apoptosis: a mechanism contributing to remodeling of skeletal muscle in response to hindlimb unweighting. *Am. J. Physiol.* 273, C579–C587.

Allen, D. L., Linderman, J. O. N. K., Roy, R., David, L., Linderman, J. K., Bigbee, J., et al. (1997b). Apoptosis: of skeletal a mechanism contributing to remodeling muscle in response to hindlimb unweighting. *J. Appl. Physiol.* 83, 1857–1861.

Allen, D. L., Monke, S. R., Talmadge, R. J., Roy, R. R., and Edgerton, V. R. (1995). Plasticity of myonuclear number in hypertrophied and atrophied mammalian skeletal muscle fibers. *J. Appl. Physiol.* 78, 1969–1976.

Allen, D. L., Roy, R. R., and Edgerton, V. R. (1999). Myonuclear domains in muscle adaptation and disease. *Muscle Nerve* 22, 1350–1360.

Allen, D. L., Yasui, W., Tanaka, T., Ohira, Y., Nagaoka, S., Sekiguchi, C., et al. (1996). Myonuclear number and myosin heavy chain expression in rat soleus single muscle fibers after spaceflight. *J. Appl. Physiol.* 81, 145–151.

Amthor, H., Otto, A., Macharia, R., McKinnell, I., and Patel, K. (2006). Myostatin imposes reversible quiescence on embryonic muscle precursors. *Dev. Dyn.* 235, 672–680. doi: 10.1002/dvdy.20680

Amthor, H., Otto, A., Vulin, A., Rochat, A., Dumonceaux, J., Garcia, L., et al. (2009). Muscle hypertrophy driven by myostatin blockade does not require stem/precursor-cell activity. *Proc. Natl. Acad. Sci. U.S.A.* 106, 7479–7484. doi: 10.1073/pnas.0811129106

Aravamudan, B., Mantilla, C. B., Zhan, W.-Z., and Sieck, G. C. (2006). Denervation effects on myonuclear domain size of rat diaphragm fibers. *J. Appl. Physiol.* 100, 1617–1622. doi: 10.1152/japplphysiol.01277.2005

Baldwin, K. M., Haddad, F., Pandorf, C. E., Roy, R. R., and Edgerton, V. R. (2013). Alterations in muscle mass and contractile phenotype in response to unloading models: role of transcriptional/pretranslational mechanisms. *Front. Physiol.* 4:284. doi: 10.3389/fphys.2013.00284

Biressi, S., and Rando, T. A. (2010). Heterogeneity in the muscle satellite cell population. *Semin. Cell Dev. Biol.* 21, 845–854. doi: 10.1016/j.semcdb.2010.09.003

Bischoff, R. (1986). A satellite cell mitogen from crushed adult muscle. *Dev. Biol.* 115, 140–147. doi: 10.1016/0012-1606(86)90235-6

Bischoff, R. (1990). Interaction between satellite cells and skeletal muscle fibers. *Development* 109, 943–952.

Blaauw, B., Canato, M., Agatea, L., Toniolo, L., Mammucari, C., Masiero, E., et al. (2009). Inducible activation of Akt increases skeletal muscle mass and force without satellite cell activation. *FASEB J.* 23, 3896–3905. doi: 10.1096/fj.09-131870

Bloomfield, S. A. (1997). Changes in musculoskeletal structure and function with prolonged bed rest. *Med. Sci. Sports Exerc.* 29, 197–206. doi: 10.1097/00005768-199702000-00006

Bodine, S. C., Latres, E., Baumhueter, S., Lai, V. K., Nunez, L., Clarke, B. A., et al. (2001). Identification of ubiquitin ligases required for skeletal muscle atrophy. *Science* 294, 1704–1708. doi: 10.1126/science.1065874

Booth, F. W., and Baldwin, K. M. (1996). *Handbook of Physiology. Exercise: Regulation and Integration of Multiple Systems.* Bethesda, MD: American Physiological Society.

Booth, F. W., and Thomason, D. B. (1991). Molecular and cellular adaptation of muscle in response to exercise: perspectives of various models. *Physiol. Rev.* 71, 541–585.

Boppart, M. D., De Lisio, M., Zou, K., and Huntsman, H. D. (2013). Defining a role for non-satellite stem cells in the regulation of muscle repair following exercise. *Front. Physiol.* 4:310. doi: 10.3389/fphys.2013.00310

Brooks, N., Cloutier, G. J., Cadena, S. M., Layne, J. E., Nelsen, C. A., Freed, A. M., et al. (2008). Resistance training and timed essential amino acids protect against the loss of muscle mass and strength during 28 days of bed rest and energy deficit. *J. Appl. Physiol.* 105, 241–248. doi: 10.1152/japplphysiol.01346.2007

Brooks, N. E., Cadena, S. M., Vannier, E., Cloutier, G., Carambula, S., Myburgh, K. H., et al. (2010). Effects of resistance exercise combined with essential amino acid supplementation and energy deficit on markers of skeletal muscle atrophy and regeneration during bed rest and active recovery. *Muscle Nerve* 42, 927–935. doi: 10.1002/mus.21780

Brooks, N. E., Myburgh, K. H., and Storey, K. B. (2011). Myostatin levels in skeletal muscle of hibernating ground squirrels. *J. Exp. Biol.* 214, 2522–2527. doi: 10.1242/jeb.055764

Brooks, N. E., Schuenke, M. D., and Hikida, R. S. (2009). Ageing influences myonuclear domain size differently in fast and slow skeletal muscle of rats. *Acta Physiol. (Oxf).* 197, 55–63. doi: 10.1111/j.1748-1716.2009.01983.x

Bruusgaard, J. C., Egner, I. M., Larsen, T. K., Dupre-Aucouturier, S., Desplanches, D., and Gundersen, K. (2012). No change in myonuclear number during muscle unloading and reloading. *J. Appl. Physiol.* 113, 290–296. doi: 10.1152/japplphysiol.00436.2012

Bruusgaard, J. C., and Gundersen, K. (2008). *In vivo* time-lapse microscopy reveals no loss of murine myonuclei during weeks of muscle atrophy. *J. Clin. Invest.* 118, 1450–1457. doi: 10.1172/JCI34022

Bruusgaard, J. C., Johansen, I. B., Egner, I. M., Rana, Z. A., and Gundersen, K. (2010). Myonuclei acquired by overload exercise precede hypertrophy and are not lost on detraining. *Proc. Natl. Acad. Sci. U.S.A.* 107, 15111–15116. doi: 10.1073/pnas.0913935107

Bruusgaard, J. C., Liestøl, K., and Gundersen, K. (2006). Distribution of myonuclei and microtubules in live muscle fibers of young, middle-aged, and old mice. *J. Appl. Physiol.* 100, 2024–2030. doi: 10.1152/japplphysiol.00913.2005

Bunn, J. A., Buford, T. W., Serra, M. C., Kreider, R. B., and Willoughby, D. S. (2011). Protein and amino acid supplementation does not alter proteolytic gene expression following immobilization. *J. Nutr. Metab.* 2011, 539690. doi: 10.1155/2011/539690

Burleigh, I. G. (1977). Observations on the number of nuclei within the fibres of some red and white muscles. *J. Cell Sci.* 23, 269–284.

Cameron-Smith, D. (2002). Exercise and skeletal muscle gene expression. *Clin. Exp. Pharmacol. Physiol.* 29, 209–213. doi: 10.1046/j.1440-1681.2002.03621.x

Carlson, C. J., Booth, F. W., and Gordon, S. E. (1999). Skeletal muscle myostatin mRNA expression is fiber-type specific and increases during hindlimb unloading. *Am. J. Physiol.* 277, R601–R606.

Carlsson, P., and Mahlapuu, M. (2002). Forkhead transcription factors: key players in development and metabolism. *Dev. Biol.* 250, 1–23. doi: 10.1006/dbio.2002.0780

Chargé, S. B. P., and Rudnicki, M. A. (2004). Cellular and molecular regulation of muscle regeneration. *Physiol. Rev.* 84, 209–238. doi: 10.1152/physrev.00019.2003

Chesley, A., MacDougall, J. D., Tarnopolsky, M. A., Atkinson, S. A., and Smith, K. (1992). Changes in human muscle protein synthesis after resistance exercise. *J. Appl. Physiol.* 73, 1383–1388.

Darr, K. C., and Schultz, E. (1989). Hindlimb suspension suppresses muscle growth and satellite cell proliferation. *J. Appl. Physiol.* 67, 1827–1834.

Day, K., Shefer, G., Richardson, J. B., Enikolopov, G., and Yablonka-Reuveni, Z. (2007). Nestin-GFP reporter expression defines the quiescent state of skeletal muscle satellite cells. *Dev. Biol.* 304, 246–259. doi: 10.1016/j.ydbio.2006.12.026

Day, M. K., Allen, D. L., Mohajerani, L., Greenisen, M. C., Roy, R. R., and Edgerton, V. R. (1995). Adaptations of human skeletal muscle fibers to spaceflight. *J. Gravit. Physiol.* 2, 47–50.

Deng, B., Wen, J., Ding, Y., Peng, J., and Jiang, S. (2012). Different regulation role of myostatin in differentiating pig ADSCs and MSCs into adipocytes. *Cell Biochem. Funct.* 30, 145–150. doi: 10.1002/cbf.1828

Dirks, M. L., Wall, B. T., Snijders, T., Ottenbros, C. L. P., Verdijk, L. B., and van Loon, L. J. C. (2014). Neuromuscular electrical stimulation prevents muscle disuse atrophy during leg immobilization in humans. *Acta Physiol. (Oxf).* 210, 628–641. doi: 10.1111/apha.12200

Dupont-Versteegden, E. E., Murphy, R. J., Houlé, J. D., Gurley, C. M., and Peterson, C. A. (1999). Activated satellite cells fail to restore myonuclear number in spinal cord transected and exercised rats. *Am. J. Physiol.* 277, C589–C597.

Dupont-Versteegden, E. E., Strotman, B. A., Gurley, C. M., Gaddy, D., Knox, M., Fluckey, J. D., et al. (2006). Nuclear translocation of EndoG at the initiation of disuse muscle atrophy and apoptosis is specific to myonuclei. *Am. J. Physiol. Regul. Integr. Comp. Physiol.* 291, R1730–R1740. doi: 10.1152/ajpregu.00176.2006

Edgerton, V. R., and Roy, R. R. (1991). Regulation of skeletal muscle fiber size, shape and function. *J. Biomech.* 24(Suppl. 1), 123–133. doi: 10.1016/0021-9290(91)90383-X

Edgerton, V. R., Zhou, M. Y., Ohira, Y., Klitgaard, H., Jiang, B., Bell, G., et al. (1995). Human fiber size and enzymatic properties after 5 and 11 days of spaceflight. *J. Appl. Physiol.* 78, 1733–1739.

Elder, G. C., and McComas, A. J. (1987). Development of rat muscle during short- and long-term hindlimb suspension. *J. Appl. Physiol.* 62, 1917–1923.

Erbay, E., Park, I.-H., Nuzzi, P. D., Schoenherr, C. J., and Chen, J. (2003). IGF-II transcription in skeletal myogenesis is controlled by mTOR and nutrients. *J. Cell Biol.* 163, 931–936. doi: 10.1083/jcb.200307158

Fauteck, S. P., and Kandarian, S. C. (1995). Sensitive detection of myosin heavy chain composition in skeletal muscle under different loading conditions. *Am. J. Physiol.* 268, C419–C424.

Ferrando, A. A., Lane, H. W., Stuart, C. A., Davis-Street, J., and Wolfe, R. R. (1996). Prolonged bed rest decreases skeletal muscle and whole body protein synthesis. *Am. J. Physiol.* 270, E627–E633.

Ferrando, A. A., Tipton, K. D., Bamman, M. M., and Wolfe, R. R. (1997). Resistance exercise maintains skeletal muscle protein synthesis during bed rest. *J. Appl. Physiol.* 82, 807–810.

Ferreira, R., Neuparth, M. J., Ascensão, A., Magalhães, J., Vitorino, R., Duarte, J. A., et al. (2006). Skeletal muscle atrophy increases cell proliferation in mice gastrocnemius during the first week of hindlimb suspension. *Eur. J. Appl. Physiol.* 97, 340–346. doi: 10.1007/s00421-006-0197-6

Fitts, R. H., Metzger, J. M., Riley, D. A., and Unsworth, B. R. (1986). Models of disuse: a comparison of hindlimb suspension and immobilization. *J. Appl. Physiol.* 60, 1946–1953.

Fitts, R. H., Riley, D. R., and Widrick, J. J. (2000). Physiology of a microgravity environment invited review: microgravity and skeletal muscle. *J. Appl. Physiol.* 89, 823–839.

Foletta, V. C., White, L. J., Larsen, A. E., Léger, B., and Russell, A. P. (2011). The role and regulation of MAFbx/atrogin-1 and MuRF1 in skeletal muscle atrophy. *Pflugers Arch.* 461, 325–335. doi: 10.1007/s00424-010-0919-9

Ge, X., McFarlane, C., Vajjala, A., Lokireddy, S., Ng, Z. H., Tan, C. K., et al. (2011). Smad3 signaling is required for satellite cell function and myogenic differentiation of myoblasts. *Cell Res.* 21, 1591–1604. doi: 10.1038/cr.2011.72

Gibson, M. C., and Schultz, E. (1982). The distribution of satellite cells and their relationship to specific fiber types in soleus and extensor digitorum longus muscles. *Anat. Rec.* 202, 329–337. doi: 10.1002/ar.1092020305

Gilson, H., Schakman, O., Kalista, S., Lause, P., Tsuchida, K., and Thissen, J.-P. (2009). Follistatin induces muscle hypertrophy through satellite cell proliferation and inhibition of both myostatin and activin. *Am. J. Physiol. Endocrinol. Metab.* 297, E157–E164. doi: 10.1152/ajpendo.00193.2009

Glass, D. J. (2003). Signalling pathways that mediate skeletal muscle hypertrophy and atrophy. *Nat. Cell Biol.* 5, 87–90. doi: 10.1038/ncb0203-87

Glover, E. I., Phillips, S. M., Oates, B. R., Tang, J. E., Tarnopolsky, M. A., Selby, A., et al. (2008). Immobilization induces anabolic resistance in human myofibrillar protein synthesis with low and high dose amino acid infusion. *J. Physiol.* 586, 6049–6061. doi: 10.1113/jphysiol.2008.160333

Goldberg, A. L., Etlinger, J. D., Goldspink, D. F., and Jablecki, C. (1975). Mechanism of work-induced hypertrophy of skeletal muscle. *Med. Sci. Sports* 7, 185–198.

Gomes, M. D., Lecker, S. H., Jagoe, R. T., Navon, A., and Goldberg, A. L. (2001). Atrogin-1, a muscle-specific F-box protein highly expressed during muscle atrophy. *Proc. Natl. Acad. Sci. U.S.A.* 98, 14440–14445. doi: 10.1073/pnas.251541198

Grobet, L., Martin, L. J., Poncelet, D., Pirottin, D., Brouwers, B., Riquet, J., et al. (1997). A deletion in the bovine myostatin gene causes the double-muscled phenotype in cattle. *Nat. Genet.* 17, 71–74. doi: 10.1038/ng0997-71

Gundersen, K., and Bruusgaard, J. C. (2008). Nuclear domains during muscle atrophy: nuclei lost or paradigm lost? *J. Physiol.* 586, 2675–2681. doi: 10.1113/jphysiol.2008.154369

Guo, B.-S., Cheung, K.-K., Yeung, S. S., Zhang, B.-T., and Yeung, E. W. (2012). Electrical stimulation influences satellite cell proliferation and apoptosis in unloading-induced muscle atrophy in mice. *PLoS ONE* 7:e30348. doi: 10.1371/journal.pone.0030348

Gustafsson, T., Osterlund, T., Flanagan, J. N., von Waldén, F., Trappe, T. A., Linnehan, R. M., et al. (2010). Effects of 3 days unloading on molecular regulators of muscle size in humans. *J. Appl. Physiol.* 109, 721–727. doi: 10.1152/japplphysiol.00110.2009

Hackney, K. J., and Ploutz-Snyder, L. L. (2012). Unilateral lower limb suspension: integrative physiological knowledge from the past 20 years (1991-2011). *Eur. J. Appl. Physiol.* 112, 9–22. doi: 10.1007/s00421-011-1971-7

Haidet, A. M., Rizo, L., Handy, C., Umapathi, P., Eagle, A., Shilling, C., et al. (2008). Long-term enhancement of skeletal muscle mass and strength by single gene administration of myostatin inhibitors. *Proc. Natl. Acad. Sci. U.S.A.* 105, 4318–4322. doi: 10.1073/pnas.0709144105

Hall, Z. W., and Ralston, E. (1989). Nuclear domains in muscle cells. *Cell* 59, 771–772. doi: 10.1016/0092-8674(89)90597-7

Han, B., Tong, J., Zhu, M. J., Ma, C., and Du, M. (2008). Insulin-like growth factor-1 (IGF-1) and leucine activate pig myogenic satellite cells through mammalian target of rapamycin (mTOR) pathway. *Mol. Reprod. Dev.* 75, 810–817. doi: 10.1002/mrd.20832

Harlow, H. J., Lohuis, T., Beck, T. D., and Iaizzo, P. A. (2001). Muscle strength in overwintering bears. *Nature* 409, 997. doi: 10.1038/35059165

Harrison, B. C., Allen, D. L., Girten, B., Stodieck, L. S., Kostenuik, P. J., Bateman, T. A., et al. (2003). Skeletal muscle adaptations to microgravity exposure in the mouse. *J. Appl. Physiol.* 95, 2462–2470. doi: 10.1152/japplphysiol.00603.2003

Hikida, R. S., Gollnick, P. D., Dudley, G. A., Convertino, V. A., and Buchanan, P. (1989). Structural and metabolic characteristics of human skeletal muscle following 30 days of simulated microgravity. *Aviat Space Environ. Med.* 60, 664–670.

Hikida, R. S., Van Nostran, S., Murray, J. D., Staron, R. S., Gordon, S. E., and Kraemer, W. J. (1997). Myonuclear loss in atrophied soleus muscle fibers. *Anat. Rec.* 247, 350–354.

Hittel, D. S., Axelson, M., Sarna, N., Shearer, J., Huffman, K. M., and Kraus, W. E. (2010). Myostatin decreases with aerobic exercise and associates with insulin resistance. *Med. Sci. Sports Exerc.* 42, 2023–2029. doi: 10.1249/MSS.0b013e3181e0b9a8

Hvid, L. G., Suetta, C., Aagaard, P., Kjaer, M., Frandsen, U., and Ørtenblad, N. (2013). Four days of muscle disuse impairs single fiber contractile function in young and old healthy men. *Exp. Gerontol.* 48, 154–161. doi: 10.1016/j.exger.2012.11.005

Jackson, J. R., Mula, J., Kirby, T. J., Fry, C. S., Lee, J. D., Ubele, M. F., et al. (2012). Satellite cell depletion does not inhibit adult skeletal muscle regrowth following unloading-induced atrophy. *Am. J. Physiol. Cell Physiol.* 303, C854–C861. doi: 10.1152/ajpcell.00207.2012

Jejurikar, S. S., and Kuzon, W. M. (2003). Satellite cell depletion in degenerative skeletal muscle. *Apoptosis* 8, 573–578. doi: 10.1023/A:1026127307457

Jejurikar, S. S., Marcelo, C. L., and Kuzon, W. M. (2002). Skeletal muscle denervation increases satellite cell susceptibility to apoptosis. *Plast. Reconstr. Surg.* 110, 160–168. doi: 10.1097/00006534-200207000-00027

Jones, S. W., Hill, R. J., Krasney, P. A., O'Conner, B., Peirce, N., and Greenhaff, P. L. (2004). Disuse atrophy and exercise rehabilitation in humans profoundly affects the expression of genes associated with the regulation of skeletal muscle mass. *FASEB J.* 18, 1025–1027. doi: 10.1096/fj.03-1228fje

Kadi, F., Johansson, F., Johansson, R., Sjöström, M., and Henriksson, J. (2004). Effects of one bout of endurance exercise on the expression of myogenin in human quadriceps muscle. *Histochem. Cell Biol.* 121, 329–334. doi: 10.1007/s00418-004-0630-z

Kambadur, R., Sharma, M., Smith, T. P., and Bass, J. J. (1997). Mutations in myostatin (GDF8) in double-muscled Belgian Blue and Piedmontese cattle. *Genome Res.* 7, 910–916.

Kandarian, S. C., and Jackman, R. W. (2006). Intracellular signaling during skeletal muscle atrophy. *Muscle Nerve* 33, 155–165. doi: 10.1002/mus.20442

Kirkland, J. L., Tchkonia, T., Pirtskhalava, T., Han, J., and Karagiannides, I. (2002). Adipogenesis and aging: does aging make fat go MAD? *Exp. Gerontol.* 37, 757–767. doi: 10.1016/S0531-5565(02)00014-1

Kohn, T. A., Essen-Gustavsson, B., and Myburgh, K. H. (2007). Exercise pattern influences skeletal muscle hybrid fibers of runners and nonrunners. *Med. Sci. Sports Exerc.* 39, 1977–1984. doi: 10.1249/mss.0b013e3181453546

Kuang, S., Kuroda, K., Le Grand, F., and Rudnicki, M. A. (2007). Asymmetric self-renewal and commitment of satellite stem cells in muscle. *Cell* 129, 999–1010. doi: 10.1016/j.cell.2007.03.044

Kujawa, M., Baran, W., and Jankowska-Steifer, E. (2005). Quantitative ultrastructural changes in satellite cells of rats immobilized after soleus muscle denervation. *Exp. Mol. Pathol.* 78, 78–85. doi: 10.1016/j.yexmp.2004.08.007

Langley, B., Thomas, M., Bishop, A., Sharma, M., Gilmour, S., and Kambadur, R. (2002). Myostatin inhibits myoblast differentiation by down-regulating MyoD expression. *J. Biol. Chem.* 277, 49831–49840. doi: 10.1074/jbc.M204291200

LeBlanc, A. D., Schneider, V. S., Evans, H. J., Pientok, C., Rowe, R., and Spector, E. (1992). Regional changes in muscle mass following 17 weeks of bed rest. *J. Appl. Physiol.* 73, 2172–2178.

Lee, S. J. (2007). Quadrupling muscle mass in mice by targeting TGF-beta signaling pathways. *PLoS ONE* 2:e789. doi: 10.1371/journal.pone.0000789

Lee, S.-J., Huynh, T. V., Lee, Y.-S., Sebald, S. M., Wilcox-Adelman, S. A., Iwamori, N., et al. (2012). Role of satellite cells versus myofibers in muscle hypertrophy induced by inhibition of the myostatin/activin signaling pathway. *Proc. Natl. Acad. Sci. U.S.A.* 109, E2353–E2360. doi: 10.1073/pnas.1206410109

Lee, S. J., and McPherron, A. C. (2001). Regulation of myostatin activity and muscle growth. *Proc. Natl. Acad. Sci. U.S.A.* 98, 9306–9311. doi: 10.1073/pnas.151270098

Leeuwenburgh, C., Gurley, C. M., Strotman, B. A., and Dupont-Versteegden, E. E. (2005). Age-related differences in apoptosis with disuse atrophy in soleus muscle. *Am. J. Physiol. Regul. Integr. Comp. Physiol.* 288, R1288–R1296. doi: 10.1152/ajpregu.00576.2004

Lexell, J., Taylor, C. C., and Sjöström, M. (1988). What is the cause of the ageing atrophy? Total number, size and proportion of different fiber types studied in whole vastus lateralis muscle from 15- to 83-year-old men. *J. Neurol. Sci.* 84, 275–294. doi: 10.1016/0022-510X(88)90132-3

Lohuis, T. D., Harlow, H. J., Beck, T. D. I., and Iaizzo, P. A. (2007). Hibernating bears conserve muscle strength and maintain fatigue resistance. *Physiol. Biochem. Zool.* 80, 257–269. doi: 10.1086/513190

Mackey, A. L., Kjaer, M., Charifi, N., Henriksson, J., Bojsen-Moller, J., Holm, L., et al. (2009). Assessment of satellite cell number and activity status in human skeletal muscle biopsies. *Muscle Nerve* 40, 455–465. doi: 10.1002/mus.21369

Malatesta, M., and Meola, G. (2010). Structural and functional alterations of the cell nucleus in skeletal muscle wasting: the evidence *in situ*. *Eur. J. Histochem.* 54, e44. doi: 10.4081/ejh.2010.e44

Manceau, M., Gros, J., Savage, K., Thomé, V., McPherron, A., Paterson, B., et al. (2008). Myostatin promotes the terminal differentiation of embryonic muscle progenitors. *Genes Dev.* 22, 668–681. doi: 10.1101/gad.454408

Marimuthu, K., Murton, A. J., and Greenhaff, P. L. (2011). Mechanisms regulating muscle mass during disuse atrophy and rehabilitation in humans. *J. Appl. Physiol.* 110, 555–560. doi: 10.1152/japplphysiol.00962.2010

Matsuba, Y., Goto, K., Morioka, S., Naito, T., Akema, T., Hashimoto, N., et al. (2009). Gravitational unloading inhibits the regenerative potential of atrophied soleus muscle in mice. *Acta Physiol. (Oxf).* 196, 329–339. doi: 10.1111/j.1748-1716.2008.01943.x

Mauro, A. (1961). Satellite cell of skeletal muscle fibers. *J. Biophys. Biochem. Cytol.* 9, 493–495. doi: 10.1083/jcb.9.2.493

McCall, G. E., Allen, D. L., Linderman, J. K., Grindeland, R. E., Roy, R. R., Mukku, V. R., et al. (1998). Maintenance of myonuclear domain size in rat soleus after overload and growth hormone/IGF-I treatment. *J. Appl. Physiol.* 84, 1407–1412.

McCarthy, J. J., Mula, J., Miyazaki, M., Erfani, R., Garrison, K., Farooqui, A. B., et al. (2011). Effective fiber hypertrophy in satellite cell-depleted skeletal muscle. *Development* 138, 3657–3666. doi: 10.1242/dev.068858

McCroskery, S., Thomas, M., Maxwell, L., Sharma, M., and Kambadur, R. (2003). Myostatin negatively regulates satellite cell activation and self-renewal. *J. Cell Biol.* 162, 1135–1147. doi: 10.1083/jcb.200207056

McFarlane, C., Hennebry, A., Thomas, M., Plummer, E., Ling, N., Sharma, M., et al. (2008). Myostatin signals through Pax7 to regulate satellite cell self-renewal. *Exp. Cell Res.* 314, 317–329. doi: 10.1016/j.yexcr.2007.09.012

McFarlane, C., Plummer, E., Thomas, M., Hennebry, A., Ashby, M., Ling, N., et al. (2006). Myostatin induces cachexia by activating the ubiquitin proteolytic system through an NF-kappaB-independent, FoxO1-dependent mechanism. *J. Cell. Physiol.* 209, 501–514. doi: 10.1002/jcp.20757

McKay, B. R., Ogborn, D. I., Bellamy, L. M., Tarnopolsky, M. A., and Parise, G. (2012). Myostatin is associated with age-related human muscle stem cell dysfunction. *FASEB J.* 26, 2509–2521. doi: 10.1096/fj.11-198663

McPherron, A. C., Lawler, A. M., and Lee, S. J. (1997). Regulation of skeletal muscle mass in mice by a new TGF-beta superfamily member. *Nature* 387, 83–90. doi: 10.1038/387083a0

McPherron, A. C., and Lee, S. J. (1997). Double muscling in cattle due to mutations in the myostatin gene. *Proc. Natl. Acad. Sci. U.S.A.* 94, 12457–12461. doi: 10.1073/pnas.94.23.12457

Mitchell, P. O., and Pavlath, G. K. (2004). Skeletal muscle atrophy leads to loss and dysfunction of muscle precursor cells. *Am. J. Physiol. Cell Physiol.* 287, C1753–C1762. doi: 10.1152/ajpcell.00292.2004

Morey-Holton, E. R., and Globus, R. K. (2002). Hindlimb unloading rodent model: technical aspects. *J. Appl. Physiol.* 92, 1367–1377. doi: 10.1152/japplphysiol.00969.2001

Morissette, M. R., Cook, S. A., Buranasombati, C., Rosenberg, M. A., and Rosenzweig, A. (2009). Myostatin inhibits IGF-I-induced myotube hypertrophy through Akt. *Am. J. Physiol. Cell Physiol.* 297, C1124–C1132. doi: 10.1152/ajpcell.00043.2009

Mourkioti, F., and Rosenthal, N. (2005). IGF-1, inflammation and stem cells: interactions during muscle regeneration. *Trends Immunol.* 26, 535–542. doi: 10.1016/j.it.2005.08.002

Mozdziak, P. E., Pulvermacher, P. M., and Schultz, E. (2000). Unloading of juvenile muscle results in a reduced muscle size 9 wk after reloading. *J. Appl. Physiol.* 88, 158–164.

Mozdziak, P. E., Pulvermacher, P. M., and Schultz, E. (2001). Muscle regeneration during hindlimb unloading results in a reduction in muscle size after reloading. *J. Appl. Physiol.* 91, 183–190.

Mozdziak, P. E., Truong, Q., Macius, A., and Schultz, E. (1998). Hindlimb suspension reduces muscle regeneration. *Eur. J. Appl. Physiol. Occup. Physiol.* 78, 136–140. doi: 10.1007/s004210050398

Nagata, Y., Kobayashi, H., Umeda, M., Ohta, N., Kawashima, S., Zammit, P. S., et al. (2006). Sphingomyelin levels in the plasma membrane correlate with the activation state of muscle satellite cells. *J. Histochem. Cytochem.* 54, 375–384. doi: 10.1369/jhc.5A6675.2006

Narici, M. V., and de Boer, M. D. (2011). Disuse of the musculo-skeletal system in space and on earth. *Eur. J. Appl. Physiol.* 111, 403–420. doi: 10.1007/s00421-010-1556-x

Nicks, D. K., Beneke, W. M., Key, R. M., and Timson, B. F. (1989). Muscle fibre size and number following immobilisation atrophy. *J. Anat.* 163, 1–5.

Oates, B. R., Glover, E. I., West, D. W., Fry, J. L., Tarnopolsky, M. A., and Phillips, S. M. (2010). Low-volume resistance exercise attenuates the decline in strength and muscle mass associated with immobilization. *Muscle Nerve* 42, 539–546. doi: 10.1002/mus.21721

Ono, Y., Masuda, S., Nam, H.-S., Benezra, R., Miyagoe-Suzuki, Y., and Takeda, S. (2012). Slow-dividing satellite cells retain long-term self-renewal ability in adult muscle. *J. Cell Sci.* 125, 1309–1317. doi: 10.1242/jcs.096198

Paddon-Jones, D., Sheffield-Moore, M., Urban, R. J., Sanford, A. P., Aarsland, A., Wolfe, R. R., et al. (2004). Essential amino acid and carbohydrate supplementation ameliorates muscle protein loss in humans during 28 days bedrest. *J. Clin. Endocrinol. Metab.* 89, 4351–4358. doi: 10.1210/jc.2003-032159

Pavlath, G. K., Rich, K., Webster, S. G., and Blau, H. M. (1989). Localization of muscle gene products in nuclear domains. *Nature* 337, 570–573. doi: 10.1038/337570a0

Petrella, J. K., Kim, J., Cross, J. M., Kosek, D. J., and Bamman, M. M. (2006). Efficacy of myonuclear addition may explain differential myofiber growth among resistance-trained young and older men and women. *Am. J. Physiol. Endocrinol. Metab.* 291, E937–E946. doi: 10.1152/ajpendo.00190.2006

Philippou, A., Halapas, A., Maridaki, M., and Koutsilieris, M. (2007). Type I insulin-like growth factor receptor signaling in skeletal muscle regeneration and hypertrophy. *J. Musculoskelet. Neuronal Interact.* 7, 208–218.

Phillips, S. M., Tipton, K. D., Aarsland, A., Wolf, S. E., and Wolfe, R. R. (1997). Mixed muscle protein synthesis and breakdown after resistance exercise in humans. *Am. J. Physiol.* 273, E99–E107.

Pitts, G. C. (1986). Cellular aspects of growth and catch-up growth in the rat: a reevaluation. *Growth* 50, 419–436.

Raffaello, A., Milan, G., Masiero, E., Carnio, S., Lee, D., Lanfranchi, G., et al. (2010). JunB transcription factor maintains skeletal muscle mass and promotes hypertrophy. *J. Cell Biol.* 191, 101–113. doi: 10.1083/jcb.201001136

Ramaswamy, S., Nakamura, N., Sansal, I., Bergeron, L., and Sellers, W. R. (2002). A novel mechanism of gene regulation and tumor suppression by the transcription factor FKHR. *Cancer Cell* 2, 81–91. doi: 10.1016/S1535-6108(02)00086-7

Reardon, K. A., Davis, J., Kapsa, R. M., Choong, P., and Byrne, E. (2001). Myostatin, insulin-like growth factor-1, and leukemia inhibitory factor mRNAs are upregulated in chronic human disuse muscle atrophy. *Muscle Nerve* 24, 893–899. doi: 10.1002/mus.1086

Reisz-Porszasz, S., Bhasin, S., Artaza, J. N., Shen, R., Sinha-Hikim, I., Hogue, A., et al. (2003). Lower skeletal muscle mass in male transgenic mice with muscle-specific overexpression of myostatin. *Am. J. Physiol. Endocrinol. Metab.* 285, E876–E888. doi: 10.1152/ajpendo.00107.2003

Rennie, M. J., Edwards, R. H., Halliday, D., Matthews, D. E., Wolman, S. L., and Millward, D. J. (1982). Muscle protein synthesis measured by stable isotope techniques in man: the effects of feeding and fasting. *Clin. Sci. (Lond).* 63, 519–523.

Riley, D. A., Ellis, S., Slocum, G. R., Satyanarayana, T., Bain, J. L., and Sedlak, F. R. (1987). Hypogravity-induced atrophy of rat soleus and extensor digitorum longus muscles. *Muscle Nerve* 10, 560–568. doi: 10.1002/mus.880100612

Rodrigues Ade, C., and Schmalbruch, H. (1995). Satellite cells and myonuclei in long-term denervated rat muscles. *Anat. Rec.* 243, 430–437. doi: 10.1002/ar.1092430405

Rourke, B. C., Qin, A., Haddad, F., Baldwin, K. M., and Caiozzo, V. J. (2004a). Cloning and sequencing of myosin heavy chain isoform cDNAs in golden-mantled ground squirrels: effects of hibernation on mRNA expression. *J. Appl. Physiol.* 97, 1985–1991. doi: 10.1152/japplphysiol.00695.2004

Rourke, B. C., Yokoyama, Y., Milsom, W. K., and Caiozzo, V. J. (2004b). Myosin isoform expression and MAFbx mRNA levels in hibernating golden-mantled ground squirrels (*Spermophilus lateralis*). *Physiol Biochem Zool* 77, 582–593. doi: 10.1086/421753

Roy, R. R., Monke, S. R., Allen, D. L., and Edgerton, V. R. (1999a). Modulation of myonuclear number in functionally overloaded and exercised rat plantaris fibers. *J. Appl. Physiol.* 87, 634–642.

Roy, R. R., Talmadge, R. J., Hodgson, J. A., Oishi, Y., Baldwin, K. M., and Edgerton, V. R. (1999b). Differential response of fast hindlimb extensor and flexor muscles to exercise in adult spinalized cats. *Muscle Nerve* 22, 230–241.

Russo, T. L., Peviani, S. M., Durigan, J. L. Q., Gigo-Benato, D., Delfino, G. B., and Salvini, T. F. (2010). Stretching and electrical stimulation reduce the accumulation of MyoD, myostatin and atrogin-1 in denervated rat skeletal muscle. *J. Muscle Res. Cell Motil.* 31, 45–57. doi: 10.1007/s10974-010-9203-z

Sandri, M., Sandri, C., Gilbert, A., Skurk, C., Calabria, E., Picard, A., et al. (2004). Foxo transcription factors induce the atrophy-related ubiquitin ligase atrogin-1 and cause skeletal muscle atrophy. *Cell* 117, 399–412. doi: 10.1016/S0092-8674(04)00400-3

Scarda, A., Franzin, C., Milan, G., Sanna, M., Dal Prà, C., Pagano, C., et al. (2010). Increased adipogenic conversion of muscle satellite cells in obese Zucker rats. *Int. J. Obes. (Lond).* 34, 1319–1327. doi: 10.1038/ijo.2010.47

Schakman, O., Kalista, S., Barbé, C., Loumaye, A., and Thissen, J. P. (2013). Glucocorticoid-induced skeletal muscle atrophy. *Int. J. Biochem. Cell Biol.* 45, 2163–2172. doi: 10.1016/j.biocel.2013.05.036

Scharner, J., and Zammit, P. S. (2011). The muscle satellite cell at 50: the formative years. *Skelet. Muscle* 1, 28. doi: 10.1186/2044-5040-1-28

Schiaffino, S., Dyar, K. A., Ciciliot, S., Blaauw, B., and Sandri, M. (2013). Mechanisms regulating skeletal muscle growth and atrophy. *FEBS J.* 280, 4294–4314. doi: 10.1111/febs.12253

Schmalbruch, H., Al-Amood, W. S., and Lewis, D. M. (1991). Morphology of long-term denervated rat soleus muscle and the effect of chronic electrical stimulation. *J. Physiol.* 441, 233–241.

Schuelke, M., Wagner, K. R., Stolz, L. E., Hübner, C., Riebel, T., Kömen, W., et al. (2004). Myostatin mutation associated with gross muscle hypertrophy in a child. *N. Engl. J. Med.* 350, 2682–2688. doi: 10.1056/NEJMoa040933

Shao, C., Liu, M., Wu, X., and Ding, F. (2007). Time-dependent expression of myostatin RNA transcript and protein in gastrocnemius muscle of mice after sciatic nerve resection. *Microsurgery* 27, 487–493. doi: 10.1002/micr.20392

Siu, P. M., and Alway, S. E. (2009). Response and adaptation of skeletal muscle to denervation stress: the role of apoptosis in muscle loss. *Front. Biosci. (Landmark Ed).* 14:432–452. doi: 10.2741/3253

Siu, P. M., Pistilli, E. E., and Alway, S. E. (2005). Apoptotic responses to hindlimb suspension in gastrocnemius muscles from young adult and aged rats. *Am. J. Physiol. Regul. Integr. Comp. Physiol.* 289, R1015–R1026. doi: 10.1152/ajpregu.00198.2005

Smith, H. K., Maxwell, L., Martyn, J. A., and Bass, J. J. (2000). Nuclear DNA fragmentation and morphological alterations in adult rabbit skeletal muscle after short-term immobilization. *Cell Tissue Res.* 302, 235–241. doi: 10.1007/s004410000280

Snijders, T., Wall, B. T., Dirks, M. L., Senden, J. M. G., Hartgens, F., Dolmans, J., et al. (2014). Muscle disuse atrophy is not accompanied by changes in skeletal muscle satellite cell content. *Clin. Sci. (Lond).* 126, 557–566. doi: 10.1042/CS20130295

Stein, T. P., and Blanc, S. (2011). Does protein supplementation prevent muscle disuse atrophy and loss of strength? *Crit. Rev. Food Sci. Nutr.* 51, 828–834. doi: 10.1080/10408398.2010.482679

Stevens-Lapsley, J. E., Ye, F., Liu, M., Borst, S. E., Conover, C., Yarasheski, K. E., et al. (2010). Impact of viral-mediated IGF-I gene transfer on skeletal muscle following cast immobilization. *Am. J. Physiol. Endocrinol. Metab.* 299, E730–E740. doi: 10.1152/ajpendo.00230.2010

Stitt, T. N., Drujan, D., Clarke, B. A., Panaro, F., Timofeyva, Y., Kline, W. O., et al. (2004). The IGF-1/PI3K/Akt pathway prevents expression of muscle atrophy-induced ubiquitin ligases by inhibiting FOXO transcription factors. *Mol. Cell* 14, 395–403. doi: 10.1016/S1097-2765(04)00211-4

Storey, K. B., and Storey, J. M. (2007). Tribute to P. L. Lutz: putting life on "pause"–molecular regulation of hypometabolism. *J. Exp. Biol.* 210, 1700–1714. doi: 10.1242/jeb.02716

Suetta, C., Frandsen, U., Jensen, L., Jensen, M. M., Jespersen, J. G., Hvid, L. G., et al. (2012). Aging affects the transcriptional regulation of human skeletal muscle disuse atrophy. *PLoS ONE* 7:e51238. doi: 10.1371/journal.pone.0051238

Suetta, C., Frandsen, U., Mackey, A. L., Jensen, L., Hvid, L. G., Bayer, M. L., et al. (2013). Ageing is associated with diminished muscle re-growth and myogenic precursor cell expansion early after immobility-induced atrophy in human skeletal muscle. *J. Physiol.* 591, 3789–3804. doi: 10.1113/jphysiol.2013.257121

Sugiura, T., Abe, N., Nagano, M., Goto, K., Sakuma, K., Naito, H., et al. (2005). Changes in PKB/Akt and calcineurin signaling during recovery in atrophied soleus muscle induced by unloading. *Am. J. Physiol. Regul. Integr. Comp. Physiol.* 288, R1273–R1278. doi: 10.1152/ajpregu.00688.2004

Sun, Y., Ge, Y., Drnevich, J., Zhao, Y., Band, M., and Chen, J. (2010). Mammalian target of rapamycin regulates miRNA-1 and follistatin in skeletal myogenesis. *J. Cell Biol.* 189, 1157–1169. doi: 10.1083/jcb.200912093

Templeton, G. H., Padalino, M., Manton, J., Glasberg, M., Silver, C. J., Silver, P., et al. (1984). Influence of suspension hypokinesia on rat soleus muscle. *J. Appl. Physiol.* 56, 278–286.

Thompson, C. B. (1995). Apoptosis in the pathogenesis and treatment of disease. *Science* 267, 1456–1462. doi: 10.1126/science.7878464

Trendelenburg, A. U., Meyer, A., Rohner, D., Boyle, J., Hatakeyama, S., and Glass, D. J. (2009). Myostatin reduces Akt/TORC1/p70S6K signaling, inhibiting myoblast differentiation and myotube size. *Am. J. Physiol. Cell Physiol.* 296, C1258–C1270. doi: 10.1152/ajpcell.00105.2009

Tseng, B. S., Kasper, C. E., and Edgerton, V. R. (1994). Cytoplasm-to-myonucleus ratios and succinate dehydrogenase activities in adult rat slow and fast muscle fibers. *Cell Tissue Res.* 275, 39–49. doi: 10.1007/BF00305374

Tsika, R. W., Herrick, R. E., and Baldwin, K. M. (1987). Interaction of compensatory overload and hindlimb suspension on myosin isoform expression. *J. Appl. Physiol.* 62, 2180–2186.

VanderMeer, S. F. T., Jaspers, R. T., Jones, D. A., and Degens, H. (2011). The time course of myonuclear accretion during hypertrophy in young adult and older rat plantaris muscle. *Ann. Anat.* 193, 56–63. doi: 10.1016/j.aanat.2010.08.004

Verdijk, L. B., Dirks, M. L., Snijders, T., Prompers, J. J., Beelen, M., Jonkers, R. A. M., et al. (2012). Reduced satellite cell numbers with spinal cord injury and aging in humans. *Med. Sci. Sports Exerc.* 44, 2322–2330. doi: 10.1249/MSS.0b013e3182667c2e

Verdijk, L. B., Snijders, T., Drost, M., Delhaas, T., Kadi, F., and van Loon, L. J. C. (2013). Satellite cells in human skeletal muscle; from birth to old age. *Age (Dordr).* doi: 10.1007/s11357-013-9583-2. [Epub ahead of print].

Vescovo, G., Zennaro, R., Sandri, M., Carraro, U., Leprotti, C., Ceconi, C., et al. (1998). Apoptosis of skeletal muscle myofibers and interstitial cells in experimental heart failure. *J. Mol. Cell. Cardiol.* 30, 2449–2459. doi: 10.1006/jmcc.1998.0807

Wada, K.-I., Takahashi, H., Katsuta, S., and Soya, H. (2002). No decrease in myonuclear number after long-term denervation in mature mice. *Am. J. Physiol. Cell Physiol.* 283, C484–C488. doi: 10.1152/ajpcell.00025.2002

Wall, B. T., Snijders, T., Senden, J. M. G., Ottenbros, C. L. P., Gijsen, A. P., Verdijk, L. B., et al. (2013). Disuse impairs the muscle protein synthetic response to protein ingestion in healthy men. *J. Clin. Endocrinol. Metab.* 98, 4872–4881. doi: 10.1210/jc.2013-2098

Wang, Q., and McPherron, A. C. (2012). Myostatin inhibition induces muscle fibre hypertrophy prior to satellite cell activation. *J. Physiol.* 590, 2151–2165. doi: 10.1113/jphysiol.2011.226001

Wang, X. D., Kawano, F., Matsuoka, Y., Fukunaga, K., Terada, M., Sudoh, M., et al. (2006). Mechanical load-dependent regulation of satellite cell and fiber size in rat soleus muscle. *Am. J. Physiol. Cell Physiol.* 290, C981–C989. doi: 10.1152/ajpcell.00298.2005

Whittemore, L.-A., Song, K., Li, X., Aghajanian, J., Davies, M., Girgenrath, S., et al. (2003). Inhibition of myostatin in adult mice increases skeletal muscle mass and strength. *Biochem. Biophys. Res. Commun.* 300, 965–971. doi: 10.1016/S0006-291X(02)02953-4

Winick, M., and Noble, A. (1966). Cellular response in rats during malnutrition at various ages. *J. Nutr.* 89, 300–306.

Yablonka-Reuveni, Z., and Rivera, A. J. (1994). Temporal expression of regulatory and structural muscle proteins during myogenesis of satellite cells on isolated adult rat fibers. *Dev. Biol.* 164, 588–603. doi: 10.1006/dbio.1994.1226

Yasuda, N., Glover, E. I., Phillips, S. M., Isfort, R. J., and Tarnopolsky, M. A. (2005). Sex-based differences in skeletal muscle function and morphology with short-term limb immobilization. *J. Appl. Physiol.* 99, 1085–1092. doi: 10.1152/japplphysiol.00247.2005

Yin, H., Price, F., and Rudnicki, M. A. (2013). Satellite cells and the muscle stem cell niche. *Physiol. Rev.* 93, 23–67. doi: 10.1152/physrev.00043.2011

Zachwieja, J. J., Smith, S. R., Sinha-Hikim, I., Gonzalez-Cadavid, N., and Bhasin, S. (1999). Plasma myostatin-immunoreactive protein is increased after prolonged bed rest with low-dose T3 administration. *J. Gravit. Physiol.* 6, 11–15.

Zammit, P. S. (2008). All muscle satellite cells are equal, but are some more equal than others? *J. Cell Sci.* 121, 2975–2982. doi: 10.1242/jcs.019661

Zammit, P. S., Heslop, L., Hudon, V., Rosenblatt, J. D., Tajbakhsh, S., Buckingham, M. E., et al. (2002). Kinetics of myoblast proliferation show that resident satellite cells are competent to fully regenerate skeletal muscle fibers. *Exp. Cell Res.* 281, 39–49. doi: 10.1006/excr.2002.5653

Zhang, B.-T., Yeung, S. S., Liu, Y., Wang, H.-H., Wan, Y.-M., Ling, S.-K., et al. (2010). The effects of low frequency electrical stimulation on satellite cell activity in rat skeletal muscle during hindlimb suspension. *BMC Cell Biol.* 11:87. doi: 10.1186/1471-2121-11-87

Zhong, H., Roy, R. R., Siengthai, B., and Edgerton, V. R. (2005). Effects of inactivity on fiber size and myonuclear number in rat soleus muscle. *J. Appl. Physiol.* 99, 1494–1499. doi: 10.1152/japplphysiol.00394.2005

Zimmers, T. A., Davies, M. V., Koniaris, L. G., Haynes, P., Esquela, A. F., Tomkinson, K. N., et al. (2002). Induction of cachexia in mice by systemically administered myostatin. *Science* 296, 1486–1488. doi: 10.1126/science.1069525

11

Diabetic myopathy: Impact of diabetes mellitus on skeletal muscle progenitor cells

Donna M. D'Souza, Dhuha Al-Sajee and Thomas J. Hawke*

Department of Pathology and Molecular Medicine, McMaster University, Hamilton, ON, Canada

***Correspondence:**
Thomas J. Hawke, Department of Pathology and Molecular Medicine, McMaster University, 1280 Main Street West, Hamilton, ON L8S 4L8, Canada
e-mail: hawke@mcmaster.ca

Diabetes mellitus is defined as a group of metabolic diseases that are associated with the presence of a hyperglycemic state due to impairments in insulin release and/or function. While the development of each form of diabetes (Type 1 or Type 2) drastically differs, resultant pathologies often overlap. In each diabetic condition, a failure to maintain healthy muscle is often observed, and is termed diabetic myopathy. This significant, but often overlooked, complication is believed to contribute to the progression of additional diabetic complications due to the vital importance of skeletal muscle for our physical and metabolic well-being. While studies have investigated the link between changes to skeletal muscle metabolic health following diabetes mellitus onset (particularly Type 2 diabetes mellitus), few have examined the negative impact of diabetes mellitus on the growth and reparative capacities of skeletal muscle that often coincides with disease development. Importantly, evidence is accumulating that the muscle progenitor cell population (particularly the muscle satellite cell population) is also negatively affected by the diabetic environment, and as such, likely contributes to the declining skeletal muscle health observed in diabetes mellitus. In this review, we summarize the current knowledge surrounding the influence of diabetes mellitus on skeletal muscle growth and repair, with a particular emphasis on the impact of diabetes mellitus on skeletal muscle progenitor cell populations.

Keywords: diabetes mellitus, muscle satellite cells, PICs, skeletal muscle, muscle regeneration, Type 1 diabetes mellitus, Type 2 diabetes mellitus

SKELETAL MUSCLE AND MUSCLE PROGENITOR CELLS

Skeletal muscle is capable of adapting to numerous stimuli, with these responses manifested through changes in muscle size, fiber-type distribution, and/or metabolism. A critical component in skeletal muscle maintenance and plasticity is the presence of muscle progenitor cells. A complex network of intrinsic and extrinsic factors mediate changes to these progenitor cells, with such factors influenced by, and influential to, skeletal muscle health. Diseases that negatively impact muscle health, such as diabetes mellitus, may do so by negatively affecting progenitor cell quantity and/or functionality. As such, these cells (or a sub-population therein) function as a primary therapeutic target to attenuate deficits in muscle health with disease progression. While the most well defined of these progenitor cells is the satellite cell (SC; Hawke and Garry, 2001; Zammit and Relaix, 2012), evidence of a number of non-satellite cell progenitor populations contributing to the maintenance of skeletal muscle in health and disease has emerged in recent years (Pannérec et al., 2012). Throughout this brief review we will use the terms "satellite cells" or "SCs" to define this heterogeneous progenitor cell population, acknowledging that as our understanding of these other unique cell populations becomes clearer, we may revisit roles once allocated specifically to the muscle satellite cells.

PATHOPHYSIOLOGY OF TYPE 1 AND 2 DIABETES MELLITUS

The onset of Type 1 diabetes mellitus (T1DM) often occurs in childhood or adolescence and is characterized by the immune-mediated destruction of pancreatic β-cells leading to insulin deficiency. While T1DM accounts for only ~10% of diabetic cases, its prevalence over the past 30 years has increased worldwide (Onkamo et al., 1999; Gale, 2002). Adolescent muscles subjected to atrophic stimuli are more likely to endure irreversible changes (Darr and Schultz, 1989; Mozdziak et al., 2000), thus the presentation of T1DM during this critical growth period can detrimentally impact long-term muscle health. In contrast, Type 2 Diabetes Mellitus (T2DM) accounts for ~90% of diabetes mellitus cases (Masso-Gonzalez et al., 2009), and is expected to affect almost 8% of the worldwide population by 2030 (Shaw et al., 2010). Adverse health behaviors, particularly sedentary lifestyles and increased adiposity, have lead to a high incidence of insulin resistance and impaired fasting glucose (American Diabetes Association, 2006). Without therapeutic intervention, the insulin-resistant state often precipitates to pancreatic β-cell death and progression to insulin-dependent T2DM.

While the etiology of T1DM and T2DM are distinct, the end result is number of common co-morbidities including nephropathy, neuropathy, and cardiovascular disease. Diabetic myopathy, characterized by reduced physical capacity, strength, and muscle mass (Andersen et al., 1996, 1997, 2004, 2005), is a relatively understudied complication of diabetes mellitus, but is believed to directly influence the rate of co-morbidity development. This is based on the fact that skeletal muscle functions as the largest site for glucose uptake (DeFronzo et al., 1981), and therefore changes to skeletal muscle health can impact whole-body glucose homeostasis. A vital component to the maintenance of skeletal muscle is its SC population. As such, changes to SC functionality with diabetes mellitus would impact skeletal muscle health. Here we review the current state of knowledge on the relationship between skeletal muscle health and diabetes mellitus, with a particular focus on the fate and function of skeletal muscle progenitor cell populations.

SKELETAL MUSCLE IN DIABETES MELLITUS

T1DM

Muscle growth and development is significantly impaired in T1DM, resulting in reduced muscle mass and myofiber size, poor metabolic control, and a switch to a glycolytic phenotype (Andersen et al., 1997, 2004; Crowther et al., 2003; Fritzsche et al., 2008; Krause et al., 2009, 2013). While initial studies in human T1DM reported no difference in capillary density (Leinonen et al., 1982), investigations in T1DM mice illustrate that the disease is associated with a decline in skeletal muscle capillarization and angiogenesis (Kivelä et al., 2006; Krause et al., 2009). These alterations to muscle structure and metabolism often are associated with reductions in muscle function, as previously demonstrated (Huttunen et al., 1984; Poortmans et al., 1986; Almeida et al., 2008; Gordon et al., 2010). In addition to growth and function, the capacity for repair from damage is also adversely affected by T1DM, as indicated by studies of muscle regeneration using chemical and genetic models of T1DM (Gulati and Swamy, 1991; Talesara and Vashishta, 2000; Vignaud et al., 2007; Krause et al., 2011, 2013). Collectively, these studies highlight the negative impact T1DM is having on skeletal muscle and its potential for growth, maintenance, and repair.

SATELLITE CELLS AND T1DM

Satellite cells from streptozotocin (STZ)-treated diabetic mice fail to activate properly, resulting in failed regeneration following chemically induced muscle injury (Jeong et al., 2013). This extreme catabolic state has previously been shown to promote the fusion of SCs to adjacent muscle fibers in T1DM mice, as this is thought to promote the release of factors that function to sustain muscle integrity in this less than favorable metabolic condition (Brannon et al., 1989). Furthermore, Aragno et al. (2004) reported reduced myogenic regulatory factor expression and impaired differentiation in T1DM-derived myoblasts. Attenuated muscle repair has also been observed in T1DM mice (Krause et al., 2011, 2013). The impaired regeneration with diabetes was attributed to an elevation in plasma PAI-1 resulting from attenuated extracellular matrix (ECM) turnover. The delay in ECM turnover inhibited macrophage and SC migration into the damaged/necrotic regions of injured muscle. Interestingly, despite systemic increases in PAI-1, the impaired regeneration occurred in a muscle-specific pattern (Krause et al., 2013), indicating that muscles are intrinsically resistant to the T1DM environment. It is becoming increasingly clear that alterations to muscle protein turnover cannot, by itself, account for diabetic myopathy. Although studies investigating SCs in T1DM remains limited, evidence indicates that functionality is affected. Clinically, it is important to appreciate that T1DM-onset almost always occurs during childhood/adolescence, a period of extensive muscle growth. Thus, understanding alterations to the SC population in T1DM is essential for the development of therapeutic strategies to maximize muscle health during this vulnerable time.

T2DM

Similar to observations in T1DM, skeletal muscle of T2DM subjects exhibit increased glycolytic fiber number (Mårin et al., 1994; Nyholm et al., 1997), muscle atrophy (Huang et al., 2010), and decreases in capillary density (Prior et al., 2009). Perturbations to muscle metabolism in T2DM are common, resulting in decreased intermyofibrillar mitochondrial content and abnormal lipid deposition (Nielsen et al., 2010; Chomentowski et al., 2011). As a consequence of these unfavorable changes, the muscle becomes "metabolically inflexible" as it cannot easily switch between fat and carbohydrate oxidation in response to insulin (Kelley and Mandarino, 2000). Functional impairments are also evident, as demonstrated by a decline in muscle strength (Andersen et al., 2004; Park et al., 2006), a finding strongly correlated with intramuscular fat storage (Hilton et al., 2008). Studies of muscle regeneration in insulin-resistance/T2DM animal models (Nguyen et al., 2011) further identify attenuated skeletal muscle plasticity, with deleterious changes to SC function theorized as a central mechanism underlying the observed outcomes.

As discussed, diabetes mellitus impinges on skeletal muscle health. Studies have noted that the diabetic environment enhances protein degradation (Price et al., 1996; Lecker et al., 1999; Mitch et al., 1999; Mastrocola et al., 2008). While these studies are well conducted, it was not within their scope to investigate all components required for skeletal muscle growth and maintenance. Indeed, SCs are indispensable for such events (Zammit and Relaix, 2012), and thus a more complete understanding of the impact of the diabetic environment on SC function is needed.

SATELLITE CELLS AND T2DM

While studies directly assessing SC function with T2DM remain limited, a number of recent investigations have evaluated SC behavior with hyperglycemia and/or lipotoxicity. For instance, 3 weeks of a high fat feeding (HFF) affected SC content and functionality, with the latter classified as the quantity of regenerating fibers present following injury (Fitzpatrick et al., 2011). Hu et al. (2010) demonstrated reduced muscle regeneration after 8-months HFF that was attributed to a delay in myofiber maturation, rather than SC activation or proliferation. *In vitro* studies have also shown that SCs incubated in high glucose medium have an increased propensity to differentiate into adipocytes (Aguiari et al., 2008), suggesting that SC myogenic capacity may be impacted by uncontrolled diabetes. This is further substantiated through the use of genetic models of obesity and diabetes. The Obese Zucker Rat (OZR), a model for the metabolic syndrome, displays reduced SC proliferative capacity though quiescent SC percentages remain unchanged (Peterson et al., 2008); findings consistent with observed alterations to Akt signaling and myogenic regulatory factor expression (Peterson et al., 2008). Similar results were obtained in transgenic (*ob/ob*, *db/db*) models of T2DM. Specifically, impaired SC proliferation and activation were observed and were reflected in measurable impairments of muscle regeneration (Nguyen et al., 2011). A critical, but as of yet unanswered, question is the role of altered leptin signaling in mediating changes to SCs in these animal models. Interestingly, these authors found no difference in SC function or regenerative capacity in HFF mice (Nguyen et al., 2011).

In addition to altered myogenic potential, SCs derived from T2DM patients were found to retain a "diabetic phenotype" upon isolation and culturing. These T2DM-derived SCs displayed reduced lipid oxidation (Gaster et al., 2004), increased secretion of inflammatory markers leading to altered cell signaling (Green et al., 2011), impaired glucose transport (Gaster et al., 2002), and insulin-resistance (Scarda et al., 2010). These modifications were based on T2DM-induced epigenetic changes to muscle cell gene programming, modifying protein expression of factors essential to myogenesis, thereby permanently affecting muscle SCs (Broholm et al., 2012). Taken together, these findings suggest that the degree of T2DM disease severity (i.e., diet vs. genetic model) will differentially influence SC function. A more severe T2DM phenotype, as is found in genetic models of T2DM, results in impairments to the early stages of myogenesis (proliferation, activation), while the HFF models will alter the differentiation potential of the SCs. Finally, long-term exposure to T2DM may promote detrimental epigenetic changes to SCs that will inevitably affect their functionality, and ultimately, overall skeletal muscle health.

MECHANISMS FOR ALTERED SATELLITE CELL FUNCTION IN DIABETES MELLITUS

The literature is clear that the uncontrolled diabetic environment is unfavorable for skeletal muscle growth and regeneration (Vignaud et al., 2007; Peterson et al., 2008; Krause et al., 2011; Nguyen et al., 2011). However, the molecular processes governing changes to the SCs are far from elucidated.

Following a period of uncontrolled diabetes mellitus in humans (i.e., pre-diagnosis), insulin administration is the therapeutic standard, and is well studied in terms of regulating muscle protein turnover (Pain et al., 1983; Price et al., 1996; Charlton and Nair, 1998; Lee et al., 2004). What remains less known is the effect of insulin therapy on SCs. Insulin has been found to stimulate both proliferation and differentiation of SCs, with such evidence derived from a handful of *in vitro* studies (Ewton and Florini, 1981; Vandenburgh et al., 1991; Cassar-Malek et al., 1999). The paucity of data available from human diabetic muscle exposed to insulin treatment merits further consideration. In the absence of insulin, or poorly managed diabetic states, there may be a myriad of factors and processes stemming from the diabetic environment that have the potential to influence SC activity. After a review of many of these mechanisms, a select few are evident in both T1DM and T2DM. The precise modifications to skeletal muscle following diabetes onset is depicted along with the predicted mechanisms of action (**Figure 1**). These include, but are not limited to: oxidative stress, chronic low-grade inflammation, and impaired ECM remodeling. Though the impact of metabolic diseases on the changing metabolic needs of the muscle satellite cells as they move from quiescence through to differentiation is certainly of note, it is beyond the scope of this mini-review. We refer the readers to some excellent recent reviews (Fulco et al., 2008; Ryall, 2013) on this topic.

OXIDATIVE STRESS

Oxidative stress is evident in both T1DM (Aragno et al., 2004) and T2DM (Henriksen et al., 2010), and has been directly associated with elevated glucose concentrations (Bonnefont-Rousselot, 2002). Dysregulation of nitric oxide (NO) production also occurs, as hyperglycemia promotes the formation of reactive nitrogen species (RNS) to further exacerbate levels of oxidative stress (Zou et al., 2002). A shift in pro-oxidant/antioxidant balance is regarded in the pathogenesis of diabetes and its complications (Evans et al., 2002). Although an emphasis of research relating oxidative stress to skeletal muscle health has been on its modulation of protein turnover (Li et al., 1998; Zhou et al., 2001; Aragno et al., 2004), it is speculated that the concomitant increase in ROS and decrease in NO hinders satellite cell function. *In vitro* work has found that acute treatment of human muscle SCs with the ROS-inducing agent hydrogen peroxide (H_2O_2) led to reduced cell viability, shortened lifespan, and decreased proliferative capacity (Renault et al., 2002). In support of oxidative stress impairing myogenesis, Aragno et al. (2004) found that in response to muscle damage, the expression of critical myogenic factors (MyoD, myogenin, and Jun D) was reduced in STZ-diabetic rodents compared to non-diabetic rodents. Muscle creatine kinase and myosin expression were also impaired, suggesting that defects in the early phases of regeneration (i.e., satellite cell functionality) led to a cascade of events to further hinder muscle repair. It is interesting to note that oxidative stress has been implicated in the adipogenic conversion of muscle SCs (Vettor et al., 2009). Now whether this occurs within diabetic muscle has yet to be defined, however, given that the demonstrated impairments in myogenesis with diabetes appear to be linked to oxidative stress, it is clear that this area requires further investigation.

CHRONIC LOW-GRADE INFLAMMATORY PROFILE (CLIP)

With diabetes progression, a multitude of pro-inflammatory factors are elevated, constituting a state of chronic low-grade inflammation, or a chronic low-grade inflammatory profile (CLIP). The presence of this condition is evident in all forms of diabetes mellitus (Llauradó et al., 2012; Osborn and Olefsky, 2012) and is believed to occur as a result of the enhanced formation of advanced glycation end-products (AGEs; Tan et al., 2004; Ramasamy et al., 2005; Yan et al., 2008). The factors associated with CLIP can collectively and/or independently influence SC activity. While examination of each of these factors on SC function is beyond the breadth of this review, it is important to highlight a select few.

Chronic elevations of circulating Interleukin-6 (IL-6) are observed in T1DM and T2DM (Pradhan et al., 2001; Reis et al., 2012). While transient increases in IL-6 are associated with SC proliferation (Toth et al., 2011), chronically elevated IL-6 is correlated with significant decrements in muscle health (e.g., cancer cachexia; Roubenoff, 1997; McKay et al., 2013). Given the chronic elevations in IL-6 with diabetes, it is reasonable to surmise that impairments to SC functionality are occurring. Consistent with

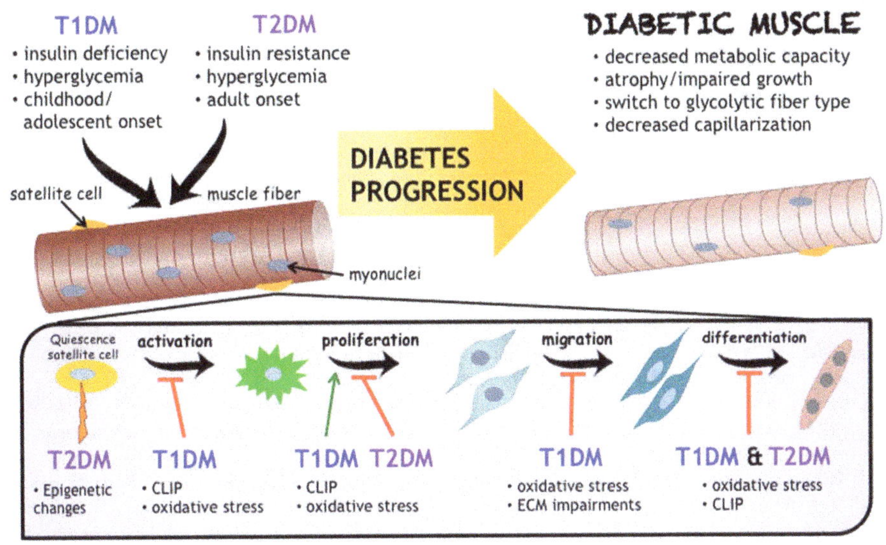

FIGURE 1 | Impact of Diabetes Mellitus on Skeletal Muscle Health. While the etiology and progression for T1DM and T2DM development are distinct, both diseases negatively influence skeletal muscle (referred to as "Diabetic Muscle") and their resident progenitor cell populations, including satellite cells. Satellite cells are critical to muscle health, and are affected by diabetes mellitus at varying stages of adult myogenesis. As outlined in this review, and schematized here, chronic low grade inflammation (also known as CLIP, or chronic low-grade inflammatory profile), oxidative stress, and impaired extracellular matrix remodeling are proposed to be common denominators for mechanisms underlying impairments to muscle health and decreased satellite cell functionality in diabetes mellitus.

this hypothesis, obese diabetic individuals displayed significant impairments in IL-6 signaling within their skeletal muscle that persisted within the satellite cells even upon removal from the diabetic environment (Nielsen et al., 2012).

Akin to IL-6, tumor necrosis factor-α (TNF-α) functions as a key mediator of the inflammatory process. Not only is TNF-α correlated with diabetes progression (Csizuadia et al., 2012; Swaroop et al., 2012), it has also been found to alter insulin-mediated glucose uptake in muscle cells *in vitro* (Yoon et al., 2011), and has been implicated in the development of insulin resistance through studies knocking out its respective receptors (Uysal et al., 1997; Romanatto et al., 2009). With respect to SCs, TNF-α is thought to exert its effects through stimulation of factors that promote entry into the cell cycle (Li et al., 2003). In support of this, TNF-α treated myoblasts displayed an increased proliferative capacity while differentiation was hindered (Alter et al., 2008).

The presence of CLIP, as found in diabetes, will undoubtedly alter skeletal muscle homeostasis. This emerging and exciting new area of interest, though still in its infancy, presents an intriguing avenue for further therapeutic investigations.

IMPAIRED EXTRACELLULAR MATRIX (ECM) REMODELING

Studies have found that central constituents of the plasminogen system are required for normal growth and repair within a variety of tissues types, including skeletal muscle (Romer et al., 1996; Lluís et al., 2001; Shimizu et al., 2001). Within muscle, inhibition of PAI-1 (a critical inhibitor of the plasminogen system) was found to increase MyoD expression and accelerate muscle repair (Koh et al., 2005). Of particular note, elevated ECM levels have been demonstrated in a variety of diabetic tissues (Berria et al., 2006; Krause et al., 2011). Excessive ECM levels are likely the result of altered protein expression (Lecker et al., 2004), especially in regards to matrix metalloproteinases (Hopps and Caimi, 2012). The improper turnover of ECM proteins may also hinder growth factor signaling, further impeding myogenesis (Gopinath and Rando, 2008). While the aforementioned studies identify that aspects of muscle health are clearly subject to modification with diabetes mellitus, one must also account for diabetic-induced changes to the environment in which the muscle SCs reside. The adverse remodeling of the ECM in diabetic muscle, as evidenced by increased collagen presence, will inevitably affect SC functionality and its capacity to migrate within regenerating muscle (Krause et al., 2013). These defects are also prevalent in senescent skeletal muscle (Franceschi, 2007; Kurtz and Oh, 2012; Vasilaki and Jackson, 2013). Thus, potential therapies to attenuate negative alterations to SC behavior with diabetes onset may also function to mitigate sarcopenia.

SIGNIFICANCE AND CONCLUSIONS

Diabetes mellitus is a global health concern. While diabetes mellitus begins as a result of an impairment in insulin signaling (deficiency/resistance), numerous other factors quickly become altered making the pathogenesis of diabetic complications multi-faceted. Here we provide an overview of the importance of the muscle SC, the impact of T1DM and T2DM on this cell population, and potential "common" mechanisms for altered SC function. Based on the limited number of studies to date, it is evident that various stages of the myogenic process are affected by diabetes mellitus and impairments to SC function are occurring. Given the vital role of these cells in the lifelong maintenance of skeletal muscle, and the importance of a physically and metabolically healthy skeletal muscle mass in attenuating the morbidity and mortality associated with diabetes mellitus, a comprehensive understanding of SC in the diabetic environment is of fundamental significance. Identifying the proponents that attenuate normal SC function in diabetes mellitus will lead to the development of therapies that restore SC activity in order to sustain muscle health, and subsequently attenuate other diabetic complications.

REFERENCES

Aguiari, P., Leo, S., Zavan, B., Vindigni, V., Rimessi, A., Bianchi, K., et al. (2008). High glucose induces adipogenic differentiation of muscle-derived stem cells. *Proc. Natl. Acad. Sci. U.S.A.* 105, 1226–1231. doi: 10.1073/pnas.0711402105

Almeida, S., Riddell, M. C., and Cafarelli, E. (2008). Slower conduction velocity and motor unit discharge frequency are associated with muscle fatigue during isometric exercise in Type 1 diabetes mellitus. *Muscle Nerve* 37, 231–240. doi: 10.1002/mus.20919

Alter, J., Rozentzweig, D., and Bengal, E. (2008). Inhibition of myoblast differentiation by tumor necrosis factor alpha is mediated by c-Jun N-terminal kinase 1 and leukemia inhibitory factor. *J. Biol. Chem.* 283, 23224–23234. doi: 10.1074/jbc.M801379200

American Diabetes Association. (2006). Diagnosis and classification of diabetes mellitus. *Diabetes Care* 29, 43–48. doi: 10.2337/dc09-S062

Andersen, H., Gadeberg, P. C., Brock, B., and Jakobsen, J. (1997). Muscular atrophy in diabetic neuropathy: a stereological magnetic resonance imaging study. *Diabetologia* 40, 1062–1069. doi: 10.1007/s001250050788

Andersen, H., Gjerstad, M. D., and Jakobsen, J. (2004). Atrophy of foot muscles: a measure of diabetic neuropathy. *Diabetes Care* 27, 2382–2385. doi: 10.2337/diacare.27.10.2382

Andersen, H., Poulsen, P. L., Mogensen, C. E., and Jakobsen, J. (1996). Isokinetic muscle strength in long-term IDDM patients in relation to diabetic complications. *Diabetes* 45, 440–445. doi: 10.2337/diab.45.4.440

Andersen, H., Schmitz, O., and Nielsen, S. (2005). Decreased isometric muscle strength after acute hyperglycaemia in Type 1 diabetic patients. *Diabet. Med.* 22, 1401–1407. doi: 10.1111/j.1464-5491.2005.01649.x

Aragno, M., Mastrocola, R., Catalano, M. G., Brignardello, E., Danni, O., and Boccuzzi, G. (2004). Oxidative stress impairs skeletal muscle repair in diabetic rats. *Diabetes* 53, 1082–1088. doi: 10.2337/diabetes.53.4.1082

Berria, R., Wang, L., Richardson, D. K., Finlayson, J., Belfort, R., Pratipanawatr, T., et al. (2006). Increased collagen content in insulin-resistant skeletal muscle. *Am. J. Physiol. Endocrinol. Metab.* 290, E560–E565. doi: 10.1152/ajpendo.00202.2005

Bonnefont-Rousselot, D. (2002). Glucose and reactive oxygen species. *Curr. Opin. Clin. Nutr. Metab. Care* 5, 561–568. doi: 10.1097/00075197-200209000-00016

Brannon, M. A., Dodson, M. V., Wheeler, B. A., Mathison, B. D., and Mathison, B. A. (1989). Satellite cells derived from streptozotocin-diabetic rats display altered fusion parameters *in vitro*. *Metab. Clin. Exp.* 38, 348–352. doi: 10.1016/0026-0495(89)90123-6

Broholm, C., Brandt, C., Schultz, N. S., Nielsen, A. R., Pedersen, B. K., and Scheele, C. (2012). Deficient leukemia inhibitory factor signaling in muscle precursor cells from patients with Type 2 diabetes. *Am. J. Physiol. Endocrinol. Metab.* 303, E283–E292. doi: 10.1152/ajpendo.00586.2011

Cassar-Malek, I., Langlois, N., Picard, B., and Geay, Y. (1999). Regulation of bovine satellite cell proliferation and differentiation by insulin and triiodothyronine. *Domest. Anim. Endocrinol.* 17, 373–388. doi: 10.1016/S0739-7240(99)00055-7

Charlton, M., and Nair, K. S. (1998). Protein metabolism in insulin-dependent diabetes mellitus. *J. Nutr.* 128, 323S–327S.

Chomentowski, P., Coen, P. M., Radiková, Z., Goodpaster, B. H., and Toledo, F. G. (2011). Skeletal muscle mitochondria in insulin resistance: differences in intermyofibrillar versus subsarcolemmal subpopulations and relationship to metabolic flexibility. *J. Clin. Endocrinol. Metab.* 96, 494–503. doi: 10.1210/jc.2010-0822

Crowther, G. J., Milstein, J. M., Jubrias, S. A., Kushmerick, M. J., Gronka, R. K., and Conley, K. E. (2003). Altered energetic properties in skeletal muscle of men with well-controlled insulin-dependent (type 1) diabetes. *Am. J. Physiol. Endocrinol. Metab.* 284, E655–E662. doi: 10.1152/ajpendo.00343.2002

Csizuadia, E., Qipo, A., Libermann, T. A., Strom, T. B., Bhasin, M., Awdeh, Z., et al. (2012). The role of TNF-α in mice with Type 1- and 2- diabetes. *PLoS ONE* 7:e33254. doi: 10.1371/journal.pone.0033254

Darr, K. C., and Schultz, E. (1989). Hindlimb suspension suppresses muscle growth and satellite cell proliferation. *J. Appl. Physiol.* 67, 1827–1834.

DeFronzo, R. A., Jacot, E., Jequier, E., Maeder, E., Wahren, J., and Felber, J. P. (1981). The effect of insulin on the disposal of intravenous glucose. results from indirect calorimetry and hepatic and femoral venous catheterization. *Diabetes* 30, 1000–1007. doi: 10.2337/diab.30.12.1000

Evans, J. L., Goldfine, I. D., Maddux, B. A., and Grodsky, G. M. (2002). Oxidative stress and stress-activated signaling pathways: a unifying hypothesis of Type 2 diabetes. *Endocr. Rev.* 23, 599–622. doi: 10.1210/er.2001-0039

Ewton, Z., and Florini, R. (1981). Effects of the somatomedins differentiation and insulin on myoblast *in vitro*. *Dev. Biol.* 39, 31–39. doi: 10.1016/0012-1606(81)90312-2

Fitzpatrick, C., Wagers, A. J., Woo, M., Jimenez-Chillaron, J., Patti, M. E., Cerletti, M., et al. (2011). Early life nutrition modulates muscle stem cell number: implications for muscle mass and repair. *Stem Cells Dev.* 20, 1763–1769. doi: 10.1089/scd.2010.0349

Franceschi, C. (2007). Inflammaging as a major characteristic of old people: can it be prevented or cured? *Nutr. Rev.* 65, S173–S176. doi: 10.1301/nr.2007.dec.S173-S176

Fritzsche, K., Blüher, M., Schering, S., Buchwalow, I. B., Kern, M., Linke, A., et al. (2008). Metabolic profile and nitric oxide synthase expression of skeletal muscle fibers are altered in patients with Type 1 diabetes. *Exp. Clin. Endocrinol. Diabetes* 116, 606–613. doi: 10.1055/s-2008-1073126

Fulco, M., Cen, Y., Zhao, P., Hoffman, E. P., McBurney, M. W., Sauve, A. A., et al. (2008). Glucose restriction inhibits skeletal myoblast differentiation by activating SIRT1 through AMPK-mediated regulation of Nampt. *Dev. Cell* 14, 661–673. doi: 10.1016/j.devcel.2008.02.004

Gale, E. A. M. (2002). A missing link in the hygiene hypothesis? *Diabetologia* 45, 588–594. doi: 10.1007/s00125-002-0801-1

Gaster, M., Petersen, I., Højlund, K., Poulsen, P., and Beck-Nielsen, H. (2002). The diabetic phenotype is conserved in myotubes established from diabetic subjects: evidence for primary defects in glucose transport and glycogen synthase activity. *Diabetes* 51, 921–927. doi: 10.2337/diabetes.51.4.921

Gaster, M., Rustan, A. C., Aas, V., and Beck-Nielsen, H. (2004). Reduced lipid oxidation in skeletal muscle from Type 2 diabetic subjects may be of genetic origin: evidence from cultured myotubes. *Diabetes* 53, 542–548. doi: 10.2337/diabetes.53.3.542

Gopinath, S. D., and Rando, T. A. (2008). Stem cell review series: aging of the skeletal muscle stem cell niche. *Aging Cell* 7, 590–598. doi: 10.1111/j.1474-9726.2008.00399.x

Gordon, C. S., Serino, A. S., Krause, M. P., Campbell, J. E., Cafarelli, E., Adegoke, O. A., et al. (2010). Impaired growth and force production in skeletal muscles of young partially pancreatectomized rats: a model of adolescent Type 1 diabetic myopathy? *PLoS ONE* 5:e14032. doi: 10.1371/journal.pone.0014032

Green, C. J., Scheele, C., Pedersen, B. K., and Pedersen, M. (2011). Elevated NF- B activation is conserved in human myocytes cultured from obese Type 2 diabetic patients and attenuated by AMP-activated protein kinase. *Diabetes* 60, 2810–2819. doi: 10.2337/db11-0263

Gulati, A. K., and Swamy, M. S. (1991). Regeneration of skeletal muscle in streptozotocin-induced diabetic rats. *Anat. Rec.* 229, 298–304. doi: 10.1002/ar.1092290303

Hawke, T. J., and Garry, D. J. (2001). Myogenic satellite cells: physiology to molecular biology. *J. Appl. Physiol.* 91, 534–551. doi: 10.1063/1.3603452

Henriksen, E. J., Diamond-Stanic, M. K., and Marchionne, E. M. (2010). Oxidative stress and the etiology of insulin resistance and Type 2 diabetes. *Free Radic. Biol. Med.* 51, 993–999. doi: 10.1016/j.freeradbiomed.2010.12.005

Hilton, T. N., Tuttle, L. J., Bohnert, K. L., Mueller, M. J., and Sinacore, D. R. (2008). Excessive adipose tissue infiltration in skeletal muscle in individuals with obesity, diabetes mellitus, and peripheral neuropathy: association with performance and function. *Phys. Ther.* 88, 1336–1344. doi: 10.2522/ptj.20080079

Hopps, E., and Caimi, G. (2012). Matrix metalloproteinases in metabolic syndrome. *Eur. J. Intern. Med.* 23, 99–104. doi: 10.1016/j.ejim.2011.09.012

Hu, Z., Wang, H., Lee, I. H., Modi, S., Wang, X., Du, J., et al. (2010). PTEN inhibition improves muscle regeneration in mice fed a high-fat diet. *Diabetes* 59, 1312–1320. doi: 10.2337/db09-1155

Huang, B. K., Monu, J. U., and Doumanian, J. (2010). Diabetic myopathy: MRI patterns and current trends. *Am. J. Roentgenol.* 195, 198–204. doi: 10.2214/AJR.09.2494

Huttunen, N. P., Kaar, M. L., Knip, M., Mustonen, A., Puukka, R., and Akerblom, H. K. (1984). Physical fitness of children and adolescents with insulin-dependent diabetes mellitus. *Ann. Clin. Res.* 16, 1–5.

Jeong, J., Conboy, M. J., and Conboy, I. M. (2013). Pharmacological inhibition of myostatin/TGF-ß receptor/pSmad 3 signaling rescues muscle regenerative responses in mouse model of type 1 diabetes. *Acta. Pharmacol. Sin.* 34, 1052–1060. doi: 10.1038/aps.2013.67

Kelley, D. E., and Mandarino, L. J. (2000). Fuel selection in human skeletal muscle in insulin resistance: a reexamination. *Diabetes* 49, 677–683. doi: 10.2337/diabetes.49.5.677

Kivelä, R., Silvennoinen, M., Touvra, A. M., Lehti, T. M., Kainulainen, H., and Vihko, V. (2006). Effects of experimental Type 1 diabetes and exercise training on angiogenic gene expression and capillarization in skeletal muscle. *FASEB J.* 20, 1570–1572. doi: 10.1096/fj.05-4780fje

Koh, T. J., Bryer, S. C., Pucci, A. M., and Sisson, T. H. (2005). Mice deficient in plasminogen activator inhibitor-1 have improved skeletal muscle regeneration. *Am. J. Physiol. Cell Physiol.* 289, C217–C223. doi: 10.1152/ajpcell.00555.2004

Krause, M. P., Al-Sajee, D., D'Souza, D. M., Rebalka, I. A., Moradi, J., Riddell, M. C., et al. (2013). Impaired macrophage and satellite cell infiltration occurs in a muscle-specific fashion following injury in diabetic skeletal muscle. *PLoS ONE* 8:e70971. doi: 10.1371/journal.pone.0070971

Krause, M. P., Moradi, J., Nissar, A. A., Riddell, M. C., and Hawke, T. J. (2011). Inhibition of plasminogen activator inhibitor-1 restores skeletal muscle regeneration in untreated Type 1 diabetic mice. *Diabetes* 60, 1964–1972. doi: 10.2337/db11-0007

Krause, M. P., Riddell, M. C., Gordon, C. S., Imam, S. A., Cafarelli, E., and Hawke, T. J. (2009). Diabetic myopathy differs between Ins2Akita+/- and streptozotocin-induced Type 1 diabetic models. *J. Appl. Physiol.* 106, 1650–1659. doi: 10.1152/japplphysiol.91565.2008

Kurtz, A., and Oh, S. J. (2012). Age related changes of the extracellular matrix and stem cell maintenance. *Prev. Med.* Suppl:S50–S56. doi: 10.1016/j.ypmed.2012.01.003

Lecker, S. H., Jagoe, R. T., Gilbert, A., Gomes, M., Baracos, V., Bailey, J., et al. (2004). Multiple types of skeletal muscle atrophy involve a common program of changes in gene expression. *FASEB J.* 18, 39–51. doi: 10.1096/fj.03-0610com

Lecker, S. H., Solomon, V., Price, S. R., Kwon, Y. T., Mitch, W. E., and Goldberg, A. L. (1999). Ubiquitin conjugation by the N-end rule pathway and mRNAs for its components increase in muscles of diabetic rats. *J. Clin. Invest.* 104, 1411–1420. doi: 10.1172/JCI7300

Lee, S. W., Dai, G., Hu, Z., Wang, X., Du, J., and Mitch, W. E. (2004). Regulation of muscle protein degradation: coordinated control of apoptotic and ubiquitin-proteasome systems by phosphatidylinositol 3 kinase. *J. Am. Soc. Nephrol.* 15, 1537–1545. doi: 10.1097/01.ASN.0000127211.86206.E1

Leinonen, H., Matikainen, E., and Juntunen, J. (1982). Permeability and morphology of skeletal muscle capillaries in Type 1 (insulin-dependent) diabetes mellitus. *Diabetologia* 22, 158–162. doi: 10.1007/BF00283744

Li, Y. P., Lecker, S. H., Chen, Y., Waddell, I. D., Goldberg, A. L., and Reid, M. B. (2003). TNF-alpha increases ubiquitin-conjugating activity in skeletal muscle by up-regulating UbcH2/E220k. *FASEB J.* 17, 1048–1057. doi: 10.1096/fj.02-0759com

Li, Y. P., Schwartz, R. J., Waddell, I. D., Holloway, B. R., and Reid, M. B. (1998). Skeletal muscle myocytes undergo protein loss and reactive oxygen-mediated NF-kappaB activation in response to tumor necrosis factor alpha. *FASEB J.* 12, 871–880.

Llauradó, G., Gallart, L., Tirado, R., Megia, A., Simón, I., Caixàs, A., et al. (2012). Insulin resistance, low-grade inflammation and Type 1 diabetes mellitus. *Acta Diabetol.* 49, 33–39. doi: 10.1007/s00592-011-0257-1

Lluís, F., Roma, J., Suelves, M., Parra, M., Aniorte, G., Gallardo, E., et al. (2001). Urokinase-dependent plasminogen activation is required for efficient skeletal muscle regeneration *in vivo*. *Blood* 97, 1703–1711. doi: 10.1182/blood.V97.6.1703

Mårin, P., Andersson, B., Krotkiewski, M., and Björntorp, P. (1994). Muscle fiber composition and capillary density in women and men with NIDDM. *Diabetes Care* 17, 382–386. doi: 10.2337/diacare.17.5.382

Masso-Gonzalez, E., Johansson, S., Wallander, M.-A., and Garcia-Rodriguez, L. (2009). Trends in the prevalence and incidence of diabetes in the UK - 1996 to 2005. *J. Epidemiol. Community Health* 63, 332–336. doi: 10.1136/jech.2008.080382

Mastrocola, R., Reffo, P., Penna, F., Tomasinelli, C. E., Boccuzzi, G., Baccino, F. M., et al. (2008). Muscle wasting in diabetic and in tumor-bearing rats: role of oxidative stress. *Free Radic. Biol. Med.* 44, 584–593. doi: 10.1016/j.freeradbiomed.2007.10.047

McKay, B. R., Ogborn, D. I., Baker, J. M., Toth, K. G., Tarnopolsky, M. A., and Parise, G. (2013). Elevated SOCS3 and altered IL-6 signaling is associated with age-related human muscle stem cell dysfunction. *Am. J. Physiol. Cell Physiol.* 304, C717–C728. doi: 10.1152/ajpcell.00305.2012

Mitch, W. E., Bailey, J. L., Wang, X., Jurkovitz, C., Newby, D., and Price, S. R. (1999). Evaluation of signals activating ubiquitin-proteasome proteolysis in a model of muscle wasting. *Am. J. Physiol.* 276, C1132–C1138.

Mozdziak, P. E., Pulvermacher, P. M., and Schultz, E. (2000). Unloading of juvenile muscle results in a reduced muscle size 9 wk after reloading. *J. Appl. Physiol.* 88, 158–164.

Nguyen, M.-H., Cheng, M., and Koh, T. J. (2011). Impaired muscle regeneration in Ob/ob and Db/db mice. *ScientificWorldJournal* 11, 1525–1535. doi: 10.1100/tsw.2011.137

Nielsen, A. R., Kelly, M., Fischer, C. P., Pedersen, M., Broholm, C., Taudorf, S., et al. (2012). Satellite cells derived from obese humans with Type 2 diabetes and differentiated into myocytes *in vitro* exhibit abnormal response to IL-6. *PLoS ONE* 7:0039657. doi: 10.1371/journal.pone.0039657

Nielsen, J., Mogensen, M., Vind, B. F., Sahlin, K., Højlund, K., Schrøder, H. D., et al. (2010). Increased subsarcolemmal lipids in Type 2 diabetes: effect of training on localization of lipids, mitochondria, and glycogen in sedentary human skeletal muscle. *Am. J. Physiol. Endocrinol. Metab.* 298, E706–E713. doi: 10.1152/ajpendo.00692.2009

Nyholm, B., Qu, Z., Kaal, A., Pedersen, S. B., Gravholt, C. H., Andersen, J. L., et al. (1997). Evidence of an increased number of Type IIb muscle fibers in insulin-resistant first-degree relatives of patients with NIDDM. *Diabetes* 46, 1822–1828. doi: 10.2337/diab.46.11.1822

Onkamo, P., Väänänen, S., Karvonen, M., and Tuomilehto, J. (1999). Worldwide increase in incidence of Type I diabetes–the analysis of the data on published incidence trends. *Diabetologia* 42, 1395–1403. doi: 10.1007/s001250051309

Osborn, O., and Olefsky, J. M. (2012). The cellular and signaling networks linking the immune system and metabolism in disease. *Nat. Med.* 18, 363–374. doi: 10.1038/nm.2627

Pain, V. M., Albertse, E. C., and Garlick, P. J. (1983). Protein metabolism in skeletal muscle, diaphragm, and heart of diabetic rats. *Am. J. Physiol.* 245, E604–E610.

Pannérec, A., Marazzi, G., and Sassoon, D. (2012). Stem cells in the hood: the skeletal muscle niche. *Trends Mol. Med.* 18, 599–606. doi: 10.1016/j.molmed.2012.07.004

Park, S. W., Goodpaster, B. H., Strotmeyer, E. S., de Rekeneire, N., Harris, T. B., Schwartz, A. V., et al. (2006). Decreased muscle strength and quality in older adults with Type 2 diabetes: the health, aging, and body composition study. *Diabetes* 55, 1813–1818. doi: 10.2337/db05-1183

Peterson, J. M., Bryner, R. W., and Alway, S. E. (2008). Satellite cell proliferation is reduced in muscles of Obese Zucker Rats but restored with loading. *Am. J. Physiol. Cell Physiol.* 295, C521–C528. doi: 10.1152/ajpcell.00073.2008

Poortmans, J. R., Saerens, P., Edelman, R., Vertongen, F., and Dorchy, H. (1986). Influence of the degree of metabolic control on physical fitness in Type I diabetic adolescents. *Int. J. Sports Med.* 7, 232–235. doi: 10.1055/s-2008-1025765

Pradhan, A. D., Manson, J. E., Rifai, N., Buring, J. E., and Ridker, P. M. (2001). C-reactive protein, interleukin 6, and risk of developing Type 2 diabetes mellitus. *J. Am. Med. Assoc.* 286, 327–334. doi: 10.1001/jama.286.3.327

Price, S. R., Bailey, J. L., Wang, X., Jurkovitz, C., England, B. K., Ding, X., et al. (1996). Muscle wasting in insulinopenic rats results from activation of the ATP-dependent, ubiquitin-proteasome proteolytic pathway by a mechanism including gene transcription. *J. Clin. Invest.* 98, 1703–1708. doi: 10.1172/JCI118968

Prior, S. J., McKenzie, M. J., Joseph, L. J., Ivey, F. M., Macko, R. F., Hafer-Macko, C. E., et al. (2009). Reduced skeletal muscle capillarization and glucose intolerance. *Microcirculation* 16, 203–212. doi: 10.1080/10739680802502423

Ramasamy, R., Vannucci, S. J., Yan, S. S., Herold, K., Yan, S. F., and Schmidt, A. M. (2005). Advanced glycation end products and RAGE: a common thread in aging, diabetes, neurodegeneration, and inflammation. *Glycobiology* 15, 16R–28R. doi: 10.1093/glycob/cwi053

Renault, V., Thornell, L. E., Eriksson, P. O., Butler-Browne, G., and Mouly, V. (2002). Regenerative potential of human skeletal muscle during aging. *Aging Cell* 1, 132–139. doi: 10.1046/j.1474-9728.2002.00017.x

Reis, J. S., Amaral, C. A., Volpe, C. M., Fernandes, J. S., Borges, E. A., Isoni, C. A., et al. (2012). Oxidative stress and interleukin-6 secretion during the progression of type 1 diabetes. *Arg. Bras. Endocrinol. Metabol.* 56, 441–448. doi: 10.1590/S0004-27302012000700006

Romanatto, T., Roman, E. A., Arruda, A. P., Denis, R. G., Solon, C., Milanski, M., et al. (2009). Deletion of tumor necrosis factor-alpha receptor 1 (TNFR1) protects against diet-induced obesity by means of increased thermogenesis. *J. Biol. Chem.* 284, 36213–36222. doi: 10.1074/jbc.M109.030874

Romer, J., Bugge, T. H., Pyke, C., Lund, L. R., Flick, M. J., Degen, J. L., et al. (1996). Impaired wound healing in mice with a disrupted plasminogen gene. *Nat. Med.* 2, 287–292. doi: 10.1038/nm0396-287

Roubenoff, R. (1997). Inflammatory and hormonal mediators of cachexia. *J. Nutr.* 127, 1014S–1016S.

Ryall, J. G. (2013). Metabolic reprogramming as a novel regulator of skeletal muscle development and regeneration. *FEBS J.* 280, 4004–4013. doi: 10.1111/febs.12189

Scarda, A., Franzin, C., Milan, G., Sanna, M., Dal Prà, C., Pagano, C., et al. (2010). Increased adipogenic conversion of muscle satellite cells in Obese Zucker Rats. *Int. J. Obes.* 34, 1319–1327. doi: 10.1038/ijo.2010.47

Shaw, J. E., Sicree, R. A., and Zimmet, P. Z. (2010). Global estimates of the prevalence of diabetes for 2010 and 2030. *Diabetes Res. Clin. Pract.* 87, 4–14. doi: 10.1016/j.diabres.2009.10.007

Shimizu, M., Hara, A., Okuno, M., Matsuno, H., Okada, K., Ueshima, S., et al. (2001). Mechanism of retarded liver regeneration in plasminogen activator-deficient mice: impaired activation of hepatocyte growth factor after fas-mediated massive hepatic apoptosis. *Hepatology* 33, 569–576. doi: 10.1053/jhep.2001.22650

Swaroop, J. J., Rajarajeswari, D., and Naidu, J. N. (2012). Association of TNF-α with insulin resistance in Type 2 diabetes mellitus. *Indian J. Med. Res.* 135, 127–130. doi: 10.4103/0971-5916.93435

Talesara, C. L., and Vashishta, N. (2000). Regenerative ability of gastrocnemius muscle under diabetic condition with special reference to SDH & m-ATPase. *Indian J. Exp. Biol.* 38, 567–574.

Tan, K. C., Chow, W. S., Tam, S., Bucala, R., and Betteridge, J. (2004). Association between acute-phase reactants and advanced glycation end products in Type 2 diabetes. *Diabetes Care* 27, 223–228. doi: 10.2337/diacare.27.1.223

Toth, K. G., McKay, B. R., De Lisio, M., Little, J. P., Tarnopolsky, M. A., and Parise, G. (2011). IL-6 induced STAT3 signalling is associated with the proliferation of human muscle satellite cells following acute muscle damage. *PLoS ONE* 6:0017392. doi: 10.1371/journal.pone.0017392

Uysal, K. T., Wiesbrock, S. M., Marino, M. W., and Hotamisligil, G. S. (1997). Protection from obesity-induced insulin-resistance in mice lacking Tnf- alpha function. *Nature* 389, 610–614. doi: 10.1038/39335

Vandenburgh, H. H., Karlisch, P., Shansky, J., and Feldstein, R. (1991). Insulin and IGF-I induce pronounced hypertrophy of skeletal myofibers in tissue culture. *Am. J. Physiol.* 260, C475–C484.

Vasilaki, A., and Jackson, M. J. (2013). Role of reactive oxygen species in the defective regeneration seen in aging muscle. *Free Radic. Biol. Med.* 65, 317–323. doi: 10.1016/j.freeradbiomed.2013.07.008

Vettor, R., Milan, G., Franzin, C., Sanna, M., De Coppi, P., Rizzuto, R., et al. (2009). The origin of intermuscular adipose tissue and its pathophysiological implications. *Am. J. Physiol. Endocrinol. Metab.* 297, E987–E998. doi: 10.1152/ajpendo.00229.2009

Vignaud, A., Ramond, F., Hourdé, C., Keller, A., Butler-Browne, G., and Ferry, A. (2007). Diabetes provides an unfavorable environment for muscle mass and function after muscle injury in mice. *Pathobiology* 74, 291–300. doi: 10.1159/000105812

Yan, S. F., Ramasamy, R., and Schmidt, A. M. (2008). Mechanisms of disease: advanced glycation end-products and their receptor in inflammation and diabetes complications. *Nat. Clin. Pract. Endocrinol. Metab.* 4, 285–293. doi: 10.1038/ncpendmet0786

Yoon, J. H., Song, P., Jang, J. H., Kim, D. K., Choi, S., Kim, J., et al. (2011). Proteomic analysis of tumor necrosis factor-alpha (TNF-alpha)-induced L6 myotube secretome reveals novel TNF-alpha-dependent myokines in diabetic skeletal muscle. *J. Proteome Res.* 10, 5315–5325. doi: 10.1021/pr200573b

Zammit, P. S., and Relaix, F. (2012). Satellite cells are essential for skeletal muscle regeneration: the cell on the edge returns centre stage. *Development* 139, 2845–2856. doi: 10.1242/dev.069088

Zhou, L. Z., Johnson, A. P., and Rando, T. A. (2001). NF Kappa B and AP-1 mediate transcriptional responses to oxidative stress in skeletal muscle cells. *Free Radic. Biol. Med.* 31, 1405–1416. doi: 10.1016/S0891-5849(01)00719-5

Zou, M.-H., Shi, C., and Cohen, R. A. (2002). Oxidation of the zinc- thiolate complex and uncoupling of endothelial nitric oxide synthase by peroxynitrite. *J. Clin. Invest.* 31, 1405–1416. doi: 10.1172/JCI14442

12

Isolation, characterization and molecular regulation of muscle stem cells

So-ichiro Fukada*, Yuran Ma, Takuji Ohtani, Yoko Watanabe, Satoshi Murakami and Masahiko Yamaguchi

Laboratory of Molecular and Cellular Physiology, Graduate School of Pharmaceutical Sciences, Osaka University, Osaka, Japan

****Correspondence:***
So-ichiro Fukada, Laboratory of Molecular and Cellular Physiology, Graduate School of Pharmaceutical Sciences, Osaka University, 1-6 Yamada-oka, Suita, Osaka 565-0871, Japan
e-mail: fukada@phs.osaka-u.ac.jp

Skeletal muscle has great regenerative capacity which is dependent on muscle stem cells, also known as satellite cells. A loss of satellite cells and/or their function impairs skeletal muscle regeneration and leads to a loss of skeletal muscle power; therefore, the molecular mechanisms for maintaining satellite cells in a quiescent and undifferentiated state are of great interest in skeletal muscle biology. Many studies have demonstrated proteins expressed by satellite cells, including Pax7, M-cadherin, Cxcr4, syndecan3/4, and c-met. To further characterize satellite cells, we established a method to directly isolate satellite cells using a monoclonal antibody, SM/C-2.6. Using SM/C-2.6 and microarrays, we measured the genes expressed in quiescent satellite cells and demonstrated that Hesr3 may complement Hesr1 in generating quiescent satellite cells. Although Hesr1- or Hesr3-single knockout mice show a normal skeletal muscle phenotype, including satellite cells, Hesr1/Hesr3-double knockout mice show a gradual decrease in the number of satellite cells and increase in regenerative defects dependent on satellite cell numbers. We also observed that a mouse's genetic background affects the regenerative capacity of its skeletal muscle and have established a line of DBA/2-background *mdx* mice that has a much more severe phenotype than the frequently used C57BL/10-*mdx* mice. The phenotype of DBA/2-*mdx* mice also seems to depend on the function of satellite cells. In this review, we summarize the methodology of direct isolation, characterization, and molecular regulation of satellite cells based on our results. The relationship between the regenerative capacity of satellite cells and progression of muscular disorders is also summarized. In the last part, we discuss application of the accumulating scientific information on satellite cells to treatment of patients with muscular disorders.

Keywords: satellite cells, skeletal muscle, maintenance, muscular diseases, quiescence, notch, microarray, cell therapies

INTRODUCTION

One of the best-known examples of regeneration is the ability of newts to regenerate limbs and tails. This process was believed to utilize specialized multipotent cells that have the potential to produce all types of cells. The existence of this type of multipotent stem cells seemed to be the reason newts, but not humans, can regenerate limbs. However, a recent study of the axotl has suggested a different model (Kragl et al., 2009). Instead of multipotent stem cells, each tissue produces progenitor cells with restricted potential. In other words, each cell keeps a memory of its tissue origin during regeneration. Humans who lose a limb cannot produce new one because most types of cells do not retain their regenerative potentials in humans. Skeletal muscle, however, seems to be an exception. Muscle stem cells, known as satellite cells, make it possible for humans and newts to regenerate, because the potential for muscle regeneration using satellite cell-like cells is maintained across species (Morrison et al., 2006). Because the ultimate goal of regenerative medicine is to rebuild lost tissue, the study of muscle regeneration and satellite cells will help us clarify the principles of regeneration.

How many times can skeletal muscle rebuild itself? In other words, how many times can satellite cells proliferate to make new myofibers in mammals? Two groups have reported a powerful regenerative capacity of skeletal muscle in rats and mice. Luz et al. reported that C57BL/10 mice regenerated muscle without loss of myofibers or gain of fibrotic areas after 50 bupivacaine injections into the TA muscle (Luz et al., 2002). Sadeh et al. showed active regeneration cycles in rats that had received weekly injections of bupivacaine for 6 months. They reported a lack of evidence for reduction or exhaustion of muscle fiber capacity to regenerate despite ongoing degeneration–regeneration cycles over a period approximating one fourth of the rat life expectancy (Sadeh et al., 1985). These results clearly indicate that the satellite cell pool is efficiently maintained during multiple degeneration–regeneration cycles in these animals. However, actually, there are many inherited and non-inherited muscle disorders that exhibit a progressive loss of muscle mass and weakness. Duchenne muscular dystrophy is a well-known inherited muscle disease that results from the lack of functional dystrophin proteins. In disease environments, satellite cells are forced to continue to proliferate and differentiate because newly formed myofibers are repeatedly damaged. This regeneration–degeneration cycle is considered to lead to exhaustion of satellite cell potentials, which is one reason why dystrophic patients exhibit progressive symptoms. In addition, the microenvironment of satellite cells in disease conditions may affect long-term survival and/or maintenance of their functions. The same genes that are responsible for inherited muscle disease might directly contribute to sustaining the satellite cell pool. Our knowledge of how to overcome and develop new therapeutic methodologies for muscle diseases based on satellite cell biology is still limited, but if we can manipulate satellite cell potential, it may lead to treatment of many muscle disorders. To accomplish this, we have to understand the molecular and cellular mechanisms of satellite cells. In this chapter, we will introduce the methodology of direct isolation of satellite cells, which was the first step to revealing the molecular and cellular mechanisms of satellite cells. Next, based on recent studies, we will show molecular regulation of satellite cells, and the relationship between the capacity of satellite cells and the progression of muscular disorders. In the last part, we discuss how to apply the accumulating scientific results on satellite cells to treating patients with muscle disorders.

A

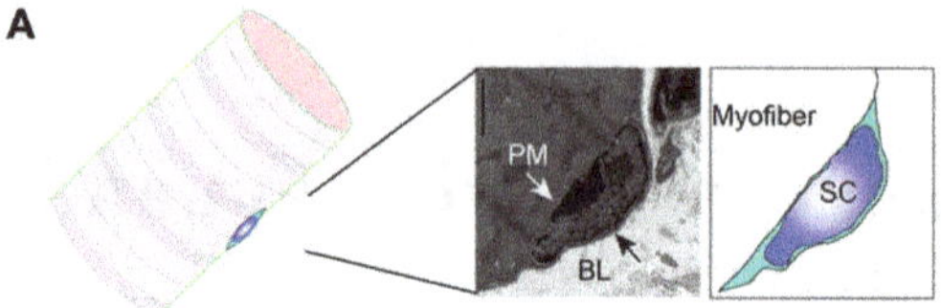

B

Nuclei	: Pax7, Pax3, Hesr3(HeyL), Rbp-J, p57
Nuclear envelope	: Lamin A/C, Emerin
Cytoplasm	: Sprouty1, C/EBPβ
Cell surface	: M-cadherin, CD34, Vcam1, Calcitonin receptor, Odz4, Integrin α7/β1, Syndecan4, Caveolin1, Cxcr4, Fzd7, Notch3

FIGURE 1 | Proteins expressed in quiescent muscle satellite cells. **(A)** Location of satellite cells. PM, plasma membrane; BL, basal lamina; SC, satellite cell. **(B)** Satellite cell molecules whose protein expressions are confirmed. Red indicates "quiescence genes."

SATELLITE CELLS

Satellite cells were discovered by Dr. Alexander Mauro as mononuclear cells attached to myofibers in frog muscle (Mauro, 1961). Subsequently, satellite cells were found in mammalian skeletal muscle. The name is derived from their location between the basal lamina and sarcolemma (plasma membrane of myofiber) (**Figure 1A**). Like other stem cells, satellite cells are maintained in an undifferentiated and quiescent state in uninjured muscles (Schultz et al., 1978), and therefore, transcriptional activity is much lower than in proliferating myoblasts. In fact, the nucleus occupies most of the cell area, and only small portions are observed as cytoplasm by electronic microscopy (**Figure 1A**). In addition, the RNA content of quiescent satellite cells is about one fourth of that of cultured myoblasts (Fukada et al., 2007). Freter et al. demonstrated global suppression of RNA polymerase II serine-2 phosphorylation, which triggers productive transcription elongation, mRNA processing, and release of the mature mRNA in adult stem cells including satellite cells (Freter et al., 2010). However, recent studies show that the quiescent state is not "passive," but rather a highly regulated cell state that is rapidly activated in response to injury or damage (Liu et al., 2013), therefore the "active" molecular regulation of stem cells is of great interest in the field of stem cell research.

In the past 15 years, many studies have reported other myogenic stem/progenitor cells, for example, bone marrow cells, side population (SP) cells, and muscle-resident interstitial cells, that seemed to function as stem cells for muscle regeneration (Ferrari et al., 1998; Gussoni et al., 1999; Jackson et al., 1999; Asakura and Rudnicki, 2002; Asakura et al., 2002; Fukada et al., 2002; LaBarge and Blau, 2002; Tamaki et al., 2002; Polesskaya et al., 2003). However, the physiological roles of these types of cells are limited, and, now there is no doubt that satellite cells play essential roles during skeletal muscle regeneration (Collins et al., 2005; Lepper et al., 2011; Sambasivan et al., 2011). In addition, a single satellite cell has potential for both myogenic differentiation and self-renewal; therefore, the functions and characteristics of satellite cells satisfy the criteria of stem cells, and satellite cells function physiologically as stem cells for skeletal muscle homeostasis (Sacco et al., 2008). Satellite cells also play essential roles in skeletal muscle development. White et al. estimated that satellite cells contribute to the increase in the number of myofiber nuclei in mice until 3 weeks after birth (White et al., 2010).

The identification and observation of satellite cells had been dependent on electronic microscopy. However, the discovery of M-cadherin expression on satellite cells has allowed us to easily identify them by conventional microscopy (Irintchev et al., 1994). Pax7 is also widely used to identify satellite cells by microscopy. In contrast to M-cadherin-null mice, Pax7-null mice show severe loss of muscle mass and satellite cell pools (Seale et al., 2000). In addition to these molecules, expression of several other proteins in quiescent satellite cells has been reported (**Figure 1B**). Above all, identification of cell surface molecules allows us to isolate living quiescent satellite cells, using a specific antibody that recognizes the extracellular domain of the protein. In the next section, we will introduce the history and methodologies of direct isolation of satellite cells.

DIRECT ISOLATION OF SATELLITE CELLS

Direct isolation of stem cells is a powerful tool to investigate their biology. Direct isolation of hematopoietic stem cells made research on hematopoietic stem cells the cutting edge of stem cell biology (Osawa et al., 1996). On the other hand, identification of stem cells by culture-based methods sometimes lacks reproducibility because culture conditions might affect it. Therefore, direct isolation of stem cells is essential for the study of stem cell biology.

When we started to study muscle satellite cells, nobody had succeeded in direct isolation of them, although Blau's group reported isolation of myogenic cells using an anti-integrin a7 antibody from crude cultured mononuclear cells derived from skeletal muscle (Blanco-Bose et al., 2001). To directly isolate satellite cells, we tried to develop a monoclonal antibody. We injected C2/4 cells (a subclone of C2C12) into rats, and produced hybridoma cells by a standard method. C2/4 cells were used for FACS-based screenings because our aim was to establish a monoclonal antibody suited to FACS analyses. In addition, skeletal muscle-derived mononuclear cells were also used for the FACS-based screening process. Finally, SM/C-2.6, a new monoclonal antibody, was established (Fukada et al., 2004), and then we established a method to isolate pure satellite cells using SM/C-2.6, anti-CD31, -CD45, and -Sca-1 antibodies (Fukada et al., 2007; Ikemoto et al., 2007). All mononuclear myogenic cells in skeletal muscle at different stages of injury as well as uninjured muscle were purified in the SM/C-2.6(+)CD31(−)CD45(−)Sca-1(−) fraction (Ikemoto et al., 2007; Segawa et al., 2008). SM/C-2.6 also contributed to the generation of myogenic cells from embryonic stem (ES) cells and induced pluripotent stem (iPS) cells (Chang et al., 2009; Mizuno et al., 2010). Furthermore, the antibody led to the identification of mesenchymal progenitors, which are the original cell sources of both the fibrosis and adipogenesis that are the hallmarks of progressed muscular dystrophies (Uezumi et al., 2010, 2011; Ito et al., 2013). In *in vitro* culture conditions, cells easily lose *in vivo* characteristics, including gene expression. In addition, a lack of purification allows contamination by other types of cells and affects the results. Therefore, the purification of isolated cells is essential for these analyses, and our methods to assure the purity are widely used in many laboratories (Israeli et al., 2007; Verma et al., 2010; Yajima et al., 2010; Tokura et al., 2011; Urciuolo et al., 2013).

There are other methods to purify muscle satellite cells. In 2004, Sherwood et al. demonstrated that the integrin α7(+)integrin β1(+)Cxcr4(+)CD34(+)CD45(−)Sca-1(−)Mac-1(−) fraction contained only myogenic cells (Sherwood et al., 2004). In 2005, Montarras et al. showed that satellite cells are highly enriched in the CD34(+)CD45(−)Sca-1(−) fraction (Montarras et al., 2005). Syndecan3/4 is also used as a positive marker of satellite cell isolation (Tanaka et al., 2009). The positive marker used depends on the laboratory, but many research groups use the same negative markers. The positive and negative markers used for directly isolating satellite cells are listed in **Table 1**. In addition to these cell surface-based methods for isolation of satellite cells, genetic modifications also allow us to directly isolate quiescent satellite cells. Green or yellow fluorescent protein expression under a Pax3 (Montarras et al., 2005; Bosnakovski et al., 2008) or Pax7 promoter is one established method for direct isolation of satellite cells. Unfortunately, although information on satellite cells in humans is still limited, SM/C-2.6 does not react with human, rat, or dog cells (unpublished data). Thus, neural cell adhesion molecules (NCAM) is used for identification of human satellite cells in tissues (Cashman et al., 1987), and a few groups have reported direct isolation of satellite cells using anti-NCAM (CD56) antibodies (Dellavalle et al., 2007).

Table 1 | Markers used in the direct isolation of muscle satellite cells.

Positive markers	Negative markers	References
SM/C-2.6	CD31, CD45, Sca-1	Fukada et al., 2004, 2007
Integrin α7, Integrin β1, Cxcr4	CD45, Sca-1, Mac-1	Sherwood et al., 2004
CD34	CD45, Sca-1	Montarras et al., 2005

FACS analyses do not provide information about the location of satellite cells. In general, immunohistochemistry studies are necessary to provide information on the location of the cells of interest (Irintchev et al., 1994), and therefore, the expression of positive markers on satellite cells must be examined by immunohistochemistry in order to isolate satellite cells. Importantly, the positive markers for isolating satellite cells described above were examined their expression on satellite cells by immunohistochemistry. Therefore, isolated cells by FACS are considered to be equivalent to the anatomically identified satellite cells (Beauchamp et al., 2000; Cornelison et al., 2001; Fukada et al., 2004).

As described above, some muscle stem cells except for satellite cells are identified by FACS. Muscle-SP cells are defined by Hoechst-efflux (Gussoni et al., 1999; Jackson et al., 1999). Satellite cells do not exist in the SP cell fraction (Fukada et al., 2004), and therefore muscle satellite cells and SP cells are considered to be different cell populations. Like muscle-SP cells, the other types of muscle stem cells are located in interstitial areas in muscle (Tamaki et al., 2002; Uezumi et al., 2006), and therefore SP cells and muscle-resident interstitial cells are completely distinct populations from satellite cells, making the study of immunohistochemistry essential for using positive markers to isolate muscle satellite cells.

However, FACS studies have many advantages in on-going studies of stem cell biology. FACS can easily elucidate the cell size, cellular granularity, and frequency of a stem cell population (Fukada et al., 2011). In addition, direct isolation assures single cell transplantation (Sacco et al., 2008), and Montarras and Ikemoto reported that freshly isolated cells have much higher muscle reconstitution potential than cultured cells (Montarras et al., 2005; Ikemoto et al., 2007). Among the benefits of direct isolation, one of the most notable is that we can perform genome-wide gene expression analyses using isolated cells and microarrays. In fact, we have identified a great number of unexpected genes in quiescent satellite cells (Fukada et al., 2007). In the next section, we will introduce genes that are specifically or highly expressed in satellite cells in the dormant state.

QUIESCENCE GENES

Cultured myoblasts and myogenic cell lines play important roles in studies of myogenic differentiation, and essential processes for myogenic differentiation have been established. Establishment of C2 cells (Yaffe and Saxel, 1977) and the subclone C2C12 (Blau et al., 1983a) has played extremely important roles in studies of myogenic cell biology. Single myofiber culture is also excellent model to investigate the differentiation and self-renewal mechanisms of satellite cells *in vitro* (Rosenblatt et al., 1995). However, little was known about the genes expressed in quiescent satellite cells until 2007 when our group first compared the genes of quiescent satellite cells and cultured myoblasts. We found that 507 genes (665 probes) were expressed in quiescent satellite cells at levels more than 5-fold higher than in activated satellite cells (Fukada et al., 2007). To date, among these genes, the physiological roles of Sprouty1 (Spry1), Notch3, and Cepbb, in satellite cells have been elucidated using gene-deleted mice (Kitamoto and Hanaoka, 2010; Shea et al., 2010; Marchildon et al., 2012).

Spry1 is an inhibitor of receptor tyrosine kinase signaling, and the lack of Spry1 leads to loss of the satellite cell pool during the regeneration process. In uninjured young and adult muscle, Spry1 is not essential for maintaining satellite cells, but in aged muscle, the loss of Spry1 leads to a decrease in the number of satellite cells due to accelerated fibroblast growth factor (FGF) signaling (Chakkalakal et al., 2012). Kitamoto et al. showed that half of satellite cells and myoblasts express Notch3, and that Notch3 expression is downregulated during myogenic differentiation (Kitamoto and Hanaoka, 2010). Intriguingly, the loss of Notch3 increases the number of satellite cells in uninjured muscle. In addition, after repetitive muscle injuries, like repeated CTX injections or dystrophic condition, Notch3-deficient mice showed remarkable overgrowth of muscle mass. Notch3-deficient myoblasts show accelerated proliferation, and Notch3-induced myoblasts exhibit decreased BrdU-uptake. Therefore, in quiescent satellite cells, Notch3 might keep the cell cycle in a quiescent state. The investigation of aged Notch3-deficient mice is expected to explain the roles of Notch3 in satellite cells over long periods. CCAAT/enhancer binding proteins (C/EBPs) form a family of basic leucine zipper (bZIP) transcription factors, of which C/EBPβ is involved in many regulatory and differentiation processes as both an activator and a repressor. The loss of *Cebpb* does not affect the number of satellite cells, but C/EBPβ has the potential to induce Pax7 expression and inhibit myogenic differentiation because loss of *Cebpb* expression in satellite cells promotes fiber hypertrophy *in vivo* and cell fusion *in vitro* (Marchildon et al., 2012). Like Spry1, loss of *Cebpb* might affect the satellite cell pool in aged mice. In addition, our transcriptome analyses have shown that *Cebpd* is also highly expressed in quiescent satellite cells. Therefore, C/EBP family genes might regulate muscle satellite cells in a physiological manner.

Bone morphogenetic proteins (BMPs) constitute a subgroup of the transforming growth factor (TGF)-β superfamily, and are known as myogenic differentiation regulators. Gamell et al. reported that Bmp2 induces phosphorylation of Akt and migration of C2C12 (Gamell et al., 2008). Wang et al. indicated that Bmp signaling positively regulates the proliferation of both fetal myogenic progenitors and satellite cells *in vivo* (Wang et al., 2010). They also indicated that BMP signaling is not active in quiescent satellite cells, but that proliferating satellite cells exhibit active BMP signaling. These results indicate that quiescent satellite cells do not respond to BMP signaling in their dormant state. Intriguingly, our microarray results showed that quiescent satellite cells express extremely high levels of *Bmp2, 4,* and *6* genes (Fukada et al., 2007). Therefore, an unknown mechanism might control BMP activity or translation of BMPs in quiescent satellite cells. In BMP signaling, Smad1, Smad5, and Smad8 are specific intracellular transducers. On the other hand, Smad2 and Smad3 transduce TGF-β signaling. Ge et al. reported that Smad3-null mice showed a decreased number of satellite cells (Ge et al., 2011). However, this study was performed using Smad3-null mice, therefore, we cannot conclude that Smad3 plays direct roles in quiescent satellite cells because myofibers of Smad3-null mice are also affected by the lack of Smad3. However, hematopoietic stem cells (Yamazaki et al., 2011) and some stem cells (Oshimori and Fuchs, 2012) are controlled by TGF-β signaling. Likewise, TGF-β might be an essential regulator for the maintenance of satellite cells. In **Table 2**, we summarized the genes that affect satellite cell numbers in uninjured adult skeletal muscle (Seale et al., 2000; Kitamoto and Hanaoka, 2010; Angione et al., 2011; Fukada et al., 2011; Ge et al., 2011; Hosoyama et al., 2011; Juan et al., 2011; Bjornson et al., 2012; Chakkalakal et al., 2012; Cheung et al., 2012; Mourikis et al., 2012).

On the other hand, 659 genes (814 probes) were upregulated (>5-fold) in the activated state in our microarray results. The most highly upregulated gene (334-fold) was *Hmga2*; Li at al. demonstrated that Hmga2 plays essential roles in myoblast proliferation and myogenesis (Li et al., 2012). Therefore, our transcriptome analyses include many functional genes that explain satellite cell states.

As mentioned above, satellite cells occupy a unique location and do not express the myogenic determination gene MyoD. Therefore, we hypothesized that the genes responsible for maintaining satellite cells are specifically expressed in quiescent satellite cells in skeletal muscle. To isolate such genes, we also prepared non-myogenic cells from skeletal muscle for comparison with quiescent and activated satellite cells, and 63 genes were finally

Table 2 | Genes known to control satellite cell number *in vivo*.

Target molecule	Experimental procedure	Result*	References
Pax7	Null	Decreased (60 days, 0–10%)	Seale et al., 2000
Hesr1 and Hesr3	Null	Decreased (20 weeks, <20%)	Fukada et al., 2011
Rbp-J	Conditional (Pax7-CreERT2)	Decreased (44 days, 20%)	Bjornson et al., 2012; Mourikis et al., 2012
Rb	Conditional (Pax7-CreERT2)	Increased (14 days, 152%)	Hosoyama et al., 2011
Notch3	Null	Increased (4 months, 140%)	Kitamoto and Hanaoka, 2010
Dicer	Conditional (Pax7-CreERT2)	Decreased (14 days, 20%)	Cheung et al., 2012
Smad3	Null	Decreased (50%)	Ge et al., 2011
Sprouty	Conditional (Pax7-CreERT2)	Decreased (22 months, 50%)	Chakkalakal et al., 2012
PPARd	Conditional (Myf5-Cre)	Decreased (2–3 months, 60%)	Angione et al., 2011
Ezh2	Conditional (Pax7-Cre)	Decreased (60 days, 60%)	Juan et al., 2011

**Percentage shows the frequency of satellite cell number compared to control mice. In the case of null mice, the period shows age of mice analyzed. In the case of Pax7-CreERT2 mice, the period after last injection of tamoxifen is indicated.*

identified as "quiescence genes," which are highly expressed in quiescent satellite cells but not in cultured myoblasts and non-myogenic cells in skeletal muscle (Fukada et al., 2007). Almost none of the genes had been previously reported in skeletal muscle biology.

Other groups also performed similar comparisons to characterize quiescent satellite cells. Pallafacchina et al. compared the gene expression profiles of quiescent satellite cells with samples of neonatal satellite cells and *mdx* mouse-derived Pax3+ cells (Pallafacchina et al., 2010). Our "quiescence genes" are expressed at higher rates in quiescent satellite cells than in neonatal satellite cells, but the ratio is not very significant. This discrepancy is dependent on the type of cells used for comparison because Pallafacchina et al. also showed significant differences between quiescent satellite cells and cultured myoblasts. Pallafacchina et al. isolated quiescent satellite cell-specific genes (e.g., *Apoe*, *Ms4a4d*, *Fgl2*, *Timp4*, *Adh1*, *Ahr*, *Osmr*), but these genes are also expressed in non-myogenic cells in skeletal muscle. Another discrepancy is the expression of Notch-related genes in quiescent satellite cells. We identified Notch signaling-related genes (*Notch3* and *HeyL/Hesr3*) as the most highly expressed genes in quiescent satellite cells, although Pallafacchina's results did not show the importance of Notch signaling in quiescent satellite cells. However, recent studies have clearly demonstrated the essential roles of Notch signaling for maintaining quiescent satellite cells *in vivo* as well as developmental stages (see below). On the other hand, quiescent satellite cells share common features in our and Pallafacchina's results, for example, some cell adhesion molecules and transcriptional factors. Although our reports had not mentioned it, Pallafacchina et al. intriguingly found up-regulation of anti-oxidative genes in quiescent satellite cells. In fact, our original data also included ant-oxidative genes in quiescent-stage specific manner. These results imply the importance of oxidative stress in quiescent satellite cells. Farina et al. analyzed gene expressions of quiescent satellite cells, activated satellite cells (ASC, 12 h after injury), and proliferating myoblasts (Prof. SC, 48 h after injury) (Farina et al., 2012). Their study focused mainly on the RNA-binding proteins that are highly expressed in quiescent satellite cells compared to ASC or Prof. SC. However, *Zfp36* was the sole common RNA-binding protein among the three microarray studies. Transcriptional and translational regulation of RNA may be essential for maintaining satellite cells in a dormant state, so quiescent satellite cell-specific expressions of RNA-binding proteins were limited in the three studies. The three microarray studies are summarized in **Table 3**. In the next sections, we would like to introduce our three "quiescence genes": Hesr3, calcitonin receptor, and Odz4, with some speculation about their roles.

NOTCH EFFECTOR GENES AND SATELLITE CELLS

Notch signaling is essential for development of diverse tissues (Lai, 2004). When Notch is activated, its intracellular domain is cleaved by γ-secretase and it translocates to the nucleus, where it activates the transcription of target genes through interaction with Rbpj. Rbpj-mediated Notch signaling is known as the canonical pathway, and the families of *Hes* (hairy and enhancer of split) and *Hesr* (hes-related, also known as Hey/Herp/Hrt/Chf) are known as primary targets of Notch signaling (Iso et al., 2003; Fischer and Gessler, 2007). Among Hes and Hesr family genes, quiescent satellite cells specifically and highly express Hesr3 in skeletal muscle. Quiescent satellite cells also express Hesr1. However, Hesr1 is not included in the 'quiescence genes' because endothelial cells in skeletal muscle, as well as other tissues, express Hesr1. In addition, when primary myoblasts or C2C12 are stimulated with Delta-like 1 or 4, respectively, Hesr1 and Hesr3 are induced in both types of cells (Buas et al., 2009; Fukada et al., 2011). Therefore, Hesr1 and Hesr3 seem to be the major downstream targets of Notch signaling in adult satellite cells (Yamaguchi and Fukada, 2013).

The roles of Notch signaling are powerful and complicated because it has opposite effects on some lineage cells. In myogenic cells, Notch signaling has two roles: one is inducing myogenic commitment and the other is inhibiting myogenesis. Dezawa et al. produced myogenic cells from bone marrow stromal cells via the transient activation of Notch signaling in the processes (Dezawa et al., 2005). Rios et al. reported that neural crest-derived delta-like 1 transiently activates Notch signaling in cells located in the medial border of the dermomyotome and that this event is essential for the induction of both Myf5 and MyoD in them (Rios et al., 2011). They also showed that sustained Notch signaling inhibits myogenic differentiation even in the medial border of the dermomyotome. These results demonstrated that transient Notch signaling works as an inducer of myogenesis. On the other hand, the myogenic inhibitory effect of Notch signaling is extremely well known (Kuroda et al., 1999). Induction of Notch signaling suppresses the expression of MyoD, and myogenic differentiation is strongly inhibited. Hesr1 and Hesr3 also seem to play roles in anti-myogenic differentiation because unusual expressions of MyoD and myogenin were observed in satellite cells derived from Hesr1/Hesr3 double-knockout mice (Fukada et al., 2011). Although Hesr1 or Hesr3 single-knockout mice did not show any defect in skeletal muscle including satellite cells and regenerative potential, Hesr1/Hesr3 double-knockout mice showed a remarkable defect in satellite cells. Therefore, in adult satellite cells, Notch signaling seems to be activated constitutively to work as a myogenic inhibitor.

Vasyutina et al. demonstrated the essential roles of canonical Notch signaling to generate the satellite cell pool during embryonic development using conditional depletion of Rbp-J (Vasyutina et al., 2007). However, in Hesr1/Hesr3 double-knockout mice, most of the satellite cell pool existed in mice by the 7th day after birth. These results suggest that the downstream target of Notch is changed during skeletal muscle development. Using Rbpj-floxed and Pax7-CreERT2 mice, two independent groups reported the essential role of Notch signaling for maintaining satellite cells in an undifferentiated state in mouse adult skeletal muscle (Bjornson et al., 2012; Mourikis et al., 2012). When Rbpj was depleted in satellite cells by injection of tamoxifen, quiescent satellite cells started to express myogenic proteins (MyoD and myogenin) and then fused with myofibers. Although further study of conditional Hesr1/Hesr3 depletion remains to be done, these results suggest that the Notch/Rbp-J/Hesr1/Hesr3 pathway is essential to maintain adult satellite cells in a quiescent and undifferentiated state (Yamaguchi and Fukada, 2013). In **Table 2**, we summarized the

Table 3 | Molecular signatures of quiescent satellite cells identified by three independent studies.

	Fukada et al. (2007)	Pallafacchina et al. (2010)	Farina et al. (2012)
Comparison	Cultured myoblasts, NON-myogenic cells	1-week neonatal SC, *mdx* SC	*In vivo* activated SC12, 48 h, Syndecan-4-null
Method			
Isolation	SM/C-2.6+CD45-	Pax3-GFP	Syndecan-3
Muscle	Limb muscles	Diaphragm, pectoralis, and abdominal muscles	Limb muscles
Microarray	MOE430A (Affymetrix)	MOE430v2 (Affymetrix)	MOE430v2 (Affymetrix)
Quiescence genes*			
Calcr	QSC>ASC (×74)	QSC>ASC (×1.8)	ND
Nap1l5	QSC>ASC (×62)	QSC>ASC (9.9)	ND
Odz4	QSC>ASC (×24)	QSC>ASC (×1.96)	ND
Pde4b	QSC>ASC (×23)	QSC>ASC (×5.77)	QSC>ASC (×11.21)
Pof1b	QSC>ASC (×23)	QSC>ASC (×2.79)	ND
RhoH	QSC>ASC (×17)	QSC>ASC (×3.9)	ND
Cebpb	QSC>ASC (×16)	QSC>ASC (×3.19)	ND
Maff	QSC>ASC (×14)	QSC>ASC (×3.19)	ND
Quiescence genes**			
Apoe	QSC>ASC (×293)	QSC>ASC (×23)	ND
Dpt	QSC>ASC (×199)	QSC>ASC (×2.2)	ND
Ms4a4d	QSC>ASC (×144)	QSC>ASC (×78)	ND
Adh1	QSC>ASC (×55)	QSC>ASC (×28)	ND
Osmr	QSC>ASC (×37)	QSC>ASC (×26)	ND
Fgl2	QSC>ASC (×23)	QSC>ASC (×42)	ND
Timp4	QSC>ASC (×12)	QSC>ASC (×49)	ND
Ahr	QSC>ASC (×8)	QSC>ASC (×48)	ND
Cell adhesion	Chodl, Eva1, CD34, Aoc3, Tek, Icam1, Pcdhb9. Efs, Esam1, Cdh5, Cldn5, Nope, Itgb5, Emcn, Cdh13, Sdc4, Dcn, Pcdh9n	Itgb1, CD24, Sdc4, Cldn1, Eva1, CD38, Esam1, Smoc2, Icam2, Cldn5, Dcn, Fgl2	Sdc4, Pak1, Pcdh18, Col3a1
Notch	QSC high (Notch3, HeyL)	QSC low	QSC high (HeyL)
Anti-oxidative stress	Cyp4b1, Gstt1, Gstt3, Sod3, Ugt1a2, Ahr, Cp, Gpx3, Cyp2d22, Cyp39a1, Cyp27a1	Sult1a1, Cyp4b1, Abcd1a, Ugt1, Fmo2, Ahr, Gstm1, Cyp26b1, Srxn1, Txnrd1, Cp, Gpx3	ND
Transcriptional factors	Sox17, Meox2, Sox7, Sox18, Klf4, 9, 15	Sox17, Meox2, Sox7, Sox18, Klf7, Dach1, Prdm16	ND
RNA-binding protein	Rnase4, Zfp36, Zfp36l1, Rnpc2, Csdc2	Rnase4, Ddx5, Sfrs3, Son, Zfp36, Ddx58, Rbpms	Cherp, Ddx5, Hnrnpc, Sfrs3, Snrpb, Snrpe, Son, Srrm1, U2af1l4, Zranb2, Eif4h, Hnrpdl, Poldip3, Rpl22, Rps23, Rps9, Khdrbs1, Rnaset2a, Zfp36, Zfp36l1, Ddx58, Mex3b, Qars, Rad21, Rbm26, Rbpms

*ND, Not described. * "Quiescence genes" of our analyses. These genes are highly expressed in quiescent satellite cells more than in non-myogenic cells in skeletal muscle. **These genes are highly expressed in quiescent satellite cells, but not listed in our "quiescence genes" because non-myogenic cells also expressed these genes.*

phenotypes of Rbp-J-null and Hesr1/Hesr3-dKO mice in adult skeletal muscle.

Melanocyte, intestinal, and neural stem cells also use canonical Notch signaling for their maintenance (Moriyama et al., 2006; Imayoshi et al., 2010; Pellegrinet et al., 2011). In these three stem cells, Hes1 is the major downstream target of Notch signaling. Although the downstream target of Notch signaling is not conserved, canonical Notch signaling seems to be a common molecular mechanism to maintain stem cells in some adult tissues. Notch signaling is essential for the differentiation of hematopoietic cells, but hematopoietic stem cells do not require Notch signaling for maintenance (Maillard et al., 2008).

As described, Notch signaling seems to be one of the essential signaling pathways for maintaining satellite cells. The activation of Notch signaling is induced by its specific ligands, Dll1, Dll4, and Jagged. Basically, direct cell–cell contact is necessary to induce Notch signaling. Until now, the ligand and its origin for maintaining the satellite cell pool have been unclear. Satellite cells are directly attached to myofibers, and therefore, myofibers may express the ligand. Another possibility is that released ligand activates Notch signaling in satellite cells. Sun et al. indicated that Dll1 can be shed and act on myoblasts in an autocrine manner (Sun et al., 2008). The other possibility is ligand-independent activation of Notch receptors. Sima protein, an ortholog of mammalian hypoxia-inducible factor-α (HIF-α), colocalizes with Notch in endocytic vesicles and enables cleavage of the intracellular domain of Notch in Drosophila blood cells (Mukherjee et al., 2011). Gustafsson et al. also demonstrated that HIF-α interacts with the Notch intracellular domain and promotes the expression of the Notch target genes (Gustafsson et al., 2005). The role of HIF-α in muscle satellite cells is still unknown, but these pathways may be used to activate Notch signaling in adult satellite cells.

NOTCH SIGNALING AND OTHER SIGNALING PATHWAYS

Cross-talk signals between Notch and other pathways in some types of cells are reported. For example, Hes proteins promote Stat3 phosphorylation and activation through association with Jak2 and Stat3 in neuroepithelial cells (Kamakura et al., 2004). BMP and Notch signaling also have synergistic effects. Dahlqvist demonstrated that BMP-induced inhibition of myogenic differentiation requires Notch signaling (Dahlqvist et al., 2003). However, phosphorylation of neither Stat3 nor Smad1/5/8 (downstream targets of BMP signaling) was observed in quiescent satellite cells (Kami and Senba, 2002; Wang et al., 2010). Therefore, these signaling pathways do not seem to work coordinately with Notch signaling to sustain the satellite cell pool, although they might work together to activate or start proliferation of satellite cells because phosphorylated Stat3 nor Smad1/5/8 are observed in activated or proliferating satellite cells.

In endothelial cells, Notch signaling inhibits the phosphorylation of Rb (a driver of cell cycle progression), which leads to a decrease in BrdU uptake (Noseda et al., 2004). Rb is a well-known tumor suppressor gene, and phosphorylation of Rb allows the cell cycle to progress. Hosoyama et al. demonstrated that Rb-conditional depletion increased the number of satellite cells in uninjured muscle (Hosoyama et al., 2011). Therefore, even in quiescent satellite cells, Notch signaling might inhibit the phosphorylation of Rb to suppress cell cycle progression. However, the expression of proliferative markers (Ki67 and phosphorylated histone-H3) was not observed in Rb-cKO satellite cells, as it was in Rbp-J cKO satellite cells. Therefore, these results suggest that Rb-independent quiescence mechanisms are regulated by Notch signaling, which plays roles in maintaining the satellite cell pool in dormant state.

Ge et al. reported that Smad3-null mice had a decreased number of satellite cells (Ge et al., 2011). Using the myogenic cell line C2C12, Blokzijl et al. indicated that TGF-β stimulation induces Hes1 expression in a Notch signaling activation-dependent manner (Blokzijl et al., 2003). Furthermore, Smad3 interacts directly with NICD and binds to the promoter regions of Notch target genes via Rbp-J. Therefore, in quiescent satellite cells, TGF-β and Notch might work cooperatively to sustain the dormant state.

CALCITONIN RECEPTOR AND Odz4 AND SATELLITE CELLS

Calcitonin is a molecule that is well known to regulate homeostasis of the calcium level in the blood (Becker et al., 2002). Calcitonin is released from the thyroid and works in bone and kidney. The action of calcitonin is mediated by its specific receptor, the calcitonin receptor. The calcitonin receptor is a G-protein-coupled seven transmembrane protein. Expression of calcitonin receptor is well known in osteoclasts, which play essential roles in bone absorption, and results in the release of calcium into the blood. The balance between osteoclasts and osteoblasts is tightly regulated to maintain bone homeostasis. When the balance is tipped toward osteoclasts, the osteoclastic process is accelerated, and osteoporosis occurs. Calcitonin receptor signaling inhibits the function of osteoclasts via protein kinase A (Suzuki et al., 1996); therefore, synthetic calcitonin is used for treatment of osteoporosis. We found specific expression of calcitonin receptors in quiescent satellite cells, but not in activated satellite cells. The expression of calcitonin receptors seems to be specific in quiescent satellite cells because the re-expression of calcitonin receptors during the regenerative process is related to the end of muscle regeneration (Fukada et al., 2007; Yamaguchi et al., 2012). Therefore, these specific expression patterns imply that calcitonin receptors play several roles in maintaining satellite cells in a quiescent state. In fact, we observed that activation of calcitonin receptors by its ligand delays activation of satellite cells *in vitro* (Fukada et al., 2007). Calcitonin receptor-null mice die *in utero*, and thus the roles of calcitonin receptors in myogenic lineage cells remain unknown. To reveal the physiological importance of calcitonin receptors in satellite cells, the study of satellite cell-specific deletion of calcitonin receptors is essential, and is one of our most important ongoing investigations.

Although the physiological importance of calcitonin receptors in satellite cells is unclear, Cheung et al. demonstrated that mir-489, which is located in intron 4 of the *calcitonin receptor* gene, is essential for satellite cell quiescence (Cheung et al., 2012). Mir-489 is also specifically expressed in quiescent satellite cells like calcitonin receptor mRNA. Because coding and non-coding genes are often transcribed simultaneously, transcription of *calcitonin receptor* genes is tightly regulated in satellite cells, and investigations of *calcitonin receptor* gene regulation might elucidate the activation or self-renewal mechanism of satellite cells.

Odz is the vertebrate homolog of the Drosophila odd Oz. Odz family proteins belonging to the type II transmembrane protein family (Levine et al., 1994). One member of the Odz family, Odz4, is highly expressed in the central nervous system, developing eyes, and somites (Zhou et al., 2003). In addition, we reported the expression of Odz4 protein in satellite cells (Yamaguchi et al., 2012). The function of Odz4 is little known, but recent reports demonstrated the importance of Odz in oligodendrocyte differentiation and process formation (Suzuki et al., 2012). They also indicated that focal adhesion kinase, a key regulator of cell adhesion, is activated downstream of Odz4. Therefore, in satellite cells, Odz4 might control cell adhesion and/or differentiation. Odz4 and calcitonin receptor are expressed in quiescent satellite cells but not in proliferating myoblasts. Intriguingly, the timings of Odz4 and calcitonin receptor re-expression during skeletal muscle regeneration are different (Yamaguchi et al., 2012). Currently, we do not know the characteristics of Pax7(+)Odz4(+)calcitonin receptor(−) cells, but we have speculated that this type of cell contributes to the maturation of myofibers because the appearance of Pax7(+)Odz4(+)calcitonin receptor(−) cells is observed during maturation of immature myofibers (**Figure 2**). Like *calcitonin receptor* genes, the *Odz4* intron contains a quiescent satellite cell-specific microRNA, mir-708 (Cheung et al., 2012). The function of mir-708 is also unknown, but the gene expression mechanism of *Odz4* might be important for efficient skeletal muscle regeneration.

BONE AND SKELETAL MUSCLE MAY USE COMMON MOLECULES FOR MAINTENANCE

Skeletal muscle works as a locomotorium in cooperation with bone. Some diseases or environmental conditions affect both skeletal muscle and bone. For instance, inactivity, as seen in a gravity-free state or bed rest, leads to the loss of muscle weight and bone density. Aging and muscular dystrophy also affect both skeletal muscle and bone states. Duchenne muscular dystrophy patients have low bone mineral density and increased risk of fractures (Bachrach, 2005). Although it has been considered that the bone impairment of DMD patients results from muscle weakness, the bone-skeletal muscle system might have direct regulatory networks via cytokines or exosomes. Otherwise, the bone and skeletal muscle systems use a similar gene network to maintain their homeostasis.

Hesr1/Hesr3 are essential for generation of quiescent satellite cells and to maintain their numbers in adult skeletal muscle. Hesr1/Hesr3 double knock-out mice have other phenotypes besides that of satellite cells. Fischer et al. reported that deletion of both Hesr1 and Hesr3 causes severe heart malformations, including membranous ventricular septal defects and dysplastic atrioventricular and pulmonary valves (Fischer et al., 2007). In addition, Tu et al. demonstrated the essential roles of Hesr1/Hesr3 in osteoblasts (Tu et al., 2012). As is well known, expression of calcitonin receptors in osteoclasts is essential to sustain the homeostasis of bone. Although the physiological importance of calcitonin receptors remains unknown, Hesr1/Hesr3 and calcitonin receptor might be common regulators for both bone and skeletal muscle systems.

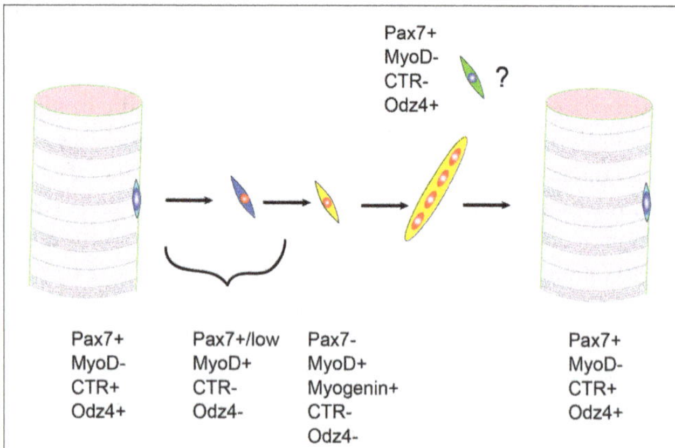

FIGURE 2 | Expressions of calcitonin receptor (CTR) and Odz4 proteins during skeletal muscle regeneration. Pax7+MyoD-CTR-Odz4+ cells are frequently observed during myofiber maturation.

QUIESCENCE GENES AND CANCER PROGRESSION

The quiescent state includes two types of cell cycles, reversible and irreversible. Myofibers are mitotically quiescent, and it is an irreversible state. The induction of msx1 in myotubes (which are also irreversibly quiescent) leads to the generation of mononuclear cells that proliferate (Odelberg et al., 2000). This phenomenon is biologically interesting, but myotubes and myofibers do not generate mononuclear cells in a physiological manner. On the other hand, stem cells, including satellite cells, are in a reversible quiescent state. The molecular mechanisms of reversible quiescence are an interest of many investigators. Reversible quiescence is conserved from yeast to human cells to maintain particular cells, including stem cells, in the body. Uncontrolled reversible quiescence mechanisms can lead to cancer. Intriguingly, Spry1, Notch3, Cebpb, calcitonin receptor, and Odz4 are reported to relate to cancer cells (Wang et al., 1999; Kwabi-Addo et al., 2004; Thomas and Shah, 2005; Park et al., 2006). Cell cycle inhibitors (cyclin-dependent kinase inhibitors) are highly expressed in stem cells, and their breakdown leads to abnormal cell cycle regulation and results in cancer development. Sang et al. indicated that Hes1 is a key transcriptional factor for reversible cellular quiescence in human fibroblasts (Sang et al., 2008). The authors also showed that Hes1 allows human rhabdomyosarcoma cells to evade differentiation and irreversible cycle arrest. As described above, melanocyte stem cells, intestinal stem cells, and neural stem cells require Hes1 downstream of Notch signaling to maintain their pool. Therefore, elucidation of the quiescence mechanisms of stem cells, including satellite cells, will shed light on the principle of the quiescent state, and may lead to the discovery of new therapeutic targets for cancers.

RELATIONSHIP BETWEEN SATELLITE CELLS AND MUSCLE DISORDERS

Muscular dystrophies are the best known muscle disorders, and investigations of them have been central to exploring skeletal muscle biology. The loss of satellite cell numbers and function is considered to be one reason why many muscular dystrophies exhibit progressive symptoms. Besides muscular dystrophies, there are many muscle disorders that exhibit a relationship with impairments of satellite cells. In addition, some reports have shown the direct contribution of satellite cells to the disease condition. For instance, the appearance of fibrosis and adipocytes had been considered to be due to satellite cell transdifferentiation into fibroblasts and adipocytes (Asakura et al., 2001; Li et al., 2004; Alexakis et al., 2007). However, recent studies have demonstrated that satellite cells cannot differentiate into adipocytes and fibroblasts (Joe et al., 2010; Uezumi et al., 2010, 2011; Starkey et al., 2011). Consistent with these observations, Crist et al. clarified that satellite cells are committed progenitor cells especially linked to myogenic cells (Crist et al., 2012). In this section, we will focus on the relationship between satellite cell myogenic potential and disease progression in three muscle disorders and discuss the contribution of satellite cell function to these disorders.

DIFFERENCE BETWEEN HUMAN MUSCULAR DYSTROPHY AND MOUSE MODEL

Duchenne muscular dystrophy (DMD) is a well-known inherited muscular disorder, and the causative gene, *Dystrophin*, is coded in the X-chromosome (Koenig et al., 1988). Patients exhibit progressive symptoms, and histologically, accumulation of fibrosis and adipocytes and loss of myofibers are observed. The *Dystrophin* gene encodes a 427-kDa cytoskeletal protein that forms the dystrophin/glycoprotein complex at the sarcolemma with α- and β-dystroglycans, α-, β-, γ-, ε-, and δ-sarcoglycans, and other molecules, and links the cytoskeleton proteins of myofibers to the extracellular matrix in skeletal muscle (Ervasti and Campbell, 1993). It is supposed that the loss of dystrophin leads to the degeneration of myofibers due to a disturbance in assembly of the dystrophin/glycoprotein complex.

The *mdx* mouse (the correct nomenclature is C57BL/10-DMDmdx) is the most widely used model animal of DMD (Bulfield et al., 1984). Although *mdx* mice have a mutation in the *dystrophin* gene and show degeneration of myofibers, the symptoms of *mdx* mice are remarkably milder than those of DMD patients. In contrast with DMD patients, accumulation of fat and fibrosis in *mdx* mice are barely observed except in the diaphragm, and neither myofibers nor muscle weight are lost throughout much of their life span. One reason for the difference between DMD and *mdx* is explained by the excellent regeneration capacity of *mdx* compared with DMD. However, *mdx* mice carrying another strain background (DBA/2) show similar phenotypes to humans; loss of muscle weight, increased fibrosis, accumulation of adipocytes, and decreased muscle force (Fukada et al., 2010). Intriguingly, satellite cell functions of DBA/2 also differ from those of C57BL/6 mice. Therefore, one of reason for the severe phenotype of DBA/2-*mdx* seems to be inferior function of satellite cells compared to C57BL/10-*mdx*.

The life spans of mice and humans are completely different. In humans, long-term proliferation of satellite cells might be necessary. However, the human telomere is much shorter than that of the mouse. Based on this, Sacco et al. hypothesized that the longer telomere allows satellite cells to proliferate repeatedly in mice. To elucidate this hypothesis, they generated *mdx* mice lacking the RNA component of telomerase (*mdx*/mTR) and demonstrated that *mdx*/mTR mice exhibit severe muscular dystrophy and a decrease in the loss of satellite cell proliferation (Sacco et al., 2010). The phenotypes of DBA/2-*mdx* are unlikely dependent on the telomere erosion because DBA/2 mice have longer telomeres than C57BL/6 (Manning et al., 2002). These results indicate that the differences between human and mouse models depend on several functions of satellite cells: one is telomere length, but the other factors are unknown.

Other dystrophic mouse models, gamma-sarcoglycan-null mice, also depend on the mouse genetic background, and DBA/2-background mice exhibit the most severe phenotype of the strains examined (Heydemann et al., 2005). Intriguingly, the aged phenotype of DBA/2 is much more severe than that of C57BL/6 (Lionikas et al., 2006). In addition, the low reconstitution potential of the DBA/2-strain is not restricted to skeletal muscle. DBA/2-derived hematopoietic stem cells (HSCs) show low reconstitution, and Liang et al. revealed the gene, latexin, responsible for this phenotype (Liang et al., 2007). These results suggest that similar analyses will also lead to the discovery of genes responsible for skeletal muscle satellite cells, which may lead to the discovery of a new therapeutic methodology for muscular disorders.

MUSCULAR DYSTROPHY AND SATELLITE CELLS

Conceptually, exhaustion of the satellite cell pool leads to the progression of muscular dystrophy. In fact, the loss of proliferative potential was observed in myoblasts derived from DMD patients (Blau et al., 1983b). One of our surprising findings was that quiescent satellite cells showed high expressions of *dystrophin* and *dystroglycan* genes compared to myoblasts (Fukada et al., 2007). Both dystrophin and dystroglycan have been considered essential proteins for stability of the myofiber membrane (sarcolemma), and it is well known that the lack of these genes leads to muscular dystrophies. The roles of these genes in satellite cells are still unknown, but these genes might be essential for cell adhesion and stability of satellite cells as well as myofibers.

Recently, Kanagawa et al. showed a functional defect of myogenic cells in the mouse model of Fukuyama-type congenital muscular dystrophy, which is caused by an ancient retrotransposal insertion in the *Fukutin* gene (Kobayashi et al., 1998; Kanagawa et al., 2013). Interestingly, fukutin-deficient myoblasts showed a significantly low potential for myotube formation, even myoblasts that originated from mice that had not started to exhibit a dystrophic phenotype. These results indicate that fukutin is necessary for myotube formation; therefore, efficient regeneration is likely to be impaired in Fukuyama-type muscular dystrophy. In addition, lamin A/C and emerin, which are expressed in quiescent satellite cells, are known as causal genes for autosomal-Emery-Dreifuss muscular dystrophy (A-EDMD) (Bonne et al., 1999) and X-EDMD (Bione et al., 1994), respectively. Therefore, some causative genes for muscular dystrophy may affect satellite cells and/or their daughter cells directly, which might determine the severity of symptoms (Gnocchi et al., 2008).

SARCOPENIA AND SATELLITE CELLS

Current progress and improvement of medical treatment prolong lives, but aging-related physical morbidity is becoming a social problem. Normal skeletal muscle also faces these problems. Most of us exhibit drastic deterioration of performance with age. One cause is sarcopenia, which is linked to the loss of muscle mass and function. Sarcopenia is inevitable, and likely to contribute to the decline of muscle strength and ability to maintain daily activities. Some researchers define sarcopenia as "an appendicular muscle mass/height^2 less than two standard deviations below the mean for that of a young healthy adult" (Iannuzzi-Sucich et al., 2002). According to this definition, the percentage of elderly suffering from sarcopenia has reached 10–25% or more (Baumgartner et al., 1999). In light of this severe phenomenon and the tendency of the global geriatric population to increase in number, sarcopenia will become a social problem. Besides sarcopenia, there are other muscle disorders accompanying the loss of muscle mass, known as atrophies. However, sarcopenia can be distinguished from other types of muscle atrophy by a decrease in the number of myofibers. Myofiber formation is based on the fusion of a large number of myoblasts (Moss and Leblond, 1970; Hawke and Garry, 2001) and requires the participation of satellite cells in the regenerative process of myofibers; a relationship between satellite cells and sarcopenia is possible, although it still remains controversial. Trendelenburg et al. demonstrated that TAK-1/p38/nNF-κB signaling pathway inhibits myoblast differentiation by increasing the level of activin A (Trendelenburg et al., 2012). Upregulation of TNF-1α and IL-1β is reported in sarcopenia, and they drive TAK-1/p38/nNF-κB. The NF-κB pathway is well known as an inducer of muscle atrophy (Cai et al., 2004). Therefore, the NF-κB pathway might be activated in both satellite cells and myofibers, which leads to suppression of myogenic differentiation and atrophy in myofibers.

In sarcopenia, direct contributions by the satellite cell pool are proposed because many studies have demonstrated the loss of satellite cell pools throughout the aging period. In contrast, some reports indicate that the number of satellite cells in muscle of elderly rats and mice is unchanged. Although it has not been fully elucidated, the discrepancy is likely to be connected to a difference in the muscle tissues analyzed (e.g., levator, soleus, vastus lateralis, and tibialis anterior, etc.) (Gibson and Schultz, 1983; Nnodim, 2000; Brack et al., 2005; Schafer et al., 2005). Based on the fact that sarcopenia mainly presents a decline in type 2 muscle fibers, some researchers have confirmed the observation of a 45% reduction in satellite cell numbers in type 2 muscle fibers in old (76 ± 1 years) vs. young (20 ± 1 years) populations (Verdijk et al., 2007). In addition, several available tests demonstrate that activated satellite cells can partially counter sarcopenia (Cutlip et al., 2009; Snijders et al., 2009; Aagaard et al., 2010). These backgrounds contribute to the maximal connection between satellite cells and sarcopenia. Intriguingly, DBA/2 strain mice exhibit a more remarkable loss of muscle mass than C57BL/6 mice, and the satellite cell pool of DBA/2 is reduced earlier in their life span than that of C57BL/6 (our unpublished data). As described in the previous section, DBA/2 satellite cells are inferior to those of C57BL/6 mice, and therefore, the investigation of DBA/2-satellite cells might lead to discovery of the central pathway for the maintenance of satellite cell pool throughout life.

CANCER CACHEXIA AND SATELLITE CELLS

Some cancers induce the loss of body weight. A decrease beyond 5% of body weight in 12 months or less can be defined as cancer cachexia. Because skeletal muscle mass occupies about 40% of body weight, cancer cachexia is generally associated with the loss of muscle weight. Although the molecular mechanism evoking muscle atrophy in cancer cachexia patients remains largely unknown, some studies have begun to reveal the molecular mechanisms of cancer cachexia. Acharyya et al. indicated that dysfunction of dystrophin in a cancer cachexia mouse model leads to weakness of the myofiber membrane (Acharyya et al., 2005). The membrane structure of myofibers is considered an important element for maintaining the satellite cell pool, and therefore, there is a possibility that a change in the myofiber membrane affects satellite cells. In fact, Penna et al. found an increased number of satellite cells in cancer cachexia model mice (Penna et al., 2010). Further, up-regulation of TNF-α and IL-6 in cachexia patients and animal models is well known. Although the relationship between these cytokines and muscle wasting is unclear, these cytokines inhibit muscle differentiation (Coletti et al., 2002, 2005; Guttridge, 2004). Zhou indicated that activation of ActRIIB (receptor for activin and myostatin) contributes to the loss of mass in cancer cachexia model mice and that an ActRIIB antagonist may be a therapeutic approach to the treatment of cancer cachexia (Zhou et al., 2010). As described for sarcopenia, the ActRII signaling pathway inhibits myogenic differentiation. Based on this information, it is possible to hypothesize that cancer cachexia involves satellite cell dysfunctions. In this case, satellite cells may be directly targeted for the treatment of cancer cachexia, and a molecular mechanism for regulation of satellite cells may solve this problem in the near future. In addition, recently it was reported that muscle stromal cells (PDGFRa+ cells, which are considered to be mesenchymal progenitors) are essential to sustain muscle mass (Roberts et al., 2013). Depletion of muscle stromal cells leads to the loss of muscle mass, and cancer cachexia induced a decrease in the number of muscle stromal cells. Therefore, muscle mesenchymal progenitors might be also a direct target of cancer cachexia as well as muscle satellite cells and myofibers.

FUTURE STRATEGIES FOR STEM CELL RESEARCH TO TREAT MUSCLE DISORDERS

Satellite cells undoubtedly have the best potential to produce new myofibers *in vivo*. However, there are obstacles to overcome. One problem is the low migration potential of satellite cells. Most muscular dystrophy patients have dystrophic symptoms in systemic skeletal muscles; therefore, satellite cells have to be transplanted via blood vessels. Unfortunately, satellite cells cannot cross blood vessels, so the use of satellite cells is considered limited to the relatively localized muscle diseases such as oculopharyngeal muscular dystrophy (OPMD). Recently, Cappellari et al. reported that Dll4 and PDGFβ signals convert myogenic cells to pericyte-like cells without erasing their myogenic memory (Cappellari et al., 2013). Unlike satellite cells, pericytes can cross blood vessel walls and migrate into skeletal muscle tissue (Dellavalle et al., 2007). Therefore, satellite cells might acquire the ability to cross blood vessels and form myofibers by using the methodology.

Another problem is the difficulty of obtaining large numbers of satellite cells from a donor. In addition, expansion of satellite cells *in vitro* reduces their regenerative activity, as described above (Montarras et al., 2005; Ikemoto et al., 2007). However, several studies have shed light on ways to improve the culture system. Gilbert et al. indicated the importance of substrate elasticity in sustaining satellite cell function *in vitro* (Gilbert et al., 2010). Notch ligand stimulation also allows the expansion of satellite cells without a decrease *in vivo* regenerative potential (Parker et al., 2012). As described above, recent studies have indicated that Notch signaling is one of the essential signaling pathways to maintain satellite cells. The reason why Notch signals improve myogenic cell transplantation is unknown, but one possibility is the down-regulation of MyoD. Asakura et al. demonstrated that the survival of MyoD-null mice-derived myoblasts is superior to that of wild-type myoblasts (Asakura et al., 2007). The authors also showed that many anti-apoptotic genes were up-regulated in MyoD-null myoblasts, whereas genes known to execute apoptosis were down-regulated. The relationship between Notch and MyoD in an improved protocol for myogenic cell transplantation must be revealed for realization of satellite cell therapy for DMD patients because Notch signaling also affects cell cycle genes in satellite cells.

Another source of cells for therapy for muscle disorders is iPS cell-derived myogenic cells (Mizuno et al., 2010; Darabi et al., 2012). A method to produce myogenic cells from iPS cells, which have some of the same features as satellite cells, might solve the problem of cell numbers. Because satellite cells are mitotically quiescent, we need to generate proliferating myogenic cells that have myogenic potential similar to satellite cells. The myogenic cell appearing in embryonic and neonatal developmental stages is one model candidate for a myogenic progenitor derived from iPS cells. However, Sakai et al. compared the regenerative potential of fetal and adult satellite cells, and found that adult satellite cells are superior to fetal satellite cells (Sakai et al., 2013). Researchers have just begun to understand the satellite cell on the molecular level. For the development of satellite cell-like cells from iPS cells, we need to understand the process of generating satellite cells during development as well as regeneration. Relaix et al. observed that Pax3(+)Pax7(+) cells derived from the central region of the dermomyotome are the origin of satellite cells (Relaix et al., 2005). In addition, satellite cells express MyoD during this process (Kanisicak et al., 2009). The Notch signaling pathway perhaps down-regulates MyoD to generate the satellite cell pool. However, before they become myogenin(+) cells, we cannot anticipate the destiny of MyoD(+) myogenic cells during the development and regeneration processes. One of the most important questions is how the satellite cell pool is established during embryonic and postnatal development. Understanding this will lead to success in the generation of satellite cell-like cells from iPS cells.

The physiological self-renewal mechanism of satellite cells during regeneration must also be revealed. Some evidences have indicated an asymmetrical model of self-renewal of satellite cells (Conboy and Rando, 2002; Shinin et al., 2006; Kuang et al., 2007). Wnt7a signaling promotes symmetrical division of Myf5- satellite cells and ameliorates the *mdx* phenotype (Le Grand et al., 2009; von Maltzahn et al., 2012). Elucidation of these processes may also lead to successful generation of satellite cell-like cells from iPS cells. Taken together, in either case (satellite cells or iPS cells), the molecular mechanisms for both generation, maintenance, and self-renewal of satellite cells must be revealed to attain our goal.

In addition, another mechanism must be understood for the successful cell transplantation for muscle disorders. To date, we have not paid attention to the fusion process between transplanted cells and myofibers. When donor cells are transplanted, they have to cross the basal lamina and fuse with myofibers. Horsley et al. indicated the myotube-myoblast fusion process requires IL4/IL-4R signaling mediated by NFATc2 (Horsley et al., 2003). However, the structure, functions, and gene expressions of myotubes differ remarkably from those of myofibers. Therefore, we need to consider the process of myoblast-with-myofiber fusion. The identification of such genes will improve the efficiency of satellite cell/iPS-derived myogenic cell therapy.

PROSPECTS

For 10 years, the isolation, characterization, and molecular regulation of satellite cells have been studied, and accumulating evidence is starting to reveal the molecular mechanisms for maintaining the satellite cell pool. In addition, recent studies are beginning to identify the roles of satellite cells in several different disorders. For instance, McCarthy et al. indicated that acute hypertrophy is not dependent on satellite cells (McCarthy et al., 2011). On the other hand, acute and chronic regenerations are required to fulfill the potential of satellite cells. These results indicate that not all muscle-related disorders depend on satellite cell function. In the aging process, the dependence on satellite cells is controversial. To develop a new therapeutic approach, we have to understand the contribution of satellite cells to each disease. In sarcopenia research, a Pax7-CreERT2::Rosa-DTA strategy might be useful to elucidate the dependency of satellite cells. In addition, until now, the genes causing muscular dystrophies have only been considered as a function of the sarcolemma in myofibers. However, some of them are expressed in quiescent satellite cells (Cohn et al., 2002; Fukada et al., 2007; Gnocchi et al., 2009). Therefore, they may regulate the quiescence and undifferentiated states of satellite cells, and additional functions of causative genes in satellite cells might explain the severity of each disease.

The generation of iPS cells has assisted the cell therapy approach to many disorders including muscular dystrophy (Takahashi and Yamanaka, 2006; Takahashi et al., 2007). The successful establishment of iPS cells was supported by studies of ES cells. Finding culture conditions that can maintain ES cells in an undifferentiated state is probably the most important contribution to the birth of iPS cells. For cell treatment of muscular disorders, we have at least two choices, satellite cells or iPS-derived myogenic cells. In either case, we would like to reiterate that understanding the molecular mechanisms of muscle satellite cells is essential to accomplish successful myogenic cell therapy.

Skeletal muscle is indispensable for motility. In addition, skeletal muscle has the potential to control other tissues. For instance, Bostrom et al. showed that a skeletal muscle-derived cytokine, irisin, converts white fat cells to brown fat-like cells (Bostrom et al., 2012). The relationship between exercise and immune function is a well-known open window theory (Nieman and Pedersen, 1999). Thus, skeletal muscle itself might be a therapeutic target for other diseases like diabetes. Much still remains to be revealed about striated muscle, but striated muscle might have many powers to control unanticipated physiologies. We hope that the study of satellite cells will open new doors of striated muscle biology and lead to a recovery of muscle power in muscle disorder patients.

ACKNOWLEDGMENTS

We thank Katherine Ono for reading this manuscript. Our work was supported by JSPS KAKENHI grant (18800023 to So-ichiro Fukada), MEXT KAKENHI grant (20700358 to So-ichiro Fukada), Intramural Research Grant (22-1 to So-ichiro Fukada) for Neurological and Psychiatric Disorders of NCNP, the Nakatomi Foundation (to So-ichiro Fukada).

REFERENCES

Aagaard, P., Suetta, C., Caserotti, P., Magnusson, S. P., and Kjaer, M. (2010). Role of the nervous system in sarcopenia and muscle atrophy with aging: strength training as a countermeasure. *Scand. J. Med. Sci. Sports* 20, 49–64. doi: 10.1111/j.1600-0838.2009.01084.x

Acharyya, S., Butchbach, M. E., Sahenk, Z., Wang, H., Saji, M., Carathers, M., et al. (2005). Dystrophin glycoprotein complex dysfunction: a regulatory link between muscular dystrophy and cancer cachexia. *Cancer Cell* 8, 421–432. doi: 10.1016/j.ccr.2005.10.004

Alexakis, C., Partridge, T., and Bou-Gharios, G. (2007). Implication of the satellite cell in dystrophic muscle fibrosis: a self-perpetuating mechanism of collagen overproduction. *Am. J. Physiol. Cell. Physiol.* 293, C661–C669. doi: 10.1152/ajpcell.00061.2007

Angione, A. R., Jiang, C., Pan, D., Wang, Y. X., and Kuang, S. (2011). PPARdelta regulates satellite cell proliferation and skeletal muscle regeneration. *Skeletal Muscle* 1, 33. doi: 10.1186/2044-5040-1-33

Asakura, A., Hirai, H., Kablar, B., Morita, S., Ishibashi, J., Piras, B. A., et al. (2007). Increased survival of muscle stem cells lacking the MyoD gene after transplantation into regenerating skeletal muscle. *Proc. Natl. Acad. Sci. U.S.A.* 104, 16552–16557. doi: 10.1073/pnas.0708145104

Asakura, A., Komaki, M., and Rudnicki, M. (2001). Muscle satellite cells are multipotential stem cells that exhibit myogenic, osteogenic, and adipogenic differentiation. *Differentiation* 68, 245–253. doi: 10.1046/j.1432-0436.2001.680412.x

Asakura, A., and Rudnicki, M. A. (2002). Side population cells from diverse adult tissues are capable of *in vitro* hematopoietic differentiation. *Exp. Hematol.* 30, 1339–1345. doi: 10.1016/S0301-472X(02)00954-2

Asakura, A., Seale, P., Girgis-Gabardo, A., and Rudnicki, M. A. (2002). Myogenic specification of side population cells in skeletal muscle. *J. Cell Biol.* 159, 123–134. doi: 10.1083/jcb.200202092

Bachrach, L. K. (2005). Taking steps towards reducing osteoporosis in Duchenne muscular dystrophy. *Neuromuscul. Disord.* 15, 86–87. doi: 10.1016/j.nmd.2004.10.011

Baumgartner, R. N., Waters, D. L., Gallagher, D., Morley, J. E., and Garry, P. J. (1999). Predictors of skeletal muscle mass in elderly men and women. *Mech. Ageing Dev.* 107, 123–136. doi: 10.1016/S0047-6374(98)00130-4

Beauchamp, J. R., Heslop, L., Yu, D. S., Tajbakhsh, S., Kelly, R. G., Wernig, A., et al. (2000). Expression of CD34 and Myf5 defines the majority of quiescent adult skeletal muscle satellite cells. *J. Cell Biol.* 151, 1221–1234. doi: 10.1083/jcb.151.6.1221

Becker, K., Muller, B., Nylen, E., Cohen, R., White, J., and Snider, J. (2002). *Calcitonin Gene Family of Peptides, 2nd Edn.*Vol. 1, (New York, NY: Academic Press).

Bione, S., Maestrini, E., Rivella, S., Mancini, M., Regis, S., Romeo, G., et al. (1994). Identification of a novel X-linked gene responsible for Emery-Dreifuss muscular dystrophy. *Nat. Genet.* 8, 323–327. doi: 10.1038/ng1294-323

Bjornson, C. R., Cheung, T. H., Liu, L., Tripathi, P. V., Steeper, K. M., and Rando, T. A. (2012). Notch Signaling is Necessary to Maintain Quiescence in Adult Muscle Stem Cells. *Stem Cells* 30, 232–242. doi: 10.1002/stem.773

Blanco-Bose, W. E., Yao, C. C., Kramer, R. H., and Blau, H. M. (2001). Purification of mouse primary myoblasts based on alpha 7 integrin expression. *Exp. Cell Res.* 265, 212–220. doi: 10.1006/excr.2001.5191

Blau, H. M., Chiu, C. P., and Webster, C. (1983a). Cytoplasmic activation of human nuclear genes in stable heterocaryons. *Cell* 32, 1171–1180. doi: 10.1016/0092-8674(83)90300-8

Blau, H. M., Webster, C., and Pavlath, G. K. (1983b). Defective myoblasts identified in Duchenne muscular dystrophy. *Proc. Natl. Acad. Sci. U.S.A.* 80, 4856–4860. doi: 10.1073/pnas.80.15.4856

Blokzijl, A., Dahlqvist, C., Reissmann, E., Falk, A., Moliner, A., Lendahl, U., et al. (2003). Cross-talk between the Notch and TGF-beta signaling pathways mediated by interaction of the Notch intracellular domain with Smad3. *J. Cell Biol.* 163, 723–728. doi: 10.1083/jcb.200305112

Bonne, G., Di Barletta, M. R., Varnous, S., Becane, H. M., Hammouda, E. H., Merlini, L., et al. (1999). Mutations in the gene encoding lamin A/C cause autosomal dominant Emery-Dreifuss muscular dystrophy. *Nat. Genet.* 21, 285–288. doi: 10.1038/6799

Bosnakovski, D., Xu, Z., Li, W., Thet, S., Cleaver, O., Perlingeiro, R. C., et al. (2008). Prospective isolation of skeletal muscle stem cells with a Pax7 reporter. *Stem Cells* 26, 3194–3204. doi: 10.1634/stemcells.2007-1017

Bostrom, P., Wu, J., Jedrychowski, M. P., Korde, A., Ye, L., Lo, J. C., et al. (2012). A PGC1-alpha-dependent myokine that drives brown-fat-like development of white fat and thermogenesis. *Nature* 481, 463–468. doi: 10.1038/nature10777

Brack, A. S., Bildsoe, H., and Hughes, S. M. (2005). Evidence that satellite cell decrement contributes to preferential decline in nuclear number from large fibres during murine age-related muscle atrophy. *J. Cell Sci.* 118, 4813–4821. doi: 10.1242/jcs.02602

Buas, M. F., Kabak, S., and Kadesch, T. (2009). Inhibition of myogenesis by Notch: evidence for multiple pathways. *J. Cell Physiol.* 218, 84–93. doi: 10.1002/jcp.21571

Bulfield, G., Siller, W. G., Wight, P. A., and Moore, K. J. (1984). X chromosome-linked muscular dystrophy (mdx) in the mouse. *Proc. Natl. Acad. Sci. U.S.A.* 81, 1189–1192. doi: 10.1073/pnas.81.4.1189

Cai, D., Frantz, J. D., Tawa, N. E. Jr., Melendez, P. A., Oh, B. C., Lidov, H. G., et al. (2004). IKKbeta/NF-kappaB activation causes severe muscle wasting in mice. *Cell* 119, 285–298. doi: 10.1016/j.cell.2004.09.027

Cappellari, O., Benedetti, S., Innocenzi, A., Tedesco, F. S., Moreno-Fortuny, A., Ugarte, G., et al. (2013). Dll4 and PDGF-BB convert committed skeletal myoblasts to pericytes without erasing their myogenic memory. *Dev. Cell* 24, 586–599. doi: 10.1016/j.devcel.2013.01.022

Cashman, N. R., Covault, J., Wollman, R. L., and Sanes, J. R. (1987). Neural cell adhesion molecule in normal, denervated, and myopathic human muscle. *Ann. Neurol.* 21, 481–489. doi: 10.1002/ana.410210512

Chakkalakal, J. V., Jones, K. M., Basson, M. A., and Brack, A. S. (2012). The aged niche disrupts muscle stem cell quiescence. *Nature* 490, 355–360. doi: 10.1038/nature11438

Chang, H., Yoshimoto, M., Umeda, K., Iwasa, T., Mizuno, Y., Fukada, S., et al. (2009). Generation of transplantable, functional satellite-like cells from mouse embryonic stem cells. *FASEB J.* 23, 1907–1919. doi: 10.1096/fj.08-123661

Cheung, T. H., Quach, N. L., Charville, G. W., Liu, L., Park, L., Edalati, A., et al. (2012). Maintenance of muscle stem-cell quiescence by microRNA-489. *Nature* 482, 524–528. doi: 10.1038/nature10834

Cohn, R. D., Henry, M. D., Michele, D. E., Barresi, R., Saito, F., Moore, S. A., et al. (2002). Disruption of DAG1 in differentiated skeletal muscle reveals a role for dystroglycan in muscle regeneration. *Cell* 110, 639–648. doi: 10.1016/S0092-8674(02)00907-8

Coletti, D., Moresi, V., Adamo, S., Molinaro, M., and Sassoon, D. (2005). Tumor necrosis factor-alpha gene transfer induces cachexia and inhibits muscle regeneration. *Genesis* 43, 120–128. doi: 10.1002/gene.20160

Coletti, D., Yang, E., Marazzi, G., and Sassoon, D. (2002). TNFalpha inhibits skeletal myogenesis through a PW1-dependent pathway by recruitment of caspase pathways. *EMBO J.* 21, 631–642. doi: 10.1093/emboj/21.4.631

Collins, C. A., Olsen, I., Zammit, P. S., Heslop, L., Petrie, A., Partridge, T. A., et al. (2005). Stem cell function, self-renewal, and behavioral heterogeneity of cells from the adult muscle satellite cell niche. *Cell* 122, 289–301. doi: 10.1016/j.cell.2005.05.010

Conboy, I. M., and Rando, T. A. (2002). The regulation of Notch signaling controls satellite cell activation and cell fate determination in postnatal myogenesis. *Dev. Cell* 3, 397–409. doi: 10.1016/S1534-5807(02)00254-X

Cornelison, D. D., Filla, M. S., Stanley, H. M., Rapraeger, A. C., and Olwin, B. B. (2001). Syndecan-3 and syndecan-4 specifically mark skeletal muscle satellite cells and are implicated in satellite cell maintenance and muscle regeneration. *Dev. Biol.* 239, 79–94. doi: 10.1006/dbio.2001.0416

Crist, C. G., Montarras, D., and Buckingham, M. (2012). Muscle satellite cells are primed for myogenesis but maintain quiescence with sequestration of Myf5 mRNA targeted by microRNA-31 in mRNP granules. *Cell Stem Cell* 11, 118–126. doi: 10.1016/j.stem.2012.03.011

Cutlip, R. G., Baker, B. A., Hollander, M., and Ensey, J. (2009). Injury and adaptive mechanisms in skeletal muscle. *J. Electromyogr. Kinesiol.* 19, 358–372. doi: 10.1016/j.jelekin.2008.06.007

Dahlqvist, C., Blokzijl, A., Chapman, G., Falk, A., Dannaeus, K., Ibanez, C. F., et al. (2003). Functional Notch signaling is required for BMP4-induced inhibition of myogenic differentiation. *Development* 130, 6089–6099. doi: 10.1242/dev.00834

Darabi, R., Arpke, R. W., Irion, S., Dimos, J. T., Grskovic, M., Kyba, M., et al. (2012). Human ES- and iPS-derived myogenic progenitors restore DYSTROPHIN and improve contractility upon transplantation in dystrophic mice. *Cell Stem Cell* 10, 610–619. doi: 10.1016/j.stem.2012.02.015

Dellavalle, A., Sampaolesi, M., Tonlorenzi, R., Tagliafico, E., Sacchetti, B., Perani, L., et al. (2007). Pericytes of human skeletal muscle are myogenic precursors distinct from satellite cells. *Nat. Cell Biol.* 9, 255–267. doi: 10.1038/ncb1542

Dezawa, M., Ishikawa, H., Itokazu, Y., Yoshihara, T., Hoshino, M., Takeda, S., et al. (2005). Bone marrow stromal cells generate muscle cells and repair muscle degeneration. *Science* 309, 314–317. doi: 10.1126/science.1110364

Ervasti, J. M., and Campbell, K. P. (1993). A role for the dystrophin-glycoprotein complex as a transmembrane linker between laminin and actin. *J. Cell Biol.* 122, 809–823. doi: 10.1083/jcb.122.4.809

Farina, N. H., Hausburg, M., Betta, N. D., Pulliam, C., Srivastava, D., Cornelison, D., et al. (2012). A role for RNA post-transcriptional regulation in satellite cell activation. *Skeletal Muscle* 2, 21. doi: 10.1186/2044-5040-2-21

Ferrari, G., Cusella-De Angelis, G., Coletta, M., Paolucci, E., Stornaiuolo, A., Cossu, G., et al. (1998). Muscle regeneration by bone marrow-derived myogenic progenitors. *Science* 279, 1528–1530. doi: 10.1126/science.279.5356.1528

Fischer, A., and Gessler, M. (2007). Delta-Notch–and then? Protein interactions and proposed modes of repression by Hes and Hey bHLH factors. *Nucleic Acids Res.* 35, 4583–4596. doi: 10.1093/nar/gkm477

Fischer, A., Steidl, C., Wagner, T. U., Lang, E., Jakob, P. M., Friedl, P., et al. (2007). Combined loss of Hey1 and HeyL causes congenital heart defects because of impaired epithelial to mesenchymal transition. *Circ. Res.* 100, 856–863. doi: 10.1161/01.RES.0000260913.95642.3b

Freter, R., Osawa, M., and Nishikawa, S. (2010). Adult stem cells exhibit global suppression of RNA polymerase II serine-2 phosphorylation. *Stem Cells* 28, 1571–1580. doi: 10.1002/stem.476

Fukada, S., Higuchi, S., Segawa, M., Koda, K., Yamamoto, Y., Tsujikawa, K., et al. (2004). Purification and cell-surface marker characterization of quiescent satellite cells from murine skeletal muscle by a novel monoclonal antibody. *Exp. Cell Res.* 296, 245–255. doi: 10.1016/j.yexcr.2004.02.018

Fukada, S., Miyagoe-Suzuki, Y., Tsukihara, H., Yuasa, K., Higuchi, S., Ono, S., et al. (2002). Muscle regeneration by reconstitution with bone marrow or fetal liver cells from green fluorescent protein-gene transgenic mice. *J. Cell Sci.* 115, 1285–1293.

Fukada, S., Morikawa, D., Yamamoto, Y., Yoshida, T., Sumie, N., Yamaguchi, M., et al. (2010). Genetic background affects properties of satellite cells and mdx phenotypes. *Am. J. Pathol.* 176, 2414–2424. doi: 10.2353/ajpath.2010.090887

Fukada, S., Uezumi, A., Ikemoto, M., Masuda, S., Segawa, M., Tanimura, N., et al. (2007). Molecular signature of quiescent satellite cells in adult skeletal muscle. *Stem Cells* 25, 2448–2459. doi: 10.1634/stemcells.2007-0019

Fukada, S., Yamaguchi, M., Kokubo, H., Ogawa, R., Uezumi, A., Yoneda, T., et al. (2011). Hesr1 and Hesr3 are essential to generate undifferentiated quiescent satellite cells and to maintain satellite cell numbers. *Development* 138, 4609–4619. doi: 10.1242/dev.067165

Gamell, C., Osses, N., Bartrons, R., Ruckle, T., Camps, M., Rosa, J. L., et al. (2008). BMP2 induction of actin cytoskeleton reorganization and cell migration requires PI3-kinase and Cdc42 activity. *J. Cell Sci.* 121, 3960–3970. doi: 10.1242/jcs.031286

Ge, X., McFarlane, C., Vajjala, A., Lokireddy, S., Ng, Z. H., Tan, C. K., et al. (2011). Smad3 signaling is required for satellite cell function and myogenic differentiation of myoblasts. *Cell Res.* 21, 1591–1604. doi: 10.1038/cr.2011.72

Gibson, M. C., and Schultz, E. (1983). Age-related differences in absolute numbers of skeletal muscle satellite cells. *Muscle Nerve* 6, 574–580. doi: 10.1002/mus.880060807

Gilbert, P. M., Havenstrite, K. L., Magnusson, K. E., Sacco, A., Leonardi, N. A., Kraft, P., et al. (2010). Substrate elasticity regulates skeletal muscle stem cell self-renewal in culture. *Science* 329, 1078–1081. doi: 10.1126/science.1191035

Gnocchi, V. F., Ellis, J. A., and Zammit, P. S. (2008). Does satellite cell dysfunction contribute to disease progression in Emery-Dreifuss muscular dystrophy? *Biochem. Soc. Trans.* 36, 1344–1349. doi: 10.1042/BST0361344

Gnocchi, V. F., White, R. B., Ono, Y., Ellis, J. A., and Zammit, P. S. (2009). Further characterisation of the molecular signature of quiescent and activated mouse muscle satellite cells. *PLoS ONE* 4:e5205. doi: 10.1371/journal.pone.0005205

Gussoni, E., Soneoka, Y., Strickland, C. D., Buzney, E. A., Khan, M. K., Flint, A. F., et al. (1999). Dystrophin expression in the mdx mouse restored by stem cell transplantation. *Nature* 401, 390–394. doi: 10.1038/43919

Gustafsson, M. V., Zheng, X., Pereira, T., Gradin, K., Jin, S., Lundkvist, J., et al. (2005). Hypoxia requires notch signaling to maintain the undifferentiated cell state. *Dev. Cell* 9, 617–628. doi: 10.1016/j.devcel.2005.09.010

Guttridge, D. C. (2004). Signaling pathways weigh in on decisions to make or break skeletal muscle. *Curr. Opin. Clin. Nutr. Metab. Care* 7, 443–450. doi: 10.1097/01.mco.0000134364.61406.26

Hawke, T. J., and Garry, D. J. (2001). Myogenic satellite cells: physiology to molecular biology. *J. Appl. Physiol.* 91, 534–551.

Heydemann, A., Huber, J. M., Demonbreun, A., Hadhazy, M., and McNally, E. M. (2005). Genetic background influences muscular dystrophy. *Neuromuscul. Disord.* 15, 601–609. doi: 10.1016/j.nmd.2005.05.004

Horsley, V., Jansen, K. M., Mills, S. T., and Pavlath, G. K. (2003). IL-4 acts as a myoblast recruitment factor during mammalian muscle growth. *Cell* 113, 483–494. doi: 10.1016/S0092-8674(03)00319-2

Hosoyama, T., Nishijo, K., Prajapati, S. I., Li, G., and Keller, C. (2011). Rb1 gene inactivation expands satellite cell and postnatal myoblast pools. *J. Biol. Chem.* 286, 19556–19564. doi: 10.1074/jbc.M111.229542

Iannuzzi-Sucich, M., Prestwood, K. M., and Kenny, A. M. (2002). Prevalence of sarcopenia and predictors of skeletal muscle mass in healthy, older men and women. *J. Gerontol. A Biol. Sci. Med. Sci.* 57, M772–M777. doi: 10.1093/gerona/57.12.M772

Ikemoto, M., Fukada, S., Uezumi, A., Masuda, S., Miyoshi, H., Yamamoto, H., et al. (2007). Autologous transplantation of SM/C-2.6(+) satellite cells transduced with micro-dystrophin CS1 cDNA by lentiviral vector into mdx mice. *Mol. Ther.* 15, 2178–2185. doi: 10.1038/sj.mt.6300295

Imayoshi, I., Sakamoto, M., Yamaguchi, M., Mori, K., and Kageyama, R. (2010). Essential roles of Notch signaling in maintenance of neural stem cells in developing and adult brains. *J. Neurosci.*30, 3489–3498. doi: 10.1523/JNEUROSCI.4987-09.2010

Irintchev, A., Zeschnigk, M., Starzinski-Powitz, A., and Wernig, A. (1994). Expression pattern of M-cadherin in normal, denervated, and regenerating mouse muscles. *Dev. Dyn.* 199, 326–337. doi: 10.1002/aja.1001990407

Iso, T., Kedes, L., and Hamamori, Y. (2003). HES and HERP families: multiple effectors of the Notch signaling pathway. *J. Cell Physiol.* 194, 237–255. doi: 10.1002/jcp.10208

Israeli, D., Ziaei, S., Gjata, B., Benchaouir, R., Rameau, P., Marais, T., et al. (2007). Expression of mdr1 is required for efficient long term regeneration of dystrophic muscle. *Exp. Cell Res.* 313, 2438–2450. doi: 10.1016/j.yexcr.2007.02.036

Ito, T., Ogawa, R., Uezumi, A., Ohtani, T., Watanabe, Y., Tsujikawa, K., et al. (2013). Imatinib attenuates severe mouse dystrophy and inhibits proliferation and fibrosis-marker expression in muscle mesenchymal progenitors. *Neuromuscul. Disord.* 23, 349–356. doi: 10.1016/j.nmd.2012.10.025

Jackson, K. A., Mi, T., and Goodell, M. A. (1999). Hematopoietic potential of stem cells isolated from murine skeletal muscle. *Proc. Natl. Acad. Sci. U.S.A.* 96, 14482–14486. doi: 10.1073/pnas.96.25.14482

Joe, A. W., Yi, L., Natarajan, A., Le Grand, F., So, L., Wang, J., et al. (2010). Muscle injury activates resident fibro/adipogenic progenitors that facilitate myogenesis. *Nat. Cell Biol.* 12, 153–163. doi: 10.1038/ncb2015

Juan, A. H., Derfoul, A., Feng, X., Ryall, J. G., Dell'Orso, S., Pasut, A., et al. (2011). Polycomb EZH2 controls self-renewal and safeguards the transcriptional identity of skeletal muscle stem cells. *Genes Dev.* 25, 789–794. doi: 10.1101/gad.2027911

Kamakura, S., Oishi, K., Yoshimatsu, T., Nakafuku, M., Masuyama, N., and Gotoh, Y. (2004). Hes binding to STAT3 mediates crosstalk between Notch and JAK-STAT signalling. *Nat. Cell Biol.* 6, 547–554. doi: 10.1038/ncb1138

Kami, K., and Senba, E. (2002). *In vivo* activation of STAT3 signaling in satellite cells and myofibers in regenerating rat skeletal muscles. *J. Histochem. Cytochem.* 50, 1579–1589. doi: 10.1177/002215540205001202

Kanagawa, M., Yu, C. C., Ito, C., Fukada, S., Hozoji-Inada, M., Chiyo, T., et al. (2013). Impaired viability of muscle precursor cells in muscular dystrophy with glycosylation defects and amelioration of its severe phenotype by limited gene expression. *Hum. Mol. Genet.* 22, 3003–3015. doi: 10.1093/hmg/ddt157

Kanisicak, O., Mendez, J. J., Yamamoto, S., Yamamoto, M., and Goldhamer, D. J. (2009). Progenitors of skeletal muscle satellite cells express the muscle determination gene, MyoD. *Dev. Biol.* 332, 131–141. doi: 10.1016/j.ydbio.2009.05.554

Kitamoto, T., and Hanaoka, K. (2010). Notch3 null mutation in mice causes muscle hyperplasia by repetitive muscle regeneration. *Stem Cells* 28, 2205–2216. doi: 10.1002/stem.547

Kobayashi, K., Nakahori, Y., Miyake, M., Matsumura, K., Kondo-Iida, E., Nomura, Y., et al. (1998). An ancient retrotransposal insertion causes Fukuyama-type congenital muscular dystrophy. *Nature* 394, 388–392. doi: 10.1038/28256

Koenig, M., Monaco, A. P., and Kunkel, L. M. (1988). The complete sequence of dystrophin predicts a rod-shaped cytoskeletal protein. *Cell* 53, 219–228. doi: 10.1016/0092-8674(88)90383-2

Kragl, M., Knapp, D., Nacu, E., Khattak, S., Maden, M., Epperlein, H. H., et al. (2009). Cells keep a memory of their tissue origin during axolotl limb regeneration. *Nature* 460, 60–65. doi: 10.1038/nature08152

Kuang, S., Kuroda, K., Le Grand, F., and Rudnicki, M. A. (2007). Asymmetric self-renewal and commitment of satellite stem cells in muscle. *Cell* 129, 999–1010. doi: 10.1016/j.cell.2007.03.044

Kuroda, K., Tani, S., Tamura, K., Minoguchi, S., Kurooka, H., and Honjo, T. (1999). Delta-induced Notch signaling mediated by RBP-J inhibits MyoD expression and myogenesis. *J. Biol. Chem.* 274, 7238–7244. doi: 10.1074/jbc.274.11.7238

Kwabi-Addo, B., Wang, J., Erdem, H., Vaid, A., Castro, P., Ayala, G., et al. (2004). The expression of Sprouty1, an inhibitor of fibroblast growth factor signal transduction, is decreased in human prostate cancer. *Cancer Res.* 64, 4728–4735. doi: 10.1158/0008-5472.CAN-03-3759

LaBarge, M. A., and Blau, H. M. (2002). Biological progression from adult bone marrow to mononucleate muscle stem cell to multinucleate muscle fiber in response to injury. *Cell* 111, 589–601. doi: 10.1016/S0092-8674(02)01078-4

Lai, E. C. (2004). Notch signaling: control of cell communication and cell fate. *Development* 131, 965–973. doi: 10.1242/dev.01074

Le Grand, F., Jones, A. E., Seale, V., Scime, A., and Rudnicki, M. A. (2009). Wnt7a activates the planar cell polarity pathway to drive the symmetric expansion of satellite stem cells. *Cell Stem Cell* 4, 535–547. doi: 10.1016/j.stem.2009.03.013

Lepper, C., Partridge, T. A., and Fan, C. M. (2011). An absolute requirement for Pax7-positive satellite cells in acute injury-induced skeletal muscle regeneration. *Development* 138, 3639–3646. doi: 10.1242/dev.067595

Levine, A., Bashan-Ahrend, A., Budai-Hadrian, O., Gartenberg, D., Menasherow, S., and Wides, R. (1994). Odd Oz: a novel Drosophila pair rule gene. *Cell* 77, 587–598. doi: 10.1016/0092-8674(94)90220-8

Li, Y., Foster, W., Deasy, B. M., Chan, Y., Prisk, V., Tang, Y., et al. (2004). Transforming growth factor-beta1 induces the differentiation of myogenic cells into fibrotic cells in injured skeletal muscle: a key event in muscle fibrogenesis. *Am. J. Pathol.* 164, 1007–1019. doi: 10.1016/S0002-9440(10)63188-4

Li, Z., Gilbert, J. A., Zhang, Y., Zhang, M., Qiu, Q., Ramanujan, K., et al. (2012). An HMGA2-IGF2BP2 axis regulates myoblast proliferation and myogenesis. *Dev. Cell* 23, 1176–1188. doi: 10.1016/j.devcel.2012.10.019

Liang, Y., Jansen, M., Aronow, B., Geiger, H., and Van Zant, G. (2007). The quantitative trait gene latexin influences the size of the hematopoietic stem cell population in mice. *Nat. Genet.* 39, 178–188. doi: 10.1038/ng1938

Lionikas, A., Blizard, D. A., Vandenbergh, D. J., Stout, J. T., Vogler, G. P., McClearn, G. E., et al. (2006). Genetic determinants of weight of fast- and slow-twitch skeletal muscles in old mice. *Mamm. Genome* 17, 615–628. doi: 10.1007/s00335-005-0177-x

Liu, L., Cheung, T. H., Charville, G. W., Hurgo, B. M., Leavitt, T., Shih, J., et al. (2013). Chromatin modifications as determinants of muscle stem cell quiescence and chronological aging. *Cell Rep.* 4, 189–204. doi: 10.1016/j.celrep.2013.05.043

Luz, M. A., Marques, M. J., and Santo Neto, H. (2002). Impaired regeneration of dystrophin-deficient muscle fibers is caused by exhaustion of myogenic cells. *Braz J. Med. Biol. Res.* 35, 691–695. doi: 10.1590/S0100-879X2002000600009

Maillard, I., Koch, U., Dumortier, A., Shestova, O., Xu, L., Sai, H., et al. (2008). Canonical notch signaling is dispensable for the maintenance of adult hematopoietic stem cells. *Cell Stem Cell* 2, 356–366. doi: 10.1016/j.stem.2008.02.011

Manning, E. L., Crossland, J., Dewey, M. J., and Van Zant, G. (2002). Influences of inbreeding and genetics on telomere length in mice. *Mamm. Genome* 13, 234–238. doi: 10.1007/s003350020027

Marchildon, F., Lala, N., Li, G., St-Louis, C., Lamothe, D., Keller, C., et al. (2012). CCAAT/enhancer binding protein beta is expressed in satellite cells and controls myogenesis. *Stem Cells* 30, 2619–2630. doi: 10.1002/stem.1248

Mauro, A. (1961). Satellite cell of skeletal muscle fibers. J Biophys Biochem Cytol 9, 493–495. doi: 10.1083/jcb.9.2.493

McCarthy, J. J., Mula, J., Miyazaki, M., Erfani, R., Garrison, K., Farooqui, A. B., et al. (2011). Effective fiber hypertrophy in satellite cell-depleted skeletal muscle. *Development* 138, 3657–3666. doi: 10.1242/dev.068858

Mizuno, Y., Chang, H., Umeda, K., Niwa, A., Iwasa, T., Awaya, T., et al. (2010). Generation of skeletal muscle stem/progenitor cells from murine induced pluripotent stem cells. *FASEB J.* 24, 2245–2253. doi: 10.1096/fj.09-137174

Montarras, D., Morgan, J., Collins, C., Relaix, F., Zaffran, S., Cumano, A., et al. (2005). Direct isolation of satellite cells for skeletal muscle regeneration. *Science* 309, 2064–2067. doi: 10.1126/science.1114758

Moriyama, M., Osawa, M., Mak, S. S., Ohtsuka, T., Yamamoto, N., Han, H., et al. (2006). Notch signaling via Hes1 transcription factor maintains survival of melanoblasts and melanocyte stem cells. *J. Cell Biol.* 173, 333–339. doi: 10.1083/jcb.200509084

Morrison, J. I., Loof, S., He, P., and Simon, A. (2006). Salamander limb regeneration involves the activation of a multipotent skeletal muscle satellite cell population. *J. Cell Biol.* 172, 433–440. doi: 10.1083/jcb.200509011

Moss, F. P., and Leblond, C. P. (1970). Nature of dividing nuclei in skeletal muscle of growing rats. *J. Cell Biol.* 44, 459–462. doi: 10.1083/jcb.44.2.459

Mourikis, P., Sambasivan, R., Castel, D., Rocheteau, P., Bizzarro, V., and Tajbakhsh, S. (2012). A Critical Requirement for Notch Signaling in Maintenance of the Quiescent Skeletal Muscle Stem Cell State. *Stem Cells* 30, 243–252. doi: 10.1002/stem.775

Mukherjee, T., Kim, W. S., Mandal, L., and Banerjee, U. (2011). Interaction between Notch and Hif-alpha in development and survival of Drosophila blood cells. *Science* 332, 1210–1213. doi: 10.1126/science.1199643

Nieman, D. C., and Pedersen, B. K. (1999). Exercise and immune function. Recent developments. *Sports Med.* 27, 73–80. doi: 10.2165/00007256-199927020-00001

Nnodim, J. O. (2000). Satellite cell numbers in senile rat levator ani muscle. *Mech. Ageing Dev.* 112, 99–111. doi: 10.1016/S0047-6374(99)00076-7

Noseda, M., Chang, L., McLean, G., Grim, J. E., Clurman, B. E., Smith, L. L., et al. (2004). Notch activation induces endothelial cell cycle arrest and participates in contact inhibition: role of p21Cip1 repression. *Mol. Cell Biol.* 24, 8813–8822. doi: 10.1128/MCB.24.20.8813-8822.2004

Odelberg, S. J., Kollhoff, A., and Keating, M. T. (2000). Dedifferentiation of mammalian myotubes induced by msx1. *Cell* 103, 1099–1109. doi: 10.1016/S0092-8674(00)00212-9

Osawa, M., Hanada, K., Hamada, H., and Nakauchi, H. (1996). Long-term lymphohematopoietic reconstitution by a single CD34-low/negative hematopoietic stem cell. *Science* 273, 242–245. doi: 10.1126/science.273.5272.242

Oshimori, N., and Fuchs, E. (2012). The harmonies played by TGF-beta in stem cell biology. *Cell Stem Cell* 11, 751–764. doi: 10.1016/j.stem.2012.11.001

Pallafacchina, G., Francois, S., Regnault, B., Czarny, B., Dive, V., Cumano, A., et al. (2010). An adult tissue-specific stem cell in its niche: a gene profiling analysis of *in vivo* quiescent and activated muscle satellite cells. *Stem Cell Res.* 4, 77–91. doi: 10.1016/j.scr.2009.10.003

Park, J. T., Li, M., Nakayama, K., Mao, T. L., Davidson, B., Zhang, Z., et al. (2006). Notch3 gene amplification in ovarian cancer. *Cancer Res.* 66, 6312–6318. doi: 10.1158/0008-5472.CAN-05-3610

Parker, M. H., Loretz, C., Tyler, A. E., Duddy, W. J., Hall, J. K., Olwin, B. B., et al. (2012). Activation of Notch signaling during *ex vivo* expansion maintains donor muscle cell engraftment. *Stem Cells* 30, 2212–2220. doi: 10.1002/stem.1181

Pellegrinet, L., Rodilla, V., Liu, Z., Chen, S., Koch, U., Espinosa, L., et al. (2011). Dll1- and dll4-mediated notch signaling are required for homeostasis of intestinal stem cells. *Gastroenterology* 140, 1230–1240; e1231–e1237. doi: 10.1053/j.gastro.2011.01.005

Penna, F., Costamagna, D., Fanzani, A., Bonelli, G., Baccino, F. M., and Costelli, P. (2010). Muscle wasting and impaired myogenesis in tumor bearing mice are prevented by ERK inhibition. *PLoS ONE* 5:e13604. doi: 10.1371/journal.pone.0013604

Polesskaya, A., Seale, P., and Rudnicki, M. A. (2003). Wnt signaling induces the myogenic specification of resident CD45+ adult stem cells during muscle regeneration. *Cell* 113, 841–852. doi: 10.1016/S0092-8674(03)00437-9

Relaix, F., Rocancourt, D., Mansouri, A., and Buckingham, M. (2005). A Pax3/Pax7-dependent population of skeletal muscle progenitor cells. *Nature* 435, 948–953. doi: 10.1038/nature03594

Rios, A. C., Serralbo, O., Salgado, D., and Marcelle, C. (2011). Neural crest regulates myogenesis through the transient activation of NOTCH. *Nature* 473, 532–535. doi: 10.1038/nature09970

Roberts, E. W., Deonarine, A., Jones, J. O., Denton, A. E., Feig, C., Lyons, S. K., et al. (2013). Depletion of stromal cells expressing fibroblast activation protein-alpha from skeletal muscle and bone marrow results in cachexia and anemia. *J. Exp. Med.* 210, 1137–1151. doi: 10.1084/jem.20122344

Rosenblatt, J. D., Lunt, A. I., Parry, D. J., and Partridge, T. A. (1995). Culturing satellite cells from living single muscle fiber explants. *In Vitro Cell. Dev. Biol. Anim.* 31, 773–779. doi: 10.1007/BF02634119

Sacco, A., Doyonnas, R., Kraft, P., Vitorovic, S., and Blau, H. M. (2008). Self-renewal and expansion of single transplanted muscle stem cells. *Nature* 456, 502–506. doi: 10.1038/nature07384

Sacco, A., Mourkioti, F., Tran, R., Choi, J., Llewellyn, M., Kraft, P., et al. (2010). Short telomeres and stem cell exhaustion model Duchenne muscular dystrophy in mdx/mTR mice. *Cell* 143, 1059–1071. doi: 10.1016/j.cell.2010.11.039

Sadeh, M., Czyewski, K., and Stern, L. Z. (1985). Chronic myopathy induced by repeated bupivacaine injections. *J. Neurol. Sci.* 67, 229–238. doi: 10.1016/0022-510X(85)90119-4

Sakai, H., Sato, T., Sakurai, H., Yamamoto, T., Hanaoka, K., Montarras, D., et al. (2013). Fetal skeletal muscle progenitors have regenerative capacity after intramuscular engraftment in dystrophin deficient mice. *PLoS ONE* 8:e63016. doi: 10.1371/journal.pone.0063016

Sambasivan, R., Yao, R., Kissenpfennig, A., Van Wittenberghe, L., Paldi, A., Gayraud-Morel, B., et al. (2011). Pax7-expressing satellite cells are indispensable for adult skeletal muscle regeneration. *Development* 138, 3647–3656. doi: 10.1242/dev.067587

Sang, L., Coller, H. A., and Roberts, J. M. (2008). Control of the reversibility of cellular quiescence by the transcriptional repressor HES1. *Science* 321, 1095–1100. doi: 10.1126/science.1155998

Schafer, R., Zweyer, M., Knauf, U., Mundegar, R. R., and Wernig, A. (2005). The ontogeny of soleus muscles in mdx and wild type mice. *Neuromuscul. Disord.* 15, 57–64. doi: 10.1016/j.nmd.2004.09.011

Schultz, E., Gibson, M. C., and Champion, T. (1978). Satellite cells are mitotically quiescent in mature mouse muscle: an EM and radioautographic study. *J. Exp. Zool.* 206, 451–456. doi: 10.1002/jez.1402060314

Seale, P., Sabourin, L. A., Girgis-Gabardo, A., Mansouri, A., Gruss, P., and Rudnicki, M. A. (2000). Pax7 is required for the specification of myogenic satellite cells. *Cell* 102, 777–786. doi: 10.1016/S0092-8674(00)00066-0

Segawa, M., Fukada, S., Yamamoto, Y., Yahagi, H., Kanematsu, M., Sato, M., et al. (2008). Suppression of macrophage functions impairs skeletal muscle regeneration with severe fibrosis. *Exp. Cell Res.* 314, 3232–3244. doi: 10.1016/j.yexcr.2008.08.008

Shea, K. L., Xiang, W., LaPorta, V. S., Licht, J. D., Keller, C., Basson, M. A., et al. (2010). Sprouty1 regulates reversible quiescence of a self-renewing adult muscle stem cell pool during regeneration. *Cell Stem Cell* 6, 117–129. doi: 10.1016/j.stem.2009.12.015

Sherwood, R. I., Christensen, J. L., Conboy, I. M., Conboy, M. J., Rando, T. A., Weissman, I. L., et al. (2004). Isolation of adult mouse myogenic progenitors: functional heterogeneity of cells within and engrafting skeletal muscle. *Cell* 119, 543–554. doi: 10.1016/j.cell.2004.10.021

Shinin, V., Gayraud-Morel, B., Gomes, D., and Tajbakhsh, S. (2006). Asymmetric division and cosegregation of template DNA strands in adult muscle satellite cells. *Nat. Cell Biol.* 8, 677–687. doi: 10.1038/ncb1425

Snijders, T., Verdijk, L. B., and van Loon, L. J. (2009). The impact of sarcopenia and exercise training on skeletal muscle satellite cells. *Ageing Res. Rev.* 8, 328–338. doi: 10.1016/j.arr.2009.05.003

Starkey, J. D., Yamamoto, M., Yamamoto, S., and Goldhamer, D. J. (2011). Skeletal muscle satellite cells are committed to myogenesis and do not spontaneously adopt nonmyogenic fates. *J. Histochem. Cytochem.* 59, 33–46. doi: 10.1369/jhc.2010.956995

Sun, D., Li, H., and Zolkiewska, A. (2008). The role of Delta-like 1 shedding in muscle cell self-renewal and differentiation. *J. Cell Sci.* 121, 3815–3823. doi: 10.1242/jcs.035493

Suzuki, H., Nakamura, I., Takahashi, N., Ikuhara, T., Matsuzaki, K., Isogai, Y., et al. (1996). Calcitonin-induced changes in the cytoskeleton are mediated by a signal pathway associated with protein kinase A in osteoclasts. *Endocrinology* 137, 4685–4690. doi: 10.1210/en.137.11.4685

Suzuki, N., Fukushi, M., Kosaki, K., Doyle, A. D., de Vega, S., Yoshizaki, K., et al. (2012). Teneurin-4 is a novel regulator of oligodendrocyte differentiation and myelination of small-diameter axons in the CNS. *J. Neurosci.* 32, 11586–11599. doi: 10.1523/JNEUROSCI.2045-11.2012

Takahashi, K., Tanabe, K., Ohnuki, M., Narita, M., Ichisaka, T., Tomoda, K., et al. (2007). Induction of pluripotent stem cells from adult human fibroblasts by defined factors. *Cell* 131, 861–872. doi: 10.1016/j.cell.2007.11.019

Takahashi, K., and Yamanaka, S. (2006). Induction of pluripotent stem cells from mouse embryonic and adult fibroblast cultures by defined factors. *Cell* 126, 663–676. doi: 10.1016/j.cell.2006.07.024

Tamaki, T., Akatsuka, A., Ando, K., Nakamura, Y., Matsuzawa, H., Hotta, T., et al. (2002). Identification of myogenic-endothelial progenitor cells in the interstitial spaces of skeletal muscle. *J. Cell Biol.* 157, 571–577. doi: 10.1083/jcb.200112106

Tanaka, K. K., Hall, J. K., Troy, A. A., Cornelison, D. D., Majka, S. M., and Olwin, B. B. (2009). Syndecan-4-expressing muscle progenitor cells in the SP engraft as satellite cells during muscle regeneration. *Cell Stem Cell* 4, 217–225. doi: 10.1016/j.stem.2009.01.016

Thomas, S., and Shah, G. (2005). Calcitonin induces apoptosis resistance in prostate cancer cell lines against cytotoxic drugs via the Akt/survivin pathway. *Cancer Biol. Ther.* 4, 1226–1233. doi: 10.4161/cbt.4.11.2093

Tokura, Y., Nakayama, Y., Fukada, S., Nara, N., Yamamoto, H., Matsuda, R., et al. (2011). Muscle injury-induced thymosin beta4 acts as a chemoattractant for myoblasts. *J. Biochem.* 149, 43–48. doi: 10.1093/jb/mvq115

Trendelenburg, A. U., Meyer, A., Jacobi, C., Feige, J. N., and Glass, D. J. (2012). TAK-1/p38/nNFkappaB signaling inhibits myoblast differentiation by increasing levels of Activin A. *Skeletal Muscle* 2:3. doi: 10.1186/2044-5040-2-3

Tu, X., Chen, J., Lim, J., Karner, C. M., Lee, S. Y., Heisig, J., et al. (2012). Physiological notch signaling maintains bone homeostasis via RBPjk and Hey upstream of NFATc1. *PLoS Genet.* 8:e1002577. doi: 10.1371/journal.pgen.1002577

Uezumi, A., Fukada, S., Yamamoto, N., Takeda, S., and Tsuchida, K. (2010). Mesenchymal progenitors distinct from satellite cells contribute to ectopic fat cell formation in skeletal muscle. *Nat. Cell Biol.* 12, 143–152. doi: 10.1038/ncb2014

Uezumi, A., Ito, T., Morikawa, D., Shimizu, N., Yoneda, T., Segawa, M., et al. (2011). Fibrosis and adipogenesis originate from a common mesenchymal progenitor in skeletal muscle. *J. Cell Sci.* 124, 3654–3664. doi: 10.1242/jcs.086629

Uezumi, A., Ojima, K., Fukada, S., Ikemoto, M., Masuda, S., Miyagoe-Suzuki, Y., et al. (2006). Functional heterogeneity of side population cells in skeletal muscle. *Biochem. Biophys. Res. Commun.* 341, 864–873. doi: 10.1016/j.bbrc.2006.01.037

Urciuolo, A., Quarta, M., Morbidoni, V., Gattazzo, F., Molon, S., Grumati, P., et al. (2013). Collagen VI regulates satellite cell self-renewal and muscle regeneration. *Nat. Commun.* 4, 1964. doi: 10.1038/ncomms2964

Vasyutina, E., Lenhard, D. C., Wende, H., Erdmann, B., Epstein, J. A., and Birchmeier, C. (2007). RBP-J (Rbpsuh) is essential to maintain muscle progenitor cells and to generate satellite cells. *Proc. Natl. Acad. Sci. U.S.A.* 104, 4443–4448. doi: 10.1073/pnas.0610647104

Verdijk, L. B., Koopman, R., Schaart, G., Meijer, K., Savelberg, H. H., and van Loon, L. J. (2007). Satellite cell content is specifically reduced in type II skeletal muscle fibers in the elderly. *Am. J. Physiol. Endocrinol. Metab.* 292, E151–E157. doi: 10.1152/ajpendo.00278.2006

Verma, M., Asakura, Y., Hirai, H., Watanabe, S., Tastad, C., Fong, G. H., et al. (2010). Flt-1 haploinsufficiency ameliorates muscular dystrophy phenotype by developmentally increased vasculature in mdx mice. *Hum. Mol. Genet.* 19, 4145–4159. doi: 10.1093/hmg/ddq334

von Maltzahn, J., Renaud, J. M., Parise, G., and Rudnicki, M. A. (2012). Wnt7a treatment ameliorates muscular dystrophy. *Proc. Natl. Acad. Sci. U.S.A.* 109, 20614–20619. doi: 10.1073/pnas.1215765109

Wang, H., Noulet, F., Edom-Vovard, F., Tozer, S., Le Grand, F., and Duprez, D. (2010). Bmp signaling at the tips of skeletal muscles regulates the number of fetal muscle progenitors and satellite cells during development. *Dev. Cell* 18, 643–654. doi: 10.1016/j.devcel.2010.02.008

Wang, X. Z., Jolicoeur, E. M., Conte, N., Chaffanet, M., Zhang, Y., Mozziconacci, M. J., et al. (1999). gamma-heregulin is the product of a chromosomal translocation fusing the DOC4 and HGL/NRG1 genes in the MDA-MB-175 breast cancer cell line. *Oncogene* 18, 5718–5721. doi: 10.1038/sj.onc.1202950

White, R. B., Bierinx, A. S., Gnocchi, V. F., and Zammit, P. S. (2010). Dynamics of muscle fibre growth during postnatal mouse development. *BMC Dev. Biol.* 10:21. doi: 10.1186/1471-213X-10-21

Yaffe, D., and Saxel, O. (1977). Serial passaging and differentiation of myogenic cells isolated from dystrophic mouse muscle. *Nature* 270, 725–727. doi: 10.1038/270725a0

Yajima, H., Motohashi, N., Ono, Y., Sato, S., Ikeda, K., Masuda, S., et al. (2010). Six family genes control the proliferation and differentiation of muscle satellite cells. *Exp. Cell Res.* 316, 2932–2944. doi: 10.1016/j.yexcr.2010.08.001

Yamaguchi, M., and Fukada, S. (2013). "Regulation of muscle stem cell quiescent and undifferentiated state: roles of Hesr1 and Hesr3 genes," in *Tumor Dormancy, Quiescence, and Senescence*, Vol. 1, ed. M. A. Hayat (Netherlands: Springer), 107–116.

Yamaguchi, M., Ogawa, R., Watanabe, Y., Uezumi, A., Miyagoe-Suzuki, Y., Tsujikawa, K., et al. (2012). Calcitonin receptor and Odz4 are differently expressed in Pax7-positive cells during skeletal muscle regeneration. *J. Mol. Histol.* 43, 581–587. doi: 10.1007/s10735-012-9421-3

Yamazaki, S., Ema, H., Karlsson, G., Yamaguchi, T., Miyoshi, H., Shioda, S., et al. (2011). Nonmyelinating Schwann cells maintain hematopoietic stem cell hibernation in the bone marrow niche. *Cell* 147, 1146–1158. doi: 10.1016/j.cell.2011.09.053

Zhou, X., Wang, J. L., Lu, J., Song, Y., Kwak, K. S., Jiao, Q., et al. (2010). Reversal of cancer cachexia and muscle wasting by ActRIIB antagonism leads to prolonged survival. *Cell* 142, 531–543. doi: 10.1016/j.cell.2010.07.011

Zhou, X. H., Brandau, O., Feng, K., Oohashi, T., Ninomiya, Y., Rauch, U., et al. (2003). The murine Ten-m/Odz genes show distinct but overlapping expression patterns during development and in adult brain. *Gene Expr. Patterns* 3, 397–405. doi: 10.1016/S1567-133X(03)00087-5

13

Muscle hypertrophy is associated with increases in proteasome activity that is independent of MuRF1 and MAFbx expression

Leslie M. Baehr[1], *Matthew Tunzi*[2] *and Sue C. Bodine*[1,2]*

[1] *Department of Physiology and Membrane Biology, University of California, Davis, Davis, CA, USA*
[2] *Department of Neurobiology, Physiology, and Behavior, University of California, Davis, Davis, CA, USA*

Correspondence:
Sue C. Bodine, Department of Neurobiology, Physiology, and Behavior, University of California, Davis, One Shields Ave., Davis, CA 95616, USA
e-mail: scbodine@ucdavis.edu

The regulation of skeletal muscle mass depends on the balance between protein synthesis and degradation. The role of protein degradation and in particular, the ubiquitin proteasome system, and increased expression of the E3 ubiquitin ligases, MuRF1 and MAFbx/atrogin-1, in the regulation of muscle size in response to growth stimuli is unclear. Thus, the aim of this study was to measure both proteasome activity and protein synthesis in mice over a 14-day period of chronic loading using the functional overload (FO) model. Further, the importance of MuRF1 and MAFbx expression in regulating muscle hypertrophy was examined by measuring muscle growth in response to FO in mice with a null deletion (KO) of either MuRF1 or MAFbx. In wild type (WT) mice, the increase in muscle mass correlated with significant increases (2-fold) in protein synthesis at 7 and 14 days. Interestingly, proteasome activity significantly increased in WT mice after one day, and continued to increase, peaking at 7 days following FO. The increase in proteasome activity was correlated with increases in the expression of the Forkhead transcription factors, FOXO1 and FOXO3a, which increased after both MuRF1 and MAFbx increased and returned to baseline. As in WT mice, hypertrophy in the MuRF1 and MAFbx KO mice was associated with significant increases in proteasome activity after 14 days of FO. The increase in plantaris mass was similar between the WT and MuRF1 KO mice following FO, however, muscle growth was significantly reduced in female MAFbx KO mice. Collectively, these results indicate that muscle hypertrophy is associated with increases in both protein synthesis and degradation. Further, MuRF1 or MAFbx expression is not required to increase proteasome activity following increased loading, however, MAFbx expression may be required for proper growth/remodeling of muscle in response to increase loading.

Keywords: ubiquitin proteasome system, protein degradation, puromycin, functional overload, forkhead transcription factors

INTRODUCTION

Skeletal muscle is a highly plastic tissue that modifies its size through the regulation of signaling pathways that control protein synthesis and protein degradation. In response to increases in mechanical loading, muscle hypertrophy, or an increase in muscle size, occurs as the result of a net increase in protein synthesis relative to degradation. It has been well demonstrated that the Akt/mTOR signaling pathway is a major regulator of muscle growth, as activation of S6K1, eIF4E, and eIF2B stimulate mRNA translation and ultimately lead to increases in protein synthesis (Bodine et al., 2001b; Rommel et al., 2001; Kubica et al., 2008). In addition, recent work has revealed that both beta adrenergic signaling (Minetti et al., 2011) and bone morphogenetic protein (BMP) signaling (Sartori et al., 2013) can regulate muscle mass and promote skeletal muscle hypertrophy. What is less understood is the role of protein degradation in the remodeling process that occurs in response to loading and leads to an increase in fiber cross-sectional area.

Increases in protein degradation are generally associated with the loss of muscle mass, i.e., atrophy, and occur in response to decreased loading, inactivity, and a variety of pathological conditions. In skeletal muscle, the ubiquitin proteasome system (UPS) is responsible for the majority of protein degradation (Rock et al., 1994), although cathepsins, calpains, caspase-3, and autophagy are also involved in the breakdown of muscle proteins (Du et al., 2004, Tisdale, 2005). Associated with muscle atrophy and the increase in protein degradation is the rapid and sustained increase in MuRF1 and MAFbx/atrogin-1 expression, two muscle-specific E3 ubiquitin ligases thought to target specific proteins for degradation by the 26S proteasome (Bodine et al., 2001a). Deletion of MuRF1 or MAFbx has been shown to spare muscle mass in a variety of atrophy-inducing conditions (Bodine et al., 2001a; Labeit et al., 2010; Baehr et al., 2011), however, the role of MuRF1 and MAFbx, as well as the UPS, in regulating increases in muscle fiber size is less clear.

A few studies have reported increases in MuRF1 and MAFbx expression following an acute bout of resistance exercise in humans, however, no studies have made concurrent measurements of protein synthesis and UPS activity following chronic mechanical loading (Yang et al., 2006; Louis et al., 2007;

Marino et al., 2008). Thus, the aim of this study was to examine both protein synthesis and proteasome activity, along with MuRF1 and MAFbx expression in mice over 14 days of chronic loading using the functional overload (FO) model. Furthermore, although we have recently shown that muscle growth is not impaired in young or old MuRF1 KO mice (Hwee et al., 2013), it remains to be seen whether growth is affected by the loss of MAFbx, and whether the loss of MuRF1 or MAFbx depresses proteasome activity under anabolic conditions.

MATERIALS AND METHODS

ANIMALS

Forty three month old male C57BL/6 wild type (WT) mice and 110 9 month old male and female MuRF1 and MAFbx null (KO) mice were used for this study. The WT mice were purchased from Jackson Laboratories and the MuRF1 ($n = 60$) and MAFbx ($n = 50$) null mice were generated from a breeding colony maintained by the UCD Mouse Biology Program in a mouse barrier facility. To induce hypertrophy of the plantaris muscle, mice were subjected to bilateral functional overload. Mice were anaesthetized with 2–3% inhaled isoflurane and using aseptic technique, the ankle extensor muscles and Achilles tendon were exposed by making a small incision to the posterior lower limb. The entire soleus and over half of the medial and lateral gastrocnemius muscles were removed from each hindlimb without damaging the plantaris neural-vascular supply. The wound was irrigated with sterile saline and the incision was closed with subcuticular sutures. Mice were given an analgesic (buprenorphine, 0.1 mg/kg) immediately following the surgery and returned to their cage once they recovered.

At 1, 3, 7, and 14 days post-surgery, the WT animals were anesthetized with 2–3% inhaled isoflurane and the plantaris muscles were removed, weighed, frozen in liquid nitrogen, and stored at −80°C for future analysis. For the MuRF1 and MAFbx KO mice, the plantaris muscles were removed and weighed following 14 days of FO. The right plantaris muscle was pinned on cork at a length approximating L_0 and frozen in isopentane cooled in liquid nitrogen for histological analysis while the left plantaris muscle was frozen in liquid nitrogen and stored at—80°C. Following tissues collection, the mice were euthanized by exsanguination. All animal procedures were approved by the Institutional Animal Care and Use Committee at the University of California, Davis.

PROTEIN SYNTHESIS MEASUREMENTS

Protein synthesis was measured *in vivo* in the WT mice using the SUnSET method as previously described (Goodman et al., 2011b). Exactly 30 min before the plantaris muscles were excised, mice were given an intraperitoneal injection of 0.04 μmol/g puromycin dissolved in 100 μl of phosphate buffered saline (PBS) ($n = 5$/group). Puromycin expression was analyzed by Western Blot as described below.

mRNA EXPRESSION ANALYSIS

Total RNA was extracted from powdered plantaris muscle using TRIzol reagent according to the manufacturer's instructions (Invitrogen). cDNA was then synthesized using a QuantiTech Reverse Transcription Kit (Qiagen) from one μg of total RNA. *MuRF1 and MAFbx* gene expression was measured by quantitative PCR (qPCR) in WT mice following 1, 3, 7, and 14 days of FO ($n = 7$/group). qPCR was performed using *Power* SYBR® Green PCR Master Mix (Life Technologies) on an ABI 7900HT thermocycler. Cycling conditions were one cycle at 94°C for 10 min followed by forty cycles at 94°C for 30 s, 59°C for 30 s, and 72°C for 30 s. Each sample was run in triplicate. Sequences of the mouse forward and reverse primers are as follows: MuRF1 forward: 5′-GCTGGTGGAAAA CATCATTGACAT-3′; reverse: 5′-CATCGGGTGGCTGCCTTT-3′; MAFbx forward: 5′-CTTTCAACAGACTGGACTTCTCGA-3′; reverse: 5′-CAGCTCCAACAGCCTTACTACGT-3′; FOXO1 forward: 5′-TTCCTTCATTCTGCACACGA-3′; reverse: 5′-GTC CTACGCCGACCTCATC-3′; FOXO3a forward: 5′-CAGGCTCCT CACTGTATTCAGCTA-3′; reverse: 5′-CATTGAACATGTCCAG GTCCAA-3′; GAPDH forward: 5′- CCAGCCTCGTCCCGTAG AC-3′; reverse: 5′- ATGGCAACAATCTCCACTTTGC-3′. All data was normalized to GAPDH expression.

PROTEASOME ACTIVITY

20S and 26S β5 proteasome activity was measured as previously described (Gomes et al., 2012). Briefly, proteasomes were collected in the supernatant after 30 min centrifugation at 12,000 *g* following homogenization in 300 μl of buffer containing 50 mM Tris, 150 mM NaCl, 5 mM MgCl2, 1 mM EDTA, and 0.5 mM DTT at pH 7.5. The chymotrypsin (β5)-like activities were assayed using 10 μg of protein and the fluorescently tagged substrate SUC-LLVY-AMC (Bachem). Both assays were carried out in a total volume of 100 μl. The 26S ATP-dependent assay was performed in homogenization buffer with the addition of 100 μM ATP. The 20S ATP-independent assay was carried out in assay buffer containing 25 mM HEPES, 0.5 mM EDTA, and 0.001% SDS (pH 7.5). Each assay was conducted in the absence and presence of the proteasome inhibitor Bortezomib at a final concentration of 2 mM. The activity of the 20S and 26S proteasome was measured by calculating the difference between fluorescence units recorded with or without the inhibitor in the reaction medium. Released AMC was measured using a Fluoroskan Ascent fluorometer (Thermo Electron) at an excitation wavelength of 390 nm and an emission wavelength of 460 nm. Fluorescence was measured at 15-min intervals for 2 h. All assays were linear in this range and each sample was assayed in triplicate.

WESTERN BLOTTING

Frozen plantaris muscles from control and FO mice were homogenized in proteasome assay lysis buffer (50 mM Tris, 150 mM NaCl, 5 mM MgCl2, 1 mM EDTA, and 0.5 mM DTT at pH 7.5). The supernatant was collected following centrifugation at 12,000 *g* for 30 min and protein concentrations were determined in triplicate using the Bradford method (Bio-Rad). Ten to twenty micrograms of protein was subjected to SDS-PAGE on 10% acrylamide gels and transferred to polyvinylidene diflouride (PVDF) membrane. Membranes were blocked in 3% nonfat dairy milk in Tris-buffered saline with 0.1% Tween-20 added (TBST) or 1% pigskin gelatin for 1 h and then probed with primary antibody overnight at 4°C. Puromycin (Millipore), BiP (BD Biosciences), PDI (Cell Signaling), and CHOP (Cell Signaling) were used at a concentration of 1:1000. The next day, membranes were washed and incubated with HRP conjugated secondary antibodies at 1:10,000 for 1 h at room temperature. Immobilon Western Chemiluminescent HRP substrate (Millipore) was then added to the membranes. Image acquisition and band quantification was performed using the ChemiDoc™ MP System and Image Lab 5.0 software (Biorad).

STATISTICS

Results are presented as mean ± standard deviation (*SD*) unless otherwise indicated. The data was analyzed by One-Way ANOVA or by Student's *t*-test (Sigma Stat). Tukey's *post-hoc* analysis was used to determine differences when interactions existed. Statistical significance was set at $p < 0.05$.

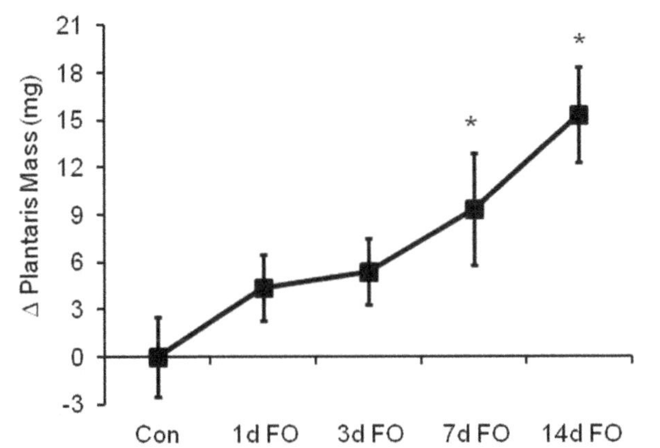

FIGURE 1 | Time course of load-induced growth in wild type (WT) mice following functional overload (FO). Growth of the plantaris muscle was calculated after 1, 3, 7, and 14 days of FO and expressed as a change in mass relative to the control group. Data are expressed as mean ± SD ($n = 8$/group). *$P < 0.05$ vs. control.

RESULTS

To determine the extent to which the ubiquitin proteasome system (UPS) is activated during a model of load-induced muscle growth, male C57BL/6 mice were subjected to bilateral functional overload for 1, 3, 7, or 14 days. As shown in **Figure 1**, the response of the plantaris to an increase in load was a swift and steady increase in size over 14 days. Significant increases in mass of 43 and 65% were observed after 7 and 14 days, respectively.

Given the significant hypertrophy of the plantaris muscle, we next looked at changes in protein synthesis in the plantaris muscle over a 14-day period of FO. Protein synthesis was measured *in vivo* using the SUrface SEnsing of Translation (SUnSET) method, a nonradioactive technique in which changes in the rate of protein synthesis are reflected by the amount of puromycin that is incorporated into newly synthesized proteins (Schmidt et al., 2009; Goodman et al., 2011b). Using this method, we found that protein synthesis increased by 58% at 3 days and was significantly elevated from 7 to 14 days of FO, reaching a level that was 100% above control within the first 14 days of FO (**Figure 2**).

Increases in ER stress can occur during high rates of protein synthesis (Rayavarapu et al., 2012). Considering that FO produces significant muscle hypertrophy, we investigated the expression of various ER stress markers in the plantaris muscle following FO. As shown in **Figure 3**, we found significant increases in BiP and PDI expression beginning at 3 days post FO, with the largest increase seen after 7 days of FO. The maladaptive ER stress marker CHOP was also found to increase over the 14 days following FO, however, the relative increase was significantly lower than that observed for BiP and PDI (**Figure 3B**).

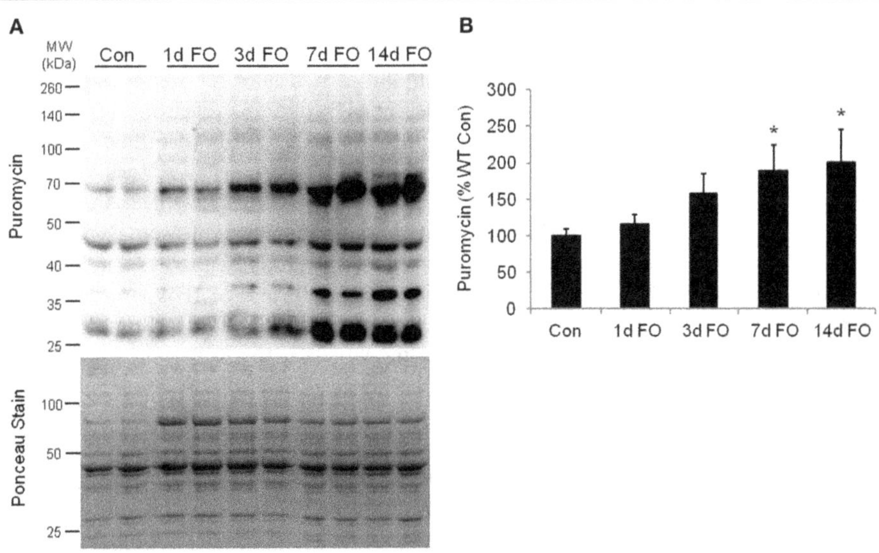

FIGURE 2 | Measurement of protein synthesis using the SUnSET method following functional overload (FO). (A) Representative image of western blot analysis for puromycin following no treatment (Con) and FO for 1, 3, 7, or 14 days in WT mice. The corresponding ponceau stain was used to verify equal loading of proteins. **(B)** Quantification of the puromycin western blots. Puromycin values are expressed as a percentage of the control muscles value (mean ± *SD*, $n = 5$/group). *$P < 0.05$ vs. control puromycin expression.

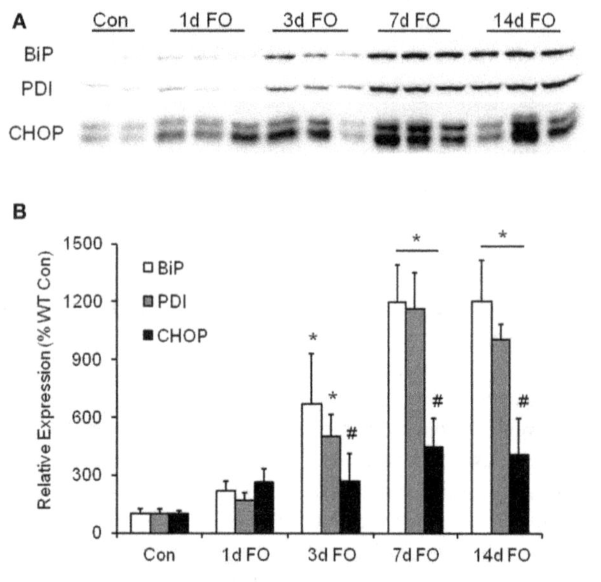

FIGURE 3 | Markers of endoplasmic reticulum (ER) stress are higher in the plantaris muscle following functional overload (FO). (A) Representative western blot of ER stress markers BiP, PDI, and CHOP in WT mice after no treatment (Con) and 1, 3, 7, and 14 days of FO. **(B)** Quantification of the western blots for BiP (open bars), PDI (gray bars), and CHOP (black bars). A ponceau stain of the membrane was used to normalize protein expression. Data are expressed as a percentage of the respective control value for each protein (mean ± *SD*, $n = 4$–6/group). $^{*}P < 0.05$ vs. control expression for each protein, $^{\#}P < 0.05$ CHOP vs. BiP, or PDI at given time point.

In humans, resistance exercise has been shown to increase protein degradation (Phillips et al., 1997), but it is unclear whether this breakdown is related to upregulation of MuRF1 and MAFbx expression or alterations in proteasome activity. Thus, we measured the time course of MuRF1 and MAFbx expression and the chymotrypsin-like (β5) proteasome activities in WT mice following FO. In addition, the time course of FOXO1 and FOXO3a expression was measured since they are known transcriptional regulators of MuRF1 and MAFbx under atrophy conditions (Sandri et al., 2004; Waddell et al., 2008). Expression of both MuRF1 and MAFbx was found to increase significantly after one day of FO, but then return to control levels by 3 days post FO (**Figures 4A,B**). After 3 days of FO, gene expression was suppressed below control levels, with significant reductions in MAFbx expression occurring after 7 and 14 days of FO (**Figure 4B**). The rapid increase in MuRF1 and MAFbx expression was mirrored by significant increases in 20S and 26S β5 proteasome activity after 1 day of FO, but unlike MuRF1 and MAFbx, proteasome activity remained elevated throughout the 14 days of chronic loading (**Figures 4D,E**). Peak activity for the 20S proteasome was found to occur at 3 days post FO, while peak activity for the 26S proteasome was found at 7 days post FO. Surprisingly, the pattern of FOXO1 and FOXO3a expression was more similar to that of the 26S β5 proteasome rather than MuRF1 and MAFbx expression. Significant increases in FOXO1 and FOXO3a expression did not occur until 3 days post FO, after which expression of both genes continued to increase through 7 days of FO before returning to baseline levels at 14 days post FO (**Figure 4C**).

Given the changes in MuRF1 and MAFbx expression and proteasome activity following functional overload, we then asked if deletion of MuRF1 or MAFbx compromised muscle growth. Fourteen days of overload produced significant growth of the plantaris in both female and male MuRF1 KO mice, which was similar to that observed in WT mice of both genders (**Figure 5**). This result is comparable to what has been previously reported for male MuRF1 KO mice (Hwee et al., 2013). In contrast, the deletion of MAFbx appeared to have a significant effect on load-induced growth, especially in female mice (**Figure 5**). In response to overload, a significant increase in plantaris mass was measured in male MAFbx KO mice, with the mean increase in mass being slightly less and more variable in the MAFbx KO (range of mass: 20–34 mg) compared to the WT (range of mass: 29–37 mg) mice. In female mice, however, MAFbx KO mice showed no significant growth in response to FO, which differed significantly from what was observed in the WT mice (**Figure 5**).

The decrease in muscle growth did not appear to be due to an inability to activate the proteasome, as both MuRF1 and MAFbx KO mice had similar increases in 26S β5 proteasome activity following 14 days of FO (**Figure 6**). Since we did not have sufficient numbers of KO mice to collect FO data at 3 and 7 days, we do not know whether proteasome activity in the KO mice increased to the same extent as the WT mice.

DISCUSSION

Proteolysis is essential for normal muscle function and routine protein turnover. Most cellular proteins are degraded by the UPS (Rock et al., 1994; Mitch and Goldberg, 1996), a highly selective system that targets proteins for breakdown via the addition of a polyubiquitin chain. The coordinated effort of three groups of enzymes, termed E1, E2, and E3s, results in the attachment of ubiquitin to a substrate protein, with multiple lysine 48-linked ubiquitin molecules serving as a signal for that protein to be degraded by the 26S proteasome (Chau et al., 1989). Both MuRF1 and MAFbx have been identified as muscle-specific E3 ubiquitin ligases, making them responsible for catalyzing the transfer of ubiquitin from the E2 enzyme to the substrate protein. In skeletal muscle, increases in proteasome activity are generally associated with muscle atrophy, a process that is characterized by the induction of MuRF1 and MAFbx (Auclair et al., 1997; Hobler et al., 1999; Bodine et al., 2001a; Gomes et al., 2001). However, little is known about the role of the UPS during muscle growth and whether MuRF1 and/or MAFbx are required for muscle hypertrophy. Thus, the purpose of this study was to examine the time course of MuRF1 and MAFbx expression along with proteasome activity in a model of load-induced muscle growth, and to determine if MuRF1 and MAFbx KO mice show an attenuated growth response following 14 days of functional overload (FO).

Functional overload is a commonly used model for studying muscle growth in rodents and results in rapid and robust increases in muscle mass as a result of chronic overload. Hypertrophy in this model is marked by significant increases in protein synthesis, which we confirmed in this study using the puromycin technique

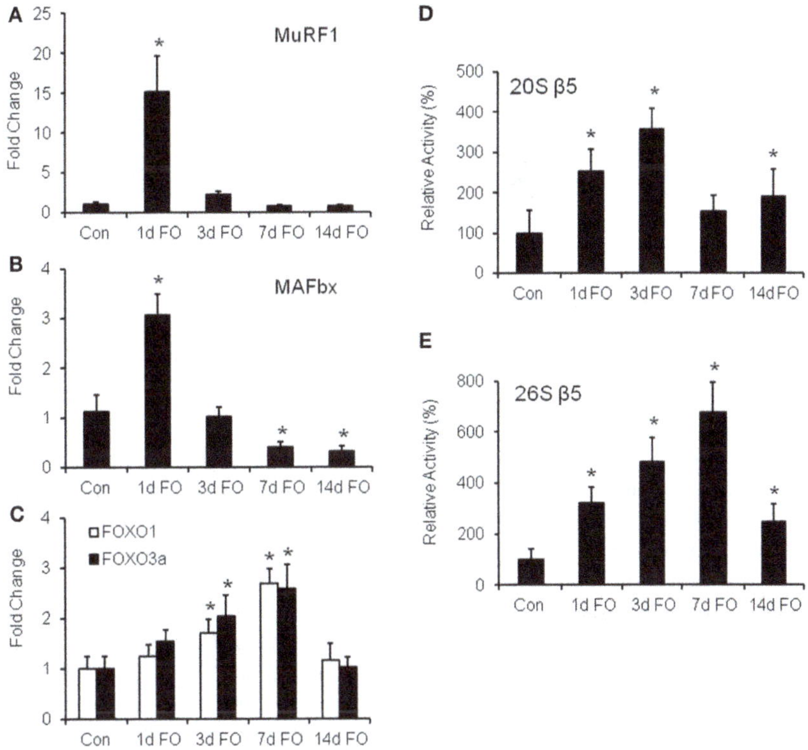

FIGURE 4 | Functional overload (FO) induces a proteolytic response in the plantaris muscle. mRNA expression of **(A)** MuRF1, **(B)** MAFbx, and **(C)** FOXO1, and FOXO3a was measured in WT mice following no treatment (Con) and FO for 1, 3, 7, or 14 days. Expression values were normalized to GAPDH and are expressed as a fold change (mean ± *SD*) relative to control ($n = 7$/group) $^{*}P < 0.05$ vs. control mRNA expression. Activity of the β5 subunit of the 20S **(D)** and 26S **(E)** proteasome was assessed by fluorometric assay in WT mice following no treatment (Con) and FO for 1, 3, 7, or 14 days. Data is expressed as a percentage of the control value (mean ± *SD*, $n = 5$–8/group). $^{*}P < 0.05$ vs. control proteolytic activity.

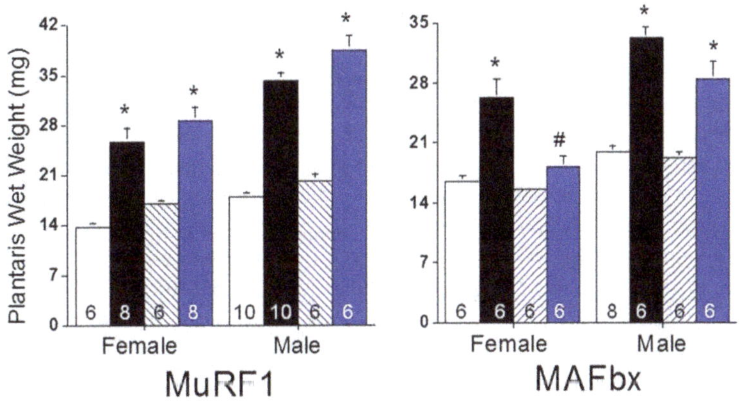

FIGURE 5 | Response of MuRF1 and MAFbx KO mice to functional overload (FO). Growth of the plantaris muscle was calculated after 14 days of FO in male and female WT, MuRF1 KO, and MAFbx KO mice and expressed as absolute wet weight (mg). Measurements were made in untreated control [white (WT) or blue hatched (KO) bars] and overloaded [black (WT) and blue (KO) bars] muscles. Data are expressed as mean ± s.e.m and group size is indicated in each bar. $^{*}P < 0.05$ vs. control; $^{\#}P < 0.05$ vs. WT FO.

(Schmidt et al., 2009; Goodman et al., 2011b). Moreover, the increase in protein synthesis was closely matched to the increase in plantaris mass in the WT mice. During this period of elevated protein synthesis, significant increases in the expression of the ER chaperone proteins BiP and PDI were also observed. An increase in BiP and PDI expression might be predicted, as an elevated rate of protein synthesis would increase the protein handling responsibilities of the endoplasmic reticulum (ER). An increase in BiP and PDI enhances the protein folding capabilities of the ER (Rayavarapu et al., 2012) and would help reduce

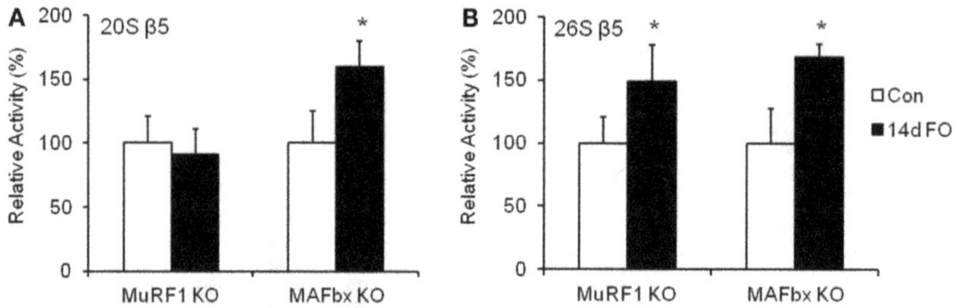

FIGURE 6 | Proteasome activity increases in MuRF1 and MAFbx null (KO) mice after 14 days of functional overload (FO). Proteolytic activity of the β5 subunit of the 20S **(A)** and 26S **(B)** proteasome was assessed by fluorometric assay in MuRF1 and MAFbx KO mice after no treatment (Con, open bars) or 14 days of functional overload (14d FO, black bars). Data are expressed as a percentage of each respective control value (mean ± *SD*, $n = 4$–6/group). $^*P < 0.05$ vs. control.

the number of misfolded proteins and keep ER stress at a minimum. An accumulation of misfolded proteins can cause the ER to activate apoptosis signaling through an increase in the expression of CHOP (Fu et al., 2008). Although FO did result in an increase in CHOP expression, the relative increase in expression was significantly lower than the increase in BiP and PDI expression, suggesting that the ER was able to implement an adaptive response to the influx of newly synthesized proteins, which ultimately get incorporated into the myofibers resulting in increases in myofiber cross-sectional area and force capacity.

A novel finding in this study was that both 20S and 26S β5 proteasome activity was increased throughout the 14 day overload period, indicating that increased loading can result in the activation of machinery involved in protein breakdown. The increase in proteasome activity occurred within the first 24 h of overload and increased to a level (4–6-fold) that was much greater than what we have observed during denervation-induced atrophy (<2-fold) (Gomes et al., 2012). Interestingly, the peak in 26S β5 activity occurred at 7 days, a time when protein synthesis was found to be significantly elevated. This finding is similar to a study by Miyazaki et al. in which protein synthesis and protein degradation rates were both found to peak at 7 days after FO (Miyazaki et al., 2011). However, it is important to note that the largest gains in muscle mass occurred between 7 and 14 days post FO, which was the time period in which protein synthesis rates were rising and proteasome activity was beginning to decrease.

An increase in MuRF1 and MAFbx expression is generally assumed to lead to an increase in proteasome activity, as a greater quantity of ubiquitin ligases should increase the number of polyubiquitinated proteins inside the cell. However, we show here that under growth conditions, proteasome activity remained elevated for a much longer time period than did the induction of MuRF1 and MAFbx. In fact, significant increases in MuRF1 and MAFbx expression were measured only at day one of FO, and by day 3 of FO, their expression had returned to baseline levels and then were suppressed below baseline levels. Our finding that MuRF1 expression is only increased at 1 day post FO differs slightly from a study by Marino et al., in which MuRF1 was found to be increased after 3 days of FO (Marino et al., 2008). However, similar results were found when comparing MAFbx expression, as we also found no induction of MAFbx at 3 days after FO followed by a significant decrease in MAFbx expression at 7 and 14 days (Marino et al., 2008). In the majority of human studies that examined proteolytic activity after an acute bout of resistance exercise, MuRF1, but not MAFbx expression has been shown to increase transiently after the exercise bout (Yang et al., 2006; Louis et al., 2007; Murton et al., 2008). However, chronic resistance training in rats resulted in decreased MuRF1 and MAFbx expression, which may be in line with this decreased expression we saw at 7 and 14 days following FO (Zanchi et al., 2009).

Our data show that MuRF1 and MAFbx are not always good markers of proteasome activity. The apparent disconnect between MuRF1 and MAFbx expression and proteasome activity has been previously observed. In a study by Vary et al., acute alcohol intoxication increased MuRF1 and MAFbx expression, but did not increase skeletal muscle proteolysis (Vary et al., 2008). Similarly, we have shown that 14 days of glucocorticoid treatment did not result in an increase in activity for any of the three catalytic subunits of the proteasome despite significant upregulation of MuRF1 and MAFbx expression (Baehr et al., 2011). Conversely, when mice were allowed to recover following 7 days of hindlimb unloading, MuRF1 and MAFbx expression was not increased at any of the time points analyzed, but 20S β5 proteasome activity was significantly increased on the first day of recovery (Lang et al., 2012). Lastly, under denervation conditions, the lack of MuRF1 resulted in greater activation of the proteasome, not less (Gomes et al., 2012).

Under atrophy conditions, the FOXOs are often implicated in the induction of MuRF1 and MAFbx, but our results clearly indicate that this is not the case in the functional overload model, as FOXO expression did not increase until after MuRF1 and MAFbx expression had returned to baseline levels. The largest increase in FOXO1 and FOXO3a expression was found to occur after 7 days of functional overload, which is consistent with the findings of Goodman et al. (2011a) who showed that both total protein and phosphorylation levels of FOXO1 and FOXO3a were significantly elevated at 7 days of FO. Our results suggest that the FOXOs may be mediating protein degradation independently of MuRF1 and MAFbx, and may be at least partially responsible for the observed increase in proteasome activity. More work is needed to determine the role of the FOXOs in regulating the ubiquitin proteasome system during skeletal muscle growth.

Mechanical loading has been shown to initiate an inflammatory response and a number of cytokines have been reported to increase during muscle hypertrophy (Huey et al., 2007). One cytokine in particular that was reported to be elevated early after FO was TNFα (Huey et al., 2007). Circulating levels of TNFα can lead to increases in both MuRF1 and MAFbx expression (Li et al., 2005; Adams et al., 2008), so it is possible that the short-lived increase in expression seen in this study was directly related to muscle inflammation. While an inflammatory response appears to be required for normal growth following FO (Marino et al., 2008), it is unclear whether induction of MuRF1 and MAFbx is critical in this response. Our results indicate that MAFbx, but not MuRF1, may be necessary for normal remodeling and growth, as the MAFbx KO mice had an attenuated growth response (especially among the female animals), whereas the MuRF1 KO mice showed no deficiencies in their ability to hypertrophy.

In skeletal muscle, a few targets of MAFbx have been identified, including eIF3f (Lagirand-Cantaloube et al., 2008), MyoD (Tintignac et al., 2005), and myogenin (Jogo et al., 2009). These targets are generally associated with protein synthesis (eIF3f), satellite cell proliferation (MyoD), and muscle-specific gene transcription (MyoD, myogenin), all of which are important for muscle hypertrophy (Ishido et al., 2004; Baar et al., 2006). In addition, recent *in vitro* work by Lokireddy et al. revealed that MAFbx preferentially degrades sarcomeric proteins following myostatin treatment, with myosin heavy chain, myosin light chain, desmin, and vimentin identified as targets of MAFbx ubiquitination (Lokireddy et al., 2011a,b). Thus, even though it appears that the lack of MAFbx should promote muscle growth, the inability to turnover key sarcomeric proteins, such as myosin heavy chain, during the remodeling process could explain why the growth response was impaired in the MAFbx KO mice. Furthermore, while MAFbx KO mice have been shown to spare muscle mass following denervation (Bodine et al., 2001a), histological analysis of denervated MAFbx muscles has revealed dystrophic and necrotic fibers. Consequently, it appears that MAFbx may be required for the proper remodeling of muscle fibers under growth and atrophy conditions. The explanation for the finding that the loss of MAFbx had a greater effect on load-induced growth in female vs. male mice is not clearly evident. In previous experiments that have examined the response of MAFbx KO mice to triggers of muscle atrophy, we have observed no gender-based differences.

Similar to MAFbx, MuRF1 has been reported to interact and ubiquitinate myofibrillar proteins (Cohen et al., 2009), suggesting that MuRF1 also plays a role in regulating protein turnover. However, given the normal hypertrophic response to FO in the MuRF1 KO mice, it seems that MuRF1 is not essential for muscle growth. Considering that protein synthesis is higher in MuRF1 KO mice under atrophy conditions (Koyama et al., 2008; Baehr et al., 2011), it may be that the major role of MuRF1 in skeletal muscle is to suppress protein synthesis. Thus, deletion of MuRF1 is advantageous to muscle growth and consequently, the MuRF1 KO mice maintain an ability to hypertrophy throughout their lifetime. The different phenotypes in the MuRF1 and MAFbx KO mice suggest that the two E3 ligases have different physiological substrates. Clearly more research is needed to determine the physiological targets of both MuRF1 and MAFbx in skeletal muscle.

In summary, our results indicate that muscle hypertrophy is associated with increases in both protein synthesis and degradation. The increase in degradation is the result of activation of the UPS, and proteasome activity remains elevated even after MuRF1 and MAFbx expression has returned to baseline levels. Interestingly, MuRF1 and MAFbx expression become suppressed below baseline even though FOXO1 and FOXO3a expression are elevated. The loss of MuRF1 or MAFbx does not appear to suppress the increase in proteasome activity in response to chronic increases in load; however, the loss of MAFbx does appear to negatively impact the remodeling process that occurs during growth. These findings highlight the need for a better understanding of the roles of MuRF1 and MAFbx in the function of skeletal muscle, which will require identification of their *in vivo* substrates.

REFERENCES

Adams, V., Mangner, N., Gasch, A., Krohne, C., Gielen, S., Hirner, S., et al. (2008). Induction of MuRF1 is essential for TNF-alpha-induced loss of muscle function in mice. *J. Mol. Biol.* 384, 48–59. doi: 10.1016/j.jmb.2008.08.087

Auclair, D., Garrel, D. R., Chaouki Zerouala, A., and Ferland, L. H. (1997). Activation of the ubiquitin pathway in rat skeletal muscle by catabolic doses of glucocorticoids. *Am. J. Physiol.* 272, C1007–C1016.

Baar, K., Nader, G., and Bodine, S. (2006). Resistance exercise, muscle loading/unloading and the control of muscle mass. *Essays Biochem.* 42, 61–74. doi: 10.1042/bse0420061

Baehr, L. M., Furlow, J. D., and Bodine, S. C. (2011). Muscle sparing in muscle RING finger 1 null mice: response to synthetic glucocorticoids. *J. Physiol.* 589, 4759–4776. doi: 10.1113/jphysiol.2011.212845

Bodine, S. C., Latres, E., Baumhueter, S., Lai, V. K.-M., Nunez, L., Clarke, B. A., et al. (2001a). Identification of ubiquitin ligases required for skeletal muscle atrophy. *Science* 294, 1704–1708. doi: 10.1126/science.1065874

Bodine, S. C., Stitt, T. N., Gonzalez, M., Kline, W. O., Stover, G. L., Bauerlein, R., et al. (2001b). Akt/mTOR pathway is a crucial regulator of skeletal muscle hypertrophy and can prevent muscle atrophy *in vivo*. *Nat. Cell Biol.* 3, 1014–1019. doi: 10.1038/ncb1101-1014

Chau, V., Tobias, J. W., Bachmair, A., Marriott, D., Ecker, D. J., Gonda, D. K., et al. (1989). A multiubiquitin chain is confined to specific lysine in a targeted short-lived protein. *Science* 243, 1576–1583. doi: 10.1126/science.2538923

Cohen, S., Brault, J. J., Gygi, S. P., Glass, D. J., Valenzuela, D. M., Gartner, C., et al. (2009). During muscle atrophy, thick, but not thin, filament components are degraded by MuRF1-dependent ubiquitylation. *J. Cell Biol.* 185, 1083–1095. doi: 10.1083/jcb.200901052

Du, J., Wang, X., Miereles, C., Bailey, J. L., Debigare, R., Zheng, B., et al. (2004). Activation of caspase-3 is an initial step triggering accelerated muscle proteolysis in catabolic conditions. *J. Clin. Invest.* 113, 115–123. doi: 10.1172/JCI18330

Fu, H. Y., Minamino, T., Tsukamoto, O., Sawada, T., Asai, M., Kato, H., et al. (2008). Overexpression of endoplasmic reticulum-resident chaperone attenuates cardiomyocyte death induced by proteasome inhibition. *Cardiovasc. Res.* 79, 600–610. doi: 10.1093/cvr/cvn128

Gomes, A. V., Waddell, D. S., Siu, R., Stein, M., Dewey, S., Furlow, J. D., et al. (2012). Upregulation of proteasome activity in muscle RING finger 1-null mice following denervation. *FASEB J.* 26, 2986–2999. doi: 10.1096/fj.12-204495

Gomes, M. D., Lecker, S. H., Jagoe, R. T., Navon, A., and Goldberg, A. L. (2001). Atrogin-1, a muscle-specific F-box protein highly expressed during muscle atrophy. *Proc. Natl. Acad. Sci. U.S.A.* 98, 14440–14445. doi: 10.1073/pnas.251541198

Goodman, C. A., Frey, J. W., Mabrey, D. M., Jacobs, B. L., Lincoln, H. C., You, J. S., et al. (2011a). The role of skeletal muscle mTOR in the regulation of mechanical load-induced growth. *J. Physiol.* 589, 5485–5501. doi: 10.1113/jphysiol.2011.218255

Goodman, C. A., Mabrey, D. M., Frey, J. W., Miu, M. H., Schmidt, E. K., Pierre, P., et al. (2011b). Novel insights into the regulation of skeletal muscle protein synthesis as revealed by a new nonradioactive *in vivo* technique. *FASEB J.* 25, 1028–1039. doi: 10.1096/fj.10-168799

Hobler, S. C., Williams, A., Fischer, D., Wang, J. J., Sun, X., Fischer, J. E., et al. (1999). Activity and expression of the 20S proteasome are increased in skeletal muscle during sepsis. *Am. J. Physiol.* 277, R434–R440.

Huey, K. A., Mccall, G. E., Zhong, H., and Roy, R. R. (2007). Modulation of HSP25 and TNF-α during the early stages of functional overload of a rat slow and fast muscle. *J. Appl. Physiol.* 102, 2307–2314. doi: 10.1152/japplphysiol.00021.2007

Hwee, D. T., Baehr, L. M., Philp, A., Baar, K., and Bodine, S. C. (2013). Maintenance of muscle mass and load-induced growth in Muscle RING Finger 1 null mice with age. *Aging Cell.* 1, 92–101. doi: 10.1111/acel.12150

Ishido, M., Kami, K., and Masuhara, M. (2004). Localization of MyoD, myogenin and cell cycle regulatory factors in hypertrophying rat skeletal muscles. *Acta Physiol. Scand.* 180, 281–289. doi: 10.1046/j.0001-6772.2003.01238.x

Jogo, M., Shiraishi, S., and Tamura, T. A. (2009). Identification of MAFbx as a myogenin-engaged F-box protein in SCF ubiquitin ligase. *FEBS Lett.* 583, 2715–2719. doi: 10.1016/j.febslet.2009.07.033

Koyama, S., Hata, S., Witt, C. C., Ono, Y., Lerche, S., Ojima, K., et al. (2008). Muscle RING-finger protein-1 (MuRF1) as a connector of muscle energy metabolism and protein synthesis. *J. Mol. Biol.* 376, 1224–1236. doi: 10.1016/j.jmb.2007.11.049

Kubica, N., Crispino, J. L., Gallagher, J. W., Kimball, S. R., and Jefferson, L. S. (2008). Activation of the mammalian target of rapamycin complex 1 is both necessary and sufficient to stimulate eukaryotic initiation factor 2B[var epsilon] mRNA translation and protein synthesis. *Int. J. Biochem. Cell Biol.* 40, 2522–2533. doi: 10.1016/j.biocel.2008.04.010

Labeit, S., Kohl, C. H., Witt, C. C., Labeit, D., Jung, J., and Granzier, H. (2010). Modulation of muscle atrophy, fatigue and MLC phosphorylation by MuRF1 as indicated by hindlimb suspension studies on MuRF1-KO mice. *J. Biomed. Biotechnol.* 2010:693741. doi: 10.1155/2010/693741

Lagirand-Cantaloube, J., Offner, N., Csibi, A., Leibovitch, M. P., Batonnet-Pichon, S., Tintignac, L. A., et al. (2008). The initiation factor eIF3-f is a major target for atrogin1/MAFbx function in skeletal muscle atrophy. *EMBO J.* 27, 1266–1276. doi: 10.1038/emboj.2008.52

Lang, S. M., Kazi, A. A., Hong-Brown, L., and Lang, C. H. (2012). Delayed recovery of skeletal muscle mass following hindlimb immobilization in mTOR heterozygous mice. *PLoS ONE* 7:e38910. doi: 10.1371/journal.pone.0038910

Li, Y.-P., Chen, Y., John, J., Moylan, J., Jin, B., Mann, D. L., et al. (2005). TNF-α acts via p38 MAPK to stimulate expression of the ubiquitin ligase atrogin1/MAFbx in skeletal muscle. *FASEB J.* 19, 362–370. doi: 10.1096/fj.04-2364com

Lokireddy, S., McFarlane, C., Ge, X., Zhang, H., Sze, S. K., Sharma, M., et al. (2011a). Myostatin induces degradation of sarcomeric proteins through a Smad3 signaling mechanism during skeletal muscle wasting. *Mol. Endocrinol.* 25, 1936–1949. doi: 10.1210/me.2011-1124

Lokireddy, S., Mouly, V., Butler-Browne, G., Gluckman, P. D., Sharma, M., Kambadur, R., et al. (2011b). Myostatin promotes the wasting of human myoblast cultures through promoting ubiquitin-proteasome pathway-mediated loss of sarcomeric proteins. *Am. J. Physiol.Cell Physiol.* 301, C1316–C1324. doi: 10.1152/ajpcell.00114.2011

Louis, E., Raue, U., Yang, Y., Jemiolo, B., and Trappe, S. (2007). Time course of proteolytic, cytokine, and myostatin gene expression after acute exercise in human skeletal muscle. *J. Appl. Physiol.* 103, 1744–1751. doi: 10.1152/japplphysiol.00679.2007

Marino, J. S., Tausch, B. J., Dearth, C. L., Manacci, M. V., Mcloughlin, T. J., Rakyta, S. J., et al. (2008). β2-Integrins contribute to skeletal muscle hypertrophy in mice. *Am. J. Physiol. Cell Physiol.* 295, C1026–C1036. doi: 10.1152/ajpcell.212.2008

Minetti, G. C., Feige, J. N., Rosenstiel, A., Bombard, F., Meier, V., Werner, A., et al. (2011). Galphai2 signaling promotes skeletal muscle hypertrophy, myoblast differentiation, and muscle regeneration. *Sci. Signal.* 4, ra80. doi: 10.1126/scisignal.2002038

Mitch, W. E., and Goldberg, A. L. (1996). Mechanisms of muscle wasting. The role of the ubiquitin-proteasome pathway. *N. Engl. J. Med.* 335, 1897–1905. doi: 10.1056/NEJM199612193352507

Miyazaki, M., McCarthy, J. J., Fedele, M. J., and Esser, K. A. (2011). Early activation of mTORC1 signalling in response to mechanical overload is independent of phosphoinositide 3-kinase/Akt signalling. *J. Physiol.* 589, 1831–1846. doi: 10.1113/jphysiol.2011.205658

Murton, A. J., Constantin, D., and Greenhaff, P. L. (2008). The involvement of the ubiquitin proteasome system in human skeletal muscle remodelling and atrophy. *Biochim. Biophys. Acta* 1782, 730–743. doi: 10.1016/j.bbadis.2008.10.011

Phillips, S. M., Tipton, K. D., Aarsland, A., Wolf, S. E., and Wolfe, R. R. (1997). Mixed muscle protein synthesis and breakdown after resistance exercise in humans. *Am. J. Physiol.* 273, E99–E107.

Rayavarapu, S., Coley, W., and Nagaraju, K. (2012). Endoplasmic reticulum stress in skeletal muscle homeostasis and disease. *Curr. Rheumatol. Rep.* 14, 238–243. doi: 10.1007/s11926-012-0247-5

Rock, K. L., Gramm, C., Rothstein, L., Clark, K., Stein, R., Dick, L., et al. (1994). Inhibitors of the proteasome block the degradation of most cell proteins and the generation of peptides presented on MHC class I molecules. *Cell* 78, 761–771. doi: 10.1016/S0092-8674(94)90462-6

Rommel, C., Bodine, S. C., Clarke, B. A., Rossman, R., Nunez, L., Stitt, T. N., et al. (2001). Mediation of IGF-1-induced skeletal myotube hypertrophy by PI(3)K/Akt/mTOR and PI(3)K/Akt/GSK3 pathways. *Nat. Cell Biol.* 3, 1009–1013. doi: 10.1038/ncb1101-1009

Sandri, M., Sandri, C., Gilbert, A., Skurk, C., Calabria, E., Picard, A., et al. (2004). Foxo transcription factors induce the atrophy-related ubiquitin ligase atrogin-1 and cause skeletal muscle atrophy. *Cell* 117, 399–412. doi: 10.1016/S0092-8674(04)00400-3

Sartori, R., Schirwis, E., Blaauw, B., Bortolanza, S., Zhao, J., Enzo, E., et al. (2013). BMP signaling controls muscle mass. *Nat. Genet.* 11, 1309–1318. doi: 10.1038/ng.2772

Schmidt, E. K., Clavarino, G., Ceppi, M., and Pierre, P. (2009). SUnSET, a nonradioactive method to monitor protein synthesis. *Nat. Methods* 6, 275–277. doi: 10.1038/nmeth.1314

Tintignac, L. A., Lagirand, J., Batonnet, S., Sirri, V., Leibovitch, M. P., and Leibovitch, S. A. (2005). Degradation of MyoD mediated by the SCF (MAFbx) ubiquitin ligase. *J. Biol. Chem.* 280, 2847–2856. doi: 10.1074/jbc.M411346200

Tisdale, M. J. (2005). The ubiquitin-proteasome pathway as a therapeutic target for muscle wasting. *J. Support. Oncol.* 3, 209–217.

Vary, T. C., Frost, R. A., and Lang, C. H. (2008). Acute alcohol intoxication increases atrogin-1 and MuRF1 mRNA without increasing proteolysis in skeletal muscle. *Am. J. Physiol. Regul. Integr. Comp. Physiol.* 294, R1777–R1789. doi: 10.1152/ajpregu.00056.2008

Waddell, D. S., Baehr, L. M., Van Den Brandt, J., Johnsen, S. A., Reichardt, H. M., Furlow, J. D., et al. (2008). The glucocorticoid receptor and FOXO1 synergistically activate the skeletal muscle atrophy-associated MuRF1 gene. *Am. J. Physiol. Endocrinol. Metab.* 295, E785–E797. doi: 10.1152/ajpendo.00646.2007

Yang, Y., Jemiolo, B., and Trappe, S. (2006). Proteolytic mRNA expression in response to acute resistance exercise in human single skeletal muscle fibers. *J. Appl. Physiol.* 101, 1442–1450. doi: 10.1152/japplphysiol.00438.2006

Zanchi, N. E., De Siqueira Filho, M. A., Lira, F. S., Rosa, J. C., Yamashita, A. S., De Oliveira Carvalho, C. R., et al. (2009). Chronic resistance training decreases MuRF-1 and Atrogin-1 gene expression but does not modify Akt, GSK-3beta and p70S6K levels in rats. *Eur. J. Appl. Physiol.* 106, 415–423. doi: 10.1007/s00421-009-1033-6

14

More than a bystander: The contributions of intrinsic skeletal muscle defects in motor neuron diseases

Justin G. Boyer*[1,2]*, Andrew Ferrier*[1,2] *and Rashmi Kothary*[1,2,3]*

[1] *Ottawa Hospital Research Institute, Regenerative Medicine Program, Ottawa, ON, Canada*
[2] *Department of Cellular and Molecular Medicine, University of Ottawa, Ottawa, ON, Canada*
[3] *Department of Medicine, University of Ottawa, Ottawa, ON, Canada*

Correspondence:
Rashmi Kothary, Ottawa Hospital Research Institute, 501 Smyth Road, Ottawa, ON K1H 8L6, Canada
e-mail: rkothary@ohri.ca

Spinal muscular atrophy (SMA), amyotrophic lateral sclerosis (ALS), and spinal-bulbar muscular atrophy (SBMA) are devastating diseases characterized by the degeneration of motor neurons. Although the molecular causes underlying these diseases differ, recent findings have highlighted the contribution of intrinsic skeletal muscle defects in motor neuron diseases. The use of cell culture and animal models has led to the important finding that muscle defects occur prior to and independently of motor neuron degeneration in motor neuron diseases. In SMA for instance, the muscle specific requirements of the SMA disease-causing gene have been demonstrated by a series of genetic rescue experiments in SMA models. Conditional ALS mouse models expressing a muscle specific mutant *SOD1* gene develop atrophy and muscle degeneration in the absence of motor neuron pathology. Treating SBMA mice by over-expressing IGF-1 in a skeletal muscle-specific manner attenuates disease severity and improves motor neuron pathology. In the present review, we provide an in depth description of muscle intrinsic defects, and discuss how they impact muscle function in these diseases. Furthermore, we discuss muscle-specific therapeutic strategies used to treat animal models of SMA, ALS, and SBMA. The study of intrinsic skeletal muscle defects is crucial for the understanding of the pathophysiology of these diseases and will open new therapeutic options for the treatment of motor neuron diseases.

Keywords: mouse models, neuromuscular disease, myofiber degeneration, fusion defect, insulin-like growth factor 1

INTRODUCTION

Everything from physical exercise to daily chores and even breathing depends on force generated by skeletal muscles. For a skeletal muscle to produce a contraction, a signal in the form of an action potential is required. The motor neuron is responsible for providing this required signal. The site where the motor neuron joins the muscle is called the neuromuscular junction and together, the motor neuron and the muscle are referred to as the motor unit.

Defects in the motor unit can seriously impact muscle contraction generation and lead to severely disabling diseases. Motor neuron diseases consist of a group of conditions characterized by motor neuron loss and atrophy of the associated musculature. Spinal muscular atrophy (SMA), amyotrophic lateral sclerosis (ALS), and spinal-bulbar muscular atrophy (SBMA) are examples of such motor neuron diseases. Although these diseases have quite different etiologies, SMA, ALS, or SBMA are all typified by progressive paralysis resulting in severe disability, and are commonly fatal.

Although the importance of motor neuron pathology is well-established in these diseases, recent work has revealed an involvement of other cell types, including myocytes, in the pathogenic process (Bricceno et al., 2012a; Hamilton and Gillingwater, 2013). Muscle weakness and atrophy are often tightly associated with motor neuron pathology. Importantly, however, use of both cell culture and conditional mouse models has revealed defects in skeletal muscle that occur in the absence of defective motor neurons. Such studies highlight a potential contribution of skeletal muscle defects to the symptoms of SMA, ALS, and SBMA patients. These findings have major implications for the development of therapeutics for these diseases. In the current review, we discuss the latest findings regarding intrinsic muscle defects as well as muscle-specific therapeutic strategies to treat SMA, ALS, and SBMA.

SPINAL MUSCULAR ATROPHY

DISEASE CHARACTERISTICS

SMA represents the leading genetic cause of infant death, affecting 1 in 10,000 live births per year (Pearn, 1978; Prior et al., 2010). Clinically, it is typified by progressive muscle weakness and loss of alpha motor neurons from the spinal cord. SMA is caused by mutations or deletions in the *SMN1* gene (Lefebvre et al., 1995). Due to a second, partially functionally copy, named *SMN2*, SMA is a disease of low SMN levels, rather than no SMN (Brzustowicz et al., 1993; Rochette et al., 2001). The clinical severity of SMA is categorized into 4 main types, which vary in their time of onset and expected prognosis (reviewed in Boyer et al., 2010). Furthermore, *SMN2* serves as a disease modifier since the copy number of the *SMN2* gene in SMA patients modulates disease severity.

The SMN protein is ubiquitously expressed and localizes to the nucleus and cytoplasm (Liu and Dreyfuss, 1996). In the nucleus, SMN is present in gemini of coiled bodies (gems) which are structures associated with Cajal bodies (Liu and Dreyfuss, 1996; Coovert et al., 1997; Lefebvre et al., 1997). Here, SMN forms a complex with Gemin 2–8 as well as with Sm proteins to regulate small nuclear ribonucleoprotein (snRNP) biogenesis (Liu and Dreyfuss, 1996; Meister et al., 2000; Pellizzoni et al., 2002; Ogawa et al., 2007). SnRNPs are essential for pre-mRNA splicing and a decrease in SMN produces a reduction in snRNP assembly in SMA patients (Will and Luhrmann, 2001; Wan et al., 2005). In additional to SMN's established role in snRNP biogenesis, it has also been suggested to have a role in transcription and mRNA transport (Pellizzoni et al., 2001; Meister et al., 2002; Paushkin et al., 2002; Rossoll et al., 2003; Kariya et al., 2008).

Since the identification of SMN as the disease-causing gene in SMA, a number of mouse models have been generated to gain insight into the pathogenic process. *Smn* knockout mice ($Smn^{-/-}$) are embryonic lethal while heterozygous ($Smn^{+/-}$) mice can be used as a model of very mild SMA (Schrank et al., 1997). Mice do not harbor the *SMN2* gene as it is unique to humans, but by introducing low copies of the human *SMN2* gene into the $Smn^{-/-}$background, researchers were able generate a mouse model ($Smn^{-/-}$;*SMN2*) mimicking the severe SMA phenotype (Monani et al., 2000). Although the $Smn^{-/-}$;*SMN2* model is genetically representative of human patients, these mutant mice are very small in size and have a short life span making them difficult models to work with, especially when assessing therapeutics. The recent creation of milder SMA model mice has led to the discovery that cell types other than motor neurons are also affected in SMA (Hammond et al., 2010; Michaud et al., 2010; Bowerman et al., 2012a,b; Osborne et al., 2012; Cobb et al., 2013). These mice will also allow for the identification of new mechanisms of disease and will facilitate testing of therapeutic approaches.

MUSCLE INTRINSIC DEFECTS

As motor neurons and skeletal muscle are both functionally and structurally connected, it is difficult to study skeletal muscle defects independently from diseased motor neurons. The use of cell culture and conditional mouse models has, however, allowed researchers to study the role of Smn in skeletal muscle. Shafey et al. (2005) generated a series of hypomorphic cell lines in which Smn expression was depleted to varying levels in C2C12 myoblasts. Upon reducing Smn levels, defects such as decreased proliferation, aberrant myoblast fusion and malformed myotubes became apparent. These findings demonstrate that low Smn levels can result in intrinsic muscle defects and suggest a role for Smn in myoblast fusion. *In vivo*, the importance of Smn has been highlighted by conditional knockout mice in which the muscle-specific knockout of *Smn* was achieved using a floxed Smn allele with Cre recombinase controlled by the *human skeletal actin* (*HSA*) muscle-specific promoter (Cifuentes-Diaz et al., 2001). These mice develop a phenotype reminiscent of that observed in mouse models of muscular dystrophy. Skeletal muscle fibers from these mice have a disorganized sarcolemma and the mice have a reduced lifespan without displaying any overt neuropathology (Cifuentes-Diaz et al., 2001; Nicole et al., 2003). Although the results from conditional mouse studies have demonstrated a need for Smn in skeletal muscle, advances in animal genetic manipulation now allows for conditional deletion of Smn with residual *SMN2* expression. Therefore, we propose that skeletal muscle conditional SMA model mice be revisited using genetics reminiscent of the human disease.

Studies demonstrating muscle intrinsic defects have also been performed using human primary myoblasts from SMA patients. Upon differentiation of human myoblasts, myotubes from SMA patients displayed a reduction in fusion (Arnold et al., 2004), a result reminiscent of what was observed in the C2C12 Smn-knockdown cells. Furthermore, skeletal muscle defects such as vacuolization and compromised sarcomere structures were reported in human SMA muscle cells co-cultured with rat spinal cord explants (Braun et al., 1995). Although these primary cell culture studies were fairly concise, they nonetheless provide valuable insight into intrinsic muscle abnormalities. Collectively, the cell culture and conditional mouse studies were the first to show muscle intrinsic defects in SMA, and establish and validate a strong rationale to study muscle defects in the context of SMA.

ABNORMAL SKELETAL MUSCLE DEVELOPMENT IN SMA MICE

A growing body of evidence suggests that Smn-depletion leads to aberrant skeletal muscle development in SMA model mice. In the $Smn^{-/-}$;*SMN*2;Δ7 mouse model, Lee et al. (2011) showed that the cross-sectional area of myofibers did not increase from P5 to P13 suggesting impaired muscle growth. Similarly, the tibialis anterior muscle from phenotype stage $Smn^{-/-}$;*SMN*2 mice show similar cross-sectional area as that in pre-symptomatic mice (Dachs et al., 2011). A study on patient samples confirms that SMA muscles demonstrate impaired growth and maturation characterized by smaller and disorganized myotubes (Martinez-Hernandez et al., 2009). Collectively, these studies point to defects in muscle growth, however, the molecular basis for this is still unclear. One possibility for the reduced myofiber size in muscles from SMA model mice is that it is due to a defect in post-natal muscle development. Delayed muscle development is supported by the increased expression of immature myosin heavy chain (MHC) isoform in SMA model mice. Sustained expression of the embryonic and perinatal MHC isoforms has been detected at the transcript and protein level in phenotype stage $Smn^{-/-}$;*SMN*2;Δ7 mice (Kong et al., 2009; Lee et al., 2011). Furthermore, reduced expression of fast MHC isoforms has been reported in skeletal muscles of SMA model mice (Biondi et al., 2008; Lee et al., 2011). The transition between developmental MHC isoforms and fast MHC isoforms occurs later in development compared to slow MHC isoforms (Schiaffino and Reggiani, 2011), therefore delayed muscle development could account for the decreased expression of type 2B and 2× fibers in SMA muscles. The aberrant MHC expression profile was also associated with a delay in postsynaptic endplate development. The expression of the immature acetylcholine receptor persists in severe SMA model mice and is accompanied by impaired postsynaptic maturation at the morphological level (Kariya et al., 2008; Kong et al., 2009; Dachs et al., 2011; Bowerman et al., 2012a). A recent study assessed the functional capacities of skeletal muscle and demonstrated muscle weakness was an early feature of pathology in multiple mouse models of SMA (Boyer et al., 2013). Moreover, the severe muscle weakness was associated with delayed expression of mature isoforms of muscle function proteins such as ryanodine receptors and sodium channels. For the moment, direct evidence demonstrating that muscle weakness in SMA model mice is due to the delayed myogenesis and aberrant expression of muscle function proteins is lacking. Nonetheless, together these results suggest a role for Smn in skeletal muscle development. Further, it suggests that low levels of Smn lead to impaired muscle maturation, and thereby causing muscle weakness.

Hayhurst et al. (2012) have provided evidence suggesting that Smn-depletion leads to accelerated muscle differentiation *in vivo*. Satellite cells, identified by the paired-box transcription factor Pax7, were increased in number and expressed myogenic markers earlier in *Smn*$^{-/-}$;*SMN2* mice compared to controls. Despite the accelerated expression of the myogenic regulatory factors in *Smn*$^{-/-}$;*SMN2* satellite cells, these cells failed to grow upon differentiation in culture (Hayhurst et al., 2012).

How low levels of Smn lead to specific developmental defects in SMA model mice is unclear at the moment. However, several possible scenarios can be envisaged. First, Smn has specific function(s) during development through its association with one or more binding partners or second that low levels of Smn disrupts a major cellular process such as splicing which could impact on the expression of multiple genes important for muscle development and function. Thirdly, as muscle development is orchestrated by activity, defects at the levels of the motor neuron may negatively impact upon the expression of factors controlling post-natal muscle maturation.

TARGETING PATHWAYS OF MUSCLE ATROPHY IN SMA

Although several attempts have been made to promote muscle growth in SMA model mice, few studies have begun addressing the underlying mechanisms leading to muscle atrophy in the disease. During skeletal muscle atrophy caused by denervation, myogenin is up-regulated and directly stimulates the expression of muscle-specific ubiquitin E3 ligases, namely atrogin 1 and muscle RING-finger protein 1 (MuRF1), collectively referred to as atrogenes (Moresi et al., 2010). Substrates for atrogin 1 include MyoD, and eIF3f, which is an activator of protein synthesis, while sarcomeric proteins such as myosins and troponins are substrates of MuRF1 (Bonaldo and Sandri, 2013). Deletion of either atrogin 1 or MuRF1 leads to complete protection from denervation-induced muscle atrophy (Bodine et al., 2001).

Recently, a study by Bricceno et al. (2012b) demonstrated that following phenotype onset, a robust increase in atrogene expression was observed in SMA model mice (**Table 1**). Increased myogenin expression correlated with the up-regulation of the atrogenes, suggesting that the atrophy was mediated by muscle denervation. The expression of myogenin and atrogenes was also increased in skeletal muscle samples from human patients. Administration of the histone deacetylase inhibitor trichostatin A (TSA) prior to muscle atrophy onset attenuated atrogene expression in a mouse model of SMA (Bricceno et al., 2012b). TSA treatment decreased atrogene expression in denervated mice in which atrophy is mediated by myogenin but had no effect in a starved model of atrophy. Thus, this result suggests that TSA directly impacts on the myogenin dependent atrogene pathway. Direct

Table 1 | Summary of pathways leading to muscle atrophy in motor neuron diseases.

	Molecular pathways leading to atrophy
SMA	- increased expression of myogenin, MuRF1 and atrogin 1 in SMA model mice and SMA human muscle samples (Bricceno et al., 2012b) - TSA administration reduced the levels of atrogenes in SMA model mice (Bricceno et al., 2012b)
ALS	- increased levels of atrogin 1 but not MuRF1 in ALS *SOD1*^{G93A} model mice and ALS human samples (Léger et al., 2006) - decreased levels of AKT in ALS human samples (Léger et al., 2006) - increased levels of FoxO3 and MuRF1 but not atrogin1 in *MLC/SOD1*^{G93A} animals (Dobrowolny et al., 2005) - increased levels of expression of autophagy genes in *MLC/SOD1*^{G93A} mice (Dobrowolny et al., 2005)

evidence supporting denervation of the muscles used in the study by Bricceno et al. (2012b) was not presented. Therefore, it is not fully understood whether the up-regulation of myogenin in SMA model mice is attributable to impaired myogenesis, muscle denervation or both. Currently, understanding mechanisms of atrophy in SMA is an understudied area of research. For instance, whether the autophagic pathway or calpain-mediated muscle breakdown contribute to muscle atrophy in SMA is not known but could be of therapeutic importance. Further dissection of the molecular pathways responsible for the muscle atrophy, and testing therapeutics to treat atrophy in SMA is definitely warranted.

A ROLE FOR SMN IN MUSCLE

By isolating single myofibrils from myofibers, Walker et al. (2008) were able to identify Smn as a sarcomeric protein in striated muscle from mice. Specifically, Smn localizes to the Z-disc where it interacts with the actin crosslinking protein α-actinin (Rajendra et al., 2007; Walker et al., 2008; Shafey et al., 2010). Interestingly, other members of the SMN complex such as Gemins 2, 3, 4, and 6 are also present at Z-discs. However, other proteins essential for snRNP assembly are absent, suggesting that Smn plays a novel role at this adhesion site.

Currently, it is unclear whether there are any overt cytoskeletal structural defects in muscles from SMA model mice. Since mature muscles require less Smn expression than developing muscle (La Bella et al., 1998), the residual full-length protein produced by *SMN2* may be sufficient to fulfill its role at the Z-disc. However, given the localization of Smn in skeletal muscle, the complete absence of full-length Smn protein in skeletal muscle may lead to cytoskeletal defects reminiscent of what was observed in Smn muscle-specific depleted mice. Given the domains present in the Smn protein, it is unlikely that Smn plays a structural role in mature myofibers. However, a role for Smn in mechanosensing may be possible.

INCREASED CELL DEATH IN SMA MUSCLE

To gain insight into intrinsic molecular changes in skeletal muscle prior to motor neuron degeneration, Mutsaers et al. (2011)

performed a proteomic screen using the rostral band of the levator auris longus muscle in pre-symptomatic severe SMA model mice. Several proteins involved in cell death pathways were aberrantly expressed, some of which were validated in skeletal muscle from human patients. Furthermore, the authors highlighted changes in protein expression that were not identified in muscle samples from denervated mice, suggesting these changes are unlikely to be due to defective muscle innervation. In a separate study, increased apoptotic cell death was observed in muscles from phenotype stage $Smn^{-/-}$;*SMN2* mice but was not detected at the pre-symptomatic P0-P1 time point. To demonstrate that the presence of apoptotic cell death was a muscle intrinsic phenomenon, Dachs et al. (2011) performed sciatic nerve denervation in neonatal mice. Forty-eight hours post-denervation, no increase in apoptotic cells was observed in the experimentally denervated muscles compared to sham controls. Therefore, the increased cell death correlates with disease progression in $Smn^{-/-}$;*SMN2* mice and is not attributed to acute muscle denervation *per se*. That said, an investigation of cell death in Smn-depleted C2C12 cells and cultured satellite cells isolated from $Smn^{-/-}$;*SMN2* mice revealed normal proportion of apoptotic cells (Shafey et al., 2005; Hayhurst et al., 2012). Furthermore, the number of apoptotic cells in type 1 human SMA muscle samples was comparable to controls (Martinez-Hernandez et al., 2009). Therefore, it would appear that increased cell death in skeletal muscle might be limited to mouse models of SMA. How the absence of Smn leads to increased apoptosis and whether apoptosis in skeletal muscle is primary or secondary to the SMA pathogenesis is unclear and requires further study.

THE THERAPEUTIC REQUIREMENTS OF SMN IN SKELETAL MUSCLE

Several therapeutic approaches currently being developed for the treatment of SMA involve increasing SMN levels. In an attempt to demonstrate the therapeutic requirements of SMN in neuronal and muscle tissue, a series of genetic rescues in mouse models were performed. In an initial study, the expression of Smn was driven by either the muscle-specific promoter *HSA* or by the neuron-specific *prion protein* promoter (*PrP*) (Gavrilina et al., 2008). Crossing *HSA* and *PrP* rescue mice onto the $Smn^{-/-}$;*SMN2* background allowed for a direct comparison between both the neuronal and muscle approaches on survival. The longest surviving *PrP* rescued line lived an average of 210 days while the best surviving *HSA* rescued line lived an average of 160 days. Thus, these results demonstrate that rescue in either neurons or muscle can offer significant improvements in survival. However, the results from this study are challenging to interpret given that both the longest surviving muscle and neuronal rescue lines demonstrated leaky Smn protein expression in the spinal cord and in muscle, respectively. Moreover, the use of the *HSA* promoter to express Smn in skeletal muscle may not be early enough in development, and may therefore not be representative of when Smn is needed in skeletal muscle. In addition, the use of the *PrP* promoter makes it difficult to conclude that Smn is required precisely in the spinal cord since this promoter targets multiple cell types in the nervous system.

More recently, a similar study was performed using conditional SMA model mice expressing tissue-specific Cre drivers, including the motor neuron-specific choline acetyltransferase promoter ($ChAT^{cre}$), and the muscle-specific myogenic determination 1 ($MyoD^{cre}$) and myogenic factor 5 ($Myf5^{cre}$). MyoD and Myf5 are myogenic regulatory factors expressed very early during myogenesis and it was therefore anticipated that they would yield more significant improvements in the survival of SMA mice (Martinez et al., 2012). Interestingly, restoring Smn expression in motor neurons of $ChAT^{cre}$ mice led to a very modest increase in survival (from 15 to 23 days) compared to the survival reported using the *PrP* promoter. The $ChAT^{cre}$ extended survival 2 days more than the muscle-specific promoters $MyoD^{cre}$ and $Myf5^{cre}$. $ChAT^{cre}$ conditional mice showed increased SMN expression in motor neurons and improved neuromuscular junction function and morphology. Despite these improvements, only the $MyoD^{cre}$ and the $Myf5^{cre}$ lines produced a robust increase in the cross-sectional area of myofibers. It should be noted that Smn expression from the $Myf5^{cre}$ driver was detectable in the neuronal tissue making it somewhat difficult to interpret the results from this particular conditional mouse model (Martinez et al., 2012). Nonetheless, the results from $MyoD^{cre}$ and $Myf5^{cre}$ demonstrate the importance of restoring Smn expression in skeletal muscle and suggest that a combinatorial expression of Smn in both myofibers and motor neurons may provide a more impressive extension of life in mouse models of SMA. These data, suggest that restoration of Smn expression in skeletal muscle should not be overlooked when developing therapeutic strategies.

INDUCING MUSCLE GROWTH PATHWAYS IN SMA MODEL MICE

In an effort to reverse the muscle atrophy phenotype in mouse models of SMA, researchers have attempted to stimulate muscle growth pathways by various means. Myostatin is a potent negative regulator of muscle mass and the modulation of the myostatin pathway leads to dramatic muscle growth (Lee and McPherron, 2001). It was therefore hypothesized that modulation of the myostatin pathway may lead to phenotypic improvements in mouse models of SMA. Interestingly, myostatin and follistatin, a myostatin antagonist, were both found to be increased in mouse models of SMA suggesting a possible compensatory attempt by the animal to minimize muscle size loss (Sumner et al., 2009). Genetic overexpression of myostatin in SMA model mice proved to have a modest effect on muscle weight but offered no improvements in motor function and survival (Rindt et al., 2012). In a similar study, the genetic overexpression of follistatin in SMA model mice did not increase myofiber size or improve lifespan (Sumner et al., 2009). However, administration of recombinant follistatin in the same SMA mouse models used as in the genetic overexpression studies had a positive effect on the disease phenotype and lifespan (Rose et al., 2009). Specifically, delivery of the recombinant follistatin increased muscle mass, body weight, improved motor function and also increased motor neuron numbers and size in SMA model mice. Collectively, these changes led to an increase in median survival time. The differences in results between both follistatin studies are unclear but are likely attributed to the different methods used to overexpress follistatin that is, genetic overexpression versus administration of recombinant protein.

Insulin-like growth factor 1 (IGF-1) is a robust positive regulator of muscle mass and the overexpression of IGF-1 in mice causes a dramatic increase in musculature (Musaro et al., 2001).

Interestingly, circulating IGF-1 levels are reduced in multiple mouse models of SMA (Hua et al., 2011; Murdocca et al., 2012). Delivery of IGF-1 to the central nervous system of type III SMA model mice using an adeno-associated virus vector proved beneficial for motor neuron health but had little effect on myofiber integrity and motor function (Tsai et al., 2012). The systemic administration of IPLEX (recombinant human IGF-1 complexed with recombinant human IGF-1 binding protein 3) by intraperitoneal injection in *Smn*$^{-/-}$;*SMN2;Δ7* animals led to increased myofiber size, reduced motor neuron cell loss but did not impact on life span and body weight of SMA model mice (Murdocca et al., 2012). Finally, combining SMN trans-splicing with an IGF-1 vector increased life span and body mass in a severe mouse model of SMA (Shababi et al., 2011). It is difficult to partial out whether the improvements in myofiber size were due to the IGF-1 protein acting on myofibers directly or rather, increased muscle size was a secondary consequence from the healthier motor neurons. The genetic muscle overexpression of IGF-1 onto the same SMA background used in the follistatin studies led to increased muscle mass as well as an increase in the median lifespan (Bosch-Marce et al., 2011). Overexpression of muscle IGF-1 had little effect on markers of muscle maturity. Therefore, IGF-1 cannot restore proper muscle development in SMA model mice. IGF-1 may prove to be of greater benefit to diseases in which myofibers have formed and matured properly and are subsequently affected by intrinsic and extrinsic pathology. In fact, promoting muscle growth using IGF-1 overexpression before the muscle has fully matured may be detrimental to the tissue. Furthermore, it should be noted that the SMA model mice were crossed to IGF-1 overexpressing heterozygotes. Therefore, the benefits of IGF-1 may have been more obvious had the mice been bred to homozygosity.

Perhaps targeting molecules more downstream where myostatin and IGF-1 pathways converge might yield more robust results. For example, Akt is downstream of both myostatin and IGF-1, and overexpression of Akt in mice has led to increased muscle size (Lai et al., 2004; Schiaffino and Mammucari, 2011). In addition to promoting muscle growth, Akt also plays an important role in inhibiting mechanisms of atrophy including inhibiting atrogenes and the autophagic pathway (Schiaffino and Mammucari, 2011).

AMYOTROPHIC LATERAL SCLEROSIS (ALS)

DISEASE CHARACTERISTICS

ALS is a progressive adult-onset fatal disease characterized by the selective degeneration of upper motor neurons in the cerebral cortex and lower motor neurons of the brain stem and spinal cord (Rowland and Shneider, 2001). Features of the disease include muscle weakness and atrophy, spasticity and paralysis. It has an incidence of two per 100,000 people per year in the United States (Rowland and Shneider, 2001).

The term "amyotrophic" refers to the muscle atrophy, weakness and fasciculation that signify disease of lower motor neurons, while "lateral sclerosis" refers to the hardening of lateral columns, where gliosis follows the degeneration of corticospinal tracts (Rowland and Shneider, 2001). The mean duration of survival for ALS patients is 3–5 years following disease onset, with denervation of the respiratory muscles and diaphragm generally representing the fatal event of the disease. Despite intense research efforts, limited therapeutic options remain in attenuating disease progression; nevertheless advances are being made in palliative therapy (Carter et al., 2012).

A vast majority of ALS cases are sporadic and have no known genetic component, except for missense mutations in the TAR-DNA binding protein (Kabashi et al., 2008). Inherited forms of ALS (fALS) have an autosomal dominant or recessive pattern of inheritance and constitute ~10% or less of the remaining ALS cases (Rowland and Shneider, 2001). In 1993, a breakthrough in ALS research was made with the discovery of missense mutations in the *Cu/Zn superoxide dismutase 1 (SOD1)* gene of a subset of fALS cases (Rosen et al., 1993). It is estimated that 15–20% of fALS patients harbor missense mutations in the *SOD1* gene (equating to 2% of all ALS cases).

SOD1 is a ubiquitously expressed cytosolic metalloprotease that non-covalently binds Cu and Zn. The enzyme functions by detoxifying and maintaining intracellular superoxide anions (O_2^-) by catalyzing the dismutation of O_2^- to molecular oxygen and hydrogen peroxide. As such, mutations in SOD1 impart oxidative stress, which has become a key mechanism underlying disease pathogenesis (Barber et al., 2006). That said, to date, a number of different pathogenic mechanisms are believed to trigger ALS pathogenesis (Ilieva et al., 2009).

Most of our current knowledge of ALS pathogenic mechanisms comes from transgenic mice expressing various forms of mutant SOD1. Studies with these mice have highlighted multiple targets of damage in disease including mitochondria, proteasomes, and secretory pathways. Furthermore, while expression of mutant SOD1 within motor neurons is a primary determinant of disease onset and of an early phase of disease progression, the expression of mutant SOD1 also affects structural, physiological, and metabolic parameters in other cell types (e.g., glia and skeletal muscle) (see reviews Boillee et al., 2006; Ilieva et al., 2009). ALS is now considered a multisystemic disease, wherein a variety of cell types act synergistically to exacerbate disease pathogenesis (Ilieva et al., 2009).

The progressive paralysis in ALS is the result of degeneration and demise of motor neurons (Rowland and Shneider, 2001). Data from multiple studies suggest that toxicity is non-cell-autonomous, meaning toxicity to motor neurons derives from damage developed within cell types beyond the motor neuron (see reviews Fuchs et al., 1994; Boillee et al., 2006; Ilieva et al., 2009). Studies supporting this notion showed that ubiquitous transgenic overexpression of SOD1 mutations causing fALS leads to an ALS phenotype in mice (Wong et al., 1995), however, restricted expression of mutant SOD1 in neurons alone is not sufficient to cause this phenotype. It is perhaps important to note, however, that levels of mutant SOD1 selectively expressed in motor neurons may have been too low to initiate disease (Pramatarova et al., 2001; Lino et al., 2002). More recent studies suggest that neuron-specific expression of human mutant SOD1 in mice triggers motor neuron degeneration (Jaarsma et al., 2008; Wang et al., 2008). These discrepant studies indicate that mutant SOD1-induced motor neuron degeneration is at least partly cell autonomous, and non-neuronal mutant SOD1 expression is also likely required for disease manifestation.

MUSCLE DEFECTS IN ALS

Numerous studies support the notion that multiple tissues outside the CNS, including skeletal muscle (Wiedemann et al., 1998; Krasnianski et al., 2005; Dupuis et al., 2006), fibroblasts (Aguirre et al., 1998; McEachern et al., 2000), and lymphocytes (Cova et al., 2006) are affected in human ALS. In both sporadic and fALS, functional aberrations and skeletal muscle pathology are present including neurogenic-induced muscle pathology and mitochondria dysfunction (Vielhaber et al., 1999; Krasnianski et al., 2005; Echaniz-Laguna et al., 2006; Corti et al., 2009). Similarly, transgenic mice expressing mutant SOD1 recapitulate functional and metabolic deficits in skeletal muscle as seen in human ALS patients (Derave et al., 2003; Dupuis et al., 2004; Mahoney et al., 2006).

Selective expression of mutant SOD1 in mouse skeletal muscle using the myosin light chain (MLC) promoter (*MCL/SOD1*^{G93A}) induced ALS-like muscle pathologies, including progressive muscle atrophy, reduced muscle strength, impaired contractility, and mitochondrial dysfunction (Dobrowolny et al., 2008). Interestingly, exclusive expression of mutant SOD1 in skeletal muscle did not trigger the degeneration of motor neurons. This finding contrasts with a similar study from Wong and Martin (2010), where human mutated SOD1 expression driven from the *HSA* promoter, resulted in pathologic phenotypes in both muscle and motor neurons reminiscent of ALS (Wong and Martin, 2010). The reasons for this discrepancy is unclear although it may be due to the fact the animals used were of a different age, being significantly younger in the work from Dobrowolny et al. (2008). Regardless of this, together these studies provide strong evidence that mutant SOD1 is toxic to skeletal muscle and challenged the accepted dogma that motor neuron degeneration, caused by the overexpression of mutant SOD1, is the principle driver of muscle atrophy.

Skeletal muscle mitochondrial defects have been reported in *MLC/SOD1*^{G93A} mice as well as in other mouse models of ALS (Dupuis et al., 2003, 2004; Dobrowolny et al., 2008). Previous studies have suggested that mitochondrial defects may lead to motor neuron degeneration in the context of ALS. This notion is supported by the study of Dupuis et al. (2009) in which they demonstrate that muscle mitochondria uncoupling leads to muscle denervation and motor neuron degeneration. Furthermore, muscle mitochondria uncoupling exacerbates disease progression and survival in a mouse model of ALS (Dupuis et al., 2009).

MYOGENESIS IN ALS

Altered expression of the myogenic program has previously been reported in a mouse model of ALS. Widespread differences in the transcript and protein levels of Pax7 and myogenic regulatory factors were reported at disease onset (Manzano et al., 2011). The up-regulation of these proteins may reflect an increase in satellite cell activation following myofiber degeneration that may occur at time of disease onset. The levels of myogenic regulatory factors were not differentially expressed in early and late presymptomatic ALS mice compared to controls. This result suggests that the aberrant expression of the myogenic program is unlikely to be a triggering event leading to skeletal muscle defects in ALS model mice. In a separate study, however, primary myoblasts isolated from ALS patients and induced to differentiate into myotubes showed decreased expression of MHC, and displayed fusion defects (Pradat et al., 2011). These results are reminiscent of what was observed in SMA and SBMA cell culture studies (Arnold et al., 2004; Shafey et al., 2005; Malena et al., 2013).

MECHANISMS OF ATROPHY IN ALS

The most overt symptom in ALS patients is muscle weakness, which ultimately leads to death. Understanding mechanisms of muscle atrophy in ALS, i.e., whether muscle atrophy in ALS is solely due to denervation or whether it is intrinsic, may offer potential therapeutic avenues able to alleviate atrophy-induced weakness. Léger et al. (2006) studied signaling pathways contributing to skeletal muscle atrophy using ALS human samples as well as ALS *SOD1*^{G93A} model mice. A dramatic increase in the expression of the E3 ubiquitin ligase atrogin 1 was detected in both mouse and human ALS samples. No changes were observed in the expression of MuRF1 (**Table 1**) (Léger et al., 2006). Changes upstream of atrogenes have also been reported. IGF-1 levels were decreased and the expression of activated Akt was down-regulated suggesting that muscle atrophy was associated in part to intrinsic defects not associated with myogenin-induced atrophy during denervation (Léger et al., 2006; Lunetta et al., 2012). Further evidence demonstrating that muscle atrophy is not entirely neurogenic in nature comes from studies with *MLC/SOD1*^{G93A} mouse models of ALS in which restricted mutated SOD1 expression to skeletal muscle leads to atrophy (Dobrowolny et al., 2008). Skeletal muscle atrophy in these mice is initiated by the Akt pathway which suppresses protein synthesis and induces FoxO3 mediated expression of atrogenes (e.g., atrogin1 and MuRF1) (Dobrowolny et al., 2011). Furthermore, transcript levels of genes in the autophagic pathway such as LC3, Bnip3, and CathepsinL (**Table 1**) are up-regulated in muscles from *MLC/SOD1*^{G93A} animals and may contribute to decreased myofiber size while caspases are likely end stage contributors to atrophy in these mice (Dobrowolny et al., 2008, 2011). These pathways altered in ALS conditional mice differ from the myogenin-induced atrophy observed following denervation. This supports the idea that intrinsic atrophy mechanisms are contributing to decreased myofiber size in ALS and that therapeutic approaches to reverse atrophy and increase myofiber size may prove beneficial in this disease. Based on these studies, it is difficult to overlook the importance of skeletal muscle as a contributor to the pathogenesis of ALS.

SKELETAL MUSCLE IGF-1 AS A THERAPEUTIC APPROACH IN ALS

The muscle-specific overexpression of IGF-1 has led to remarkable improvement in ALS model mice. Using the muscle *MLC* promoter, Dobrowolny et al. (2005) overexpressed IGF-1 onto the *SOD1*^{G93A} mouse model of ALS (*SOD1*^{G93A}*/mIgf-1*). This delayed disease onset and increased survival. Muscle atrophy was attenuated and satelitte cell activation was enhanced in *SOD1*^{G93A}*/mIgf-1* mice (Dobrowolny et al., 2005). Importantly, IGF-1 overexpression in muscle also preserved neuromuscular junction integrity and protected motor neurons from degeneration.

It has also been reported that viral delivery of IGF-1 to skeletal muscles leads to increased survival and protected motor neurons in ALS model mice (Kaspar et al., 2003). Interestingly, muscle viral delivery of IGF-1 in ALS model mice combined with exercise has a remarkable synergistic effect leading to an increase in survival beyond what was obseved following gene therarpy or exercise alone (Kaspar et al., 2005). It remains to been seen whether the adminstration of IGF-1 gene therapy combined with treatment of exercise mimetics such as AICAR and GW501516, can yeild similar results since exercise is likely not a feasable longterm option in severe ALS patients. Despite significant improvements in ALS model mice achieved by genetic or viral overexpression of IGF-1, to date efficacy studies of recombiant IGF-1 have yeilded positvie results in two human trials while a third trial reported no improvements in muscle strength. However, no trial has demonstated any imporovments regarding patient survival (Beauverd et al., 2012).

SPINAL AND BULBAR MUSCULAR ATROPHY (SBMA)

DISEASE CHARACTERISTICS

Spinal and bulbar muscular atrophy (SBMA), also known as Kennedy's disease, is an adult onset neuromuscular disease characterized by the degeneration and loss of lower motor neurons leading to muscle wasting. The initial phase of the disease presents as muscle cramping, hand tremors and fatigue, with muscle weakness considered a late manifestation of disease (Sambataro and Pennuto, 2012). In addition to muscle weakness, SBMA patients display other symptoms such as fasciculations that are especially prevalent in the face, neck and tongue. The disease affects an estimated 1–2 per 100,000 people (Katsuno et al., 2012).

At the molecular level, SBMA is caused by the expansion of a polyglutamine (polyQ)-encoding CAG trinucleotide repeat in the first exon of the gene coding for the androgen receptor (AR). These repeats are toxic and lead to motor neuron death causing respiratory weakness in SBMA patients (Bricceno et al., 2012a). Motor neurons express high levels of the AR relative to other neuronal populations, and the loss of AR function attributed to the expanded polyQ tract is believed to contribute to SBMA pathogenesis. However, the predominant disease mechanism involves a gain-of-toxic function that accompanies the expanded polyQ tract AR in motor neurons (Katsuno et al., 2012).

A correlation exists between the number of repeats and the age at onset of muscle weakness (Igarashi et al., 1992). Full disease manifestations are observed in men only while heterozygous females are mostly asymptomatic and women homozygous for the mutation are rare and show only mild symptoms (Schmidt et al., 2002). The AR gene is located on the proximal arm of chromosome Xq11-12 (Katsuno et al., 2012). The AR is a nuclear receptor and is part of the steroid/thyroid hormone receptor family. Upon binding to its natural ligands testosterone and dihydrotestosterone, the AR is translocated to the nucleus where it binds DNA as well as transcriptional co-regulators to control the expression of a subset of genes. However, pathological CAG triplet repeats in the AR lead to the nuclear accumulation of the receptor and this disrupts its transactivation domain's ability to interact with transcriptional co-activators. The AR is required for androgen dependent changes including proper male pubertal sexual development. SBMA patients demonstrate subtle androgen sensitivity highlighted by gynecomastia, fertility complications and atrophy of the gonads (Sambataro and Pennuto, 2012). Castration of SBMA model mice prevents any phenotype while treating female animals with testosterone exacerbates the phenotype (Katsuno et al., 2002). These results demonstrate that disease manifestations are androgen-dependent and this explains the gender bias observed in SBMA patients.

MUSCLE DEFECTS IN SBMA PATIENTS

Although SBMA is believed to be primarily a motor neuron disease, increasing evidence suggests that myogenic defects contribute significantly to the disease pathogenesis. Studies performed on SBMA patients report very high levels of serum creatine kinase (CK), which are often 10 times higher than normal (Lee et al., 2005). It has been demonstrated that CK levels are higher in SBMA than any other motor neuron or myopathic disease and the increase can be detected prior to the onset of SBMA clinical symptoms (Chahin and Sorenson, 2009). Elevated serum CK levels are indicative of muscle damage and often seen in muscular dystrophy patients.

Histological studies performed on SBMA patients' muscle biopsies have revealed the presence of both neurogenic and primary myogenic defects. With muscle samples from SBMA patients, Soraru et al. (2008), demonstrate the presence of fiber type grouping, atrophic fibers and angulated fibers, which are defects observed following chronic denervation. Necrotic myofibers as well as myofibers with centrally located nuclei, which are indicative of regenerating fibers, are also observed in SBMA muscle biopsies and are associated with primary myogenic changes (Soraru et al., 2008; Chahin and Sorenson, 2009).

Studies using primary myoblasts isolated from SBMA patients have demonstrated that these cells proliferate and differentiate normally (Malena et al., 2013). Furthermore, primary SBMA myoblasts express myogenic regulatory factors such as MyoD and myogenin at levels comparable to controls. These results are androgen-dependent and suggest that early myogenesis is not affected in SBMA. However, defects such as cytoskeletal perturbations as well as aberrant myotube fusion were observed in primary myoblasts isolated from SBMA patients.

MUSCLE DEFECTS IN MOUSE MODELS OF SBMA

The use of mouse models has significantly contributed to our understanding of the myogenic defects in the SBMA phenotype. Yu et al. (2006) used gene targeting to generate a mouse model in which they converted the mouse AR sequence to the human sequence and in the process introduced 113 CAG repeats to recapitulate the human phenotype. These knock-in mice, designated *AR113Q*, are smaller, weaker compared to control counterparts, and die at 2–4 months of age. Histologically, muscles from *AR113Q* mice have atrophic and angulated fibers. At the molecular level, myogenin and acetylcholine receptor expression were up-regulated in *AR113Q* mice while MyoD expression was unchanged compared to controls. These morphological and gene expression changes are reflective of those observed following denervation (Moresi et al., 2010). Furthermore, myogenin was not mis-regulated in primary SBMA myoblasts supporting the idea that myogenin-dependent atrophy is present in *AR113Q* mice (Malena et al., 2013). However, the skeletal muscle pathology in *AR113Q* animals was thought to be cell-autonomous because it was detected prior to overt polyQ tract-induced pathology in the spinal cord. These results raise the possibility that the AR toxicity occurs in muscle prior to motor neurons, and may be the initiating factor leading to denervation-induced atrophy.

Other histological changes such as myofibers with centrally located nuclei present in *AR113Q* mice are more reflective of intrinsic myopathic defects. The expression of genes important for muscle function, such as the muscle chloride channel 1 (CLCN-1) and the muscle-specific sodium channel SCN4A, were decreased in *AR113Q* animals. The levels of CLCN-1 and SCN4A have previously been shown to decrease following experimental denervation (Kallen et al., 1993; Klocke et al., 1994). However, subsequent analyses in *AR113Q* animals demonstrated that the mis-regulation of CLCN-1 and SCN4A was not due to denervation (Yu et al., 2006). Furthermore, the down-regulation of CLCN-1 is attributed to the mis-splicing of the gene, which is reminiscent of what is observed in the muscle disease myotonic dystrophy (Yu et al., 2009). Therefore, SBMA model mice show muscle defects that are both intrinsic and motor neuron dependent. The denervation-like defects in *AR113Q* skeletal muscles can either be associated with intrinsic muscle toxicity-induced denervation, or to a secondary consequence linked to muscle denervation since the innervation status of skeletal muscles was not directly assessed.

Perhaps more compelling evidence supporting muscle contributions to SBMA pathogenesis comes from a mouse model in which a wild type AR was overexpressed in skeletal muscle and recapitulated the phenotypic features observed in other mouse models of SBMA (Monks et al., 2007). In this model, the AR overexpression in skeletal muscle was achieved using the *HSA* promoter (*AR-HSA*). *AR-HSA* animals showed muscle pathology and molecular changes such as increased levels of myogenin and AChR that are reminiscent of those observed following denervation. Interestingly, *AR-HSA* transgenic mice did not display motor neuron cell body loss but rather exhibited axonopathy. Again, these data suggest that the AR muscle toxicity may lead to motor neuron axon loss that in turn leads to denervation-induced pathology in skeletal muscles. Moreover, this result indicates that motor neuron defects occur distally first and eventually lead to cell body loss, a dying back phenomena, and may therefore explain the phenotype observed in the *AR113Q* mouse model of SBMA. The authors demonstrate that the toxicity to muscle occurred upon the activation of the AR-HSA by its ligand rather than the overexpression of the AR-HSA *per se*. However, it is difficult to conclude that the results observed from the *AR-HSA* mouse model can be directly generalized to SBMA, especially considering that the molecular pathogenesis of the *AR-HSA* model, which lacks the expanded polyQ tract, is very different.

Table 2 | Summary of defects observed in muscle in motor neuron diseases.

		SMA	ALS	SBMA
Muscle physiology	Muscle atrophy	✓	✓	✓
	Reduced strength	✓	✓	✓
	Mitochondrial dysfunction		✓ *	
	Atrogene expression	✓	✓ *	
	Sarcomere defects	✓ *		
Development	Reduced Proliferation	✓ *		
	Fusion defects	✓ *	✓ *	✓ *
	Aberrant expression of proteins important for muscle function	✓		✓
	Change in satellite cell number	✓ *		
	Impaired postnatal growth	✓ *		
Cell death	Increase in satellite cell apoptosis	✓ *		
	Increase in cell death pathway expression	✓ *		
	Myofiber degeneration			✓ *

**Denotes defects that have been shown to be muscle intrinsic.*

SKELETAL MUSCLE AS A THERAPEUTIC TARGET IN SBMA

It has long been known that AR translocation to the nucleus is ligand-mediated and that this process is intensified in men given that the AR ligand is testosterone. Modifying testosterone levels in SBMA model mice is a ligand-targeted therapy that has proven very successful. In a mouse model of SBMA in which 97 CAG repeats were introduced into the *AR* gene (*AR97Q*), reduction of testosterone by way of castration prevented the appearance of the phenotype in male mice (Katsuno et al., 2002). In *AR97Q* female animals, administration of testosterone induced aberrant motor phenotypes and neuropathology. Treatment of *AR-HSA* female mice with testosterone provoked denervation-like symptoms similar to *AR-HSA* males. However, upon testosterone treatment cessation, *AR-HSA* females recovered normal motor function and expressed muscle genes at usual levels (Johansen et al., 2009). In agreement with these findings, survival and muscle pathology of *AR-HSA* mice is significantly ameliorated by prenatal treatment with flutamide, an AR antagonist. These data reveal that the AR expression restricted to muscle alone can lead to SBMA symptoms in mice and that these defects can be improved by blocking androgen binding. Thus, the SBMA phenotype strongly correlates with androgen expression and skeletal muscle may be an important target for SBMA treatment.

Although the use of anti-androgens is effective in treating mouse models of SBMA, it may prove to have unwanted side effects in humans. In an attempt to better understand how the AR is endogenously regulated, Palazzolo et al. (2007) uncovered a role for Akt in regulating AR function. Phosphorylation of the AR by Akt represses the AR activity through a ligand-dependent manner, thus preventing androgen from activating the AR. Modulation of Akt in cell culture models of SBMA rescued the polyQ associated cell toxicity indicating that manipulating the Akt pathway might provide phenotypic improvements in SBMA model mice (Palazzolo et al., 2007). Indeed, skeletal muscle overexpression of IGF-1, a protein that acts upstream of Akt, delayed disease onset and extended survival in SBMA model mice (Palazzolo et al., 2009). IGF-1 activates Akt and thus increases AR phosphorylation, which in turn reduces AR nuclear accumulation in muscles from SBMA model mice. A striking observation was that overexpression of IGF-1 in skeletal muscle improved motor behavior and reduced motor neuron cell loss in SBMA model mice. IGF-1 overexpression in skeletal muscle ameliorated both myofiber and motor neuron health by reducing AR nuclear aggregates. IGF-1 has previously been shown to benefit motor neurons by promoting sprouting and axonal growth, therefore IGF-1 may improve motor neuron health via its trophic properties in addition to its effects on mutant AR (Caroni and Grandes, 1990). Furthermore, overexpression of IGF-1 in skeletal muscle of wild type mice leads to gross muscle hypertrophy (Musaro et al., 2001). Therefore, IGF-1 might ameliorate muscle pathology independently of AR even though gene array data suggest that the IGF-1 signaling pathway is largely unaffected in skeletal muscle of multiple mouse models of SBMA (Mo et al., 2010).

Taken together, muscle defects are evident in SBMA and for the most part, were believed to be a secondary response to muscle denervation. However, a growing body of evidence supports the notion that muscle is the primary target of polyQ-AR toxicity and that muscle defects lead to motor neuron abnormalities. Results from various mouse models and muscle-specific targeted therapies support this idea.

CONCLUSION

Although considered motor neuron diseases, the use of conditional mouse models as well cell culture systems have highlighted the contributions of intrinsic skeletal muscle defects in SMA, ALS and SBMA (**Table 2**). The nature of the skeletal muscle defects differs between these three diseases. For instance, the most notable muscle defects in SMA are associated primarily with impaired development but defects neurogenic in origin are also observed. While in ALS, muscle defects are due to intrinsic and neurogenic factors, and appear to be present in mature myofibers rather than in developing muscle. In SBMA, cell-autonomous muscle degeneration is an overt contributor to the phenotype as are denervation-induced defects. However, results from ALS and SBMA mouse models suggest that in these diseases, skeletal muscle defects can initiate motor neuron defects. Such evidence to support this notion in SMA is currently lacking, indeed the complete absence of Smn in skeletal muscle was not associated with motor neuron defects (Cifuentes-Diaz et al., 2001). The use of appropriate conditional animals models will serve to explore this possibility further.

A common therapeutic approach used in all three diseases involves the muscle-specific overexpression of IGF-1. This approach has led to remarkable improvements in mouse models of ALS and SBMA, and to a lesser degree in SMA. The reason for this may be associated to the type of muscle defects in these diseases. The IGF-1 therapeutic approach may prove to be more beneficial in the context of mature muscle that is diseased, and may not be as efficient in SMA where muscle development is impaired.

It has always been assumed that muscle defects in SMA, ALS, and SBMA were a secondary consequence of motor neuron pathology. However, the studies described in this review shed light onto the importance of intrinsic muscle defects as a primary contributor to the pathogenesis of these diseases. As such, more research should be focused on treating intrinsic skeletal muscle defects. Indeed, regardless of whether muscle is a primary or secondary contributor to the pathogenesis of these diseases, muscle defects are present and therefore muscle is still an important therapeutic target to consider.

ACKNOWLEDGMENTS

We thank Dr. Lyndsay M. Murray for providing valuable comments during the preparation of the manuscript. Work in the Kothary laboratory is funded by grants from the Canadian Institutes of Health Research (CIHR). Justin G. Boyer was a recipient of a Frederick Banting and Charles Best CIHR Doctoral Research Award, Andrew Ferrier was supported by an Ontario Graduate Scholarship, and Rashmi Kothary is a recipient of a University Health Research Chair from the University of Ottawa.

REFERENCES

Aguirre, T., Van Den Bosch, L., Goetschalckx, K., Tilkin, P., Mathijs, G., Cassiman, J. J., et al. (1998). Increased sensitivity of fibroblasts from amyotrophic lateral sclerosis patients to oxidative stress. *Ann. Neurol.* 43, 452–457. doi: 10.1002/ana.410430407

Arnold, A. S., Gueye, M., Guettier-Sigrist, S., Courdier-Fruh, I., Coupin, G., Poindron, P., et al. (2004). Reduced expression of nicotinic AChRs in myotubes from spinal muscular atrophy I patients. *Lab. Invest.* 84, 1271–1278. doi: 10.1038/labinvest.3700163

Barber, S. C., Mead, R. J., and Shaw, P. J. (2006). Oxidative stress in ALS: a mechanism of neurodegeneration and a therapeutic target. *Biochim. Biophys. Acta* 1762, 1051–1067. doi: 10.1016/j.bbadis.2006.03.008

Beauverd, M., Mitchell, J. D., Wokke, J. H., and Borasio, G. D. (2012). Recombinant human insulin-like growth factor I (rhIGF-I) for the treatment of amyotrophic lateral sclerosis/motor neuron disease. *Cochrane Database Syst. Rev.* 11:CD002064. doi: 10.1002/14651858.CD002064.pub3

Biondi, O., Grondard, C., Lecolle, S., Deforges, S., Pariset, C., Lopes, P., et al. (2008). Exercise-induced activation of NMDA receptor promotes motor unit development and survival in a type 2 spinal muscular atrophy model mouse. *J. Neurosci.* 28, 953–962. doi: 10.1523/JNEUROSCI.3237-07.2008

Bodine, S. C., Latres, E., Baumhueter, S., Lai, V. K., Nunez, L., Clarke, B. A., et al. (2001). Identification of ubiquitin ligases required for skeletal muscle atrophy. *Science* 294, 1704–1708. doi: 10.1126/science.1065874

Boillee, S., Vande Velde, C., and Cleveland, D. W. (2006). ALS: a disease of motor neurons and their nonneuronal neighbors. *Neuron* 52, 39–59. doi: 10.1016/j.neuron.2006.09.018

Bonaldo, P., and Sandri, M. (2013). Cellular and molecular mechanisms of muscle atrophy. *Dis. Model. Mech.* 6, 25–39. doi: 10.1242/dmm.010389

Bosch-Marce, M., Wee, C. D., Martinez, T. L., Lipkes, C. E., Choe, D. W., Kong, L., et al. (2011). Increased IGF-1 in muscle modulates the phenotype of severe SMA mice. *Hum. Mol. Genet.* 20, 1844–1853. doi: 10.1093/hmg/ddr067

Bowerman, M., Murray, L. M., Beauvais, A., Pinheiro, B., and Kothary, R. (2012a). A critical smn threshold in mice dictates onset of an intermediate spinal muscular atrophy phenotype associated with a distinct neuromuscular junction pathology. *Neuromuscul. Disord.* 22, 263–276. doi: 10.1016/j.nmd.2011.09.007

Bowerman, M., Swoboda, K. J., Michalski, J. P., Wang, G. S., Reeks, C., Beauvais, A., et al. (2012b). Glucose metabolism and pancreatic defects in spinal muscular atrophy. *Ann. Neurol.* 72, 256–268. doi: 10.1002/ana.23582

Boyer, J. G., Bowerman, M., and Kothary, R. (2010). The many faces of SMN: deciphering the function critical to spinal muscular atrophy pathogenesis. *Future Neurol.* 5, 873–890. doi: 10.2217/fnl.10.57

Boyer, J. G., Murray, L. M., Scott, K., De Repentigny, Y., Renaud, J. M., and Kothary, R. (2013). Early onset muscle weakness and disruption of muscle proteins in mouse models of spinal muscular atrophy. *Skelet. Muscle* 3, 24. doi: 10.1186/2044-5040-3-24

Braun, S., Croizat, B., Lagrange, M. C., Warter, J. M., and Poindron, P. (1995). Constitutive muscular abnormalities in culture in spinal muscular atrophy. *Lancet* 345, 694–695. doi: 10.1016/S0140-6736(95)90869-2

Bricceno, K. V., Fischbeck, K. H., and Burnett, B. G. (2012a). Neurogenic and myogenic contributions to hereditary motor neuron disease. *Neurodegener. Dis.* 9, 199–209. doi: 10.1159/000335311

Bricceno, K. V., Sampognaro, P. J., Van Meerbeke, J. P., Sumner, C. J., Fischbeck, K. H., and Burnett, B. G. (2012b). Histone deacetylase inhibition suppresses myogenin-dependent atrogene activation in spinal muscular atrophy mice. *Hum. Mol. Genet.* 21, 4448–4459. doi: 10.1093/hmg/dds286

Brzustowicz, L. M., Mérette, C., Kleyn, P. W., Lehner, T., Castilla, L. H., Penchaszadeh, G. K., et al. (1993). Assessment of nonallelic genetic heterogeneity of chronic (type II and III) spinal muscular atrophy. *Hum. Hered.* 43, 380–387. doi: 10.1159/000154164

Caroni, P., and Grandes, P. (1990). Nerve sprouting in innervated adult skeletal muscle induced by exposure to elevated levels of insulin-like growth factors. *J. Cell Biol.* 110, 1307–1317. doi: 10.1083/jcb.110.4.1307

Carter, G. T., Joyce, N. C., Abresch, A. L., Smith, A. E., and Vandekeift, G. K. (2012). Using palliative care in progressive neuromuscular disease to maximize quality of life. *Phys. Med. Rehabil. Clin. N. Am.* 23, 903–909. doi: 10.1016/j.pmr.2012.08.002

Chahin, N., and Sorenson, E. J. (2009). Serum creatine kinase levels in spinobulbar muscular atrophy and amyotrophic lateral sclerosis. *Muscle Nerve* 40, 126–129. doi: 10.1002/mus.21310

Cifuentes-Diaz, C., Frugier, T., Tiziano, F. D., Lacene, E., Roblot, N., Joshi, V., et al. (2001). Deletion of murine SMN exon 7 directed to skeletal muscle leads to severe muscular dystrophy. *J. Cell Biol.* 152, 1107–1114. doi: 10.1083/jcb.152.5.1107

Cobb, M. S., Rose, F. F., Rindt, H., Glascock, J. J., Shababi, M., Miller, M. R., et al. (2013). Development and characterization of an SMN2-based intermediate mouse model of Spinal Muscular Atrophy. *Hum. Mol. Genet.* 22, 1843–1855. doi: 10.1093/hmg/ddt037

Coovert, D. D., Le, T. T., McAndrew, P. E., Strasswimmer, J., Crawford, T. O., Mendell, J. R., et al. (1997). The survival motor neuron protein in spinal muscular atrophy. *Hum. Mol. Genet.* 6, 1205–1214. doi: 10.1093/hmg/6.8.1205

Corti, S., Donadoni, C., Ronchi, D., Bordoni, A., Fortunato, F., Santoro, D., et al. (2009). Amyotrophic lateral sclerosis linked to a novel SOD1 mutation with muscle mitochondrial dysfunction. *J. Neurol. Sci.* 276, 170–174. doi: 10.1016/j.jns.2008.09.030

Cova, E., Cereda, C., Galli, A., Curti, D., Finotti, C., Di Poto, C., et al. (2006). Modified expression of Bcl-2 and SOD1 proteins in lymphocytes from sporadic ALS patients. *Neurosci. Lett.* 399, 186–190. doi: 10.1016/j.neulet.2006.01.057

Dachs, E., Hereu, M., Piedrafita, L., Casanovas, A., Caldero, J., and Esquerda, J. E. (2011). Defective neuromuscular junction organization and postnatal myogenesis in mice with severe spinal muscular atrophy. *J. Neuropathol. Exp. Neurol.* 70, 444–461. doi: 10.1097/NEN.0b013e31821cbd8b

Derave, W., Van Den Bosch, L., Lemmens, G., Eijnde, B. O., Robberecht, W., and Hespel, P. (2003). Skeletal muscle properties in a transgenic mouse model for amyotrophic lateral sclerosis: effects of creatine treatment. *Neurobiol. Dis.* 13, 264–272. doi: 10.1016/S0969-9961(03)00041-X

Dobrowolny, G., Aucello, M., and Musaro, A. (2011). Muscle atrophy induced by SOD1G93A expression does not involve the activation of caspase in the absence of denervation. *Skelet. Muscle* 1, 3. doi: 10.1186/2044-5040-1-3

Dobrowolny, G., Aucello, M., Rizzuto, E., Beccafico, S., Mammucari, C., Boncompagni, S., et al. (2008). Skeletal muscle is a primary target of SOD1G93A-mediated toxicity. *Cell Metab.* 8, 425–436. doi: 10.1016/j.cmet.2008.09.002

Dobrowolny, G., Giacinti, C., Pelosi, L., Nicoletti, C., Winn, N., Barberi, L., et al. (2005). Muscle expression of a local Igf-1 isoform protects motor neurons in an ALS mouse model. *J. Cell Biol.* 168, 193–199. doi: 10.1083/jcb.200407021

Dupuis, L., Di Scala, F., Rene, F., De Tapia, M., Oudart, H., Pradat, P. F., et al. (2003). Up-regulation of mitochondrial uncoupling protein 3 reveals an early muscular metabolic defect in amyotrophic lateral sclerosis. *FASEB J.* 17, 2091–2093. doi: 10.1096/fj.02-1182fje

Dupuis, L., Gonzalez De Aguilar, J. L., Echaniz-Laguna, A., Eschbach, J., Rene, F., Oudart, H., et al. (2009). Muscle mitochondrial uncoupling dismantles neuromuscular junction and triggers distal degeneration of motor neurons. *PLoS ONE* 4:e5390. doi: 10.1371/journal.pone.0005390

Dupuis, L., Gonzalez De Aguilar, J. L., Echaniz-Laguna, A., and Loeffler, J. P. (2006). Mitochondrial dysfunction in amyotrophic lateral sclerosis also affects skeletal muscle. *Muscle Nerve* 34, 253–254. doi: 10.1002/mus.20566

Dupuis, L., Oudart, H., Rene, F., Gonzalez De Aguilar, J. L., and Loeffler, J. P. (2004). Evidence for defective energy homeostasis in amyotrophic lateral sclerosis: benefit of a high-energy diet in a transgenic mouse model. *Proc. Natl. Acad. Sci. U.S.A.* 101, 11159–11164. doi: 10.1073/pnas.0402026101

Echaniz-Laguna, A., Zoll, J., Ponsot, E., N'guessan, B., Tranchant, C., Loeffler, J. P., et al. (2006). Muscular mitochondrial function in amyotrophic lateral sclerosis is progressively altered as the disease develops: a temporal study in man. *Exp. Neurol.* 198, 25–30. doi: 10.1016/j.expneurol.2005.07.020

Fuchs, C. S., Giovannucci, E. L., Colditz, G. A., Hunter, D. J., Speizer, F. E., and Willett, W. C. (1994). A prospective study of family history and the risk of colorectal cancer. *N. Engl. J. Med.* 331, 1669–1674. doi: 10.1056/NEJM199412223312501

Gavrilina, T. O., McGovern, V. L., Workman, E., Crawford, T. O., Gogliotti, R. G., Didonato, C. J., et al. (2008). Neuronal SMN expression corrects spinal muscular atrophy in severe SMA mice while muscle-specific SMN expression has no phenotypic effect. *Hum. Mol. Genet.* 17, 1063–1075. doi: 10.1093/hmg/ddm379

Hamilton, G., and Gillingwater, T. H. (2013). Spinal muscular atrophy: going beyond the motor neuron. *Trends Mol. Med.* 19, 40–50. doi: 10.1016/j.molmed.2012.11.002

Hammond, S. M., Gogliotti, R. G., Rao, V., Beauvais, A., Kothary, R., and Didonato, C. J. (2010). Mouse survival motor neuron alleles that mimic SMN2 splicing and are inducible rescue embryonic lethality early in development but not late. *PLoS ONE* 5:e15887. doi: 10.1371/journal.pone.0015887

Hayhurst, M., Wagner, A. K., Cerletti, M., Wagers, A. J., and Rubin, L. L. (2012). A cell-autonomous defect in skeletal muscle satellite cells expressing low levels of survival of motor neuron protein. *Dev. Biol.* 368, 323–334. doi: 10.1016/j.ydbio.2012.05.037

Hua, Y., Sahashi, K., Rigo, F., Hung, G., Horev, G., Bennett, C. F., et al. (2011). Peripheral SMN restoration is essential for long-term rescue of a severe spinal muscular atrophy mouse model. *Nature* 478, 123–126. doi: 10.1038/nature10485

Igarashi, S., Tanno, Y., Onodera, O., Yamazaki, M., Sato, S., Ishikawa, A., et al. (1992). Strong correlation between the number of CAG repeats in androgen receptor genes and the clinical onset of features of spinal and bulbar muscular atrophy. *Neurology* 42, 2300–2302. doi: 10.1212/WNL.42.12.2300

Ilieva, H., Polymenidou, M., and Cleveland, D. W. (2009). Non-cell autonomous toxicity in neurodegenerative disorders: ALS and beyond. *J. Cell Biol.* 187, 761–772. doi: 10.1083/jcb.200908164

Jaarsma, D., Teuling, E., Haasdijk, E. D., De Zeeuw, C. I., and Hoogenraad, C. C. (2008). Neuron-specific expression of mutant superoxide dismutase is sufficient to induce amyotrophic lateral sclerosis in transgenic mice. *J. Neurosci.* 28, 2075–2088. doi: 10.1523/JNEUROSCI.5258-07.2008

Johansen, J. A., Yu, Z., Mo, K., Monks, D. A., Lieberman, A. P., Breedlove, S. M., et al. (2009). Recovery of function in a myogenic mouse model of spinal bulbar muscular atrophy. *Neurobiol. Dis.* 34, 113–120. doi: 10.1016/j.nbd.2008.12.009

Kabashi, E., Valdmanis, P. N., Dion, P., Spiegelman, D., McConkey, B. J., Vande Velde, C., et al. (2008). TARDBP mutations in individuals with sporadic and familial amyotrophic lateral sclerosis. *Nat. Genet.* 40, 572–574. doi: 10.1038/ng.132

Kallen, R. G., Cohen, S. A., and Barchi, R. L. (1993). Structure, function and expression of voltage-dependent sodium channels. *Mol. Neurobiol.* 7, 383–428. doi: 10.1007/BF02769184

Kariya, S., Park, G. H., Maeno-Hikichi, Y., Leykekhman, O., Lutz, C., Arkovitz, M. S., et al. (2008). Reduced SMN protein impairs maturation of the neuromuscular junctions in mouse models of spinal muscular atrophy. *Hum. Mol. Genet.* 17, 2552–2569. doi: 10.1093/hmg/ddn156

Kaspar, B. K., Frost, L. M., Christian, L., Umapathi, P., and Gage, F. H. (2005). Synergy of insulin-like growth factor-1 and exercise in amyotrophic lateral sclerosis. *Ann. Neurol.* 57, 649–655. doi: 10.1002/ana.20451

Kaspar, B. K., Llado, J., Sherkat, N., Rothstein, J. D., and Gage, F. H. (2003). Retrograde viral delivery of IGF-1 prolongs survival in a mouse ALS model. *Science* 301, 839–842. doi: 10.1126/science.1086137

Katsuno, M., Adachi, H., Kume, A., Li, M., Nakagomi, Y., Niwa, H., et al. (2002). Testosterone reduction prevents phenotypic expression in a transgenic mouse model of spinal and bulbar muscular atrophy. *Neuron* 35, 843–854. doi: 10.1016/S0896-6273(02)00834-6

Katsuno, M., Tanaka, F., Adachi, H., Banno, H., Suzuki, K., Watanabe, H., et al. (2012). Pathogenesis and therapy of spinal and bulbar muscular atrophy (SBMA). *Prog. Neurobiol.* 99, 246–256. doi: 10.1016/j.pneurobio.2012.05.007

Klocke, R., Steinmeyer, K., Jentsch, T. J., and Jockusch, H. (1994). Role of innervation, excitability, and myogenic factors in the expression of the muscular chloride channel ClC-1. A study on normal and myotonic muscle. *J. Biol. Chem.* 269, 27635–27639.

Kong, L., Wang, X., Choe, D. W., Polley, M., Burnett, B. G., Bosch-Marce, M., et al. (2009). Impaired synaptic vesicle release and immaturity of neuromuscular junctions in spinal muscular atrophy mice. *J. Neurosci.* 29, 842–851. doi: 10.1523/JNEUROSCI.4434-08.2009

Krasnianski, A., Deschauer, M., Neudecker, S., Gellerich, F. N., Muller, T., Schoser, B. G., et al. (2005). Mitochondrial changes in skeletal muscle in amyotrophic lateral sclerosis and other neurogenic atrophies. *Brain* 128, 1870–1876. doi: 10.1093/brain/awh540

La Bella, V., Cisterni, C., Salaun, D., and Pettmann, B. (1998). Survival motor neuron (SMN) protein in rat is expressed as different molecular forms and is developmentally regulated. *Eur. J. Neurosci.* 10, 2913–2923. doi: 10.1111/j.1460-9568.1998.00298.x

Lai, K. M., Gonzalez, M., Poueymirou, W. T., Kline, W. O., Na, E., Zlotchenko, E., et al. (2004). Conditional activation of akt in adult skeletal muscle induces rapid hypertrophy. *Mol. Cell. Biol.* 24, 9295–9304. doi: 10.1128/MCB.24.21.9295-9304.2004

Lee, J. H., Shin, J. H., Park, K. P., Kim, I. J., Kim, C. M., Lim, J. G., et al. (2005). Phenotypic variability in Kennedy's disease: implication of the early diagnostic features. *Acta Neurol. Scand.* 112, 57–63. doi: 10.1111/j.1600-0404.2005.00428.x

Lee, S. J., and McPherron, A. C. (2001). Regulation of myostatin activity and muscle growth. *Proc. Natl. Acad. Sci. U.S.A.* 98, 9306–9311. doi: 10.1073/pnas.151270098

Lee, Y. I., Mikesh, M., Smith, I., Rimer, M., and Thompson, W. (2011). Muscles in a mouse model of spinal muscular atrophy show profound defects in neuromuscular development even in the absence of failure in neuromuscular transmission or loss of motor neurons. *Dev. Biol.* 356, 432–444. doi: 10.1016/j.ydbio.2011.05.667

Lefebvre, S., Burlen, L., Reboullet, S., Clermont, O., Burlet, P., Viollet, L., et al. (1995). Identification and characterization of a spinal muscular atrophy-determining gene. *Cell* 80, 155–165. doi: 10.1016/0092-8674(95)90460-3

Lefebvre, S., Burlet, P., Liu, Q., Bertrandy, S., Clermont, O., Munnich, A., et al. (1997). Correlation between severity and SMN protein level in spinal muscular atrophy. *Nat. Genet.* 16, 265–269. doi: 10.1038/ng0797-265

Léger, B., Vergani, L., Soraru, G., Hespel, P., Derave, W., Gobelet, C., et al. (2006). Human skeletal muscle atrophy in amyotrophic lateral sclerosis reveals a reduction in Akt and an increase in atrogin-1. *FASEB J.* 20, 583–585. doi: 10.1096/fj.05-5249fje

Lino, M. M., Schneider, C., and Caroni, P. (2002). Accumulation of SOD1 mutants in postnatal motoneurons does not cause motoneuron pathology or motoneuron disease. *J. Neurosci.* 22, 4825–4832.

Liu, Q., and Dreyfuss, G. (1996). A novel nuclear structure containing the survival of motor neurons protein. *EMBO J.* 15, 3555–3565.

Lunetta, C., Serafini, M., Prelle, A., Magni, P., Dozio, E., Ruscica, M., et al. (2012). Impaired expression of insulin-like growth factor-1 system in skeletal muscle of amyotrophic lateral sclerosis patients. *Muscle Nerve* 45, 200–208. doi: 10.1002/mus.22288

Mahoney, D. J., Kaczor, J. J., Bourgeois, J., Yasuda, N., and Tarnopolsky, M. A. (2006). Oxidative stress and antioxidant enzyme upregulation in SOD1-G93A mouse skeletal muscle. *Muscle Nerve* 33, 809–816. doi: 10.1002/mus.20542

Malena, A., Pennuto, M., Tezze, C., Querin, G., D'ascenzo, C., Silani, V., et al. (2013). Androgen-dependent impairment of myogenesis in spinal and bulbar muscular atrophy. *Acta Neuropathol.* 126, 109–121. doi: 10.1007/s00401-013-1122-9

Manzano, R., Toivonen, J. M., Olivan, S., Calvo, A. C., Moreno-Igoa, M., Munoz, M. J., et al. (2011). Altered expression of myogenic regulatory factors in the mouse model of amyotrophic lateral sclerosis. *Neurodegener. Dis.* 8, 386–396. doi: 10.1159/000324159

Martinez, T. L., Kong, L., Wang, X., Osborne, M. A., Crowder, M. E., Van Meerbeke, J. P., et al. (2012). Survival motor neuron protein in motor neurons determines synaptic integrity in spinal muscular atrophy. *J. Neurosci.* 32, 8703–8715. doi: 10.1523/JNEUROSCI.0204-12.2012

Martinez-Hernandez, R., Soler-Botija, C., Also, E., Alias, L., Caselles, L., Gich, I., et al. (2009). The developmental pattern of myotubes in spinal muscular atrophy indicates prenatal delay of muscle maturation. *J. Neuropathol. Exp. Neurol.* 68, 474–481. doi: 10.1097/NEN.0b013e3181a10ea1

McEachern, G., Kassovska-Bratinova, S., Raha, S., Tarnopolsky, M. A., Turnbull, J., Bourgeois, J., et al. (2000). Manganese superoxide dismutase levels are elevated in a proportion of amyotrophic lateral sclerosis patient cell lines. *Biochem. Biophys. Res. Commun.* 273, 359–363. doi: 10.1006/bbrc.2000.2933

Meister, G., Buhler, D., Laggerbauer, B., Zobawa, M., Lottspeich, F., and Fischer, U. (2000). Characterization of a nuclear 20S complex containing the survival of motor neurons (SMN) protein and a specific subset of spliceosomal Sm proteins. *Hum. Mol. Genet.* 9, 1977–1986. doi: 10.1093/hmg/9.13.1977

Meister, G., Eggert, C., and Fischer, U. (2002). SMN-mediated assembly of RNPs: a complex story. *Trends Cell Biol.* 12, 472–478. doi: 10.1016/S0962-8924(02)02371-1

Michaud, M., Arnoux, T., Bielli, S., Durand, E., Rotrou, Y., Jablonka, S., et al. (2010). Neuromuscular defects and breathing disorders in a new mouse model of spinal muscular atrophy. *Neurobiol. Dis.* 38, 125–135. doi: 10.1016/j.nbd.2010.01.006

Mo, K., Razak, Z., Rao, P., Yu, Z., Adachi, H., Katsuno, M., et al. (2010). Microarray analysis of gene expression by skeletal muscle of three mouse models of Kennedy disease/spinal bulbar muscular atrophy. *PLoS ONE* 5:e12922. doi: 10.1371/journal.pone.0012922

Monani, U. R., Sendtner, M., Coovert, D. D., Parsons, D. W., Andreassi, C., Le, T. T., et al. (2000). The human centromeric survival motor neuron gene (SMN2) rescues embryonic lethality in Smn(-/-) mice and results in a mouse with spinal muscular atrophy. *Hum. Mol. Genet.* 9, 333–339. doi: 10.1093/hmg/9.3.333

Monks, D. A., Johansen, J. A., Mo, K., Rao, P., Eagleson, B., Yu, Z., et al. (2007). Overexpression of wild-type androgen receptor in muscle recapitulates polyglutamine disease. *Proc. Natl. Acad. Sci. U.S.A.* 104, 18259–18264. doi: 10.1073/pnas.0705501104

Moresi, V., Williams, A. H., Meadows, E., Flynn, J. M., Potthoff, M. J., McAnally, J., et al. (2010). Myogenin and class II HDACs control neurogenic muscle atrophy by inducing E3 ubiquitin ligases. *Cell* 143, 35–45. doi: 10.1016/j.cell.2010.09.004

Murdocca, M., Malgieri, A., Luchetti, A., Saieva, L., Dobrowolny, G., De Leonibus, E., et al. (2012). IPLEX administration improves motor neuron survival and ameliorates motor functions in a severe mouse model of spinal muscular atrophy. *Mol. Med.* 18, 1076–1085. doi: 10.2119/molmed.2012.00056

Musaro, A., McCullagh, K., Paul, A., Houghton, L., Dobrowolny, G., Molinaro, M., et al. (2001). Localized Igf-1 transgene expression sustains hypertrophy and regeneration in senescent skeletal muscle. *Nat. Genet.* 27, 195–200. doi: 10.1038/84839

Mutsaers, C. A., Wishart, T. M., Lamont, D. J., Riessland, M., Schreml, J., Comley, L. H., et al. (2011). Reversible molecular pathology of skeletal muscle in spinal muscular atrophy. *Hum. Mol. Genet.* 20, 4334–4344. doi: 10.1093/hmg/ddr360

Nicole, S., Desforges, B., Millet, G., Lesbordes, J., Cifuentes-Diaz, C., Vertes, D., et al. (2003). Intact satellite cells lead to remarkable protection against Smn gene defect in differentiated skeletal muscle. *J. Cell Biol.* 161, 571–582. doi: 10.1083/jcb.200210117

Ogawa, C., Usui, K., Aoki, M., Ito, F., Itoh, M., Kai, C., et al. (2007). Gemin2 plays an important role in stabilizing the survival of motor neuron complex. *J. Biol. Chem.* 282, 11122–11134. doi: 10.1074/jbc.M609297200

Osborne, M., Gomez, D., Feng, Z., McEwen, C., Beltran, J., Cirillo, K., et al. (2012). Characterization of behavioral and neuromuscular junction phenotypes in a novel allelic series of SMA mouse models. *Hum. Mol. Genet.* 21, 4431–4447. doi: 10.1093/hmg/dds285

Palazzolo, I., Burnett, B. G., Young, J. E., Brenne, P. L., La Spada, A. R., Fischbeck, K. H., et al. (2007). Akt blocks ligand binding and protects against expanded polyglutamine androgen receptor toxicity. *Hum. Mol. Genet.* 16, 1593–1603. doi: 10.1093/hmg/ddm109

Palazzolo, I., Stack, C., Kong, L., Musaro, A., Adachi, H., Katsuno, M., et al. (2009). Overexpression of IGF-1 in muscle attenuates disease in a mouse model of spinal and bulbar muscular atrophy. *Neuron* 63, 316–328. doi: 10.1016/j.neuron.2009.07.019

Paushkin, S., Gubitz, A. K., Massenet, S., and Dreyfuss, G. (2002). The SMN complex, an assemblyosome of ribonucleoproteins. *Curr. Opin. Cell Biol.* 14, 305–312. doi: 10.1016/S0955-0674(02)00332-0

Pearn, J. (1978). Incidence, prevalence, and gene frequency studies of chronic childhood spinal muscular atrophy. *J. Med. Genet.* 15, 409–413. doi: 10.1136/jmg.15.6.409

Pellizzoni, L., Charroux, B., Rappsilber, J., Mann, M., and Dreyfuss, G. (2001). A functional interaction between the survival motor neuron complex and RNA polymerase II. *J. Cell Biol.* 152, 75–85. doi: 10.1083/jcb.152.1.75

Pellizzoni, L., Yong, J., and Dreyfuss, G. (2002). Essential role for the SMN complex in the specificity of snRNP assembly. *Science* 298, 1775–1779. doi: 10.1126/science.1074962

Pradat, P. F., Barani, A., Wanschitz, J., Dubourg, O., Lombes, A., Bigot, A., et al. (2011). Abnormalities of satellite cells function in amyotrophic lateral sclerosis. *Amyotroph. Lateral Scler.* 12, 264–271. doi: 10.3109/17482968.2011.566618

Pramatarova, A., Laganiere, J., Roussel, J., Brisebois, K., and Rouleau, G. A. (2001). Neuron-specific expression of mutant superoxide dismutase 1 in transgenic mice does not lead to motor impairment. *J. Neurosci.* 21, 3369–3374.

Prior, T. W., Snyder, P. J., Rink, B. D., Pearl, D. K., Pyatt, R. E., Mihal, D. C., et al. (2010). Newborn and carrier screening for spinal muscular atrophy. *Am. J. Med. Genet. A* 152A, 1608–1616. doi: 10.1002/ajmg.a.33474

Rajendra, T. K., Gonsalvez, G. B., Walker, M. P., Shpargel, K. B., Salz, H. K., and Matera, A. G. (2007). A Drosophila melanogaster model of spinal muscular atrophy reveals a function for SMN in striated muscle. *J. Cell Biol.* 176, 831–841. doi: 10.1083/jcb.200610053

Rindt, H., Buckley, D. M., Vale, S. M., Krogman, M., Rose, F. F. Jr., Garcia, M. L., et al. (2012). Transgenic inactivation of murine myostatin does not decrease the severity of disease in a model of Spinal Muscular Atrophy. *Neuromuscul. Disord.* 22, 277–285. doi: 10.1016/j.nmd.2011.10.012

Rochette, C. F., Gilbert, N., and Simard, L. R. (2001). SMN gene duplication and the emergence of the SMN2 gene occurred in distinct hominids: SMN2 is unique to Homo sapiens. *Hum. Genet.* 108, 255–266. doi: 10.1007/s004390100473

Rose, F. F. Jr., Mattis, V. B., Rindt, H., and Lorson, C. L. (2009). Delivery of recombinant follistatin lessens disease severity in a mouse model of spinal muscular atrophy. *Hum. Mol. Genet.* 18, 997–1005. doi: 10.1093/hmg/ddn426

Rosen, D. R., Siddique, T., Patterson, D., Figlewicz, D. A., Sapp, P., Hentati, A., et al. (1993). Mutations in Cu/Zn superoxide dismutase gene are associated with familial amyotrophic lateral sclerosis. *Nature* 362, 59–62. doi: 10.1038/362059a0

Rossoll, W., Jablonka, S., Andreassi, C., Kroning, A. K., Karle, K., Monani, U. R., et al. (2003). Smn, the spinal muscular atrophy-determining gene product, modulates axon growth and localization of beta-actin mRNA in growth cones of motoneurons. *J. Cell Biol.* 163, 801–812. doi: 10.1083/jcb.200304128

Rowland, L. P., and Shneider, N. A. (2001). Amyotrophic lateral sclerosis. *N. Engl. J. Med.* 344, 1688–1700. doi: 10.1056/NEJM200105313442207

Sambataro, F., and Pennuto, M. (2012). Cell-autonomous and non-cell-autonomous toxicity in polyglutamine diseases. *Prog. Neurobiol.* 97, 152–172. doi: 10.1016/j.pneurobio.2011.10.003

Schiaffino, S., and Mammucari, C. (2011). Regulation of skeletal muscle growth by the IGF1-Akt/PKB pathway: insights from genetic models. *Skelet Muscle* 1, 4. doi: 10.1186/2044-5040-1-4

Schiaffino, S., and Reggiani, C. (2011). Fiber types in mammalian skeletal muscles. *Physiol. Rev.* 91, 1447–1531. doi: 10.1152/physrev.00031.2010

Schmidt, B. J., Greenberg, C. R., Allingham-Hawkins, D. J., and Spriggs, E. L. (2002). Expression of X-linked bulbospinal muscular atrophy (Kennedy disease) in two homozygous women. *Neurology* 59, 770–772. doi: 10.1212/WNL.59.5.770

Schrank, B., Gotz, R., Gunnersen, J. M., Ure, J. M., Toyka, K. V., Smith, A. G., et al. (1997). Inactivation of the survival motor neuron gene, a candidate gene for human spinal muscular atrophy, leads to massive cell death in early mouse embryos. *Proc. Natl. Acad. Sci. U.S.A.* 94, 9920–9925. doi: 10.1073/pnas.94.18.9920

Shababi, M., Glascock, J., and Lorson, C. L. (2011). Combination of SMN trans-splicing and a neurotrophic factor increases the life span and body mass in a severe model of spinal muscular atrophy. *Hum. Gene Ther.* 22, 135–144. doi: 10.1089/hum.2010.114

Shafey, D., Boyer, J. G., Bhanot, K., and Kothary, R. (2010). Identification of novel interacting protein partners of SMN using tandem affinity purification. *J. Proteome Res.* 9, 1659–1669. doi: 10.1021/pr9006987

Shafey, D., Cote, P. D., and Kothary, R. (2005). Hypomorphic Smn knockdown C2C12 myoblasts reveal intrinsic defects in myoblast fusion and myotube morphology. *Exp. Cell Res.* 311, 49–61. doi: 10.1016/j.yexcr.2005.08.019

Sorarù, G., D'ascenzo, C., Polo, A., Palmieri, A., Baggio, L., Vergani, L., et al. (2008). Spinal and bulbar muscular atrophy: skeletal muscle pathology in male patients and heterozygous females. *J. Neurol. Sci.* 264, 100–105. doi: 10.1016/j.jns.2007.08.012

Sumner, C. J., Wee, C. D., Warsing, L. C., Choe, D. W., Ng, A. S., Lutz, C., et al. (2009). Inhibition of myostatin does not ameliorate disease features of severe spinal muscular atrophy mice. *Hum. Mol. Genet.* 18, 3145–3152. doi: 10.1093/hmg/ddp253

Tsai, L. K., Chen, Y. C., Cheng, W. C., Ting, C. H., Dodge, J. C., Hwu, W. L., et al. (2012). IGF-1 delivery to CNS attenuates motor neuron cell death but does not improve motor function in type III SMA mice. *Neurobiol. Dis.* 45, 272–279. doi: 10.1016/j.nbd.2011.06.021

Vielhaber, S., Winkler, K., Kirches, E., Kunz, D., Buchner, M., Feistner, H., et al. (1999). Visualization of defective mitochondrial function in skeletal muscle fibers of patients with sporadic amyotrophic lateral sclerosis. *J. Neurol. Sci.* 169, 133–139. doi: 10.1016/S0022-510X(99)00236-1

Walker, M. P., Rajendra, T. K., Saieva, L., Fuentes, J. L., Pellizzoni, L., and Matera, A. G. (2008). SMN complex localizes to the sarcomeric Z-disc and is a proteolytic target of calpain. *Hum. Mol. Genet.* 17, 3399–3410. doi: 10.1093/hmg/ddn234

Wan, L., Battle, D. J., Yong, J., Gubitz, A. K., Kolb, S. J., Wang, J., et al. (2005). The survival of motor neurons protein determines the capacity for snRNP assembly: biochemical deficiency in spinal muscular atrophy. *Mol. Cell. Biol.* 25, 5543–5551. doi: 10.1128/MCB.25.13.5543-5551.2005

Wang, L., Sharma, K., Deng, H. X., Siddique, T., Grisotti, G., Liu, E., et al. (2008). Restricted expression of mutant SOD1 in spinal motor neurons and interneurons induces motor neuron pathology. *Neurobiol. Dis.* 29, 400–408. doi: 10.1016/j.nbd.2007.10.004

Wiedemann, F. R., Winkler, K., Kuznetsov, A. V., Bartels, C., Vielhaber, S., Feistner, H., et al. (1998). Impairment of mitochondrial function in skeletal muscle of patients with amyotrophic lateral sclerosis. *J. Neurol. Sci.* 156, 65–72. doi: 10.1016/S0022-510X(98)00008-2

Will, C. L., and Luhrmann, R. (2001). Spliceosomal UsnRNP biogenesis, structure and function. *Curr. Opin. Cell Biol.* 13, 290–301. doi: 10.1016/S0955-0674(00)00211-8

Wong, M., and Martin, L. J. (2010). Skeletal muscle-restricted expression of human SOD1 causes motor neuron degeneration in transgenic mice. *Hum. Mol. Genet.* 19, 2284–2302. doi: 10.1093/hmg/ddq106

Wong, P. C., Pardo, C. A., Borchelt, D. R., Lee, M. K., Copeland, N. G., Jenkins, N. A., et al. (1995). An adverse property of a familial ALS-linked SOD1 mutation causes motor neuron disease characterized by vacuolar degeneration of mitochondria. *Neuron* 14, 1105–1116. doi: 10.1016/0896-6273(95)90259-7

Yu, Z., Dadgar, N., Albertelli, M., Gruis, K., Jordan, C., Robins, D. M., et al. (2006). Androgen-dependent pathology demonstrates myopathic contribution to the Kennedy disease phenotype in a mouse knock-in model. *J. Clin. Invest.* 116, 2663–2672. doi: 10.1172/JCI28773

Yu, Z., Wang, A. M., Robins, D. M., and Lieberman, A. P. (2009). Altered RNA splicing contributes to skeletal muscle pathology in Kennedy disease knock-in mice. *Dis. Model Mech.* 2, 500–507. doi: 10.1242/dmm.003301
developmentally increased vasculature in mdx mice. *Hum. Mol. Genet.* 19, 4145–4159. doi: 10.1093/hmg/ddq334

von Maltzahn, J., Renaud, J. M., Parise, G., and Rudnicki, M. A. (2012). Wnt7a treatment ameliorates muscular dystrophy. *Proc. Natl. Acad. Sci. U.S.A.* 109, 20614–20619. doi: 10.1073/pnas.1215765109

Wang, H., Noulet, F., Edom-Vovard, F., Tozer, S., Le Grand, F., and Duprez, D. (2010). Bmp signaling at the tips of skeletal muscles regulates the number of fetal muscle progenitors and satellite cells during development. *Dev. Cell* 18, 643–654. doi: 10.1016/j.devcel.2010.02.008

Wang, X. Z., Jolicoeur, E. M., Conte, N., Chaffanet, M., Zhang, Y., Mozziconacci, M. J., et al. (1999). gamma-heregulin is the product of a chromosomal translocation fusing the DOC4 and HGL/NRG1 genes in the MDA-MB-175 breast cancer cell line. *Oncogene* 18, 5718–5721. doi: 10.1038/sj.onc.1202950

White, R. B., Bierinx, A. S., Gnocchi, V. F., and Zammit, P. S. (2010). Dynamics of muscle fibre growth during postnatal mouse development. *BMC Dev. Biol.* 10:21. doi: 10.1186/1471-213X-10-21

Yaffe, D., and Saxel, O. (1977). Serial passaging and differentiation of myogenic cells isolated from dystrophic mouse muscle. *Nature* 270, 725–727. doi: 10.1038/270725a0

Yajima, H., Motohashi, N., Ono, Y., Sato, S., Ikeda, K., Masuda, S., et al. (2010). Six family genes control the proliferation and differentiation of muscle satellite cells. *Exp. Cell Res.* 316, 2932–2944. doi: 10.1016/j.yexcr.2010.08.001

Yamaguchi, M., and Fukada, S. (2013). "Regulation of muscle stem cell quiescent and undifferentiated state: roles of Hesr1 and Hesr3 genes," in *Tumor Dormancy, Quiescence, and Senescence*, Vol. 1, ed. M. A. Hayat (Netherlands: Springer), 107–116.

Yamaguchi, M., Ogawa, R., Watanabe, Y., Uezumi, A., Miyagoe-Suzuki, Y., Tsujikawa, K., et al. (2012). Calcitonin receptor and Odz4 are differently expressed in Pax7-positive cells during skeletal muscle regeneration. *J. Mol. Histol.* 43, 581–587. doi: 10.1007/s10735-012-9421-3

Yamazaki, S., Ema, H., Karlsson, G., Yamaguchi, T., Miyoshi, H., Shioda, S., et al. (2011). Nonmyelinating Schwann cells maintain hematopoietic stem cell hibernation in the bone marrow niche. *Cell* 147, 1146–1158. doi: 10.1016/j.cell.2011.09.053

Zhou, X., Wang, J. L., Lu, J., Song, Y., Kwak, K. S., Jiao, Q., et al. (2010). Reversal of cancer cachexia and muscle wasting by ActRIIB antagonism leads to prolonged survival. *Cell* 142, 531–543. doi: 10.1016/j.cell.2010.07.011

Zhou, X. H., Brandau, O., Feng, K., Oohashi, T., Ninomiya, Y., Rauch, U., et al. (2003). The murine Ten-m/Odz genes show distinct but overlapping expression patterns during development and in adult brain. *Gene Expr. Patterns* 3, 397–405. doi: 10.1016/S1567-133X(03)00087-5

15

Docosahexaenoyl ethanolamide improves glucose uptake and alters endocannabinoid system gene expression in proliferating and differentiating C2C12 myoblasts

Jeffrey Kim*, *Morgan E. Carlson* and *Bruce A. Watkins*

Center on Aging, University of Connecticut Health Center, Farmington, CT, USA

Correspondence:
Bruce A. Watkins, Department of Nutrition, University of California, Davis, Davis, CA 95616-5270, USA
e-mail: baw@purdue.edu

Skeletal muscle is a major storage site for glycogen and a focus for understanding insulin resistance and type-2-diabetes. New evidence indicates that overactivation of the peripheral endocannabinoid system (ECS) in skeletal muscle diminishes insulin sensitivity. Specific n-6 and n-3 polyunsaturated fatty acids (PUFA) are precursors for the biosynthesis of ligands that bind to and activate the cannabinoid receptors. The function of the ECS and action of PUFA in skeletal muscle glucose uptake was investigated in proliferating and differentiated C2C12 myoblasts treated with either 25 μM of arachidonate (AA) or docosahexaenoate (DHA), 25 μM of EC [anandamide (AEA), 2-arachidonoylglycerol (2-AG), docosahexaenoylethanolamide (DHEA)], 1 μM of CB1 antagonist NESS0327, and CB2 inverse agonist AM630. Compared to the BSA vehicle control cell cultures in both proliferating and differentiated myoblasts those treated with DHEA, the EC derived from the n-3 PUFA DHA, had higher 24 h glucose uptake, while AEA and 2-AG, the EC derived from the n-6 PUFA AA, had lower basal glucose uptake. Adenylyl cyclase mRNA was higher in myoblasts treated with DHA in both proliferating and differentiated states while those treated with AEA or 2-AG were lower compared to the control cell cultures. Western blot and qPCR analysis showed higher expression of the cannabinoid receptors in differentiated myoblasts treated with DHA while the opposite was observed with AA. These findings indicate a compensatory effect of DHA and DHEA compared to AA-derived ligands on the ECS and associated ECS gene expression and higher glucose uptake in myoblasts.

Keywords: endocannabinoid system, C2C12 myoblasts, cannabinoid receptors, glucose uptake, gene expression, DHEA, polyunsaturated fatty acids

INTRODUCTION

Skeletal muscle serves as a major target organ for glucose removal from circulation and the relevancy of this tissue is bolstered by the disease states of insulin resistance and diabetes. Under euglycemic conditions in healthy subjects, approximately 75% of glucose removal is mediated by non-insulin stimulated glucose uptake primarily by the brain and to a lesser extent in other tissues such as skeletal muscle (Baron et al., 1988). However, under hyperglycemic conditions, glucose uptake mediated via non-insulin stimulated glucose uptake increases considerably (Capaldo et al., 1986). Moreover, the importance of basal glucose uptake is apparent during insulin resistance and diabetes when close to 80% of glucose uptake is achieved postprandially (Best et al., 1996).

In recent years, researchers have identified a physiologic mechanism that regulates the balance of macronutrient metabolism. The endocannabinoid system (ECS) is a complex network encompassing various physiological systems in the body that is comprised of the G-protein-coupled receptors, CB1 and CB2, their lipid-derived endogenous ligands termed endocannabinoids, and the enzymes that are involved in the biosynthesis/degradation of the endocannabinoids. While the ECS has been shown to influence several physiological activities, such as hunger, pain modulation, mood, and inflammation, the primary function appears to impact energy homeostasis, as activation of the ECS appears to shift energy balance toward energy storage (De Petrocellis et al., 1999; Soderstrom et al., 2004; Valenti et al., 2005; Piazza et al., 2007).

Previous findings confirm the role of the ECS in food intake and energy homeostasis. Reduced food intake was reported in mice (Despres et al., 2005) by pharmacologically antagonizing CB1 as well as in CB1 knockout mice (Pi-Sunyer et al., 2006). The interest in targeting this specific cannabinoid receptor is supported by several key findings. Importantly, antagonism of CB1

Abbreviations: 2-AG, 2-arachidonoylglycerol; 2-NBDG, 2-deoxy-2-[(7-nitro-2,1,3-benzoxadiazol-4-yl) amino]-D-glucose; AA, arachidonic acid; AEA, N-arachidonoylethanolamine; anandamide; ALA, α-linolenic acid; AMPK, AMP-activated protein kinase; BSA, bovine serum albumin; CB1, cannabinoid receptor 1; CB2, cannabinoid receptor 2; DAGLα, diacylglycerol lipase-α; DAGLβ, diacylglycerol lipase-β; DHA, docosahexaenoic acid; DHEA, docosahexaenoyl ethanolamide; DM, differentiation media; EC, endocannabinoid; ECS, endocannabinoid system; EPA, eicosapentaenoic acid; EPEA, eicosapentaenoyl ethanolamide; FAAH, fatty acid amide hydrolase; FACS, fluorescence activated cell sorting; FAME, fatty acid methyl ester; GM, growth media; IL, interleukin; IRS-1, insulin receptor substrate-1; LA, linoleic acid; MAPK, mitogen-activated protein kinase; NAPE-PLD, N-acyl phosphatidylethanolamine phospholipase; PUFA, polyunsaturated fatty acid; qPCR, quantitative polymerase chain reaction; TNF-α, tumor necrosis factor-α.

reduced food intake and body weight (Cota et al., 2003; Ravinet Trillou et al., 2003). However, the reduced food intake did not account for the total reduction in body weight, suggesting an ulterior means of energy expenditure. Furthermore, in both obese subjects and in leptin deficient mice, reduced glucose uptake and fatty acid oxidation were observed to be reversed by antagonizing CB1 (Liu et al., 2005; Cavuoto et al., 2007). Along with this, blood concentrations of the two chiefly studied endocannabinoids, anandamide (AEA) and 2-arachidonoylglycerol (2-AG) both derived from arachidonic acid (AA), are elevated in obese compared to lean individuals (Bluher et al., 2006; Matias et al., 2006).

In support of CB1 exerting a role on energy balance, evidence from several studies in animal models as well as in humans revealed that in conditions of obesity and hyperglycemia the ECS is in an overactivated state (Engeli et al., 2005; Bluher et al., 2006; Matias et al., 2006). This phenomenon is referred to as ECS tone, which is the collective actions of ligands, receptors, and enzymes of endocannabinoid synthesis and degradation. In other words, the ECS is overactivated in the state of obesity. Thus in the overactivated state a dysregulated ECS observed in both the obese and an insulin resistive state contributes to greater lipid accumulation and insulin resistance in muscle. Targeting the ECS to improve signaling for maintaining healthy muscle glucose sensitivity and reduce excessive lipid accumulation is an attractive application. Moreover findings that the ECS plays an active role in macronutrient metabolism we propose that directing endogenous agonist actions on the ECS to improve glucose homeostasis has implications for diabetes and obesity.

Recognizing that dietary sources of fatty acids and more specifically the polyunsaturated fatty acids (PUFA) can alter tissue composition of membrane phospholipids, dietary manipulation permits indirect control of the ECS on cellular functions. It is well known that the amount and type of dietary n-6 and n-3 PUFA changes the PUFA composition of membrane phospholipids in various tissues including muscle and bone compartments (Brown et al., 1991; Watkins et al., 2003; Hutchins-Wiese et al., 2012). Additionally, studies on mouse adipocytes demonstrated that cultures incubated with AA or docosahexaenoic acid (DHA) for 72 h elevated levels of these PUFA in phospholipids compared to the vehicle controls (Matias et al., 2008). Furthermore, AA treatment in the adipocyte cultures led to an increase of 2-AG concentrations while DHA treatment significantly decreased both AEA and 2-AG concentrations compared to the vehicle control.

Various studies on feeding rodents different dietary PUFA resulted in alterations in the levels of endocannabinoids of brain (Watanabe et al., 2003), adipose (Batetta et al., 2009), and liver (Artmann et al., 2008; Batetta et al., 2009). Mice fed a high fat diet supplemented with krill oil for 8 weeks were found to have reduced levels of AA-derived endocannabinoids in various peripheral tissue, including gastrocnemius (Piscitelli et al., 2011). Changes were reported in ECS genes of muscle when different dietary PUFA were fed to mice. For example, in our laboratory, analysis of quadriceps muscle from male ND4 Swiss Webster mice fed either a control diet (AIN-93G with safflower oil) or a high n-3 PUFA diet (EPA+DHA 17.6 g/kg) for 26 days revealed changes in several ECS genes (Hutchins-Wiese et al., 2012). We reported that the mRNA for AEA synthesis enzyme, N-acyl phosphatidylethanolamine phospholipase (NAPE-PLD), and 2-AG synthesis enzyme, diacylglycerol lipase (DAGL)α and DAGLβ, were higher in muscle of mice fed the n-3 PUFA diet compared to the controls. Furthermore, in this study the mRNA expression of CB1 and CB2 were both higher in muscle of mice fed the high n-3 PUFA diet. Collectively, these findings strongly suggest that dietary n-3 PUFA treatment can alter mRNA expression of key ECS genes to influence ECS signaling.

Since cellular membranes participate in numerous physiological and biochemical processes, changing the PUFA composition of cell membranes through diet can alter signaling and receptor functions associated with the ECS. Based on these findings that ECS gene expression changed upon exposure to different amounts and families of PUFA, the ECS is likely to adapt and change accordingly to these nutrients that serve as EC precursors. Therefore, an investigation exploring the adaptations from dietary PUFA enrichment on the skeletal muscle ECS is warranted as this signaling system is actively involved in energy homeostasis.

To investigate the role of the ECS on basal glucose uptake, our overall research hypothesis was that dietary long chain n-3 PUFA, DHA, and EPA, enrichment of C2C12 myoblasts restores endocannabinoid tone (action of ligands, receptors, and enzymes of the ECS synthesis and degradation) and signaling of this system to improve glucose homeostasis with potential applications to reduce obesity and diabetes. Since ECS receptor activation likely plays a role in impacting glucose uptake, the investigation also evaluated the consequences of PUFA treatment with cannabinoid receptor agonists and antagonists. The specific aim of this research was to describe the effects of PUFA enrichment on endocannabinoid gene expression and agonist/antagonist actions on glucose homeostasis in the myoblast cell line C2C12. Herein, C2C12 myoblast cell cultures were enriched with 25 μM levels of PUFA and the mRNA (qPCR) and protein expression (Western blot) of endocannabinoid enzymes and cannabinoid receptors were quantified. The expression of these enzymes and receptors were studied in myoblast cell cultures in both the proliferative and differentiation committed states. Additionally, insulin signaling/glucose uptake was measured as a consequent outcome.

MATERIALS AND METHODS

CELL CULTURES AND TREATMENTS

C2C12 cells were purchased from American Type Culture Collection (ATCC, Manassas, VA, USA) and routinely cultured in growth media (GM) consisting of Dulbecco's Modified Eagles Medium (DMEM; Thermo Fisher Scientific, Waltham, MA, USA) supplemented in 10% fetal bovine serum (FBS, Thermo Fisher Scientific, Waltham, MA, USA), and 1% antibiotic solution or in differentiation media (DM), consisting of DMEM with 2% horse serum (Thermo Fisher Scientific, Waltham, MA, USA) in place of FBS. Cultures were maintained in vented 75 cm^2 tissue culture flasks (Becton Dickinson and Company, Franklin Lakes, NJ, USA) at a density of 1×10^6 cells per flask as determined by automated TC-10 cell counter (Bio-Rad laboratories, Inc., Hercules, CA, USA). Seeded at this density, cultures became 80–85% confluent after 72 h, at which time the cells were passed onto new flasks containing fresh GM. C2C12 cell cultures in all experiments were from passages 5–9.

Proliferating and differentiated cells were used to model skeletal muscle, such as within an *ex vivo* model or whole organism. Skeletal muscle found in mammals contains a mix of both proliferating and differentiating myoblasts (during active regeneration from injury, in addition to routine organ maintenance and homeostasis). Differentiated C2C12 were chosen to mimic mature myofibers. Myogenin and MyoD1, markers of differentiation, were used to verify that myoblasts had committed toward differentiation.

CHEMICALS AND REAGENTS

The treatment media contained PUFA AA, EPA, and DHA all from Nu-Chek-Prep, Inc. (Elysian, MN, USA) and endocannabinoids (AEA and 2-AG from Abcam, PLC., Cambridge, MA, USA) that were dissolved in 100% ethanol at a final concentration of 100 mg/mL, flushed with N_2 and stored in glass amber vials at −20°C until needed. The PUFA containing media were prepared by adding fatty acid stock aliquots to either serum free GM containing endotoxin/fatty acid free BSA (Sigma Chemical Company, Saint Louis, MO, USA) that was used at a concentration dependent of PUFA concentration (2:1, PUFA:BSA). Working concentrations of the PUFA stock solutions were diluted as appropriate to achieve the necessary final concentrations. Cell cultures were treated for 24 h in 37°C at 5% CO_2. 24 h prior to cell collection then treated with varying physiologic concentrations of AA, EPA, DHA, AEA, or 2-AG at 25 μM while 5, 10, and 25 μM for the glucose uptake experiments. Additionally, NESS0327, a CB1 antagonist, or AM630, a CB2 inverse agonist were used to pretreat cells at concentrations of 1, 2, or 5 μM.

FATTY ACID METHYL ESTERS ANALYSIS OF C2C12 CELL CULTURES

Fatty acid methyl esters (FAME) analysis was performed to measure fatty acid composition in C2C12 myoblast cultures, which were washed with calcium/magnesium-free phosphate buffered saline (PBS; 137 mM NaCl, 2.7 mM KCl, 9.9 mM Na_2HPO_4, 1.8 mM KH_2PO_4; Thermo Fisher Scientific, Waltham, MA, USA) and removed by scraping with a Teflon scraper. Cells were sonicated and extracted for lipids with chloroform/methanol (2:1, vol/vol) (Thermo Fisher Scientific, Waltham, MA, USA). Extracted lipids were treated with 0.5 N NaOH in methanol, and FAME prepared by esterification using boron trifluoride (BF3) in methanol (10% w/w, Supelco Inc., Bellefonte, PA, USA). The FAME were concentrated in isooctane (HPLC grade, Fisher Scientific, Pittsburg, PA, USA) and analyzed by gas chromatography (GC) (HP 7890A series, autosampler 7693, GC ChemStation Rev.B.04.03, Agilent Technologies, Palo Alto, CA, USA) with a DB-225 column (30 m, 0.25 mm i.d., 0.15 mm film thickness, Agilent Technologies, Palo Alto, CA, USA) equipped with a flame ionization detector (Li et al., 2010). Sample peaks were identified by comparison to authentic FAME standards (Nu-Chek-Prep Inc., Elysian, MN, USA). Sample injection volume was 3 μL and split ratio 10:1. Results for FAME analysis were obtained by weight percentage reports based on the response values for authentic standards of known concentrations to determine weight percentages values. This approach facilitates lipid and subsequent FAME recovery to minimize losses in peak responses at lower concentrations of components.

QUANTITATIVE REAL-TIME POLYMERASE CHAIN REACTION (qPCR)

Analysis of mRNA expression of genes of interest was measured to understand changes in ECS and glucose-related genes after PUFA or endocannabinoid treatment. C2C12 cells were cultured in 75 cm^2 flasks until 85–90% confluent, followed by treatment with fatty acid or endocannabinoid. Afterwards, cells were washed twice with cold PBS, followed by RNA extraction with TRIzol (Invitrogen Corp., Carlsbad, CA, USA) reagent. RNA samples were then treated with DNase I (Ambion, Carlsbad, CA, USA) to remove any DNA contamination. Total RNA (1 μg) was reverse transcribed to cDNA in a reaction mixture using RNA transcriptase superscript III (Invitrogen Corp., Carlsbad, CA, USA). Briefly, 9 μL of the following were combined for each sample: 4 μL 5X VILO reaction mix containing random hexamers and dNTPs, 2 μL 10X Superscript enzyme mix® (BioRad Laboratories, Hercules, CA, USA) containing RNA inhibitors, and 3 μL of DEPC treated water for a total volume of 20 μL. Samples were heated as specified for superscript RT: 25°C for 10 min, 42°C for 60 min, and 85°C for 5 min. Synthesized cDNA product was then used for quantitative RT-PCR. A master mix for RT-PCR was prepared with SsoFast EvaGreen® Supermix (BioRad Laboratories, Hercules, CA, USA). Briefly, 10 μL SsoFast EvaGreen® was mixed with 6 μL DEPC treated water, 1 μL of 10 μM forward primer, and 1 μL of 10 μM reverse primer. A total of 18 μL of master mix was added to wells of unskirted 96-well plates with 2 μL of cDNA. All samples were analyzed in triplicate. Fluorescence emission was detected and cycle threshold (CT) values were calculated in the linear range automatically. Relative CT amounts were calculated from the standard curve for each gene, which were normalized to the reference gene, GAPDH, afterwards. The primers sequences used in this work are shown in **Table 1**. ΔΔCT values for each sample were determined by calculating the difference between the CT value of the target gene and the CT value of the reference gene, GAPDH. The normalized level of expression of the target gene in each sample was calculated using the formula $2^{-\Delta\Delta CT}$. Values were expressed as fold of the control.

WESTERN BLOT ANALYSIS

Protein expressions of genes were analyzed by collecting whole cell lysates after incubation with PUFA treatments. Cells were washed twice with cold PBS followed by scraping to dislodge from surface and transferred to 1.5 mL microfuge tubes to be lysated using a lysis buffer (100 mM Tris-HCl + 0.1% Triton X-100, pH 7.5). Lysates were then centrifuged at 12,000 g for 5 min at 4°C, after in which the supernatant was collected and stored at −80°C. Proteins were then separated by polyacrylamide gel (gradient 4–15%) electrophoresis then transferred to a PVDF membrane, to be followed by antibody incubation against the protein of interest (α-mouse-CB1, α-mouse-CB2, α-rabbit-GLUT4, α-rabbit-Insulin-R, Abcam, PLC., Cambridge, MA, USA). Protein expression was detected using Westpico horseradish peroxidase chemiluminescence and imaged using a Chemidoc XRS+ system

Table 1 | Primer sequences used for quantitative polymerase chain reaction (qPCR).

Gene	Forward	Reverse	Accession
GAPDH	TGTGATGGGTGTGAACCACGAGAA	GAGCCCTTCCACAATGCCAAAGTT	GU214026.1
CB1	TCACACCTCAGAAGATGGCAAGGT	AGCAGATGATCAACACCACCAGGA	AY522554.1
CB2	TGAAGATCGGCAGTGTGACCATGA	AATGCTGAGAGGACCCACATGACA	U21681.1
NAPE-PLD	TGGCATTGTGCATGAAAGCCCTAC	AGTGGGCATGGTGTAGTTGTCAGT	AB112350.1
FAAH	TGGCATTGTGCATGAAAGCCCTAC	AGTGGGCATGGTGTAGTTGTCAGT	NM_010173.4
DAGL-α	CGACCACCAAGTGCAACCATTGAA	AACTCGGCGAATTCTAGCACCTGA	BC148308.2
DAGL-β	TGTGTGTCAGCATGAGAGGAACCA	GTGGCGATGATGCCAATGACAACT	BC016105.1
Akt-1	GTAGCCATTGTGAAGGAG	TCTTGAGGAGGAAGTAGC	AF124142.1
Insulin-R	TCCTGGAAATCGTCAACCTGCTCA	ACGATCCAACGGGACATTCTCCAT	J05149.1
IRS-1	GGCACATCTCCTACCATT	CATCATCTCTGTATATTCCTCAAT	NM_010570.4
GLUT4	TCGTGGCCATATTTGGCTTTGTGG	TAAGGACCCATAGCATCCGCAACA	AB008453.1
GLUT1	CATCGCCCTGGCCCTGCAGGAGC	GGCACCCCCCTGCCGGAAGCCGGA	D10229.1
Adiponectin	AATGACAGGAGCTGAAGGGC	AGGTGAAGAGAACGGCCTTG	NM_009605.4
Myogenin	CGTGGGCATGTAAGGTGTGTAAGA	CATTCACTTTCTTGAGCCTGCGCT	M95800.1
MyoD1	TGAGCAAAGTGAATGAGGCCTTCG	AGAGCCTGCAGACCTTCGATGTA	M18779.1
IL-6	ATCCAGTTGCCTTCTTGGGACTGA	TAAGCCTCCGACTTGTGAAGTGGT	M20572.1
TNF-α	AGCCGATGGGTTGTACCTTGTCTA	TGAGATAGCAAATCGGCTGACGGT	D84199.2
MCP-1	TGAGCCATGGGAACAAGGAAGTCT	TGTGCTGGTCTGTGATAGGCACAT	BC055070.1
AMPK-α2	TCCTGAAGACCCCTCCTACG	GAGTGGTTCTCAGCTGTGCT	NM_178143.2
Adenylyl cyclase	GAAAGTGCGAACCCAGAGGA	ACTTGCGGACGTGTTCAGAT	AF458089.1
p42/p44 (MAPK)	AGCCACACGTTGGTACAGAG	CCAGAGCTTTGGAGTCAGCA	X58712.1
p38 (MAPK)	GGCTGATGAGGAGATGACCG	ATGGGAGGCAGAGACTGGAT	AF135185.1
JNK (MAPK)	AGTGGGTTGCATCATGGGAG	CTGCATCTGAAGGCTGGTCT	NM_016700.4

and Image Lab software (BioRad Laboratories, Hercules, CA, USA) (Tsang et al., 1989).

FLOW CYTOMETRY

In addition to Western blot analysis, FACS flow cytometry was also used to measure expression of cannabinoid receptors. C2C12 cultures were washed twice with cold PBS followed by scraping to dislodge from surface and transferred to 1.5 mL microfuge tubes to be incubated with primary antibodies (α-goat-CB1 and α-rabbit-CB2, Abcam, PLC., Cambridge, MA, USA) diluted in FACS buffer (1:250) for 1 h in 4°C. Afterwards, cells were centrifuged at 500 g for 5 min (4°C) and washed 3 times. Following washing, secondary antibodies (goat α-rabbit 488 and donkey α-goat FITC; Thermo Scientific, Abcam, PLC, Cambridge, MA, USA) were diluted in FACS buffer (1:500) for 1 h in 4°C in the dark. Cells were then centrifuged at 500 g for 5 min (4°C) and washed 3 times. Cells were resuspended in 1 mL of FACS buffer for FACS flow cytometry. Cell acquisition was performed on a FACSCalibur flow cytometer (BD Biosciences, San Jose, CA). 10,000 events were processed for each measurement. Data was analyzed using FlowJo software (Tree Star Inc., Ashland, OR).

GLUCOSE UPTAKE ASSAY

Glucose uptake assay kits (Caymen Chem, Ann Harbor, MI) were used to assess and quantify glucose uptake capacity after fatty acid, endocannabinoid, or ECS receptor inhibitor treatment. Glucose is taken up by the majority of cells via the action of glucose transporters, which facilitate glucose movement down a concentration gradient, in contrast to energy-dependent uptake of glucose in the gut or kidney. Use of a recently developed fluorescent glucose analog, 2-deoxy-2-[(7-nitro-2,1,3-benzoxadiazol-4-yl) amino]-D-glucose) (2-NBDG), allows for the target investigation of glucose uptake without having to account for glucose metabolism or conversion to glycogen once taken up by cells. 2-NBDG is a fluorescently-labeled deoxyglucose analog and is used as the sole probe for detection.

Proliferating and differentiating C2C12 cells were seeded at $\sim 5 \times 10^4$ cells/well in black walled/clear bottom 96-well plates (Corning, Inc., Corning, NY, USA) in DMEM (+1% Pen/Strep and 10% FBS). Upon reaching a confluency of 50%, differentiation was induced with differentiating media consisting of high glucose DMEM, 2% Horse Serum (HS), and 1% Pen/Strep. After 48 h, media was changed to specific PUFA or EC containing media at a concentration of 5, 10, or 25 μM or cannabinoid receptor inhibitor (1, 2, or 5 μM) for 24 h. Following PUFA enrichment, media was removed from wells and treated with 100 μg/mL 2-NBDG for 1 h. Afterwards plates were centrifuged for 5 min at 500 g at room temperature and washed twice with the provided cell-based assay. 2-NBDG taken up by the cells was then measured at a wavelength of 485/535 nm (excitation/emission) on a BioTek Synergy HT plate reader (BioTek Instruments, Inc., Winooski, VT, USA).

STATISTICAL ANALYSES

The results from experiments on gene expression and glucose uptake in proliferating and differentiated C2C12 cell cultures were analyzed for significance by One-Way ANOVA at $P < 0.05$. Where significant differences were found, a Tukey's Multiple

Comparison Test was performed at a probability of $\alpha = 0.05$ (SAS for Windows version 9.3, SAS Institute Inc., Cary, NC). The data are presented as means ± s.e.m. as well as means ± *SD* where indicated with $n = 3$ for each treatment group. These data were also expressed as standardized differences calculated from the difference between values of treatment and control divided by the mean of the control replicates [(treatment—BSA)/BSA ∗ 100, BSA is the mean of 3 BSAs]. The results from experiments on CB1 and CB2 receptor expression in proliferating and differentiated C2C12 cell cultures were performed via FACS flow cytometry were analyzed for significance by One-Way ANOVA at $P < 0.05$. Where significant differences were found, a Tukey's Multiple Comparison Test was performed at a probability of $\alpha = 0.05$. These data were also expressed as standardized differences calculated from the difference between values of treatment and control divided by the mean of the control replicates [(treatment—BSA)/BSA ∗ 100, BSA is the mean of 3 BSA values]. Flow cytometry data were also compared among three concentrations for the same treatment by One-Way ANOVA. A Two-Way ANOVA analysis was further performed on flow cytometry data to detect any interactions between the various treatments and the three tested concentrations of each treatment. Results from the analysis of fatty acid methyl esters (FAME) by gas chromatography to reflect the fatty acid composition of enriched C2C12 cell cultures (proliferating and differentiated) were analyzed by a One-Way ANOVA at $P < 0.05$. Where significant differences were found, a Tukey's Multiple Comparison Test was performed at a probability of $\alpha = 0.05$. The FAME data are expressed as means ± s.e.m. Each treatment group was comprised of three replicates.

Results from experiments on glucose uptake assay were performed in proliferating and differentiated C2C12 after PUFA or EC and inhibitor treatments (expressed as relative units of fluorescence). The collected data were analyzed for significance by one-way ANOVA at $P < 0.05$. Where significant differences were found, a Tukey's Multiple Comparison Test was performed at a probability of $\alpha = 0.05$. These data are presented as means ± s.e.m. as well as means ± *SD* with $n = 3$ for each treatment group. Glucose uptake data were also adjusted by cell numbers expressed as relative units of fluorescence/5000 cells and same statistical procedures were applied to this set of data. Glucose uptake data were further expressed as standardized differences calculated from the difference between values of treatment and control divided by the mean of the control replicates [(treatment—BSA)/BSA ∗ 100, BSA is the mean of 3 BSAs]. The same statistical procedure was applied to the adjusted and standardized data for the evaluation of results.

RESULTS

FATTY ACID ANALYSIS OF LIPIDS FROM C2C12 CELL CULTURES

C2C12 myoblasts were cultured for 24 h following subculturing to allow cells to attach to flasks. Following 24 h, cells designated for differentiation were exposed to DM for 48 h, when myotubes formation was present and levels of myogenin and MyoD1 mRNA were elevated verified by RT-PCR. Both differentiated and proliferating cells were treated with either 25 μM of AA, EPA, DHA, AEA, 2-AG, or the no-fatty acid vehicle control, BSA. The fatty acid composition of total lipids extracted from differentiated C2C12 cells after enrichment is shown in **Table 2** and for proliferating cells supplemental **Table S1**. The PUFA enrichment of cell cultures demonstrated a multiple fold increase in the respective PUFA enrichment and n-3 PUFA decreased the levels of AA. Likewise AA treatment resulted in lower levels of EPA and DHA in myoblast cultures. Treatment of cultures with AEA resulted in lower 18:2n6 but higher 20:1n9 in differentiated cells compared to the BSA vehicle control cell cultures. 2-AG treatment of differentiated myoblast cultures resulted in lower t16:1, 16:1n7, 18:1n9, 18:1n7, 18:2n6, and 20:5n3 and higher 20:1n9, 20:4n6, 22:4n6, and 22:5n3 (**Table 2**). Proliferating C2C12 cell cultures treated with 2-AG had lower t16:1, 16:1n7, 18:1n9, 18:1n7, and 18:2n6 and higher 20:4n6, 22:4n6 (**Table S1**).

DHA TREATMENT LEADS TO A COMPENSATORY EXPRESSION OF ECS-RELATED GENES SUGGESTING A DAMPENING OF ECS ACTIVATION

Analysis of mRNA by quantitative RT-PCR from proliferating and differentiated C2C12 myoblasts that were treated with 25 μM of either AA, EPA, DHA, AEA, 2-AG or a no-fatty acid BSA vehicle control revealed several changes on ECS- and glucose uptake - related mRNA expression when normalized to the housekeeping gene GAPDH. These data were pooled for analysis from two separate experiments (**Table 3** differentiated cell cultures and **Table S2** proliferating cell cultures).

Cannabinoid receptors CB1 and CB2

Compared to the BSA vehicle control cell cultures a higher expression of both CB1 and CB2 was observed with DHA, EPA, DHA, EPEA, and DHEA treatment of differentiated cells (**Table 3**). A lower expression of CB1 and CB2 was observed with AA, AEA, and 2-AG treatment of differentiated cell cultures. Treatment with AA, DHA, EPA, EPEA, and DHEA resulted in a higher amount of mRNA for CB1 and CB2 in proliferating myoblasts (**Table S2**). In these experiments n-3 PUFA and EPEA and DHEA resulted in the highest amount of cannabinoid receptor mRNA.

Synthesis and degradation enzymes

The treatment of differentiated C2C12 cell cultures with AA or AEA resulted in lower mRNA expression of NAPE-PLD while higher expression occurred with EPA treatment (**Table 3**). Expression of the synthesizing enzymes for 2-AG, DAGLα and DAGLβ, were also measured. DAGLα and DAGLβ were both observed to have higher expression with AA or EPA enrichment while 2-AG had an opposite effect and lowered mRNA expression of both enzymes. The enzyme responsible for degradation of AEA and 2-AG through hydrolysis is FAAH. This enzyme was found to be higher with AA, EPA, and AEA treatment of C2C12 cell cultures.

Similar to the differentiated cells, proliferating C2C12 cell cultures treated with AA or AEA, NAPE-PLD, which is the synthesizing enzyme for AEA, was lower compared to the no-fatty acid BSA vehicle control (**Table S2**). A higher expression of NAPE-PLD mRNA was observed with EPA and DHA treatment. AA, DHA, and AEA resulted in a higher expression of DAGLα, while

Table 2 | Fatty acid composition of total lipids from differentiated C2C12 cell cultures.

Fatty acid	Treatments						Pooled s.e.m	ANOVA *p* value
	BSA	AA	EPA	DHA	AEA	2-AG		
14:0	1.07^{a}	0.68^{b}	0.65^{b}	0.71^{b}	1.02^{a}	1.05^{a}	0.05	<0.0001
14:1n5								
15:0								
16:0	13.70^{a}	11.39^{c}	11.97^{b}	12.21^{b}	13.42^{a}	13.32^{a}	0.10	<0.0001
t16:1	2.31^{a}	1.42^{d}	1.49^{d}	1.74^{c}	2.29^{a}	2.09^{b}	0.03	<0.0001
16:1n7	4.64^{a}	2.49^{d}	2.70^{cd}	2.88^{c}	4.65^{a}	3.81^{b}	0.05	<0.0001
17:0	0^{b}	0^{b}	0.37^{a}	0.18^{ab}	0.08^{b}	0.07^{b}	0.06	0.0066
18:0	13.74^{ab}	12.44^{b}	13.56^{ab}	13.05^{ab}	14.15^{a}	14.05^{a}	0.31	0.018
18:1n9	19.80^{a}	11.67^{e}	12.90^{d}	13.95^{c}	19.69^{a}	16.50^{b}	0.15	<0.0001
18:1n7	7.04^{a}	4.91^{d}	5.06^{cd}	5.27^{c}	7.12^{a}	6.32^{b}	0.05	<0.0001
18:2n6	4.28^{a}	2.11^{e}	3.49^{d}	3.70^{c}	4.01^{b}	3.52^{d}	0.03	<0.0001
18:3n6	0.11^{b}	0.70^{a}	0.29^{b}	0^{b}	0.19^{b}	0.16^{b}	0.07	0.0002
18:3n3								
20:0								
20:1n9	0^{b}	0^{b}	0^{b}	0^{b}	0.32^{a}	0.19^{a}	0.04	0.0002
20:2n6								
20:3n6	1.79^{a}	0.28^{c}	1.04^{b}	1.34^{ab}	1.68^{a}	1.39^{ab}	0.12	<0.0001
20:4n6	9.31^{c}	33.94^{a}	6.37^{e}	7.06^{d}	9.20^{c}	15.58^{b}	0.18	<0.0001
20:3n3								
20:5n3	1.87^{c}	0.69^{e}	21.57^{a}	4.41^{b}	1.75^{c}	1.66^{d}	0.22	<0.0001
22:0	0	0	0.08	0	0	0	0.03	0.46
22:1n9								
22:4n6	0.83^{c}	4.09^{a}	0.67^{d}	0.48^{e}	0.84^{c}	1.22^{b}	0.01	<0.0001
22:5n6								
22:5n3	3.17^{c}	2.45^{d}	7.03^{a}	1.94^{e}	3.18^{c}	3.40^{b}	0.04	<0.0001
22:6n3	3.68^{b}	2.23^{c}	2.29^{c}	22.09^{a}	3.84^{b}	3.73^{b}	0.06	<0.0001
24:0	0.10	0	0	0	0.08	0.17	0.06	0.35
24:1n9	0.22	0	0.10	0.13	0.20	0.21	0.10	0.61
Saturated	28.61^{ab}	24.51^{d}	26.62^{bc}	26.15^{cd}	28.75^{a}	28.67^{ab}	0.43	<0.0001
Monounsaturated	31.70^{a}	19.08^{e}	20.76^{d}	22.23^{c}	31.98^{a}	27.03^{b}	0.18	<0.0001
Total PUFA	25.04^{d}	46.49^{a}	42.76^{b}	41.01^{b}	24.69^{d}	30.65^{c}	0.42	<0.0001
n-6 PUFA	16.32^{c}	41.11^{a}	11.87^{d}	12.58^{d}	15.92^{c}	21.87^{b}	0.19	<0.0001
n-3 PUFA	8.72^{c}	5.37^{d}	30.89^{a}	28.44^{b}	8.77^{c}	8.79^{c}	0.28	<0.0001
Ratio of n-6/n-3	1.87^{c}	7.65^{a}	0.38^{d}	0.44^{d}	1.81^{c}	2.49^{b}	0.01	<0.0001

Data represent means of $n = 3$ for each group and the pooled s.e.m. Values within rows having different superscripts are significantly different by One-way ANOVA and Tukey's mean separation test at $\alpha = 0.05$. BSA, bovine serum albumin; AA, arachidonic acid; EPA, eicosapentaenoic acid; DHA, docosahexaenoic acid; AEA, anandamide; 2AG, 2-arachidonoyl glycerol

AA, EPA, and AEA led to a higher DAGLβ expression. FAAH was observed here to be lower with AEA and AA treatment of proliferating C2C12 cell cultures.

ECS Confirmation (MAPK + Adenylyl cyclase)

In order to determine potential ECS receptor activity, several downstream events known to occur with activation were analyzed (Felder et al., 1993; Rolli-Derkinderen et al., 2003; Howlett, 2005). Here we see a lower expression of adenylyl cyclase and a higher expression of the MAPK enzymes, p42/p44, p38, and Jun N-terminal kinase (JNK) with only AEA and 2-AG in both proliferating and differentiated myoblasts (**Tables 3**, **S2**), which is consistent with the literature in confirming activation of the cannabinoid receptors (Felder et al., 1993; Howlett, 2005).

Glucose aspects

In proliferating C2C12 cultures, AA led to lower mRNA expression of insulin-R, GLUT1, and IRS-1. Contrastingly, DHA was found to have higher insulin-R, GLUT4, GLUT1, and IRS-1 mRNA expression. EPA was observed to have no significant changes to any of the genes involved in glucose uptake. AEA was observed to lower the mRNA expression of Akt-1, insulin-R, GLUT4, GLUT1, and IRS-1. 2-AG was also observed to have a negative effect on these glucose-related genes as Akt-1, GLUT1, and

Table 3 | mRNA expression in differentiated C2C12 myoblast cultures treated with PUFA and EC.

Measurement	BSA	AA	DHA	EPA	AEA	2-AG	EPEA	DHEA	Pooled s.e.m.	ANOVA *p* value
CB1	1.0^{e}	0.7^{f}	2.1^{b}	1.5^{d}	0.8^{f}	0.8^{f}	1.8^{c}	2.3^{a}	0.02	<0.0001
CB2	1.0^{d}	0.6^{e}	2.3^{a}	1.5^{c}	0.7^{e}	0.8^{de}	1.8^{b}	0.8^{de}	0.1	<0.0001
NAPE-PLD	1.0^{c}	0.7^{e}	0.8^{de}	1.6^{a}	0.5^{f}	0.9^{cd}	1.7^{a}	1.2^{b}	0.03	<0.0001
FAAH	1.0^{d}	1.5^{c}	0.9^{d}	2.8^{a}	2.4^{b}	1.1^{d}	1.6^{c}	1.5^{c}	0.1	<0.0001
DAGL-α	1.0^{c}	2.4^{b}	0.9^{cd}	3.4^{a}	1.0^{c}	0.7^{d}	1.1^{c}	1.0^{c}	0.0	<0.0001
DAGL-β	1.0^{cd}	2.1^{b}	0.8^{de}	3.4^{a}	1.1^{c}	0.6^{e}	1.1^{c}	1.1^{cd}	0.1	<0.0001
Akt-1	1.0^{de}	0.9^{ef}	1.7^{b}	1.3^{c}	0.8^{f}	1.0^{d}	1.0^{de}	2.6^{a}	0.03	<0.0001
Insulin r	1.0^{c}	0.8^{d}	1.7^{b}	1.1^{c}	0.7^{d}	0.8^{d}	1.1^{c}	2.4^{a}	0.04	<0.0001
IRS-1	1.0^{c}	0.8^{d}	1.5^{b}	1.1^{c}	0.1^{e}	0.1^{e}	1.1^{c}	1.7^{a}	0.02	<0.0001
GLUT4	1.0^{bc}	0.9^{cd}	3.1^{a}	1.0^{bc}	0.8^{d}	0.8^{d}	1.1^{b}	3.3^{a}	0.05	<0.0001
GLUT1	1.0^{c}	0.7^{d}	1.5^{b}	1.1^{c}	0.2^{e}	0.3^{e}	1.1^{c}	3.8^{a}	0.02	<0.0001
Myogenin	1.0^{b}	1.2^{b}	1.6^{a}	1.1^{b}	1.1^{b}	1.1^{b}	1.1^{b}	1.0^{b}	0.04	<0.0001
MyoD1	1.0^{b}	1.2^{b}	1.5^{a}	1.2^{b}	1.2^{b}	1.1^{b}	1.0^{b}	1.0^{b}	0.04	<0.0001
IL-6	1.0^{c}	1.5^{b}	0.5^{d}	1.1^{c}	1.9^{a}	1.6^{b}	0.6^{d}	0.5^{d}	0.02	<0.0001
TNF-α	1.0^{a}	0.7^{bc}	0.7^{b}	1.0^{a}	0.6^{cd}	0.5^{cd}	1.0^{a}	0.5^{d}	0.03	<0.0001
AMPK α2	1.0^{d}	1.0^{d}	1.6^{b}	1.1^{d}	0.7^{e}	0.7^{e}	1.3^{c}	1.8^{a}	0.02	<0.0001
Adenylyl Cyclase	1.0^{a}	1.0^{a}	1.0^{a}	1.0^{a}	0.3^{d}	0.2^{d}	0.8^{b}	0.6^{c}	0.02	<0.0001
p42/p44 (MAPK)	1.0^{e}	1.4^{d}	0.8^{f}	0.7^{f}	1.7^{c}	1.6^{c}	1.9^{b}	2.9^{a}	0.03	<0.0001
p38 (MAPK)	1.0^{cd}	1.2^{bcd}	0.8^{d}	0.9^{d}	$1.5b^{c}$	1.3^{bcd}	1.6^{b}	3.8^{a}	0.12	<0.0001
JNK (MAPK)	1.0^{e}	1.1^{d}	0.8^{f}	0.9^{ef}	1.4^{c}	1.3^{cd}	1.9^{b}	3.5^{a}	0.03	<0.0001
STANDARD DEVIATION										
CB1	0.01	0.1	0.00001	0.04	0.01	0.1	0.02	0.1		
CB2	0.03	0.01	0.2	0.2	0.02	0.02	0.02	0.02		
NAPE-PLD	0.03	0.03	0.03	0.04	0.05	0.1	0.1	0.03		
FAAH	0.03	0.1	0.1	0.1	0.2	0.04	0.02	0.1		
DAGL-α	0.04	0.1	0.1	0.2	0.1	0.05	0.1	0.03		
DAGL-β	0.1	0.1	0.1	0.2	0.04	0.04	0.1	0.1		
Akt-1	0.1	0.001	0.02	0.1	0.04	0.04	0.04	0.1		
Insulin r	0.1	0.03	0.1	0.1	0.02	0.03	0.03	0.1		
GLUT4	0.05	0.1	0.04	0.2	0.04	0.03	0.01	0.1		
Myogenin	0.1	0.04	0.1	0.1	0.002	0.1	0.001	0.03		
MyoD1	0.04	0.1	0.1	0.1	0.1	0.05	0.05	0.03		
GLUT1	0.02	0.01	0.02	0.1	0.01	0.01	0.1	0.1		
IRS-1	0.02	0.01	0.04	0.1	0.001	0.001	0.03	0.05		
IL-6	0.03	0.1	0.01	0.1	0.02	0.1	0.01	0.01		
TNF-α	0.1	0.01	0.03	0.1	0.01	0.02	0.04	0.01		
AMPK α2	0.02	0.02	0.05	0.1	0.1	0.03	0.03	0.03		
Adenylyl Cyclase	0.02	0.03	0.1	0.1	0.01	0.01	0.04	0.02		
p42/p44 (MAPK)	0.04	0.04	0.03	0.03	0.02	0.1	0.1	0.1		
p38 (MAPK)	0.02	0.02	0.02	0.1	0.0005	0.05	0.4	0.4		
JNK (MAPK)	0.01	0.04	0.02	0.1	0.04	0.02	0.04	0.1		

Data in the upper section of the table represent means of $n = 3$ for each cell culture group. qPCR output expressed in $\Delta\Delta Ct$ normalized to BSA control. Values within rows having different superscripts are significantly different by One-Way ANOVA and Tukey's mean separation test at $\alpha = 0.05$. Values in the lower section of the table are the standard deviations of all means.

BSA, bovine serum albumin; AA, arachidonic acid; EPA, eicosapentaenoic acid; DHA, docosahexaenoic acid; AEA, anandamide; 2AG, 2-arachidonoyl glycerol; CB1, cannabinoid receptor 1; CB2, cannabinoid receptor 2; NAPE-PLD, N-acyl phosphatidylethanolamine phospholipase D; FAAH, fatty acid amide hydrolase; DAGLα, diacylglycerol lipase-α; DAGLβ, diacylglycerol lipase-β; Akt1, RAC-alpha serine/threonine-protein kinase (protein kinase B); INS-R, insulin receptor; GLUT4, glucose transporter type 4; MyoD1, myogenic differentiation interleukin-6, IL-6; tumor necrosis factor-α, TNF-α.

IRS-1 were all lower compared to the no-fatty acid vehicle control.

Many of the observations found in the proliferating cells were found to be the same in the differentiated C2C12 myoblasts. AA was found to lower the expression of Akt-1, insulin-R, GLUT1, and IRS-1. Again, DHA resulted in higher mRNA expression of Akt-1, insulin-R, GLUT4, GLUT1, and IRS-1. EPA led to higher Akt-1 expression. AEA resulted in lower Akt-1, insulin-R, GLUT4,

GLUT1, and IRS-1 expression while 2-AG had a lowering effect on insulin-R, GLUT4, GLUT1, and IRS-1 mRNA.

Inflammation

In proliferating C2C12 myoblasts, inflammatory cytokine mRNA expression were analyzed and showed a higher IL-6 and TNF-α with AA, AEA, and 2-AG treatments while DHA enrichment led to a lower expression of the two inflammatory maker mRNA. In differentiated C2C12 myoblasts, IL-6 expression was shown to be lower by DHA enrichment and higher after AA, AEA, and 2-AG treatment. TNF-α expression was found to be lower with AA, DHA, AEA, and 2-AG treatment while EPA enrichment had no effect.

PUFA AND EC TREATMENT RESULTED IN VARYING CB1 AND CB2 EXPRESSION

Western blot analysis followed by densitometry was performed to measure CB1 and CB2 expression in differentiated and proliferating C2C12 myoblasts after being treated with either 25 μM of AA, EPA, DHA, AEA, 2-AG or a no-fatty acid vehicle control (**Figure 1**). In differentiated C2C12 myoblasts, AA, EPA, and DHA resulted in higher protein expression of CB1 compared to the BSA control group. CB2 protein expression was higher for AA, EPA, DHA, AEA, and 2-AG treated differentiated C2C12 myoblasts. Compared to the BSA vehicle control, EPA and DHA enrichment showed higher expression of CB1 and CB2 in proliferating C2C12 myoblasts while AEA treatment had lower expression.

FACS-flow cytometry was performed to measure CB1 and CB2 expression in differentiated and proliferating C2C12 myoblasts after being treated with either 25 μM of AA, EPA, DHA, AEA, 2-AG or a no-fatty acid vehicle control (**Figure 2**). A One-Way ANOVA revealed in differentiated C2C12 myoblasts, that DHA enrichment resulted in a higher expression of CB1 while AEA and 2-AG lower CB1 expression. CB2 expression was higher with DHA alone, while a lower amount was found with AA, AEA, and 2-AG treatment. A significant decrease in both CB1 and CB2 expression was observed with AA, EPA, DHA, AEA, or 2-AG treatment compared to the BSA control in proliferating cells.

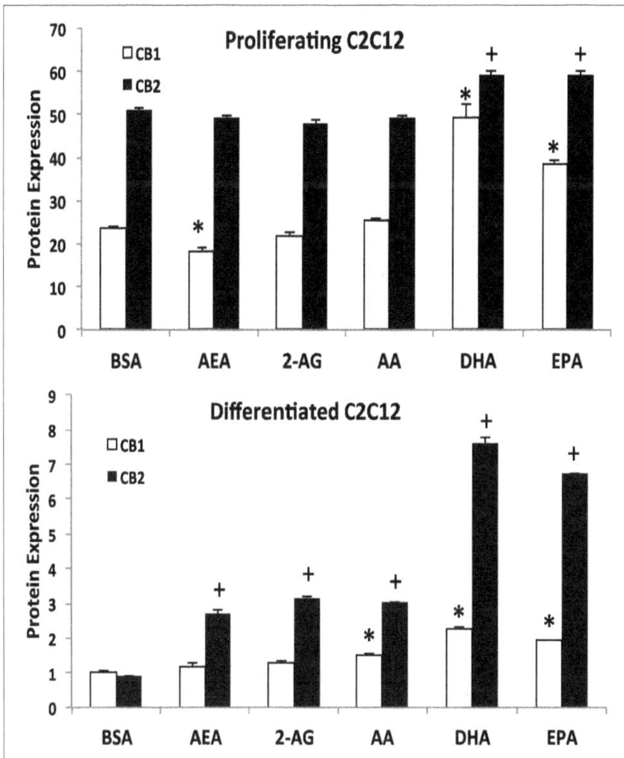

FIGURE 1 | Western blot analysis of CB1 and CB2 expression in proliferating and differentiated C2C12 myoblast cultures treated with PUFA and EC. C2C12 cultures were treated with 25 μM of respective treatments for 24 h. The bars are the means ± *SD* (error bars) of 2 experiments performed in triplicate. The asterisk (*) signifies difference compared to the BSA control for CB1 while the plus sign (+) indicates difference compared to the BSA control for CB2. In proliferating cells compared to the BSA vehicle control, DHA and EPA values for both receptors were higher; CB1 was lower in the AEA treatment. In differentiating cells compared to the BSA vehicle control, all treatments showed higher CB2 protein expression but only AA, DHA and EPA treatments were higher for CB1.

GLUCOSE UPTAKE IS ENHANCED WITH DHEA TREATMENT

Non-insulin stimulated glucose uptake was assessed in differentiated and proliferating C2C12 myoblasts after treatment with either 25 μM of AA, EPA, DHA, AEA, 2-AG, or 1 μM NESS0327 (CB1 inhibitor), 1 μM AM630 (CB2 inhibitor) or a BSA no-fatty acid vehicle control (**Figure 3**). In both differentiated and proliferating C2C12 cell cultures, AEA and 2-AG were found to result in lower glucose uptake compared to the BSA vehicle control cell cultures. However, EPEA, DHEA, NESS0327, and AM630 treatments showed higher glucose uptake. The results are presented as means ± *SD* in **Table S3**.

DISCUSSION

Enrichment of proliferating and differentiated C2C12 myoblasts with AA resulted in an increase in n-6 PUFA and the ratio of n-6/n-3 with a decrease in n-3 PUFA. Conversely, EPA or DHA treatment resulted in the opposite effect of the AA enrichment as an increase in n-3 PUFA with a decrease in n-6 PUFA was observed, resulting in a lower ratio of n-6/n-3 PUFA. These results are in accordance with previous findings in muscle and bone compartments of rodents fed n-6 or n-3 PUFA enriched diets (Watkins et al., 2000; Li et al., 2003; Watkins et al., 2006; Hutchins-Wiese et al., 2012). An aspect that differed from other fatty acid enrichment studies is the exclusion of FBS in enriching media. This exclusion allows for greater control of availing specific fatty acid exposure to cultures.

Our findings are the first to demonstrate that differentiated and proliferating C2C12 myoblasts cell cultures express key ECS-related components. Furthermore, the ECS-related components can be altered with PUFA or endocannabinoid exposure. An interesting finding was the observed increase in AA with 2-AG enrichment in both differentiated and proliferating cells. While this observation is the first to report this finding, it is very likely a result of 2-AG hydrolysis leading to the liberation and elevation of AA in cell lipids.

Several recent studies have demonstrated that endocannabinoid concentrations in tissues and in circulation are responsive to the types of dietary n-6 and n-3 PUFA when fed to animals or

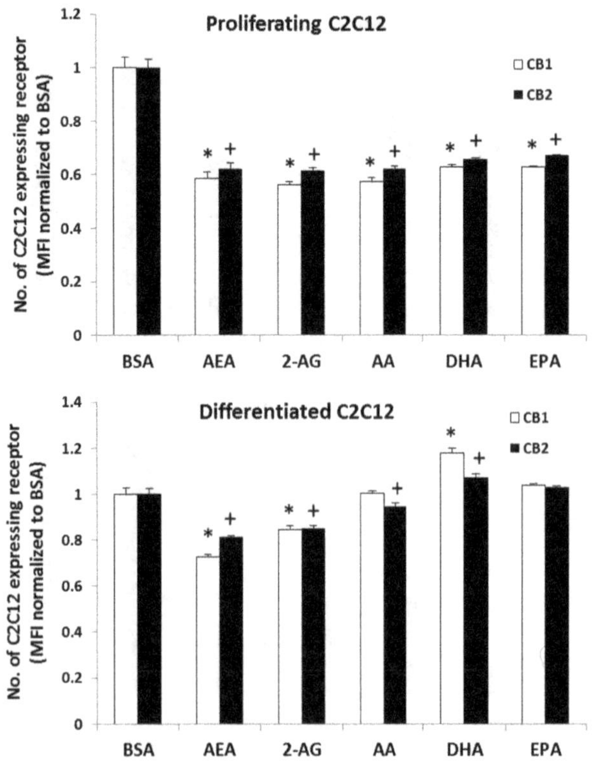

FIGURE 2 | FACS flow cytometry analysis of CB1 and CB2 expression in proliferating and differentiated C2C12 myoblast cultures treated with PUFA and EC. C2C12 cultures were treated with 25 μM concentrations of respective treatments for 24 h. The bars are the means ± *SD* (error bars) of 3 experiments performed in triplicate. The asterisk (*) signifies difference compared to the BSA control for CB1 while the plus sign (+) indicates difference compared to the BSA control for CB2. In proliferating cells all treatments were different compared to the BSA vehicle control. In differentiating cells compared to the BSA vehicle control, DHA had higher CB1 and CB2 values and AEA and 2-AG were lower values but CB2 was lower in the AA cells.

in cell cultures. Studies with mouse adipocytes incubated with AA or DHA (100 μM) for 72 h showed elevated levels of these PUFA in phospholipids (Matias et al., 2008). AA treatment in these cells led to an increase in 2-AG concentrations. Moreover, DHA treatment significantly decreased both AEA and 2-AG concentrations compared to the control. This study demonstrated that fatty acid enrichment of adipocytes in culture could also modify endocannabinoid concentrations with specificity. Several studies showed that dietary PUFA altered the levels of endocannabinoids in tissues including brain (Watanabe et al., 2003) adipose (Batetta et al., 2009), and liver (Artmann et al., 2008; Batetta et al., 2009). Aside from the ligands of the ECS, our laboratory (Hutchins et al., 2011) reported that EPA enrichment reduced the mRNA levels for the AEA synthesizing enzyme, NAPE-PLD, compared to AA and the vehicle control groups in MC3T3-E1 osteoblast-like cell cultures. While it isn't clear whether PUFA directly affect the cannabinoid receptors, CB2 mRNA was also reduced with EPA treatment. If and how long chain n-3 PUFA affect different cell types in a similar fashion, that is by impacting the ECS receptor expression, in culture or at different stages (differentiated or proliferating) and if similar responses occur *in vivo*, has not been investigated.

Our findings provide new evidence that the C2C12 myoblast cell line expresses ECS receptors and both synthesis and degradation enzymes. Further we report that treatment with PUFA or endocannabinoids were able to influence ECS tone and ultimately, signaling potential of the ECS in these cells. It is evident from the data presented here that with 24 h n-3 PUFA treatment, either EPA or DHA, the ECS tone is potentially upregulated. The mRNA and Western blot analysis for both CB1 and CB2 expression in proliferating and differentiated myoblast cultures were found to be higher than in the BSA vehicle control cell cultures. These findings are illustrated in **Figure 4**. The cannabinoid receptors were also found to be higher in differentiated cultures when analyzed by flow cytometry. Both EPA and DHA enrichment also resulted in higher endocannabinoid synthesis enzymes, NAPE-PLD and DAGLα/β, in proliferating while only EPA demonstrated the effect in differentiated C2C12 cell cultures.

Identification of components of the ECS in our cell system validates the model and was consistent with the literature, in which CB1 and CB2 was found in human skeletal muscle (Cavuoto et al., 2007; Eckardt et al., 2009) and differentiated L6 myotubes (Esposito et al., 2008). While the majority of ECS studies in muscle have focused on pharmacological interventions to monitor energy expenditure (Liu et al., 2005), mainly dealing with the short-lived antiobesity drug, Rimonabant (SR141716) (Esposito et al., 2008; Eckardt et al., 2009), the current investigation is the first to interrogate the ECS in muscle cells using dietary PUFA.

In proliferating C2C12 treated with AA, a decrease of NAPE-PLD was observed, the enzyme for AEA biosynthesis. It is possible that because of the abundant availability of the PUFA precursor, the synthesizing enzyme is being maximally saturated and less synthesis of AEA is required by the cell, resulting in a downregulation at the mRNA level of the enzyme. This is supported by the results with DHA and EPA treatments and both are potential precursors of endocannabinoids, DHEA and EPEA, respectively that were found to result in higher NAPE-PLD mRNA compared to the BSA control cells. The n-3 PUFA ethanolamides, docosahexaenoyl ethanolamide (DHEA) and eicosapentaenoyl ethanolamide (EPEA), have been previously shown to be weak ligands to cannabinoid receptors when compared to AEA (Sheskin et al., 1997), suggesting that the upregulation of ECS-related synthesis enzymes observed in this study are attributed to a compensatory response. Structure activity relationships suggest that the n-pentyl chain in AEA is necessary for optimal binding to the CB1 receptor (Felder et al., 1993); however, data relating to CB2 is inadequate. In addition, DHEA also binds to other receptors including PPARs (Artmann et al., 2008), highlighting the complexity of NAE signaling. Even with lower affinity to the cannabinoid receptors, perhaps the n-3 PUFA-derived ethanolamides are synthesized at a greater propensity leading to an inflated competition with other endocannabinoids resulting in the higher CB1 and CB2 expression seen in this study.

To confirm expression of activation of the ECS by AEA and 2-AG, the signaling pathway leading to the sequential activation of mitogen-activated protein kinase (MAPK) were also

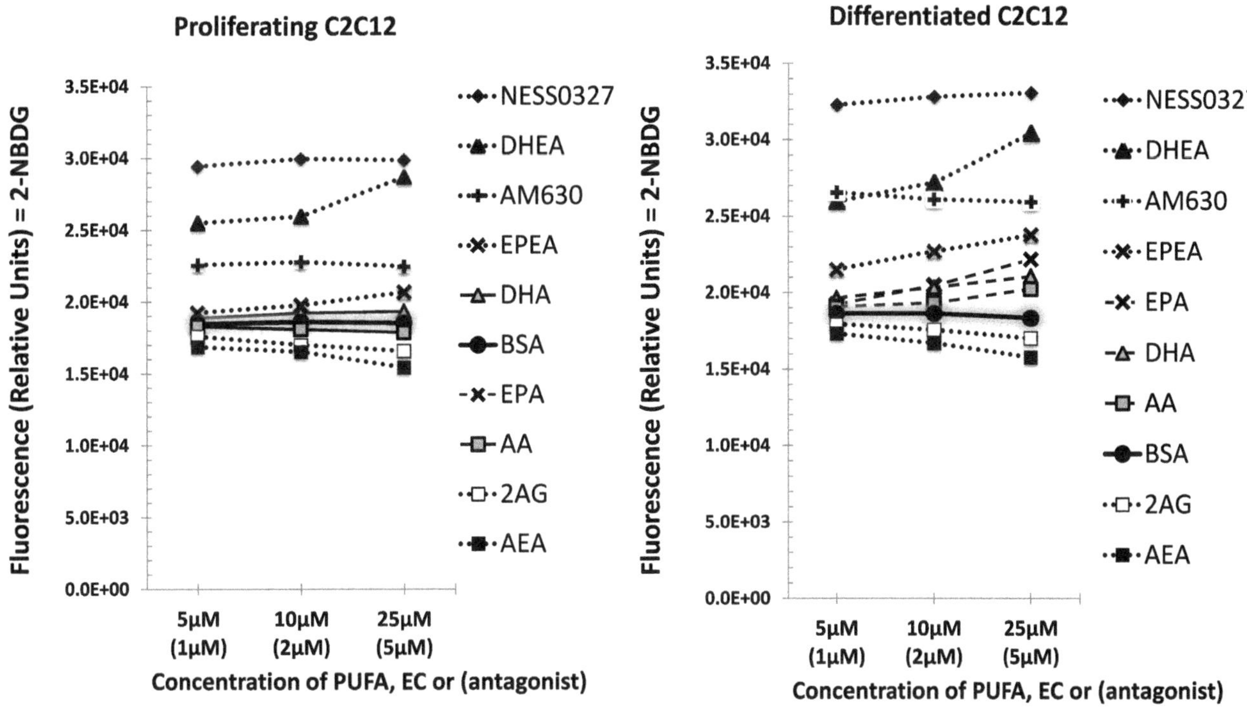

FIGURE 3 | Glucose uptake analysis of proliferating and differentiated C2C12 myoblast cultures treated with either three concentrations (5, 10, or 25 μM) of PUFA (AA, EPA, or DHA) or endocannabinoid (AEA, 2-AG, EPEA or DHEA) or with three concentrations (1, 2, or 5 μM) of cannabinoid receptor antagonist (AM630 or NESS0327) for 24 h. Values shown are means of 3 experiments performed in triplicate. In proliferating cells compared to the BSA vehicle control **(gray shaded line)**, DHA, DHEA, EPEA, AM630, and NESS0327 had higher glucose uptake while AA, AEA, and 2-AG had lower glucose uptake. In differentiated cells compared to the BSA vehicle control, glucose uptake was lower for AEA and 2-AG treatments while all other treatments were higher. Data were analyzed by a One-Way ANOVA and Tukey's mean separation test at $\alpha = 0.05$.The mean values and pooled s.e.m are shown in the supplemental materials **Table S3**.

investigated here. Stimulation of either CB1 or CB2 has previously been shown to lead to the phosphorylation and activation of p42/p44 MAPK, p38 MAPK, and Jun N-terminal kinase (JNK) (Rolli-Derkinderen et al., 2003; Howlett, 2005; Eckardt et al., 2009). The endocannabinoids AEA, 2-AG, EPEA, and DHEA were all shown to increase the mRNA expression of these signaling pathways markers that regulate nuclear transcription factors. Additionally, a lowered expression of adenylyl cyclase mRNA with the endocannabinoid treatments was observed, concurring with observations of cannabinoid receptor activation (Felder et al., 1993; Howlett, 2005). Conversely, EPA and DHA showed a decrease in mRNA expression in p42/p44 MAPK, p38MAPK, and JNK in differentiated C2C12 with proliferating cells only being affected by DHA enrichment. Previously, it has been reported that fish oil decreased these MAPK-family signaling molecules (Lo et al., 2000). From the mRNA analysis, DHEA and EPEA had the highest fold change in p38 MAPK. p38 MAPK has been found to be lower in the liver of obese and type II diabetic mice (Lee et al., 2011). Activation of p38 MAPK was found to reduce endoplasmic reticulum stress and establish euglycemia in these severely obese mice. The MAPK/ERK signaling pathway has also been found to regulate insulin sensitivity into moderate glucose metabolism in *Drosophila* (Zhang et al., 2011). Further investigations of the ECS should focus on this pathway to ascertain the potential of restoring proper glucose homeostasis in obese and type II diabetics.

Signal transduction pathways involving MAPKs as well as the phosphatidylinositol 3-kinase (PI3-K) have been previously found to be key signaling cascades involved in the differentiation process of myoblasts (Zetser et al., 1999; Li and Johnson, 2006). However, the results of studies on the role of MAPKs in regulating skeletal muscle differentiation have been controversial. For example, activation of the ERK pathway seems to be important for mediating the repressive effect of growth factors on myogenesis. One study has suggested that ERK activation positively regulates myogenesis (Weyman and Wolfman, 1998). JNK has been involved in controlling diverse cellular functions, including cell proliferation, differentiation, and apoptosis (Garrington and Johnson, 1999). The activity of JNK has been reported to be activated during differentiation of C2 myoblasts and essential for survival (Bennett and Tonks, 1997; Khurana and Dey, 2004). Additionally, the role of MAPKs in the proliferation of skeletal muscle has not yet been fully studied, although inhibition of their activation is known to lead growth arrest in many cells, including myoblasts. Lipina et al. (2010) has also examined the effects of targeting CB1 and its downstream effects, finding that impeding CB1 activation enhanced both insulin-stimulated ERK1/2 and PI3-K/protein kinase-B activity in L6 myotubes. To

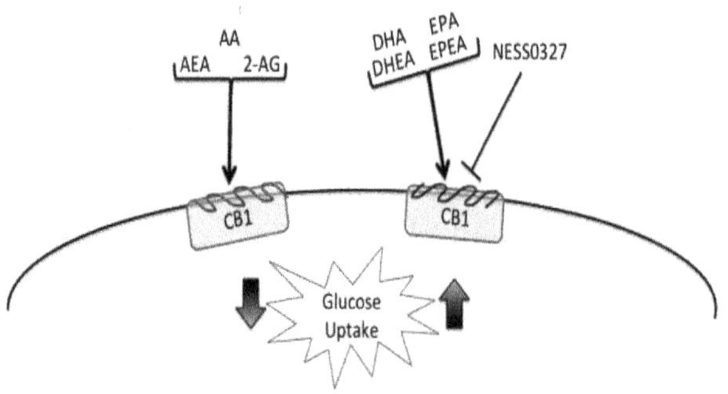

FIGURE 4 | The illustration summarizes the actions of PUFA, endocannabinoids, and cannabinoid antagonist and inverse agonist on glucose uptake and ECS gene expression in differentiated C2C12 myoblast cell cultures. Differentiated C2C12 cultures treated with AA and its derived ligands, AEA and 2-AG, led to lower basal glucose uptake compared to the BSA vehicle control group. Treatment with DHA, DHEA, EPA, and EPEA resulted in higher basal glucose uptake compared to the BSA control group. The higher levels of glucose uptake were comparable to the uptake observed with the CB1 antagonist, NESS0327. The figure is developed from the key observations found by treatment of C2C12 myoblast cell cultures with PUFA, endocannabinoids, and cannabinoid receptor antagonism on CB1, inverse agonist on CB2, and the measurement of GLUT1, insulin-R mRNA, and glucose uptake in differentiated C2C12. In the table below upward arrows represent higher expression/activity compared to the BSA vehicle control while downward arrows signify lower expression/activity compared to the BSA control. Differentiated C2C12 cultures treated with AA and its derived ligands, AEA and 2-AG, led to lower CB1, GLUT1, and insulin-R mRNA expression as well as a reduction of basal glucose uptake compared to the BSA control group. Treatment with DHA, DHEA, EPA, and EPEA resulted in higher CB1, and DHA or DHEA higher GLUT1 and insulin-R mRNA expression as well as a greater level of glucose uptake compared to the BSA control group. NS indicates not significant from the BSA control group.

	CB1 mRNA	CB2 mRNA	GLUT1 mRNA	Insulin-R mRNA	Glucose Uptake
AA	↓	↓	↓	↓	↓
AEA	↓	↓	↓	↓	↓
2-AG	↓	NS	↓	↓	↓
DHA	↑	↑	↑	↑	↑
DHEA	↑	NS	↑	↑	↑
EPA	↑	↑	NS	NS	↑
EPEA	↑	↑	NS	NS	↑
NESS0327	--	--	--	--	↑
AM630	--	--	--	--	↑

add to these findings of insulin-sensitization in skeletal muscle cells, our study demonstrates that antagonizing CB1 resulted in increasing non-insulin stimulated glucose uptake.

The expression of the transcription factor myogenin is essential for the development of functional skeletal muscle as it is required for the proper fusion of myogenic precursor cells during myogenesis (Braun et al., 1989; Wright et al., 1989) Myogenin-deficient myoblasts, however, are unable to undergo efficient fusion to form functional muscle fibers *in vivo*. This result suggests that myogenin plays an essential role in the differentiation of myoblasts into myotubes (Hasty et al., 1993; Nabeshima et al., 1993). Similarly, MyoD1 is one of the earliest markers of myogenic commitment from the mesoderm and is expressed in activated satellite cells (Edmondson and Olson, 1989). Myogenin and MyoD1 have been shown to be expressed in regenerating skeletal muscle of mice (Fuchtbauer and Westphal, 1992). While there were no differences between treatments in the proliferating C2C12, DHA enrichment led to a higher expression of myogenin and MyoD1 in the differentiated cultures. Other findings in the literature suggest that DHA increases proliferation in C2C12 cells (Lee et al., 2009). However, the mechanism behind the ability of DHA to modulate skeletal muscle differentiation, whether it is via MAPK phosphorylation, has yet to be explained.

Some have reported that endocannabinoids are involved in the hypothalamic regulation of food intake and in peripheral lipogenesis in rodents (Di Marzo et al., 2001; Osei-Hyiaman et al., 2005). Thus the ECS has become a promising target for a pharmacological approach to obesity and diabetes. Antagonism of CB1 in rodents (Liu et al., 2005), primary myoblasts (Eckardt et al., 2009), and L6 myoblasts (Esposito et al., 2008) using Rimonabant (SR141716) have demonstrated effects on energy expenditure, targeting improved glucose metabolism, however, no information is available, thus far, in directing this endogenous machinery by dietary means, specifically with PUFA.

The key findings for glucose uptake in myoblasts are summarized in **Figure 4.** Enrichment of proliferating C2C12 myoblasts with EPA and DHA N-acylethanolamides, EPEA and DHEA, respectively, NESS0327, and AM630 resulted in higher basal glucose uptake in proliferating C2C12 cultures compared to the BSA control. In differentiated myoblasts, AA, EPA, DHA, EPEA, DHEA, NESS0327, and AM630 were all found to have higher basal glucose uptake compared to the control cultures (**Figure 4**). AEA and 2-AG both showed lower basal glucose uptake in both proliferating and differentiated C2C12 (**Figure 4**), which is consistent with the findings of elevated AEA and 2-AG in type II diabetic patients (Engeli et al., 2005; Bluher et al., 2006; Matias et al., 2006). Because of the elevated levels of endocannabinoids found in obese animals (Di Marzo et al., 2001) and diabetic humans (Engeli et al., 2005), activation of CB1 may be augmented resulting in an interference with glucose metabolism in muscle cells leading to a downregulation of glucose uptake. Several studies have demonstrated that skeletal muscle is responsive to ECS manipulation in mice (Liu et al., 2005). In a study in leptin deficient obese mice, treatment with the CB1 antagonist SR141716 induced a significant increase in glucose uptake in isolated soleus muscle after 7 days of treatment. In this study GLUT1 was thought to be a possible factor responsible for the response with SR141716 of increased glucose uptake in mouse muscle. In our study of C2C12 cultures the CB1 antagonist NESS0327 resulted in the greatest uptake of glucose, validating previous findings of the negative effects of CB1 on basal glucose uptake (Liu et al., 2005; Esposito et al., 2008; Eckardt et al., 2009). Higher expression of insulin-R, IRS-1, and GLUT4 with DHA treatment is in contrast to the lower glucose uptake with AEA and 2-AG. Our findings suggest that DHA and DHEA have a positive role in improving insulin-stimulated glucose uptake in myoblasts (**Figure 4**).

Additionally, AMPK activation has previously been found to improve glucose tolerance (Buhl et al., 2002). Long-term administration of 5-aminoimidazole-4-carboxamide ribonucleoside, a drug that activates AMPK, to insulin-resistant Zucker rats was shown to improve glucose tolerance and other reduce lipid accumulation. An increase in GLUT4 translocation in skeletal muscle is mainly responsible for the observed improved glucose tolerance (Holmes et al., 1999). Additionally, AMPK is activated during exercise at intensities >60% VO_{2max} in human subjects and rats (Fujii et al., 2000; Takekoshi et al., 2006). An interesting and relevant finding in our study was that both DHA and DHEA were the only treatments that resulted in higher GLUT4 mRNA levels. DHA has previously been shown to increase intestinal glucose absorption (Gabler et al., 2009). Most recently, DHA enrichment has been shown to interact with AMPK in C2C12 myoblasts to enhance uncoupling protein expression (Lee et al., 2013). DHEA was shown in the current investigation to improve basal glucose uptake. Whether DHEA is able to activate AMPK to effect GLUT1 remains to be determined. In addition, the observed increase in glucose-related mRNA suggests that DHEA may be a potential target in improving glucose clearance by muscle. Based on our findings future experiments must be conducted to investigate specific mechanisms on how PUFA affect signaling of the ECS in muscle and glucose utilization.

Based on the data presented herein, EPA and DHA enrichment of differentiated and proliferating C2C12 myoblasts led to a decrease in downstream markers of cannabinoid receptor activation. Conversely, endocannabinoids were all shown to increase downstream markers of cannabinoid receptor activation. While AEA and 2-AG treatment caused a marked decrease in adenylyl cyclase, indicating potential activation of the cannabinoid receptors, DHEA and EPEA resulted in a significantly higher mRNA expression, suggesting secondary messenger signaling to be moderated. Further, DHEA demonstrated an increase in basal glucose uptake at levels comparable to the CB1 antagonist, NESS0327 in myoblasts. Thus the current investigation demonstrates that long chain n-3 PUFA can mediate ECS gene expression and cellular activity in proliferating and differentiated myoblast cultures.

ACKNOWLEDGMENTS

This research was supported by funds to Bruce A. Watkins for the metabolomics collaborations at the University of Connecticut, Storrs and the University of Connecticut Health Center, Center on Aging.

SUPPLEMENTARY MATERIAL

Table S1 | Fatty acid composition of total lipids from proliferating C2C12 cell cultures.

Table S2 | mRNA expression in proliferating C2C12 myoblast cultures treated with PUFA and EC.

Table S3 | Glucose uptake assay in proliferating and differentiated C2C12 after FA or EC/inhibitor treatments (expressed as relative units of fluorescence).

REFERENCES

Artmann, A., Petersen, G., Hellgren, L. I., Boberg, J., Skonberg, C., Nellemann, C., et al. (2008). Influence of dietary fatty acids on endocannabinoid and N-acylethanolamine levels in rat brain, liver and small intestine. *Biochim. Biophys. Acta* 1781, 200–212. doi: 10.1016/j.bbalip.2008.01.006

Baron, A. D., Brechtel, G., Wallace, P., and Edelman, S. V. (1988). Rates and tissue sites of non-insulin- and insulin-mediated glucose uptake in humans. *Am. J. Physiol.* 255, E769–E774.

Batetta, B., Griinari, M., Carta, G., Murru, E., Ligresti, A., Cordeddu, L., et al. (2009). Endocannabinoids may mediate the ability of (n-3) fatty acids to reduce ectopic fat and inflammatory mediators in obese Zucker rats. *J. Nutr.* 139, 1495–1501. doi: 10.3945/jn.109.104844

Bennett, A. M., and Tonks, N. K. (1997). Regulation of distinct stages of skeletal muscle differentiation by mitogen-activated protein kinases. *Science* 278, 1288–1291. doi: 10.1126/science.278.5341.1288

Best, J. D., Kahn, S. E., Ader, M., Watanabe, R. M., Ni, T. C., and Bergman, R. N. (1996). Role of glucose effectiveness in the determination of glucose tolerance. *Diabetes Care* 19, 1018–1030.

Bluher, M., Engeli, S., Kloting, N., Berndt, J., Fasshauer, M., Batkai, S., et al. (2006). Dysregulation of the peripheral and adipose tissue endocannabinoid system in human abdominal obesity. *Diabetes* 55, 3053–3060. doi: 10.2337/db06-0812

Braun, T., Bober, E., Buschhausen-Denker, G., Kohtz, S., Grzeschik, K. H., and Arnold, H. H. (1989). Differential expression of myogenic determination genes in muscle cells: possible autoactivation by the Myf gene products. *EMBO J.* 8, 3617–3625.

Brown, A. J., Pang, E., and Roberts, D. C. (1991). Persistent changes in the fatty acid composition of erythrocyte membranes after moderate intake of n-3 polyunsaturated fatty acids: study design implications. *Am. J. Clin. Nutr.* 54, 668–673.

Buhl, E. S., Jessen, N., Pold, R., Ledet, T., Flyvbjerg, A., Pedersen, S. B., et al. (2002). Long-term AICAR administration reduces metabolic disturbances and lowers blood pressure in rats displaying features of the insulin resistance syndrome. *Diabetes* 51, 2199–2206. doi: 10.2337/diabetes.51.7.2199

Capaldo, B., Santoro, D., Riccardi, G., Perrotti, N., and Sacca, L. (1986). Direct evidence for a stimulatory effect of hyperglycemia *per se* on peripheral glucose disposal in type II diabetes. *J. Clin. Invest.* 77, 1285–1290. doi: 10.1172/JCI112432

Cavuoto, P., McAinch, A. J., Hatzinikolas, G., Cameron-Smith, D., and Wittert, G. A. (2007). Effects of cannabinoid receptors on skeletal muscle oxidative pathways. *Mol. Cell. Endocrinol.* 267, 63–69. doi: 10.1016/j.mce.2006.12.038

Cota, D., Marsicano, G., Lutz, B., Vicennati, V., Stalla, G. K., Pasquali, R., et al. (2003). Endogenous cannabinoid system as a modulator of food intake. *Int. J. Obes. Relat. Metab. Disord.* 27, 289–301. doi: 10.1038/sj.ijo.0802250

De Petrocellis, L., Melck, D., Bisogno, T., Milone, A., and Di Marzo, V. (1999). Finding of the endocannabinoid signalling system in Hydra, a very primitive organism: possible role in the feeding response. *Neuroscience* 92, 377–387. doi: 10.1016/S0306-4522(98)00749-0

Despres, J. P., Golay, A., and Sjostrom, L. (2005). Effects of rimonabant on metabolic risk factors in overweight patients with dyslipidemia. *N. Engl. J. Med.* 353, 2121–2134. doi: 10.1056/NEJMoa044537

Di Marzo, V., Goparaju, S. K., Wang, L., Liu, J., Batkai, S., Jarai, Z., et al. (2001). Leptin-regulated endocannabinoids are involved in maintaining food intake. *Nature* 410, 822–825. doi: 10.1038/35071088

Eckardt, K., Sell, H., Taube, A., Koenen, M., Platzbecker, B., Cramer, A., et al. (2009). Cannabinoid type 1 receptors in human skeletal muscle cells participate in the negative crosstalk between fat and muscle. *Diabetologia* 52, 664–674. doi: 10.1007/s00125-008-1240-4

Edmondson, D. G., and Olson, E. N. (1989). A gene with homology to the myc similarity region of MyoD1 is expressed during myogenesis and is sufficient to activate the muscle differentiation program. *Genes Dev.* 3, 628–640. doi: 10.1101/gad.3.5.628

Engeli, S., Bohnke, J., Feldpausch, M., Gorzelniak, K., Janke, J., Batkai, S., et al. (2005). Activation of the peripheral endocannabinoid system in human obesity. *Diabetes* 54, 2838–2843. doi: 10.2337/diabetes.54.10.2838

Esposito, I., Proto, M. C., Gazzerro, P., Laezza, C., Miele, C., Alberobello, A. T., et al. (2008). The cannabinoid CB1 receptor antagonist rimonabant stimulates 2-deoxyglucose uptake in skeletal muscle cells by regulating the expression of phosphatidylinositol-3-kinase. *Mol. Pharmacol.* 74, 1678–1686. doi: 10.1124/mol.108.049205

Felder, C. C., Briley, E. M., Axelrod, J., Simpson, J. T., Mackie, K., and Devane, W. A. (1993). Anandamide, an endogenous cannabimimetic eicosanoid, binds to the cloned human cannabinoid receptor and stimulates receptor-mediated signal transduction. *Proc. Natl. Acad. Sci. U.S.A.* 90, 7656–7660. doi: 10.1073/pnas.90.16.7656

Fuchtbauer, E. M., and Westphal, H. (1992). MyoD and myogenin are coexpressed in regenerating skeletal muscle of the mouse. *Dev. Dyn.* 193, 34–39. doi: 10.1002/aja.1001930106

Fujii, N., Hayashi, T., Hirshman, M. F., Smith, J. T., Habinowski, S. A., Kaijser, L., et al. (2000). Exercise induces isoform-specific increase in 5′AMP-activated protein kinase activity in human skeletal muscle. *Biochem. Biophys. Res. Commun.* 273, 1150–1155. doi: 10.1006/bbrc.2000.3073

Gabler, N. K., Radcliffe, J. S., Spencer, J. D., Webel, D. M., and Spurlock, M. E. (2009). Feeding long-chain n-3 polyunsaturated fatty acids during gestation increases intestinal glucose absorption potentially via the acute activation of AMPK. *J. Nutr. Biochem.* 20, 17–25. doi: 10.1016/j.jnutbio.2007.11.009

Garrington, T. P., and Johnson, G. L. (1999). Organization and regulation of mitogen-activated protein kinase signaling pathways. *Curr. Opin. Cell Biol.* 11, 211–218. doi: 10.1016/S0955-0674(99)80028-3

Hasty, P., Bradley, A., Morris, J. H., Edmondson, D. G., Venuti, J. M., Olson, E. N., et al. (1993). Muscle deficiency and neonatal death in mice with a targeted mutation in the myogenin gene. *Nature* 364, 501–506. doi: 10.1038/364501a0

Holmes, B. F., Kurth-Kraczek, E. J., and Winder, W. W. (1999). Chronic activation of 5′-AMP-activated protein kinase increases GLUT-4, hexokinase, and glycogen in muscle. *J. Appl. Physiol. (1985)* 87, 1990–1995.

Howlett, A. C. (2005). Cannabinoid receptor signaling. *Handb. Exp. Pharmacol.* 53–79. doi: 10.1007/3-540-26573-2_2

Hutchins-Wiese, H. L., Li, Y., Hannon, K., and Watkins, B. A. (2012). Hind limb suspension and long-chain omega-3 PUFA increase mRNA endocannabinoid system levels in skeletal muscle. *J. Nutr. Biochem.* 23, 986–993. doi: 10.1016/j.jnutbio.2011.05.005

Hutchins, H. L., Li, Y., Hannon, K., and Watkins, B. A. (2011). Eicosapentaenoic acid decreases expression of anandamide synthesis enzyme and cannabinoid receptor 2 in osteoblast-like cells. *J. Nutr. Biochem.* 22, 195–200. doi: 10.1016/j.jnutbio.2010.06.001

Khurana, A., and Dey, C. S. (2004). Involvement of c-Jun N-terminal kinase activities in skeletal muscle differentiation. *J. Muscle Res. Cell Motil.* 25, 645–655. doi: 10.1007/s10974-004-7099-1

Lee, J., Sun, C., Zhou, Y., Gokalp, D., Herrema, H., Park, S. W., et al. (2011). p38 MAPK-mediated regulation of Xbp1s is crucial for glucose homeostasis. *Nat. Med.* 17, 1251–1260. doi: 10.1038/nm.2449

Lee, J. H., Tachibana, H., Morinaga, Y., Fujimura, Y., and Yamada, K. (2009). Modulation of proliferation and differentiation of C2C12 skeletal muscle cells by fatty acids. *Life Sci.* 84, 415–420. doi: 10.1016/j.lfs.2009.01.004

Lee, M. S., Kim, I. H., and Kim, Y. (2013). Effects of eicosapentaenoic acid and docosahexaenoic acid on uncoupling protein 3 gene expression in C(2)C(12) muscle cells. *Nutrients* 5, 1660–1671. doi: 10.3390/nu5051660

Li, J., and Johnson, S. E. (2006). ERK2 is required for efficient terminal differentiation of skeletal myoblasts. *Biochem. Biophys. Res. Commun.* 345, 1425–1433. doi: 10.1016/j.bbrc.2006.05.051

Li, Y., Greiner, R. S., Salem, N. Jr., and Watkins, B. A. (2003). Impact of dietary n-3 FA deficiency on rat bone tissue FA composition. *Lipids* 38, 683–686. doi: 10.1007/s11745-003-1115-8

Li, Y., Seifert, M. F., Lim, S. Y., Salem, N. Jr., and Watkins, B. A. (2010). Bone mineral content is positively correlated to n-3 fatty acids in the femur of growing rats. *Br. J. Nutr.* 104, 674–685. doi: 10.1017/S0007114510001133

Lipina, C., Stretton, C., Hastings, S., Hundal, J. S., Mackie, K., Irving, A. J., et al. (2010). Regulation of MAP Kinase–directed mitogenic and protein kinase B–mediated signaling by cannabinoid receptor type 1 in skeletal muscle cells. *Diabetes* 59, 375–385. doi: 10.2337/db09-0979

Liu, Y. L., Connoley, I. P., Wilson, C. A., and Stock, M. J. (2005). Effects of the cannabinoid CB1 receptor antagonist SR141716 on oxygen consumption and soleus muscle glucose uptake in Lep(ob)/Lep(ob) mice. *Int. J. Obes. (Lond.)* 29, 183–187. doi: 10.1038/sj.ijo.0802847

Lo, C. J., Chiu, K. C., Fu, M., Chu, A., and Helton, S. (2000). Fish oil modulates macrophage P44/P42 mitogen-activated protein kinase activity induced by lipopolysaccharide. *J. Parenter. Enteral Nutr.* 24, 159–163. doi: 10.1177/0148607100024003159

Matias, I., Carta, G., Murru, E., Petrosino, S., Banni, S., and Di Marzo, V. (2008). Effect of polyunsaturated fatty acids on endocannabinoid and N-acyl-ethanolamine levels in mouse adipocytes. *Biochim. Biophys. Acta* 1781, 52–60. doi: 10.1016/j.bbalip.2007.11.001

Matias, I., Gonthier, M. P., Orlando, P., Martiadis, V., De Petrocellis, L., Cervino, C., et al. (2006). Regulation, function, and dysregulation of endocannabinoids in models of adipose and beta-pancreatic cells and in obesity and hyperglycemia. *J. Clin. Endocrinol. Metab.* 91, 3171–3180. doi: 10.1210/jc.2005-2679

Nabeshima, Y., Hanaoka, K., Hayasaka, M., Esumi, E., Li, S., and Nonaka, I. (1993). Myogenin gene disruption results in perinatal lethality because of severe muscle defect. *Nature* 364, 532–535. doi: 10.1038/364532a0

Osei-Hyiaman, D., DePetrillo, M., Pacher, P., Liu, J., Radaeva, S., Batkai, S., et al. (2005). Endocannabinoid activation at hepatic CB1 receptors stimulates fatty acid synthesis and contributes to diet-induced obesity. *J. Clin. Invest.* 115, 1298–1305. doi: 10.1172/JCI200523057

Pi-Sunyer, F. X., Aronne, L. J., Heshmati, H. M., Devin, J., and Rosenstock, J. (2006). Effect of rimonabant, a cannabinoid-1 receptor blocker, on weight and cardiometabolic risk factors in overweight or obese patients: RIO-North America: a randomized controlled trial. *JAMA* 295, 761–775. doi: 10.1001/jama.295.7.761

Piazza, P. V., Lafontan, M., and Girard, J. (2007). Integrated physiology and pathophysiology of CB1-mediated effects of the endocannabinoid system. *Diabetes Metab.* 33, 97–107. doi: 10.1016/j.diabet.2007.02.002

Piscitelli, F., Carta, G., Bisogno, T., Murru, E., Cordeddu, L., Berge, K., et al. (2011). Effect of dietary krill oil supplementation on the endocannabinoidome of metabolically relevant tissues from high-fat-fed mice. *Nutr. Metab. (Lond.)* 8:51. doi: 10.1186/1743-7075-8-51

Ravinet Trillou, C., Arnone, M., Delgorge, C., Gonalons, N., Keane, P., Maffrand, J. P., et al. (2003). Anti-obesity effect of SR141716, a CB1 receptor antagonist, in diet-induced obese mice. *Am. J. Physiol. Regul. Integr. Comp. Physiol.* 284, R345–R353. doi: 10.1152/ajpregu.00545.2002

Rolli-Derkinderen, M., Machavoine, F., Baraban, J. M., Grolleau, A., Beretta, L., and Dy, M. (2003). ERK and p38 inhibit the expression of 4E-BP1 repressor of translation through induction of Egr-1. *J. Biol. Chem.* 278, 18859–18867. doi: 10.1074/jbc.M211696200

Sheskin, T., Hanus, L., Slager, J., Vogel, Z., and Mechoulam, R. (1997). Structural requirements for binding of anandamide-type compounds to the brain cannabinoid receptor. *J. Med. Chem.* 40, 659–667. doi: 10.1021/jm960752x

Soderstrom, K., Tian, Q., Valenti, M., and Di Marzo, V. (2004). Endocannabinoids link feeding state and auditory perception-related gene expression. *J. Neurosci.* 24, 10013–10021. doi: 10.1523/JNEUROSCI.3298-04.2004

Takekoshi, K., Fukuhara, M., Quin, Z., Nissato, S., Isobe, K., Kawakami, Y., et al. (2006). Long-term exercise stimulates adenosine monophosphate-activated protein kinase activity and subunit expression in rat visceral adipose tissue and liver. *Metab. Clin. Exp.* 55, 1122–1128. doi: 10.1016/j.metabol.2006.04.007

Tsang, V. C., Brand, J. A., and Boyer, A. E. (1989). An enzyme-linked immunoelectrotransfer blot assay and glycoprotein antigens for diagnosing human cysticercosis (*Taenia solium*). *J. Infect. Dis.* 159, 50–59. doi: 10.1093/infdis/159.1.50

Valenti, M., Cottone, E., Martinez, R., De Pedro, N., Rubio, M., Viveros, M. P., et al. (2005). The endocannabinoid system in the brain of Carassius auratus and its possible role in the control of food intake. *J. Neurochem.* 95, 662–672. doi: 10.1111/j.1471-4159.2005.03406.x

Watanabe, S., Doshi, M., and Hamazaki, T. (2003). n-3 Polyunsaturated fatty acid (PUFA) deficiency elevates and n-3 PUFA enrichment reduces brain 2-arachidonoylglycerol level in mice. *Prostaglandins Leukot. Essent. Fatty Acids* 69, 51–59. doi: 10.1016/S0952-3278(03)00056-5

Watkins, B. A., Li, Y., Allen, K. G., Hoffmann, W. E., and Seifert, M. F. (2000). Dietary ratio of (n-6)/(n-3) polyunsaturated fatty acids alters the fatty acid composition of bone compartments and biomarkers of bone formation in rats. *J. Nutr.* 130, 2274–2284.

Watkins, B. A., Li, Y., Lippman, H. E., and Feng, S. (2003). Modulatory effect of omega-3 polyunsaturated fatty acids on osteoblast function and bone metabolism. *Prostaglandins Leukot. Essent. Fatty Acids* 68, 387–398. doi: 10.1016/S0952-3278(03)00063-2

Watkins, B. A., Li, Y., and Seifert, M. F. (2006). Dietary ratio of n-6/n-3 PUFAs and docosahexaenoic acid: actions on bone mineral and serum biomarkers in ovariectomized rats. *J. Nutr. Biochem.* 17, 282–289. doi: 10.1016/j.jnutbio.2005.05.012

Weyman, C. M., and Wolfman, A. (1998). Mitogen-activated protein kinase kinase (MEK) activity is required for inhibition of skeletal muscle differentiation by insulin-like growth factor 1 or fibroblast growth factor 2. *Endocrinology* 139, 1794–1800.

Wright, W. E., Sassoon, D. A., and Lin, V. K. (1989). Myogenin, a factor regulating myogenesis, has a domain homologous to MyoD. *Cell* 56, 607–617. doi: 10.1016/0092-8674(89)90583-7

Zetser, A., Gredinger, E., and Bengal, E. (1999). p38 mitogen-activated protein kinase pathway promotes skeletal muscle differentiation. Participation of the Mef2c transcription factor. *J. Biol. Chem.* 274, 5193–5200. doi: 10.1074/jbc.274.8.5193

Zhang, W., Thompson, B. J., Hietakangas, V., and Cohen, S. M. (2011). MAPK/ERK signaling regulates insulin sensitivity to control glucose metabolism in Drosophila. *PLoS Genet.* 7:e1002429. doi: 10.1371/journal.pgen.1002429

16

Roles of nonmyogenic mesenchymal progenitors in pathogenesis and regeneration of skeletal muscle

Akiyoshi Uezumi[1]*, Madoka Ikemoto-Uezumi[2] and Kunihiro Tsuchida[1]

[1] *Division for Therapies against Intractable Diseases, Institute for Comprehensive Medical Science, Fujita Health University, Aichi, Japan*
[2] *Department of Regenerative Medicine, National Center for Geriatrics and Gerontology, National Institute for Longevity Sciences, Aichi, Japan*

***Correspondence:**
Akiyoshi Uezumi, Division for Therapies against Intractable Diseases, Institute for Comprehensive Medical Science, Fujita Health University, 1-98 Dengakugakubo, Kutsukake, Toyoake, Aichi 470-1192, Japan
e-mail: uezumi@fujita-hu.ac.jp

Adult skeletal muscle possesses a remarkable regenerative ability that is dependent on satellite cells. However, skeletal muscle is replaced by fatty and fibrous connective tissue in several pathological conditions. Fatty and fibrous connective tissue becomes a major cause of muscle weakness and leads to further impairment of muscle function. Because the occurrence of fatty and fibrous connective tissue is usually associated with severe destruction of muscle, the idea that dysregulation of the fate switch in satellite cells may underlie this pathological change has emerged. However, recent studies identified nonmyogenic mesenchymal progenitors in skeletal muscle and revealed that fatty and fibrous connective tissue originates from these progenitors. Later, these progenitors were also demonstrated to be the major contributor to heterotopic ossification in skeletal muscle. Because nonmyogenic mesenchymal progenitors represent a distinct cell population from satellite cells, targeting these progenitors could be an ideal therapeutic strategy that specifically prevents pathological changes of skeletal muscle, while preserving satellite cell-dependent regeneration. In addition to their roles in pathogenesis of skeletal muscle, nonmyogenic mesenchymal progenitors may play a vital role in muscle regeneration by regulating satellite cell behavior. Conversely, muscle cells appear to regulate behavior of nonmyogenic mesenchymal progenitors. Thus, these cells regulate each other reciprocally and a proper balance between them is a key determinant of muscle integrity. Furthermore, nonmyogenic mesenchymal progenitors have been shown to maintain muscle mass in a steady homeostatic condition. Understanding the nature of nonmyogenic mesenchymal progenitors will provide valuable insight into the pathophysiology of skeletal muscle. In this review, we focus on nonmyogenic mesenchymal progenitors and discuss their roles in muscle pathogenesis, regeneration, and homeostasis.

Keywords: mesenchymal progenitors, satellite cells, PDGFRα, adipogenesis, fibrosis, heterotopic ossification, muscle regeneration, muscle atrophy

INTRODUCTION

The most fundamental roles of skeletal muscle are the generation of force and the control of body movement by contraction. In addition, skeletal muscle serves as physical safeguard for other organs as it is anatomically located immediately beneath the skin. Because of its functional roles, skeletal muscle represents one of the most frequently damaged organs in the body. Therefore, regeneration from the damage is an essential property of skeletal muscle. One of the best examples of remarkable regeneration capacity of skeletal muscle is the study that showed myofiber regeneration after more than 20 repeated injuries (Sadeh et al., 1985). The high regeneration capacity of skeletal muscle is attributed to satellite cells, which reside between the sarcolemma and the basal lamina of myofibers. M-cadherin and Pax7 are the most reliable markers for mouse satellite cells (Irintchev et al., 1994; Seale et al., 2000). An essential role for satellite cells in adult myogenesis was exquisitely demonstrated by studies using genetically-engineered mice in which Pax7-expressing satellite cells are ablated (Lepper et al., 2011; Murphy et al., 2011; Sambasivan et al., 2011). These mice showed complete loss of regenerative response and severe fatty and fibrous degeneration after muscle injury, indicating that nonsatellite cells cannot compensate for satellite cell-dependent myogenesis. In addition to contributing to new myofiber formation, a subset of satellite cells have been shown to be capable of self-renewal (Collins et al., 2005; Montarras et al., 2005; Sacco et al., 2008; Rocheteau et al., 2012). Thus, satellite cells act as adult muscle stem cells.

Despite the presence of well-established stem cells that underlie the exceptional regeneration potential, skeletal muscle is replaced by ectopic tissues such as adipose tissue, fibrous connective tissue, and bone in several pathological conditions. These ectopic tissues become an aggravating factor in muscle weakness because they lack contractile ability and hinder the supply of nutrients to myofibers. In most cases, ectopic tissue formation within skeletal muscle is associated with severe destruction of myofibers, leading to the concept that dysregulation of the fate switch in satellite cells may underlie these degeneration processes. However, this concept was refuted by recent studies describing the identification of nonmyogenic mesenchymal progenitors in skeletal muscle. These studies established the pathological relevance of nonmyogenic mesenchymal progenitors to muscle diseases. In addition to their roles in disease conditions, nonmyogenic mesenchymal progenitors appear to play roles in muscle regeneration and in steady-state muscle homeostasis. This review focuses on nonmyogenic mesenchymal progenitors and describes their roles in the pathogenesis, regeneration, and homeostasis of skeletal muscle.

FAT INFILTRATION, FIBROSIS, AND HETEROTOPIC OSSIFICATION IN SKELETAL MUSCLE

In normal healthy muscle, especially in the gastrocnemius, occasional adipocytes can be encountered in connective tissue septa (Carpenter and Karpati, 2001). Physiological significance of these occasional adipocytes in normal muscle is largely unknown. Disease in which there is loss of muscle cells without efficient regeneration leads to an increase of ectopic adipocytes within fascicles (Carpenter and Karpati, 2001). In myopathic disorders accompanied by myofiber destruction, endomysial fibrous connective tissue increases from the onset of the disease, but the increase in endomysial fatty connective tissue is observed only after there has been an extensive loss of myofibers (Banker and Engel, 2004). The most striking accumulation of adipocytes is seen in advanced cases of Duchenne muscular dystrophy (DMD) or myotonic dystrophy, where a muscle may be almost entirely replaced by adipose tissue (Carpenter and Karpati, 2001; Banker and Engel, 2004). Fat infiltration in skeletal muscle is also pronounced in other disease conditions including obesity (Goodpaster et al., 2000; Greco et al., 2002; Sinha et al., 2002), type II diabetes (Goodpaster et al., 2000; Hilton et al., 2008), unloading (Manini et al., 2007), hemiparetic stroke (Ryan et al., 2002), and spinal cord injury (Gorgey and Dudley, 2007). Aging is accompanied by deterioration in muscle function, and fat infiltration in skeletal muscle increases with age Visser et al., 2002, 2005; Kim et al., 2009; Marcus et al., 2010; Kragstrup et al., 2011. It is not known whether adipocytes within skeletal muscle would disappear if the disease conditions could be reversed.

Fibrosis is a pathological feature associated with many chronic inflammatory diseases. Fibrosis is defined by the excessive accumulation of extracellular matrix (ECM) components, which can lead to permanent scarring and organ malfunction. Although ECM deposition is an indispensable and, typically, reversible part of wound healing, the repair process can produce a progressively irreversible fibrosis if the tissue injury is severe or repetitive or if there is a defect in the repair machinery. Fibrosis in skeletal muscle can be seen in most conditions where there is chronic muscle damage or insufficient regeneration but is most prominent in muscular dystrophy (Carpenter and Karpati, 2001; Banker and Engel, 2004). A possible exception is myotonic dystrophy, where fat infiltration appears to proceed without much fibrosis (Carpenter and Karpati, 2001). Sports injuries such as lacerations, contusions or strains can also elicit irreversible fibrotic response and lead to scar formation depending on the severity of injuries (Jarvinen et al., 2000; Beiner and Jokl, 2001). Although myofibroblasts are cells responsible for fibrosis of other organs such as liver and kidney, one should keep in mind that these cells have not been identified in most skeletal muscle diseases except for nodular fasciitis (Wirman, 1976) and pseudomalignant myositis ossificans (Povysil and Matejovsky, 1979).

Heterotopic ossification (HO) is defined as the abnormal formation of mature, lamellar bone in soft tissues outside the skeletal periosteum. The most commonly affected site is skeletal muscle. HO has been thought to result from inappropriate differentiation of progenitor cells that is induced by a pathological imbalance of local or systemic factors. There are three recognized etiologies of HO: traumatic, neurogenic, and genetic (Balboni et al., 2006). Traumatic HO is the most common type of HO and typically recognized after fractures, severe burns, and surgical trauma, especially after total hip arthroplasty (Nilsson and Persson, 1999). Neurogenic HO can be frequently seen after injuries to central nervous system (Garland et al., 1980). Other neurologic conditions have also been implicated in the development of HO, including meningitis (Lorber, 1953), myelitis (Stoikovic et al., 1955), and tetanus (Ishikawa et al., 1982). Genetic disorders in which HO arises in skeletal muscle are fibrodysplasia ossificans progressiva (FOP) and progressive osseous heteroplasia (POH) (Kaplan and Shore, 2000; Pignolo et al., 2011). FOP is a severely disabling heritable disorder of connective tissue characterized by congenital malformations of the great toes and progressive extraskeletal ossification. Mutation of the *ALK-2* gene, a BMP type I receptor, was identified in FOP patients (Shore et al., 2006) and has been shown to contribute to the pathogenesis of FOP (Chakkalakal et al., 2012). POH is a genetic disorder of mesenchymal differentiation characterized by dermal ossification during infancy and progressive HO of cutaneous, subcutaneous, and deep connective tissues including skeletal muscle during childhood. An inactivating mutation of *GNAS1* gene was reported to be the cause of POH (Shore et al., 2002).

IDENTIFICATION OF NONMYOGENIC MESENCHYMAL PROGENITORS AND THEIR CONTRIBUTION TO PATHOGENESIS OF SKELETAL MUSCLE

To clarify the origin of cell populations involved in the fatty degeneration of skeletal muscle, we conducted a comprehensive survey of cells that reside in skeletal muscle using a FACS-based cell isolation technique. As a consequence, we found that only cells expressing PDGFRα can differentiate into adipocytes. In addition to adipogenic potential, PDGFRα$^+$ cells can differentiate into osteoblastic or smooth muscle-like cells but scarcely differentiate into skeletal muscle lineage cells. Therefore, we termed these cells mesenchymal progenitors (Uezumi et al., 2010). Mesenchymal progenitors reside in the muscle interstitium and therefore represent a cell population that is distinct from satellite cells (**Figure 1**). These cells are more frequently observed in the perimysium than in the endomysium, particularly in the perivascular space. But they are distinct from pericytes because they reside outside the vessel wall and outside the capillary basement membrane. They do not originate from bone marrow, but instead represent a cell population that is resident in skeletal muscle. Importantly, only mesenchymal progenitors can participate in

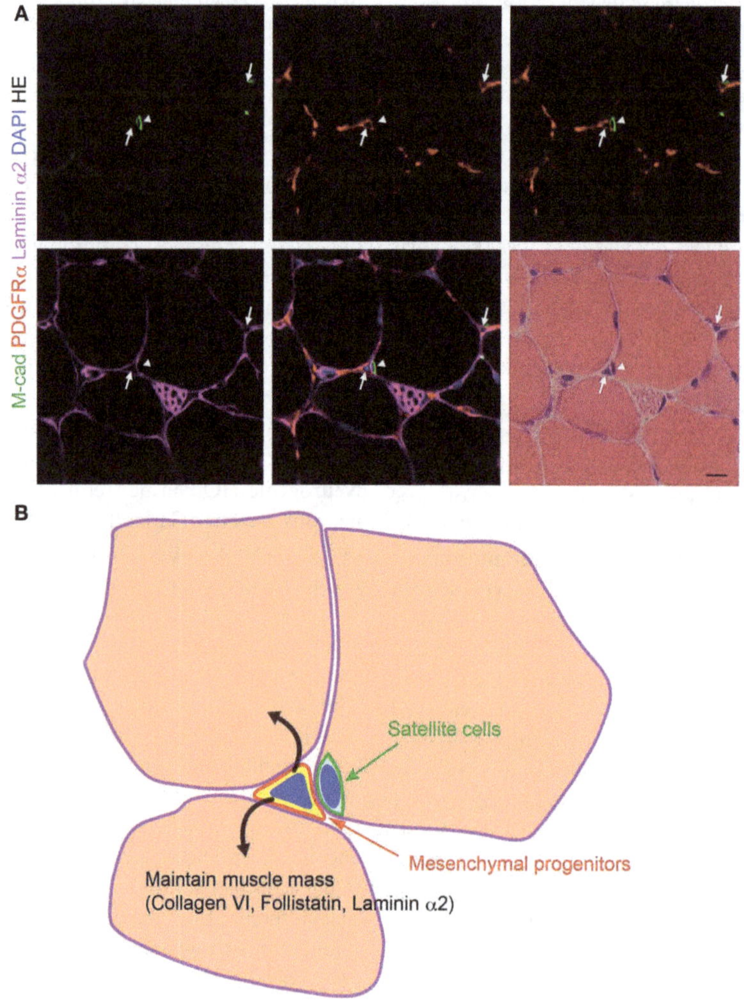

FIGURE 1 | Localization of PDGFRα$^+$ mesenchymal progenitors in normal muscle. (A) Fresh frozen section of mouse TA muscle subjected to immunofluorescence staining for M-cadherin (M-cad), PDGFRα, and laminin α2, and subsequently to HE staining. Arrows indicate PDGFRα$^+$ mesenchymal progenitors and arrowhead indicates satellite cells. Scale bar: 10 μm. **(B)** Schematic view of **(A)**. Mesenchymal progenitors that reside in muscle interstitium express collagen VI, follistatin, and laminin α2, and maintain muscle mass in a normal physiological condition.

ectopic fat cell formation when transplanted into fatty degenerating muscle, while other cells residing within skeletal muscle do not have such an activity (Uezumi et al., 2010). Another group also identified cells with adipogenic potential on the basis of Sca-1 and CD34 expression (Joe et al., 2010). Sca-1$^+$CD34$^+$ cells were referred to as fibro/adipogenic progenitors (FAPs), because these cells have the potential to produce both adipocytes and fibroblasts but fail to differentiate into osteogenic cells *in vitro*. PDGFRα$^+$ mesenchymal progenitors express Sca-1, and complementally FAPs express PDGFRα (Joe et al., 2010; Uezumi et al., 2010); thus both cell types seem to represent the same cell population. Adipocytes that emerge in skeletal muscle show unilocular morphology and PDGFRα$^+$ cell-derived adipocytes express high level of *Leptin* (Uezumi et al., 2010), indicating that mesenchymal progenitors have a high propensity to differentiate into white adipose lineage. However, brown adipogenic potential of Sca-1$^+$ progenitors was also demonstrated (Schulz et al., 2011). Thus, mesenchymal progenitors appear to possess the capacity to differentiate into both white and brown adipocytes.

In the subsequent study, we revealed that mesenchymal progenitors also contribute to skeletal muscle fibrosis (Uezumi et al., 2011). A striking increase in the number of PDGFRα$^+$ cells is conspicuous in fibrotic areas of the diaphragm from mdx mice (**Figure 2**). Using an irradiation-induced muscle fibrosis model, we further demonstrated that transplanted PDGFRα$^+$ cells directly participate in fibrotic scar tissue formation with negligible myogenic activity (Uezumi et al., 2011). In contrast, satellite cell-derived myoblasts exclusively participate in myofiber formation but do not contribute to fibrous connective tissue formation. A study by Dulauroy et al. provided further details. By inducible lineage tracing, Dulauroy et al. showed that a subset of PDGFRα$^+$ cells begin to express ADAM12 during muscle injury and an ADAM12$^+$PDGFRα$^+$ subset accumulates fibrotic regions of injured muscle (Dulauroy et al., 2012).

This study sophisticatedly demonstrated that endogenous mesenchymal progenitors are indeed the origin of profibrotic cells. However, the study utilized a CTX muscle injury model. Because skeletal muscle regenerates almost completely without development of fibrotic scar tissue after CTX injection (Hawke and Garry, 2001; Harris, 2003), this model reflects a reversible repair process rather than irreversible fibrosis. Therefore, the behavior of ADAM12$^+$PDGFRα^+ cells in a more pathologically relevant model would be of considerable interest. Using single myofibers isolated from Pax7-CreER/ROSA26 mice, a strain in which tamoxifen administration leads to permanent β-galactosidase expression only in Pax7$^+$ satellite cells, satellite cells were shown to become fibrogenic under the influence of aged serum (Brack et al., 2007). The conversion ratio was around 10% in this context. In contrast, nearly 100% of PDGFRα^+ mesenchymal progenitors were converted to fibrogenic cells when treated with TGF-β at a concentration that had no effect on satellite cell myogeneity (Uezumi et al., 2011). Although different experimental conditions used in those studies make direct comparisons difficult, mesenchymal progenitors seem to be more prone to fibrogenic conversion than satellite cells. However, further studies are needed to elucidate which cell type—satellite cells or PDGFRα^+ mesenchymal progenitors—is the main source of fibrogenic cells in an aged environment *in vivo*. The link between fibrogenesis and PDGFRα signaling has been demonstrated by several studies. Olson and Soriano generated mice in which mutant PDGFRα with increased kinase activity was knocked into a PDGFRα locus (Olson and Soriano, 2009). Thus, constitutively active PDGFRα signaling is operative only in cells that express PDGFRα endogenously in the mutant mice. The mice with mutant PDGFRα showed progressive fibrosis in multiple organs including skeletal muscle. We showed that stimulation of PDGFRα signaling in PDGFRα^+ mesenchymal progenitors promotes cell proliferation and upregulates the expression of fibrosis-related genes (Uezumi et al., 2011). Imatinib, an inhibitor of several tyrosine kinases including PDGFR, c-kit, and bcr-abl oncogene, was shown to ameliorate the dystrophic symptoms of mdx mice (Bizario et al., 2009; Huang et al., 2009; Ito et al., 2013). Importantly, imatinib treatment decreased the phosphorylation level of PDGFRα in the dystrophic muscle (Huang et al., 2009), and treatment of PDGFRα^+ mesenchymal progenitors with imatinib inhibited PDGFRα-induced proliferation and expression of fibrotic genes (Ito et al., 2013). Taking these findings into account, the therapeutic effect of imatinib exerted on dystrophic mice seems to be achieved at least in part through targeting PDGFRα^+ mesenchymal progenitors.

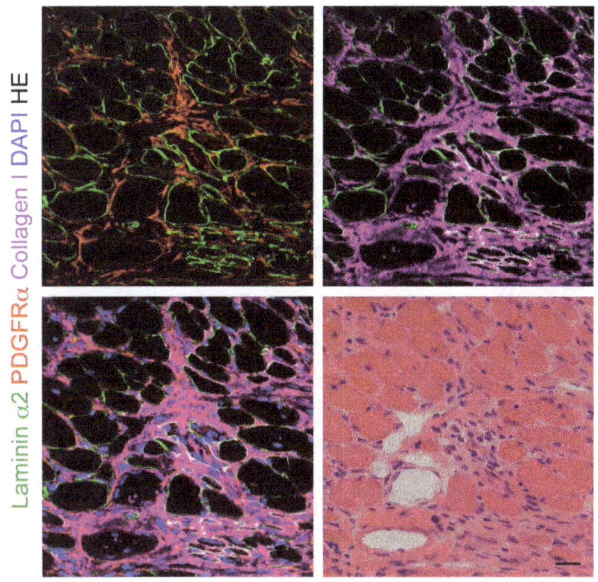

FIGURE 2 | The behavior of PDGFRα^+ mesenchymal progenitors in dystrophic muscle. Fresh frozen section of mdx diaphragm subjected to immunofluorescence staining for laminin α2, PDGFRα, and collagen I, and subsequently to HE staining. Scale bar: 20 μm.

The contribution of mesenchymal progenitors to HO in skeletal muscle was exquisitely demonstrated by Goldhamer and colleagues. By crossing lineage-specific Cre mice with Cre-dependent reporter mice, they generated several mouse lines in which specific lineage cells were permanently labeled, and showed that skeletal myogenic cells including satellite cells or smooth muscle cells do not contribute to BMP-induced HO. Instead, they found a significant contribution of Tie2-lineage cells to HO in two mouse models of dysregulated BMP signaling (Lounev et al., 2009). Tie2 is usually used as a marker of endothelial cells, but expression of the *Tie2* gene is also recognized in mesenchymal progenitors (Uezumi et al., 2010). To clarify which cell type labeled by Tie2-Cre contributes to the development of HO, Wosczyna et al. conducted further detailed research. Although endothelial cells constitute a large part of the Tie2$^+$ fraction, they did not detectably contribute to HO. After careful cell fractionation by FACS, PDGFRα^+Sca-1$^+$ cells within Tie2$^+$ fraction were found to be the predominant source of progenitors that give rise to ectopic cartilage and bone (Wosczyna et al., 2012). Clonal analysis revealed that Tie2$^+$PDGFRα^+Sca-1$^+$ progenitors are multipotent as colonies derived from single Tie2$^+$PDGFRα^+Sca-1$^+$ cells exhibited both osteogenic and adipogenic differentiation potentials.

As described above, several studies independently reported nonmyogenic mesenchymal progenitors that contribute to the pathogenesis of skeletal muscle. Progenitor cells described by different groups share a common cell surface phenotype: CD31$^-$CD45$^-$Sca-1$^+$PDGFRα^+, and therefore seem to be closely related to each other or represent the same cell population. FAPs were so named because they did not differentiate into osteogenic cells (Joe et al., 2010). But it is obvious that these progenitors possess osteo/chondrogenic potential as demonstrated in the studies by Goldhamer and colleagues. Because osteogenic potential of FAPs was assessed only in *in vitro* condition without BMP (Joe et al., 2010), their differentiation potential was probably underestimated. Therefore, the name FAPs does not represent the nature of these progenitors adequately. Although Sca-1 is widely used to identify progenitor populations in mice, it is also highly expressed in nonprogenitor cells such as endothelial cells. Furthermore, there is no human homolog of Sca-1 (Holmes and Stanford, 2007). Thus, this marker lacks relevance to the pathophysiology of human skeletal muscle. In contrast, PDGFRα is highly specific to mesenchymal progenitors (Uezumi et al., 2010) and is conserved in humans. In fact, cells equivalent to mouse PDGFRα$^+$ mesenchymal progenitors can be isolated from human muscle using PDGFRα as the marker (Oishi et al., 2013). As we have consistently used this marker since we described PDGFRα as the specific marker of mesenchymal progenitors for the first time, we believe that PDGFRα is the best marker to identify mesenchymal progenitors in skeletal muscle.

SATELLITE CELLS: MUSCLE STEM CELLS OR MULTIPOTENT STEM CELLS?

Although satellite cells have been considered as monopotential precursors that give rise only to cells of myogenic lineage (Bischof, 2004), several studies have shown that satellite cells can differentiate into cells of nonmyogenic lineages using satellite cell-derived myoblast culture or single myofiber culture (Asakura et al., 2001; Wada et al., 2002; Shefer et al., 2004). In myoblast culture, cells are usually purified by a preplating method or by culturing muscle-derived cells at a density that selectively promotes myogenic colony formation while nonmyogenic cells grow poorly. These methods require relatively long culture periods to obtain a pure culture. However, long-term culture or clonal expansion can elicit spontaneous transformations that lead to generation of the differentiation-defective cells often observed in myogenic cell lines (Lim and Hauschka, 1984). Moreover, only a few passages significantly reduce the muscle reconstitution ability of satellite cells (Montarras et al., 2005; Ikemoto et al., 2007). Therefore, the cells obtained may have undergone considerable changes during long culture periods, and thus cannot be considered equivalent to satellite cells. Single myofiber culture is a method to isolate single myofibers with their associated satellite cells by appropriate enzymatic treatment. Because each single myofiber carries a small number of satellite cells (approximately 10–20 satellite cells depending on the muscle from which the myofiber is derived) (Collins et al., 2005), contamination with only a few nonsatellite cells will have a considerable impact. In fact, it has been demonstrated that all the adipocytes that emerge in a single myofiber culture are derived from contaminated nonsatellite cells (Starkey et al., 2011).

The studies describing nonmyogenic mesenchymal progenitors showed that satellite cells do not adopt nonmyogenic fates but exclusively contribute to myogenesis even when transplanted into degenerating muscle that facilitate adipogenic, fibrogenic, or osteo/chondrogenic differentiation (Uezumi et al., 2010, 2011; Wosczyna et al., 2012). These findings suggest that satellite cells are committed to the myogenic lineage. This was further supported by the studies showing the expression of myogenic determination genes in satellite cells or progenitors of satellite cells. Using lineage tracing or selective cell ablation strategies, it has been shown that essentially all adult satellite cells originate from progenitors that had expressed MyoD, a key muscle determination gene, prenatally, and these MyoD-expressing progenitors are essential for skeletal myogenesis and satellite cell development (Kanisicak et al., 2009; Wood et al., 2013). Myf5, another muscle determination gene, is expressed at the mRNA level in the majority of satellite cells, but its translation was shown to be repressed by miR-31, leading to a model in which posttranscriptional mechanisms hold quiescent satellite cells poised to enter the myogenic program (Crist et al., 2012). Taken together, satellite cells should be considered as muscle stem cells committed to myogenic lineage. Although recent study showed that satellite cells can differentiate into brown adipocytes, this differentiation pathway is inhibited by miR-133 in a physiological context (Yin et al., 2013).

ROLES FOR NONMYOGENIC MESENCHYMAL PROGENITORS IN MUSCLE REGENERATION

The pathological relevance of nonmyogenic mesenchymal progenitors to muscle diseases leads to the idea that targeting these cells can be an excellent therapeutic strategy for the treatment of muscle disorders. However, this idea should be considered carefully, because nonmyogenic mesenchymal progenitors are also present in normal healthy muscle. In fact, we found that the number of these cells significantly increased during the muscle regeneration induced by CTX injection (Uezumi et al., 2010). As described earlier, CTX injection elicits successful muscle regeneration that is not accompanied by fat infiltration and fibrosis. Thus, mesenchymal progenitors decreased in number without making fatty and fibrous connective tissue as muscle regeneration proceeded. Intriguingly, they encircled the sheath of the basement membrane in which satellite cells undergo active myogenesis during muscle regeneration (Uezumi et al., 2010) (**Figure 3**). These findings suggest the interaction between mesenchymal progenitors and activated satellite cells. To gain insight into the interaction between them, we employed a co-culture system and found that adipogenesis of mesenchymal progenitors was strongly inhibited by the presence of myogenic cells derived from satellite cells (Uezumi et al., 2010). Rossi and co-workers demonstrated the complementary effect of this interaction. They showed that satellite cell-dependent myogenesis is promoted by mesenchymal progenitors in the co-culture (Joe et al., 2010).

The *in vivo* significance of the interaction between two types of cells was elegantly demonstrated by Kardon and colleagues. They first found that the transcription factor Tcf4 is expressed in lateral plate-derived limb mesodermal cells distinct from myogenic cells (Kardon et al., 2003). They explored the identity of Tcf4$^+$ cells and revealed that Tcf4 identifies connective tissue fibroblasts that are closely associated with skeletal muscles during development and in adulthood. By utilizing Tcf4-Cre mice, which allow genetic manipulation of connective tissue fibroblasts, fibroblasts were shown to promote slow myogenesis, the switch from fetal to adult muscle, and myoblast fusion (Mathew et al., 2011). This study clearly indicated that connective tissue fibroblasts are a critical regulator of muscle development. Roles for connective tissue fibroblasts have been further explored in adult muscle regeneration. Tcf4$^+$ fibroblasts were specifically ablated using Tcf4-CreER^{T2} knock-in mice that allow conditional gene manipulation in connective tissue fibroblasts. Fibroblast-ablated mice showed impaired muscle regeneration with premature satellite cell differentiation, depletion of the early pool of satellite cells, and smaller regenerated myofibers (Murphy et al., 2011). This was the first *in vivo* demonstration of the importance of connective tissue fibroblasts as the niche regulating satellite cell expansion during regeneration. Connective tissue fibroblasts appear to have more impact in regulating muscle regeneration because the ablation efficiency of Tcf4$^+$ cells was about 40% in

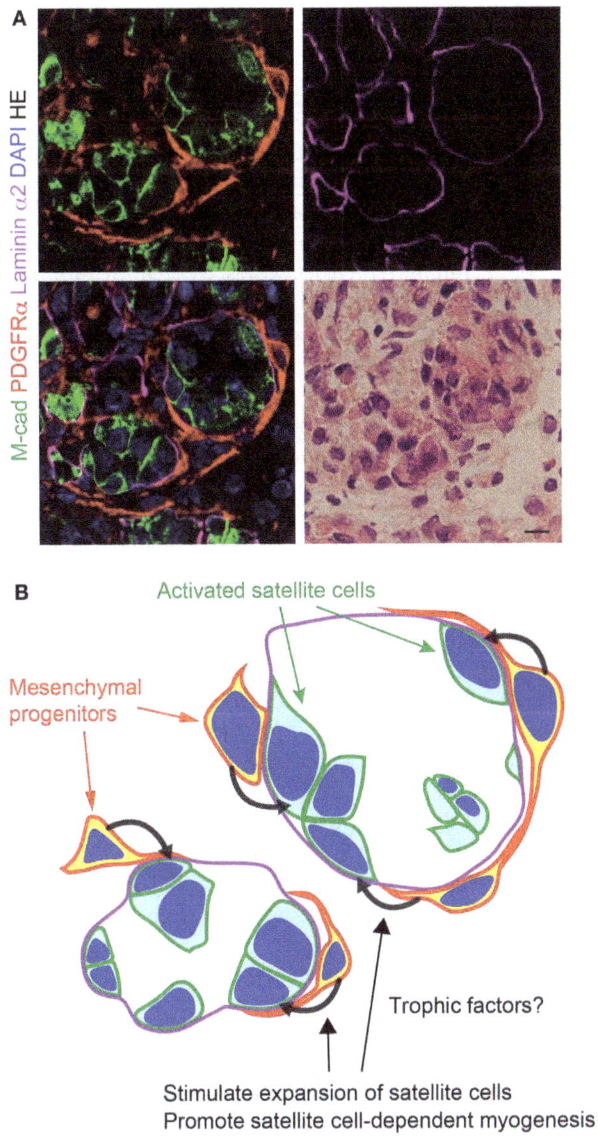

FIGURE 3 | Localization of PDGFRα$^+$ mesenchymal progenitors in regenerating muscle. (A) Fresh frozen section of regenerating muscle subjected to immunofluorescence staining for M-cadherin (M-cad), PDGFRα, and laminin α2, and subsequently to HE staining. Scale bar: 10 μm. **(B)** Schematic view of **(A)**. Mesenchymal progenitors encircle the sheath of basement membrane in which satellite cells undergo active myogenesis. Mesenchymal progenitors stimulate satellite cell expansion and promote satellite cell-dependent myogenesis. Factors responsible for these effects remain to be identified.

this study. The authors also showed that specific ablation of satellite cells resulted in a complete loss of regenerated myofibers, and, importantly, misregulation of fibroblasts, leading to a dramatic increase in fatty and fibrous connective tissue (Murphy et al., 2011). Thus, reciprocal interaction between the two types of cells is critical for efficient and effective muscle regeneration. A direct relationship between mesenchymal progenitors and Tcf4$^+$ fibroblasts remains to be demonstrated. However, Tcf4$^+$ fibroblasts express PDGFRα (Murphy et al., 2011), a marker of mesenchymal progenitors, and accumulating evidence suggests that mesenchymal progenitors and so-called fibroblasts share much more in common than previously recognized (Sudo et al., 2007; Haniffa et al., 2009). Therefore, these cells might be largely overlapping.

Heredia et al. reported that IL-4 signaling inhibits adipogenesis and stimulates the support function of mesenchymal progenitors for successful muscle regeneration (Heredia et al., 2013). IL-4 signaling also elicited phagocytic activity in mesenchymal progenitors and promoted the clearance of necrotic fibers by mesenchymal progenitors (Heredia et al., 2013). This study provided the regulatory mechanism of mesenchymal progenitors during muscle regeneration. IL-4 is also probably best known as the canonical Th2 effector cytokine and a critical developmental determinant that promotes Th2 response but inhibits Th1 response (Swain et al., 1990). Genetic background is known to greatly affect the nature of the Th cell response. BALB/c and DBA/2 mice are well known as strains with a high Th2 bias and as high producers of IL-4, and conversely, C57BL/6 and C57BL/10 mice are well known as the strains with low Th2 bias and as low producers of IL-4 (Reiner and Locksley, 1995; Bix et al., 1998; Yagi et al., 2002; Okamoto et al., 2009). Genetic background is also known to affect muscle regeneration potential. Importantly, BALB/c and DBA/2 mice show impaired muscle regeneration with adipocyte infiltration even in the CTX model that never induces fatty degeneration in C57BL/6 or C57BL/10 mice (Fukada et al., 2010). Therefore, muscle regeneration ability appears to correlate inversely with IL-4 production ability. Although self-renewal capacity of satellite cells was diminished in DBA/2 mice (Fukada et al., 2010), it still remains a mystery why high IL-4-producing strains, BALB/c and DBA/2 mice, readily develop fatty connective tissue after CTX-induced injury. Elucidation of the detailed mechanisms by which the phenotype of mesenchymal progenitors is regulated during muscle regeneration requires further investigation.

ROLES FOR NONMYOGENIC MESENCHYMAL PROGENITORS IN STEADY STATE HOMEOSTASIS OF SKELETAL MUSCLE

Nonmyogenic mesenchymal progenitors may have roles in steady state homeostasis of skeletal muscle. Collagen type VI, along with the fibrillins, is one of the microfibrillar components of the ECM. Collagen VI is found in a wide variety of extracellular matrices, including muscle, skin, tendon, cartilage, intervertebral discs, lens, internal organs, and blood vessels. Collagen VI consists of three products encoded by *COL6A1*, *COL6A2*, and *COL6A3*. One of each of the three α-chain subunits encoded by *COL6A1*, *COL6A2*, and *COL6A3* combine to form the collagen VI monomer. Within the cells, these monomers associate to form dimers, which pair up into tetramers. These tetramers are then secreted into the ECM, where they assemble to form the microfibrillar structures (Bonnemann, 2011). Collagen VI microfibrils interact with collagen I, collagen IV, and with a variety of proteoglycans such as biglycan and decorin (Voermans et al., 2008). Collagen VI occurs in both the basal lamina and the reticular lamina of muscle, and therefore is an important component of endomysium and perimysium of skeletal muscle. The functional significance of collagen VI in skeletal muscle is evident as mutations in collagen VI genes cause Ullrich congenital muscular dystrophy (UCMD) and Bethlem myopathy (Bonnemann,

2011). Disease symptoms are typically more severe in UCMD than in Bethlem myopathy. UCMD patients show progressive loss of individual muscle fibers and muscle mass, and proliferation of connective and adipose tissue. The precise mechanisms leading to reduced fiber size are currently unknown. One of the unique features of collagen VI is its regulated expression. It has been demonstrated that collagen VI is largely generated by interstitial mesenchymal cells but not by myogenic cells (Zou et al., 2008). An enhancer region of the *Col6a1* gene that is required for activation of transcription in interstitial mesenchymal cells associated skeletal muscle was identified (Braghetta et al., 2008). Using reporter mice that carry this enhancer region, the expression *Col6a1* in interstitial mesenchymal cells but not in myogenic cells was confirmed. Interestingly, it has been demonstrated that the expression of Col6a1 in mesenchymal cells associated with skeletal muscle is a consequence of an inductive process whereby myogenic cells activate a specific enhancer region in mesenchymal cells by releasing a diffusible factor; in addition, only mesenchymal cells from skeletal muscle can respond to this inductive signal (Braghetta et al., 2008). Although detailed characterization of collagen VI-producing cells has not been done, their interstitial localization and mesenchymal nature suggest that these cells are closely related to mesenchymal progenitors. Thus, it is highly possible that mesenchymal progenitors play a key role in supporting muscle fibers by producing collagen VI under the inductive cue from muscle cells. Recent study extended the importance of collagen VI by demonstrating that collagen VI also works as a key component of the satellite cell niche (Urciuolo et al., 2013).

The roles for mesenchymal progenitors in the maintenance of muscle fibers have been directly demonstrated by ablating fibroblast activation protein-α (FAP)-expressing stromal cells (Roberts et al., 2013). FAP is the type II membrane dipeptidylpeptidase, and its expression has been reported to associate with fibroblasts in the tumor stroma (Garin-Chesa et al., 1990). Note that FAP differs from FAPs, fibro/adipogenic progenitors, described earlier. FAP$^+$ stromal fibroblasts suppress the immune response to tumors, and elimination of FAP$^+$ fibroblasts from tumor stroma unmasks the immune response to cancer and allows the immune system to attack tumors (Kraman et al., 2010). Therefore, targeting FAP$^+$ stromal cells may be a promising strategy to combat cancer. However, a contraindication to any potential cancer therapy that indiscriminately depletes FAP$^+$ cells might be their presence in normal tissues. To investigate the occurrence and function of FAP$^+$ stromal cells in normal tissues, Roberts et al. generated transgenic mice that permit both the bioluminescent imaging of FAP$^+$ cells and their conditional ablation (Roberts et al., 2013). Using this mouse line, FAP$^+$ cells were found to reside in almost all tissues of the adult mouse. Surprisingly, ablation of FAP$^+$ cells caused significant loss of muscle mass and hypocellularity of the bone marrow, revealing their essential functions in maintaining normal muscle mass and hematopoiesis, respectively. The loss of skeletal muscle mass was attributed to the atrophy of myofibers, and was accompanied by a persistent decrease in follistatin (Fst) and laminin α2 expression and a transient increase in atrogin-1 and MuRF1 mRNA levels. Fst is an inhibitor of myostatin (Mstn), a negative regulator of muscle mass (McPherron et al., 1997). Systemic overexpression of Mstn was reported to induce cachexia (Zimmers et al., 2002), and conversely, Fst overexpression led to dramatic increase in muscle mass (Lee and McPherron, 2001). Fst has been shown to inhibit other TGF-β family members in addition to myostatin to regulate muscle size (Lee, 2007; Lee et al., 2010). Laminin α2 is a component of muscle basal lamina and mutations in the laminin α2 gene cause congenital muscular dystrophy, in which impaired anchoring of myofibers in the ECM results in impaired membrane stability and massive muscle fiber degeneration during early infancy (Hayashi et al., 2001). Laminin α2 deficiency was also reported to induce the upregulation of key ubiquitin ligases atrogin-1 and MuRF1 (Carmignac et al., 2011). Gene expression analysis of sorted cells confirmed that FAP$^+$ stromal cells are the major source of both Fst and laminin α2 in skeletal muscle (Roberts et al., 2013). Therefore, the ablation of FAP$^+$ stromal cells was directly responsible for the decrease in the expression of Fst and laminin α2 in muscle, which can be considered to be the basis of the loss of muscle mass and the increase of atrogin-1 and MuRF1. Intriguingly, FAP$^+$ stromal cells in muscle uniformly express PDGFRα, Sca-1 and CD90 (Roberts et al., 2013), which are shared cell surface markers with mesenchymal progenitors (Uezumi et al., 2010), and both cells are localized to the interstitial spaces of muscle tissue (Uezumi et al., 2010; Roberts et al., 2013). Thus, FAP$^+$ stromal cells appear nearly identical to mesenchymal progenitors. A further important finding was that these cells undergo considerable alterations in a cachectic condition (Roberts et al., 2013). Under a cachectic condition, the FAP-dependent bioluminescence in skeletal muscle was significantly reduced, and the downregulation of Fst and laminin α2 and the upregulation of atrogin-1 and MuRF1 again accompanied dramatic loss of muscle mass. Decreased FAP-dependent bioluminescence suggests that mesenchymal progenitors decreased in number or mesenchymal progenitors lost the expression of FAP in cachectic muscle. The latter should be the case because PDGFRα$^+$Sca-1$^+$ cells were shown to increase in number in cachectic muscle (He et al., 2013). Collectively, mesenchymal progenitors can play vital roles in the maintenance of muscle fibers by producing trophic factors such as collagen VI, Fst, and laminin α2 in a steady physiological condition (**Figure 1**), and their support functions can be severely deteriorated in cancer cachexia.

LESSONS FROM BONE MARROW

Mesenchymal stem cells (MSCs) or mesenchymal progenitors were initially identified in bone marrow. Due to the ease of their isolation and their extensive proliferation and differentiation potentials, bone marrow MSCs have been expected as a source of cells for potential use in cell-based therapy and are being introduced into a clinical setting (Abdallah and Kassem, 2008). Nevertheless, the actual identity of bone marrow MSCs remains largely unknown.

Several recent studies documented *in vivo* functions of MSCs for constructing the niche of hematopoietic stem cells (HSCs). Although several cell types in bone marrow are suggested to play a role in forming the HSC niche (Frenette et al., 2013), we focus on MSCs in this article. MSCs were reported to support hematopoiesis and colocalize with HSCs throughout ontogeny (Mendes et al., 2005). In adult bone marrow, the expression of intermediate filament nestin has been shown to identify MSCs in close contact with the vasculature and HSCs (Mendez-Ferrer et al., 2010). Perivascular nestin^{+} MSCs highly express HSC maintenance genes such as *Cxcl12*, *Scf*, and *Angpt1*, and ablation of nestin^{+} MSCs rapidly reduces the concentration of HSCs in the bone marrow. A chemokine Cxcl12 plays a crucial role in maintaining HSC function and Stem cell factor (Scf), a c-kit ligand, is required to sustain hematopoiesis. Cxcl12 is produced mainly by reticular cells scattered throughout the bone marrow, and these reticular cells were termed Cxcl12-abundant reticular (CAR) cells (Sugiyama et al., 2006). Using genetically engineered mice in which a transgene encoding the diphtheria toxin receptor-GFP fusion protein is knocked into the *Cxcl12* locus, CAR cells were shown to be required for proliferation of HSCs and lymphoid and erythroid progenitors, as well as maintenance of HSCs in an undifferentiated state (Omatsu et al., 2010). CAR cells were also shown to produce most of the Scf and Cxcl12 in the bone marrow. Interestingly, CAR cells possess the potential to differentiate into adipocytes and osteoblasts (Omatsu et al., 2010), indicating that cells with MSC activity possess HSC niche activity. FAP is expressed in multipotent bone marrow stromal cells that express PDGFRα, Sca-1, Cxcl12, and Scf (Roberts et al., 2013; Tran et al., 2013). Elimination of FAP^{+} cells has been shown to induce severe bone marrow hypocellularity (Roberts et al., 2013; Tran et al., 2013). FAP^{+} cell-depleted mice showed anemia and suppressed B-lymphopoiesis and erythropoiesis although HSC frequency was not changed in these mice (Roberts et al., 2013). Leptin receptor (*Lepr*)–expressing perivascular stromal cells were shown to be one of the major sources of Scf and required to maintain HSCs (Ding et al., 2012). However, MSC activity of *Lepr*$^{+}$ cells was not examined. The *Cxcl12* gene was knocked out conditionally using several Cre lines to clarify the importance of Cxcl12 expression in several different candidate niche cells (Greenbaum et al., 2013). As a consequence, it was demonstrated that HSCs and common lymphoid progenitors are maintained by Cxcl12 produced from Prx1-Cre-targeted cells. The paired-related homeobox gene-1 (Prx1) is expressed in the early limb bud mesenchyme and Prx1-Cre targets all mesenchymal cells in the limb bud (Logan et al., 2002). As in muscle, MSCs are enriched in PDGFRα^{+}Sca-1^{+} cells in bone marrow (Morikawa et al., 2009). Importantly, only Prx1-targeted PDGFRα^{+}Sca-1^{+} cells exhibited colony-forming unit-fibroblast activity and showed osteogenic and adipogenic differentiation, indicating that this subset is a highly enriched population of MSCs. Maintenance of committed B cell precursors is dependent on Cxcl12 from CAR cells and/or osteoblasts, and retention of hematopoietic progenitor cells in the bone marrow is dependent on Cxcl12 from CAR cells. These results showed the complexity of the niche microenvironment in the bone marrow and suggest that distinct stromal niche cells regulate specific hematopoietic stem/progenitor populations. Naveiras et al. reported an interesting finding. They showed that adipocyte-rich vertebrae of the mouse tail have reduced HSC frequency compared with adipocyte-free vertebrae of the thorax (Naveiras et al., 2009). Tail vertebrae of lipodystrophic mice showed normal HSC frequency, indicating that adipocytes act as negative regulators of the hematopoietic microenvironment. Because MSCs can produce adipocytes, this finding suggests the notion that their aberrant differentiation can negatively affect homeostasis of parenchymal cells. Among secretory proteins from adipocytes, adiponectin has been demonstrated to suppress the growth of myelomonocytic progenitors and the functions of macrophages (Yokota et al., 2000). Pinho et al. extended these findings to humans (Pinho et al., 2013). PDGFRα^{+}CD51^{+} cells in human bone marrow represent a cell population enriched for MSCs and capable of expanding human hematopoietic stem and progenitor cells. These lines of evidence suggest that the intrinsic function of MSCs in bone marrow is to act as a niche for HSCs.

CONCLUDING REMARKS

Mesenchymal stem/progenitor cells are reported to exist in almost all organs of both mice and humans (Da Silva Meirelles et al., 2006; Crisan et al., 2008). Although *in vitro* multipotency toward adipogenic, osteogenic, and chondrogenic lineages is a hallmark of MSCs, there is no evidence that fat, bone, or cartilage are continuously generated in most organs where MSCs reside. Therefore, it seems unlikely that differentiating into a certain lineage is an intrinsic *in vivo* function of MSCs. Instead, it is tempting to speculate that these cells exert support functions for parenchymal cells of the tissue where they reside, as reviewed in this paper. Their differentiation might be undesired in most cases because adipogenic differentiation has a negative impact on hematopoiesis in bone marrow (Naveiras et al., 2009). Interestingly, pancreas-derived mesenchymal cells have a greater ability to support ES cell-derived pancreatic progenitors than the mesenchymal cells derived from other organs (Sneddon et al., 2012). Thus, mesenchymal stem/progenitor cells in certain tissues might be specialized to suitably sustain the parenchyma of that tissue. Because specific expression of collagen VI in muscle mesenchymal cells requires induction cues from myogenic cells (Braghetta et al., 2008), such a specialization might be reciprocally conducted by parenchymal cells. Exploring the detailed mechanism of parenchymal-mesenchymal interactions is an important task in a future study.

ACKNOWLEDGMENTS

We thank K. Ono for proofreading the paper. Akiyoshi Uezumi was supported by JSPS KAKENHI Grant Number 24659687, Kato Memorial Bioscience Foundation, ONO Medical Research Foundation, and The Nakatomi Foundation.

REFERENCES

Abdallah, B. M., and Kassem, M. (2008). Human mesenchymal stem cells: from basic biology to clinical applications. *Gene Ther.* 15, 109–116. doi: 10.1038/sj.gt.3303067

Asakura, A., Komaki, M., and Rudnicki, M. (2001). Muscle satellite cells are multipotential stem cells that exhibit myogenic, osteogenic, and adipogenic differentiation. *Differentiation* 68, 245–253. doi: 10.1046/j.1432-0436.2001.680412.x

Balboni, T. A., Gobezie, R., and Mamon, H. J. (2006). Heterotopic ossification: pathophysiology, clinical features, and the role of radiotherapy for prophylaxis. *Int. J. Radiat. Oncol. Biol. Phys.* 65, 1289–1299. doi: 10.1016/j.ijrobp.2006.03.053

Banker, B. Q., and Engel, A. G. (2004). "Basic reactions of muscle," in *Myology, 3rd Edn*, eds A. G. Engel and C. Franzini-Armstrong (New York, NY: McGraw-Hill), 691–747.

Beiner, J. M., and Jokl, P. (2001). Muscle contusion injuries: current treatment options. *J. Am. Acad. Orthop. Surg.* 9, 227–237.

Bischof, R. (2004). "Satellite and stem cells in muscle regeneration," in *Myology, 3rd Edn,* eds A. G. Engel and C. Franzini-Armstrong (New York, NY: McGraw-Hill), 66–86.

Bix, M., Wang, Z. E., Thiel, B., Schork, N. J., and Locksley, R. M. (1998). Genetic regulation of commitment to interleukin 4 production by a CD4(+) T cell-intrinsic mechanism. *J. Exp. Med.* 188, 2289–2299. doi: 10.1084/jem.188.12.2289

Bizario, J. C., Cerri, D. G., Rodrigues, L. C., Oliveira, G. L., Nomizo, A., De Araujo, D. D., et al. (2009). Imatinib mesylate ameliorates the dystrophic phenotype in exercised mdx mice. *J. Neuroimmunol.* 212, 93–101. doi: 10.1016/j.jneuroim.2009.05.006

Bonnemann, C. G. (2011). The collagen VI-related myopathies: muscle meets its matrix. *Nat. Rev. Neurol.* 7, 379–390. doi: 10.1038/nrneurol.2011.81

Brack, A. S., Conboy, M. J., Roy, S., Lee, M., Kuo, C. J., Keller, C., et al. (2007). Increased Wnt signaling during aging alters muscle stem cell fate and increases fibrosis. *Science* 317, 807–810. doi: 10.1126/science.1144090

Braghetta, P., Ferrari, A., Fabbro, C., Bizzotto, D., Volpin, D., Bonaldo, P., et al. (2008). An enhancer required for transcription of the Col6a1 gene in muscle connective tissue is induced by signals released from muscle cells. *Exp. Cell Res.* 314, 3508–3518. doi: 10.1016/j.yexcr.2008.08.006

Carmignac, V., Quere, R., and Durbeej, M. (2011). Proteasome inhibition improves the muscle of laminin alpha2 chain-deficient mice. *Hum. Mol. Genet.* 20, 541–552. doi: 10.1093/hmg/ddq499

Carpenter, S., and Karpati, G. (2001). "Cells and structures other than skeletal muscle fibers," in *Pathology of Skeletal Muscle, 2nd Edn.* eds S. Carpenter and G. Karpati (New York, NY: Oxford), 314–369.

Chakkalakal, S. A., Zhang, D., Culbert, A. L., Convente, M. R., Caron, R. J., Wright, A. C., et al. (2012). An Acvr1 R206H knock-in mouse has fibrodysplasia ossificans progressiva. *J. Bone Miner. Res.* 27, 1746–1756. doi: 10.1002/jbmr.1637

Collins, C. A., Olsen, I., Zammit, P. S., Heslop, L., Petrie, A., Partridge, T. A., et al. (2005). Stem cell function, self-renewal, and behavioral heterogeneity of cells from the adult muscle satellite cell niche. *Cell* 122, 289–301. doi: 10.1016/j.cell.2005.05.010

Crisan, M., Yap, S., Casteilla, L., Chen, C. W., Corselli, M., Park, T. S., et al. (2008). A perivascular origin for mesenchymal stem cells in multiple human organs. *Cell Stem Cell* 3, 301–313. doi: 10.1016/j.stem.2008.07.003

Crist, C. G., Montarras, D., and Buckingham, M. (2012). Muscle satellite cells are primed for myogenesis but maintain quiescence with sequestration of Myf5 mRNA targeted by microRNA-31 in mRNP granules. *Cell Stem Cell* 11, 118–126. doi: 10.1016/j.stem.2012.03.011

Da Silva Meirelles, L., Chagastelles, P. C., and Nardi, N. B. (2006). Mesenchymal stem cells reside in virtually all post-natal organs and tissues. *J. Cell Sci.* 119, 2204–2213. doi: 10.1242/jcs.02932

Ding, L., Saunders, T. L., Enikolopov, G., and Morrison, S. J. (2012). Endothelial and perivascular cells maintain haematopoietic stem cells. *Nature* 481, 457–462. doi: 10.1038/nature10783

Dulauroy, S., Di Carlo, S. E., Langa, F., Eberl, G., and Peduto, L. (2012). Lineage tracing and genetic ablation of ADAM12(+) perivascular cells identify a major source of profibrotic cells during acute tissue injury. *Nat. Med.* 18, 1262–1270. doi: 10.1038/nm.2848

Frenette, P. S., Pinho, S., Lucas, D., and Scheiermann, C. (2013). Mesenchymal stem cell: keystone of the hematopoietic stem cell niche and a stepping-stone for regenerative medicine. *Annu. Rev. Immunol.* 31, 285–316. doi: 10.1146/annurev-immunol-032712-095919

Fukada, S., Morikawa, D., Yamamoto, Y., Yoshida, T., Sumie, N., Yamaguchi, M., et al. (2010). Genetic background affects properties of satellite cells and mdx phenotypes. *Am. J. Pathol.* 176, 2414–2424. doi: 10.2353/ajpath.2010.090887

Garin-Chesa, P., Old, L. J., and Rettig, W. J. (1990). Cell surface glycoprotein of reactive stromal fibroblasts as a potential antibody target in human epithelial cancers. *Proc. Natl. Acad. Sci. U.S.A.* 87, 7235–7239. doi: 10.1073/pnas.87.18.7235

Garland, D. E., Blum, C. E., and Waters, R. L. (1980). Periarticular heterotopic ossification in head-injured adults. Incidence and location. *J. Bone Joint Surg. Am.* 62, 1143–1146.

Goodpaster, B. H., Thaete, F. L., and Kelley, D. E. (2000). Thigh adipose tissue distribution is associated with insulin resistance in obesity and in type 2 diabetes mellitus. *Am. J. Clin. Nutr.* 71, 885–892.

Gorgey, A. S., and Dudley, G. A. (2007). Skeletal muscle atrophy and increased intramuscular fat after incomplete spinal cord injury. *Spinal Cord* 45, 304–309. doi: 10.1038/sj.sc.3101968

Greco, A. V., Mingrone, G., Giancaterini, A., Manco, M., Morroni, M., Cinti, S., et al. (2002). Insulin resistance in morbid obesity: reversal with intramyocellular fat depletion. *Diabetes* 51, 144–151. doi: 10.2337/diabetes.51.1.144

Greenbaum, A., Hsu, Y. M., Day, R. B., Schuettpelz, L. G., Christopher, M. J., Borgerding, J. N., et al. (2013). CXCL12 in early mesenchymal progenitors is required for haematopoietic stem-cell maintenance. *Nature* 495, 227–230. doi: 10.1038/nature11926

Haniffa, M. A., Collin, M. P., Buckley, C. D., and Dazzi, F. (2009). Mesenchymal stem cells: the fibroblasts' new clothes? *Haematologica* 94, 258–263. doi: 10.3324/haematol.13699

Harris, J. B. (2003). Myotoxic phospholipases A2 and the regeneration of skeletal muscles. *Toxicon* 42, 933–945. doi: 10.1016/j.toxicon.2003.11.011

Hawke, T. J., and Garry, D. J. (2001). Myogenic satellite cells: physiology to molecular biology. *J. Appl. Physiol.* 91, 534–551.

Hayashi, Y. K., Tezak, Z., Momoi, T., Nonaka, I., Garcia, C. A., Hoffman, E. P., et al. (2001). Massive muscle cell degeneration in the early stage of merosin-deficient congenital muscular dystrophy. *Neuromuscul. Disord.* 11, 350–359. doi: 10.1016/S0960-8966(00)00203-0

He, W. A., Berardi, E., Cardillo, V. M., Acharyya, S., Aulino, P., Thomas-Ahner, J., et al. (2013). NF-kappaB-mediated Pax7 dysregulation in the muscle microenvironment promotes cancer cachexia. *J. Clin. Invest.* 123, 4821–4835. doi: 10.1172/JCI68523

Heredia, J. E., Mukundan, L., Chen, F. M., Mueller, A. A., Deo, R. C., Locksley, R. M., et al. (2013). Type 2 innate signals stimulate fibro/adipogenic progenitors to facilitate muscle regeneration. *Cell* 153, 376–388. doi: 10.1016/j.cell.2013.02.053

Hilton, T. N., Tuttle, L. J., Bohnert, K. L., Mueller, M. J., and Sinacore, D. R. (2008). Excessive adipose tissue infiltration in skeletal muscle in individuals with obesity, diabetes mellitus, and peripheral neuropathy: association with performance and function. *Phys. Ther.* 88, 1336–1344. doi: 10.2522/ptj.20080079

Holmes, C., and Stanford, W. L. (2007). Concise review: stem cell antigen-1: expression, function, and enigma. *Stem Cells* 25, 1339–1347. doi: 10.1634/stemcells.2006-0644

Huang, P., Zhao, X. S., Fields, M., Ransohoff, R. M., and Zhou, L. (2009). Imatinib attenuates skeletal muscle dystrophy in mdx mice. *FASEB J.* 23, 2539–2548. doi: 10.1096/fj.09-129833

Ikemoto, M., Fukada, S., Uezumi, A., Masuda, S., Miyoshi, H., Yamamoto, H., et al. (2007). Autologous transplantation of SM/C-2.6(+) satellite cells transduced with micro-dystrophin CS1 cDNA by lentiviral vector into mdx mice. *Mol. Ther.* 15, 2178–2185. doi: 10.1038/sj.mt.6300295

Irintchev, A., Zeschnigk, M., Starzinski-Powitz, A., and Wernig, A. (1994). Expression pattern of M-cadherin in normal, denervated, and regenerating mouse muscles. *Dev. Dyn.* 199, 326–337. doi: 10.1002/aja.1001990407

Ishikawa, K., Izumi, K., and Kitagawa, T. (1982). Heterotopic ossification of the hip as a complication of tetanus. *Clin. Orthop. Relat. Res.* 166, 249–255.

Ito, T., Ogawa, R., Uezumi, A., Ohtani, T., Watanabe, Y., Tsujikawa, K., et al. (2013). Imatinib attenuates severe mouse dystrophy and inhibits proliferation and fibrosis-marker expression in muscle mesenchymal progenitors. *Neuromuscul. Disord.* 23, 349–356. doi: 10.1016/j.nmd.2012.10.025

Jarvinen, T. A., Kaariainen, M., Jarvinen, M., and Kalimo, H. (2000). Muscle strain injuries. *Curr. Opin. Rheumatol.* 12, 155–161. doi: 10.1097/00002281-200003000-00010

Joe, A. W., Yi, L., Natarajan, A., Le Grand, F., So, L., Wang, J., et al. (2010). Muscle injury activates resident fibro/adipogenic progenitors that facilitate myogenesis. *Nat. Cell Biol.* 12, 153–163. doi: 10.1038/ncb2015

Kanisicak, O., Mendez, J. J., Yamamoto, S., Yamamoto, M., and Goldhamer, D. J. (2009). Progenitors of skeletal muscle satellite cells express the muscle determination gene, MyoD. *Dev. Biol.* 332, 131–141. doi: 10.1016/j.ydbio.2009.05.554

Kaplan, F. S., and Shore, E. M. (2000). Progressive osseous heteroplasia. *J. Bone Miner. Res.* 15, 2084–2094. doi: 10.1359/jbmr.2000.15.11.2084

Kardon, G., Harfe, B. D., and Tabin, C. J. (2003). A Tcf4-positive mesodermal population provides a prepattern for vertebrate limb muscle patterning. *Dev. Cell* 5, 937–944. doi: 10.1016/S1534-5807(03)00360-5

Kim, J. Y., Kim, D. H., Choi, J., Park, J. K., Jeong, K. S., Leeuwenburgh, C., et al. (2009). Changes in lipid distribution during aging and its modulation by calorie restriction. *Age (Dordr.)* 31, 127–142. doi: 10.1007/s11357-009-9089-0

Kragstrup, T. W., Kjaer, M., and Mackey, A. L. (2011). Structural, biochemical, cellular, and functional changes in skeletal muscle extracellular matrix with aging. *Scand. J. Med. Sci. Sports* 21, 749–757. doi: 10.1111/j.1600-0838.2011.01377.x

Kraman, M., Bambrough, P. J., Arnold, J. N., Roberts, E. W., Magiera, L., Jones, J. O., et al. (2010). Suppression of antitumor immunity by stromal cells expressing fibroblast activation protein-alpha. *Science* 330, 827–830. doi: 10.1126/science.1195300

Lee, S. J. (2007). Quadrupling muscle mass in mice by targeting TGF-beta signaling pathways. *PLoS ONE* 2:e789. doi: 10.1371/journal.pone.0000789

Lee, S. J., Lee, Y. S., Zimmers, T. A., Soleimani, A., Matzuk, M. M., Tsuchida, K., et al. (2010). Regulation of muscle mass by follistatin and activins. *Mol. Endocrinol.* 24, 1998–2008. doi: 10.1210/me.2010-0127

Lee, S. J., and McPherron, A. C. (2001). Regulation of myostatin activity and muscle growth. *Proc. Natl. Acad. Sci. U.S.A.* 98, 9306–9311. doi: 10.1073/pnas.151270098

Lepper, C., Partridge, T. A., and Fan, C. M. (2011). An absolute requirement for Pax7-positive satellite cells in acute injury-induced skeletal muscle regeneration. *Development* 138, 3639–3646. doi: 10.1242/dev.067595

Lim, R. W., and Hauschka, S. D. (1984). EGF responsiveness and receptor regulation in normal and differentiation-defective mouse myoblasts. *Dev. Biol.* 105, 48–58. doi: 10.1016/0012-1606(84)90260-4

Logan, M., Martin, J. F., Nagy, A., Lobe, C., Olson, E. N., and Tabin, C. J. (2002). Expression of Cre Recombinase in the developing mouse limb bud driven by a Prxl enhancer. *Genesis* 33, 77–80. doi: 10.1002/gene.10092

Lorber, J. (1953). Ectopic ossification in tuberculous meningitis. *Arch. Dis. Child.* 28, 98–103. doi: 10.1136/adc.28.138.98

Lounev, V. Y., Ramachandran, R., Wosczyna, M. N., Yamamoto, M., Maidment, A. D., Shore, E. M., et al. (2009). Identification of progenitor cells that contribute to heterotopic skeletogenesis. *J. Bone Joint Surg. Am.* 91, 652–663. doi: 10.2106/JBJS.H.01177

Manini, T. M., Clark, B. C., Nalls, M. A., Goodpaster, B. H., Ploutz-Snyder, L. L., and Harris, T. B. (2007). Reduced physical activity increases intermuscular adipose tissue in healthy young adults. *Am. J. Clin. Nutr.* 85, 377–384.

Marcus, R. L., Addison, O., Kidde, J. P., Dibble, L. E., and Lastayo, P. C. (2010). Skeletal muscle fat infiltration: impact of age, inactivity, and exercise. *J. Nutr. Health Aging* 14, 362–366. doi: 10.1007/s12603-010-0081-2

Mathew, S. J., Hansen, J. M., Merrell, A. J., Murphy, M. M., Lawson, J. A., Hutcheson, D. A., et al. (2011). Connective tissue fibroblasts and Tcf4 regulate myogenesis. *Development* 138, 371–384. doi: 10.1242/dev.057463

McPherron, A. C., Lawler, A. M., and Lee, S. J. (1997). Regulation of skeletal muscle mass in mice by a new TGF-beta superfamily member. *Nature* 387, 83–90. doi: 10.1038/387083a0

Mendes, S. C., Robin, C., and Dzierzak, E. (2005). Mesenchymal progenitor cells localize within hematopoietic sites throughout ontogeny. *Development* 132, 1127–1136. doi: 10.1242/dev.01615

Mendez-Ferrer, S., Michurina, T. V., Ferraro, F., Mazloom, A. R., MacArthur, B. D., Lira, S. A., et al. (2010). Mesenchymal and haematopoietic stem cells form a unique bone marrow niche. *Nature* 466, 829–834. doi: 10.1038/nature09262

Montarras, D., Morgan, J., Collins, C., Relaix, F., Zaffran, S., Cumano, A., et al. (2005). Direct isolation of satellite cells for skeletal muscle regeneration. *Science* 309, 2064–2067. doi: 10.1126/science.1114758

Morikawa, S., Mabuchi, Y., Kubota, Y., Nagai, Y., Niibe, K., Hiratsu, E., et al. (2009). Prospective identification, isolation, and systemic transplantation of multipotent mesenchymal stem cells in murine bone marrow. *J. Exp. Med.* 206, 2483–2496. doi: 10.1084/jem.20091046

Murphy, M. M., Lawson, J. A., Mathew, S. J., Hutcheson, D. A., and Kardon, G. (2011). Satellite cells, connective tissue fibroblasts and their interactions are crucial for muscle regeneration. *Development* 138, 3625–3637. doi: 10.1242/dev.064162

Naveiras, O., Nardi, V., Wenzel, P. L., Hauschka, P. V., Fahey, F., and Daley, G. Q. (2009). Bone-marrow adipocytes as negative regulators of the haematopoietic microenvironment. *Nature* 460, 259–263. doi: 10.1038/nature08099

Nilsson, O. S., and Persson, P. E. (1999). Heterotopic bone formation after joint replacement. *Curr. Opin. Rheumatol.* 11, 127–131. doi: 10.1097/00002281-199903000-00008

Oishi, T., Uezumi, A., Kanaji, A., Yamamoto, N., Yamaguchi, A., Yamada, H., et al. (2013). Osteogenic differentiation capacity of human skeletal muscle-derived progenitor cells. *PLoS ONE* 8:e56641. doi: 10.1371/journal.pone.0056641

Okamoto, M., Van Stry, M., Chung, L., Koyanagi, M., Sun, X., Suzuki, Y., et al. (2009). Mina, an Il4 repressor, controls T helper type 2 bias. *Nat. Immunol.* 10, 872–879. doi: 10.1038/ni.1747

Olson, L. E., and Soriano, P. (2009). Increased PDGFRalpha activation disrupts connective tissue development and drives systemic fibrosis. *Dev. Cell* 16, 303–313. doi: 10.1016/j.devcel.2008.12.003

Omatsu, Y., Sugiyama, T., Kohara, H., Kondoh, G., Fujii, N., Kohno, K., et al. (2010). The essential functions of adipo-osteogenic progenitors as the hematopoietic stem and progenitor cell niche. *Immunity* 33, 387–399. doi: 10.1016/j.immuni.2010.08.017

Pignolo, R. J., Shore, E. M., and Kaplan, F. S. (2011). Fibrodysplasia ossificans progressiva: clinical and genetic aspects. *Orphanet J. Rare Dis.* 6, 80. doi: 10.1186/1750-1172-6-80

Pinho, S., Lacombe, J., Hanoun, M., Mizoguchi, T., Bruns, I., Kunisaki, Y., et al. (2013). PDGFRalpha and CD51 mark human nestin+ sphere-forming mesenchymal stem cells capable of hematopoietic progenitor cell expansion. *J. Exp. Med.* 210, 1351–1367. doi: 10.1084/jem.20122252

Povysil, C., and Matejovsky, Z. (1979). Ultrastructural evidence of myofibroblasts in pseudomalignant myositis ossificans. *Virchows Arch. A Pathol. Anat. Histol.* 381, 189–203. doi: 10.1007/BF01257884

Reiner, S. L., and Locksley, R. M. (1995). The regulation of immunity to Leishmania major. *Annu. Rev. Immunol.* 13, 151–177. doi: 10.1146/annurev.iy.13.040195.001055

Roberts, E. W., Deonarine, A., Jones, J. O., Denton, A. E., Feig, C., Lyons, S. K., et al. (2013). Depletion of stromal cells expressing fibroblast activation protein-alpha from skeletal muscle and bone marrow results in cachexia and anemia. *J. Exp. Med.* 210, 1137–1151. doi: 10.1084/jem.20122344

Rocheteau, P., Gayraud-Morel, B., Siegl-Cachedenier, I., Blasco, M. A., and Tajbakhsh, S. (2012). A subpopulation of adult skeletal muscle stem cells retains all template DNA strands after cell division. *Cell* 148, 112–125. doi: 10.1016/j.cell.2011.11.049

Ryan, A. S., Dobrovolny, C. L., Smith, G. V., Silver, K. H., and Macko, R. F. (2002). Hemiparetic muscle atrophy and increased intramuscular fat in stroke patients. *Arch. Phys. Med. Rehabil.* 83, 1703–1707. doi: 10.1053/apmr.2002.36399

Sacco, A., Doyonnas, R., Kraft, P., Vitorovic, S., and Blau, H. M. (2008). Self-renewal and expansion of single transplanted muscle stem cells. *Nature* 456, 502–506. doi: 10.1038/nature07384

Sadeh, M., Czyewski, K., and Stern, L. Z. (1985). Chronic myopathy induced by repeated bupivacaine injections. *J. Neurol. Sci.* 67, 229–238. doi: 10.1016/0022-510X(85)90119-4

Sambasivan, R., Yao, R., Kissenpfennig, A., Van Wittenberghe, L., Paldi, A., Gayraud-Morel, B., et al. (2011). Pax7-expressing satellite cells are indispensable for adult skeletal muscle regeneration. *Development* 138, 3647–3656. doi: 10.1242/dev.067587

Schulz, T. J., Huang, T. L., Tran, T. T., Zhang, H., Townsend, K. L., Shadrach, J. L., et al. (2011). Identification of inducible brown adipocyte progenitors residing in skeletal muscle and white fat. *Proc. Natl. Acad. Sci. U.S.A.* 108, 143–148. doi: 10.1073/pnas.1010929108

Seale, P., Sabourin, L. A., Girgis-Gabardo, A., Mansouri, A., Gruss, P., and Rudnicki, M. A. (2000). Pax7 is required for the specification of myogenic satellite cells. *Cell* 102, 777–786. doi: 10.1016/S0092-8674(00)00066-0

Shefer, G., Wleklinski-Lee, M., and Yablonka-Reuveni, Z. (2004). Skeletal muscle satellite cells can spontaneously enter an alternative mesenchymal pathway. *J. Cell Sci.* 117, 5393–5404. doi: 10.1242/jcs.01419

Shore, E. M., Ahn, J., Jan De Beur, S., Li, M., Xu, M., Gardner, R. J., et al. (2002). Paternally inherited inactivating mutations of the GNAS1 gene in progressive osseous heteroplasia. *N. Engl. J. Med.* 346, 99–106. doi: 10.1056/NEJMoa011262

Shore, E. M., Xu, M., Feldman, G. J., Fenstermacher, D. A., Cho, T. J., Choi, I. H., et al. (2006). A recurrent mutation in the BMP type I receptor ACVR1 causes inherited and sporadic fibrodysplasia ossificans progressiva. *Nat. Genet.* 38, 525–527. doi: 10.1038/ng1783

Sinha, R., Dufour, S., Petersen, K. F., Lebon, V., Enoksson, S., Ma, Y. Z., et al. (2002). Assessment of skeletal muscle triglyceride content by (1)H nuclear magnetic resonance spectroscopy in lean and obese adolescents: relationships to insulin sensitivity, total body fat, and central adiposity. *Diabetes* 51, 1022–1027. doi: 10.2337/diabetes.51.4.1022

Sneddon, J. B., Borowiak, M., and Melton, D. A. (2012). Self-renewal of embryonic-stem-cell-derived progenitors by organ-matched mesenchyme. *Nature* 491, 765–768. doi: 10.1038/nature11463

Starkey, J. D., Yamamoto, M., Yamamoto, S., and Goldhamer, D. J. (2011). Skeletal muscle satellite cells are committed to myogenesis and do not spontaneously adopt nonmyogenic fates. *J. Histochem. Cytochem.* 59, 33–46. doi: 10.1369/jhc.2010.956995

Stoikovic, J. P., Bonfiglio, M., and Paul, W. D. (1955). Myositis ossificans complicating poliomyelitis. *Arch. Phys. Med. Rehabil.* 36, 236–243.

Sudo, K., Kanno, M., Miharada, K., Ogawa, S., Hiroyama, T., Saijo, K., et al. (2007). Mesenchymal progenitors able to differentiate into osteogenic, chondrogenic, and/or adipogenic cells in vitro are present in most primary fibroblast-like cell populations. *Stem Cells* 25, 1610–1617. doi: 10.1634/stemcells.2006-0504

Sugiyama, T., Kohara, H., Noda, M., and Nagasawa, T. (2006). Maintenance of the hematopoietic stem cell pool by CXCL12-CXCR4 chemokine signaling in bone marrow stromal cell niches. *Immunity* 25, 977–988. doi: 10.1016/j.immuni.2006.10.016

Swain, S. L., Weinberg, A. D., English, M., and Huston, G. (1990). IL-4 directs the development of Th2-like helper effectors. *J. Immunol.* 145, 3796–3806.

Tran, E., Chinnasamy, D., Yu, Z., Morgan, R. A., Lee, C. C., Restifo, N. P., et al. (2013). Immune targeting of fibroblast activation protein triggers recognition of multipotent bone marrow stromal cells and cachexia. *J. Exp. Med.* 210, 1125–1135. doi: 10.1084/jem.20130110

Uezumi, A., Fukada, S., Yamamoto, N., Takeda, S., and Tsuchida, K. (2010). Mesenchymal progenitors distinct from satellite cells contribute to ectopic fat cell formation in skeletal muscle. *Nat. Cell Biol.* 12, 143–152. doi: 10.1038/ncb2014

Uezumi, A., Ito, T., Morikawa, D., Shimizu, N., Yoneda, T., Segawa, M., et al. (2011). Fibrosis and adipogenesis originate from a common mesenchymal progenitor in skeletal muscle. *J. Cell Sci.* 124, 3654–3664. doi: 10.1242/jcs.086629

Urciuolo, A., Quarta, M., Morbidoni, V., Gattazzo, F., Molon, S., Grumati, P., et al. (2013). Collagen VI regulates satellite cell self-renewal and muscle regeneration. *Nat. Commun.* 4, 1964. doi: 10.1038/ncomms2964

Visser, M., Goodpaster, B. H., Kritchevsky, S. B., Newman, A. B., Nevitt, M., Rubin, S. M., et al. (2005). Muscle mass, muscle strength, and muscle fat infiltration as predictors of incident mobility limitations in well-functioning older persons. *J. Gerontol. A Biol. Sci. Med. Sci.* 60, 324–333. doi: 10.1093/gerona/60.3.324

Visser, M., Kritchevsky, S. B., Goodpaster, B. H., Newman, A. B., Nevitt, M., Stamm, E., et al. (2002). Leg muscle mass and composition in relation to lower extremity performance in men and women aged 70 to 79: the health, aging and body composition study. *J. Am. Geriatr. Soc.* 50, 897–904. doi: 10.1046/j.1532-5415.2002.50217.x

Voermans, N. C., Bonnemann, C. G., Huijing, P. A., Hamel, B. C., Van Kuppevelt, T. H., De Haan, A., et al. (2008). Clinical and molecular overlap between myopathies and inherited connective tissue diseases. *Neuromuscul. Disord.* 18, 843–856. doi: 10.1016/j.nmd.2008.05.017

Wada, M. R., Inagawa-Ogashiwa, M., Shimizu, S., Yasumoto, S., and Hashimoto, N. (2002). Generation of different fates from multipotent muscle stem cells. *Development* 129, 2987–2995.

Wirman, J. A. (1976). Nodular fasciitis, a lesion of myofibroblasts: an ultrastructural study. *Cancer* 38, 2378–2389.

Wood, W. M., Etemad, S., Yamamoto, M., and Goldhamer, D. J. (2013). MyoD-expressing progenitors are essential for skeletal myogenesis and satellite cell development. *Dev. Biol.* 384, 114–127. doi: 10.1016/j.ydbio.2013.09.012

Wosczyna, M. N., Biswas, A. A., Cogswell, C. A., and Goldhamer, D. J. (2012). Multipotent progenitors resident in the skeletal muscle interstitium exhibit robust BMP-dependent osteogenic activity and mediate heterotopic ossification. *J. Bone Miner. Res.* 27, 1004–1017. doi: 10.1002/jbmr.1562

Yagi, R., Suzuki, W., Seki, N., Kohyama, M., Inoue, T., Arai, T., et al. (2002). The IL-4 production capability of different strains of naive CD4(+) T cells controls the direction of the T(h) cell response. *Int. Immunol.* 14, 1–11. doi: 10.1093/intimm/14.1.1

Yin, H., Pasut, A., Soleimani, V. D., Bentzinger, C. F., Antoun, G., Thorn, S., et al. (2013). MicroRNA-133 controls brown adipose determination in skeletal muscle satellite cells by targeting Prdm16. *Cell Metab.* 17, 210–224. doi: 10.1016/j.cmet.2013.01.004

Yokota, T., Oritani, K., Takahashi, I., Ishikawa, J., Matsuyama, A., Ouchi, N., et al. (2000). Adiponectin, a new member of the family of soluble defense collagens, negatively regulates the growth of myelomonocytic progenitors and the functions of macrophages. *Blood* 96, 1723–1732.

Zimmers, T. A., Davies, M. V., Koniaris, L. G., Haynes, P., Esquela, A. F., Tomkinson, K. N., et al. (2002). Induction of cachexia in mice by systemically administered myostatin. *Science* 296, 1486–1488. doi: 10.1126/science.1069525

Zou, Y., Zhang, R. Z., Sabatelli, P., Chu, M. L., and Bonnemann, C. G. (2008). Muscle interstitial fibroblasts are the main source of collagen VI synthesis in skeletal muscle: implications for congenital muscular dystrophy types Ullrich and Bethlem. *J. Neuropathol. Exp. Neurol.* 67, 144–154. doi: 10.1097/nen.0b013e3181634ef7

17

Molecular and cell-based therapies for muscle degenerations: A road under construction

Emanuele Berardi[1,2], Daniela Annibali[3], Marco Cassano[2,4], Stefania Crippa[2,5] and Maurilio Sampaolesi[1,2,6]*

[1] Translational Cardiomyology Laboratory, Department of Development and Reproduction, KUL University of Leuven, Leuven, Belgium
[2] Interuniversity Institute of Myology, Italy
[3] Laboratory of Cell Metabolism and Proliferation, Vesalius Research Center, Vlaamse Institute voor Biotechnologie, Leuven, Belgium
[4] School of Life Sciences, Ecole Polytechnique Fédérale de Lausanne, Lausanne, Switzerland
[5] Department of Medicine, University of Lausanne Medical School, Lausanne, Switzerland
[6] Division of Human Anatomy, Department of Public Health, Experimental and Forensic Medicine, University of Pavia, Pavia, Italy

***Correspondence:**
Maurilio Sampaolesi, Translational Cardiomyology Laboratory, Department of Development and Reproduction, KUL University of Leuven, Stem Cell Research Institute, 49 Herestraat B-3000 Leuven, Belgium e-mail: maurilio.sampaolesi@med.kuleuven.be

Despite the advances achieved in understanding the molecular biology of muscle cells in the past decades, there is still need for effective treatments of muscular degeneration caused by muscular dystrophies and for counteracting the muscle wasting caused by cachexia or sarcopenia. The corticosteroid medications currently in use for dystrophic patients merely help to control the inflammatory state and only slightly delay the progression of the disease. Unfortunately, walkers and wheel chairs are the only options for such patients to maintain independence and walking capabilities until the respiratory muscles become weak and the mechanical ventilation is needed. On the other hand, myostatin inhibition, IL-6 antagonism and synthetic ghrelin administration are examples of promising treatments in cachexia animal models. In both dystrophies and cachectic syndrome the muscular degeneration is extremely relevant and the translational therapeutic attempts to find a possible cure are well defined. In particular, molecular-based therapies are common options to be explored in order to exploit beneficial treatments for cachexia, while gene/cell therapies are mostly used in the attempt to induce a substantial improvement of the dystrophic muscular phenotype. This review focuses on the description of the use of molecular administrations and gene/stem cell therapy to treat muscular degenerations. It reviews previous trials using cell delivery protocols in mice and patients starting with the use of donor myoblasts, outlining the likely causes for their poor results and briefly focusing on satellite cell studies that raise new hope. Then it proceeds to describe recently identified stem/progenitor cells, including pluripotent stem cells and in relationship to their ability to home within a dystrophic muscle and to differentiate into skeletal muscle cells. Different known features of various stem cells are compared in this perspective, and the few available examples of their use in animal models of muscular degeneration are reported. Since non coding RNAs, including microRNAs (miRNAs), are emerging as prominent players in the regulation of stem cell fates we also provides an outline of the role of microRNAs in the control of myogenic commitment. Finally, based on our current knowledge and the rapid advance in stem cell biology, a prediction of clinical translation for cell therapy protocols combined with molecular treatments is discussed.

Keywords: muscle degeneration, molecular treatments, stem cells, gene and cell therapies, cachexia

INTRODUCTION

Muscular dystrophies are heterogeneous genetic diseases caused by progressive degeneration of skeletal muscle fibers (Emery, 2002). Mutations in genes encoding for crucial skeletal muscle proteins located either at the plasma membrane (i.e., dystrophin-glycoprotein complex) or, less frequently, within internal cellular membranes are responsible for those disorders. The lack of those proteins increases the probability of damage during contraction and eventually leads to fiber degeneration (Blake et al., 2002; Gumerson and Michele, 2011). Despite the extensive literature reported on this topic, the molecular mechanisms responsible for the progressive muscular degeneration are not yet understood in detail. Physiologically, muscular fiber degeneration is counterbalanced by the regeneration of new fibers formed at the expense of resident myogenic cells and usually each degeneration process is followed by a new regenerative cycle. Skeletal muscle regeneration is mainly sustained by satellite cells (Mauro, 1961), local myogenic progenitors localized underneath the basal lamina of muscle fibers (Tedesco et al., 2010).

When it is damaged, a muscle undergoes a remodeling process and the resident myogenic cells differentiate into myofibroblasts to produce extracellular matrix (ECM), which is required for the adequate tissue repair. Following repeated cycles of degeneration/regeneration, such myofibroblasts accumulate in the muscle producing large amounts of ECM proteins and thus ultimately leading to fibrosis. However, after repeated injuries, the satellite cells in the muscles become exhausted, losing their regenerative capacity. In this view, the genetic manipulation of satellite cells could potentially guarantee an improved muscle regeneration and function. In this review we provide information about the different sources of myogenic stem cells, highlighting their common features and characteristics as well as their controversies in the therapeutic approaches. Advantage and disadvantage for autologous and heterologous cell therapy will be discussed, considering the different sources of myogenic stem cells.

Alterations in skeletal muscle homeostasis can result in either atrophy or hypo-metabolism. Etiologically, the molecular determinants responsible for such metabolic changes are known as common players in different muscular wasting diseases. In this view, they represent promising therapeutic targets common to the wide range of the known muscular diseases that could determine a strong impact in terms of prognosis, clinical setting and management. Pharmacotherapy still represents the most common strategy adopted to counteract muscle wasting for a large spectrum of muscular diseases such as cancer mediated cachexia, Rheumatoid Arthritis (RA) and sarcopenia, while muscular dystrophies can also be potentially treated by a multi-therapeutic approach based on gene/cell therapies combined with molecular treatments.

PATHOPHYSIOLOGY AND CLINICAL RELEVANCE OF MUSCLE WASTING

The state of progressive loss of muscular and fat mass known as cachexia syndrome is a condition associated with several chronic diseases such as AIDS, cancer, chronic obstructive lung disease, multiple sclerosis, congestive heart failure, sepsis, diabetes, RA and tuberculosis (Laviano et al., 2003; Fearon et al., 2011). According to its multifactorial and complex nature, as well as to both the pathophysiologic and epidemiologic features of its primary-related disease, such syndrome depicts a worse global epidemiologic scenario if compared with the other musculoskeletal disorders. The dramatic effects that cachexia have on the prognosis are well-known in clinical management of cancer diseases. According with the Global Burden Diseases (GBD) estimations, up to 50% of the oncologic patients suffer from cachexia and up to 80% of them show clear signs of cachexia in the late stages of cancer progression (Laviano et al., 2003; Fearon et al., 2011; Suzuki et al., 2013). Moreover, cancer-related cachexia counteracts the efficacy of radio- and chemotherapeutic treatments by increasing their side effects and decreasing patient's quality of life (Tisdale, 2002). Such complications are directly reliable for a high percentage of mortality in cancer patients, about 20–40%, accounting for more than 2 million of global premature deaths for year (Bruera, 1997).

Among the wide range of the muscular diseases that affect musculoskeletal system by hampering respiratory and locomotive functions, RA, dystrophies and cachexia syndrome represent the most common and are considered as a serious problem for human health. In 2010 GBD estimates showed that musculoskeletal disorders accounted for more than 150,000 deaths, with an increment of 121% between 1990 and 2010 (Lim et al., 2012).

The progressive skeletal muscle weakness and wasting are the main prognostic features exhibited by the heterogeneous musculoskeletal disorders (Leung and Wagner, 2013) (**Figure 1**). Although musculoskeletal diseases and cachexia have different origins (due to genetic alterations the first and to complications of several chronic diseases the latter), body weight loss, muscle atrophy, fatigue, weakness and loss of appetite are common clinical features observed in both. Nevertheless, while many autoimmune diseases ultimately result in a cachectic state of the patients, they are often associated with unintentional weight loss. RA is an autoimmune disease where the energetic balance is normal and eventually fat mass is increased. Thus, RA is a unique example of autoimmune disease in which cachexia is not associated with a general body-wide wasting and depends exclusively on the reduction in the muscle mass that might be responsible in lowering the average survival of the patients. Therefore, muscle wasting is the key player responsible for the induction of muscle atrophy in musculoskeletal disorders, which is triggered by catabolic events occurring into the affected skeletal muscle tissue (**Figure 1**). At the molecular level, this is due to an unbalance between protein anabolism and catabolism in favor of proteolysis of some crucial proteins occurring into the muscle fibers, mediated by the expression of muscle-specific ubiquitin ligase (E3 protein) atrogin1/MAFbx and MuRF1 (Bodine et al., 2001; Gomes et al., 2001).

Beyond the basic action of mechanic contraction, the skeletal muscle is a tissue involved in many other metabolic activities such as glucose, glycogen and lipid metabolism (Jensen and Richter, 2012), as well as endocrine (Pedersen and Febbraio, 2008) and immunogenic activities (Nielsen and Pedersen, 2008). Such biological heterogeneity reflects the histological diversity observed into the skeletal muscle tissue and, in turn, highlights multifaceted possibilities for the therapeutic interventions. It has been recently demonstrated that the microenvironment outside the myofibers can actively participate to the cancer-mediated muscle wasting. This happens when circulating tumor factors induce muscle damage by activation of both satellite and non-satellite muscle progenitor cells, and such process is followed by inhibition of their myogenic differentiation due to a persistent expression of Pax7 (He et al., 2013). On the other hand, the metabolic complexity of the skeletal muscle also renders it susceptible to environmental stimuli. Epidemiological studies show indeed the potential role of environmental and lifestyle factors (i.e., physical activity, diet and sun exposure) on the increasing susceptibility of the insurgence of sarcopenia (Scott et al., 2011). Overall, studies focused on the investigation of the general molecular mechanisms responsible for muscle wasting identified some potential therapeutic targets involved in the main catabolic pathways and that could be inhibited by pharmacological and by gene- or cell-therapy based approaches. Specifically, we will discuss pharmacological strategies aimed to counteract the effects of pro-inflammatory stimuli (i.e., TNF-α, IL-6) in cachexia, sarcopenia and RA, as well vector-based micro-dystrophin transfer, oligonucleotide-induced exon-skipping and cell therapy strategy based on the use of healthy myogenic cell precursors [i.e.,

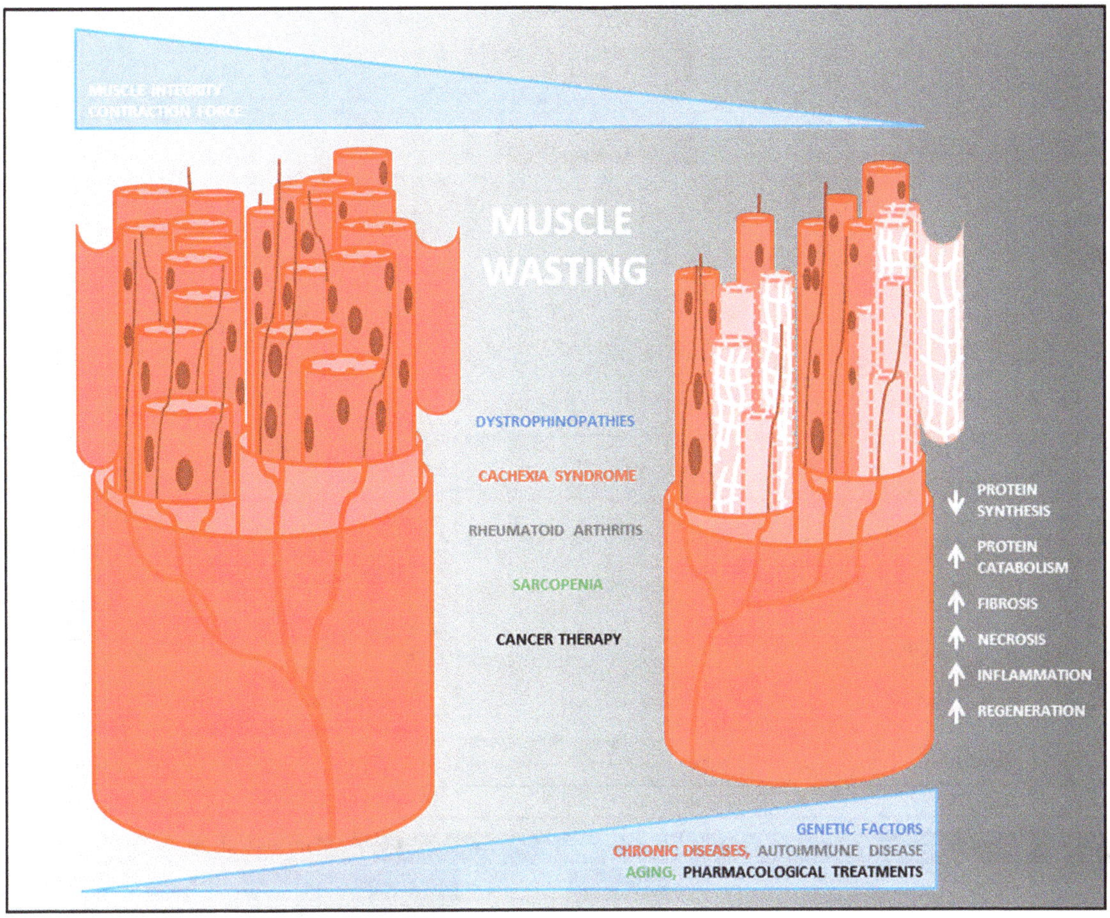

FIGURE 1 | Pathological heterogeneity of muscle wasting. Descriptive model of muscle degeneration in chronic diseases. Loss of muscle mass, decrease of fiber size and myonuclear content, reduction of contraction force and increase of fibrosis (white net) are common pathophysiological features of muscle degeneration mediated by changes into the biological process (white arrows) triggered by muscle diseases.

satellite cells, side population (SP), fibro-adipogenic progenitors (FAPs), mesoangioblasts, ES, and iPS cells] in dystrophinopathies (**Figure 2**).

PHARMACOLOGICAL APPROACH

Lack or alteration of structural proteins into the musculoskeletal system causes chronic inflammation. Although there are no specific cures for muscle wasting mediated by the different forms of muscular dystrophies and cachexia, pharmacotherapy has been the first historical clinical approach used to modulate the progression of such diseases (Abdel-Hamid and Clemens, 2012) by counteracting chronic inflammation (**Figure 2**). Because dystrophin plays a crucial role in preserving the integrity of the muscular membrane by permitting the anchorage of the dystrophin-associated protein complex, lack or genetic mutations of dystrophin result in a chronic influx of calcium into the myofibers, causing cellular death and inflammatory responses. In addition, fibrosis can occur to replace the damaged muscular fibers, causing muscle weakness (**Figure 1**). Pilot studies performed in patients affected by Duchenne/Becker and Limb-Girdle muscular dystrophies (DMD, BMD, and LGMD respectively) based on the administration of non-steroidal anti-inflammatory drugs, such as ibuprofen and nabumetone, or on the use of isosorbide dinitrate, a NO donor vasodilator, showed an improvement of the general pathophysiologic conditions (**Figure 2**). This effect was mediated by a deregulation of circulating level of TGF-β (D'Angelo et al., 2012), a known mediator of fibrosis in dystrophinopathies (Goldstein and Mcnally, 2010). Corticosteroids have been proposed as a pharmacological therapy for dystrophinopathies, in order to counteract muscle necrosis, inflammation and to reduce the muscle membrane susceptibility to damage (Abdel-Hamid and Clemens, 2012). In particular, prednisone (Griggs et al., 1991, 1993; Bonifati et al., 2000) and deflazacort (Bonifati et al., 2000) induce improvement and a long-term stabilization of the muscle strength (Bonifati et al., 2000), as well as a substantial reduction of weakness progression in DMD patients (Moxley et al., 2005). Moreover, since the elevation of cytosolic calcium concentration can trigger apoptotic and/or necrosis events in the dystrophic muscles, such physiological alteration represents another important glucocorticoid-based therapeutic target. Recently, studies in preclinical models proposed α-methylprednisolone, administrated either alone (Ruegg et al.,

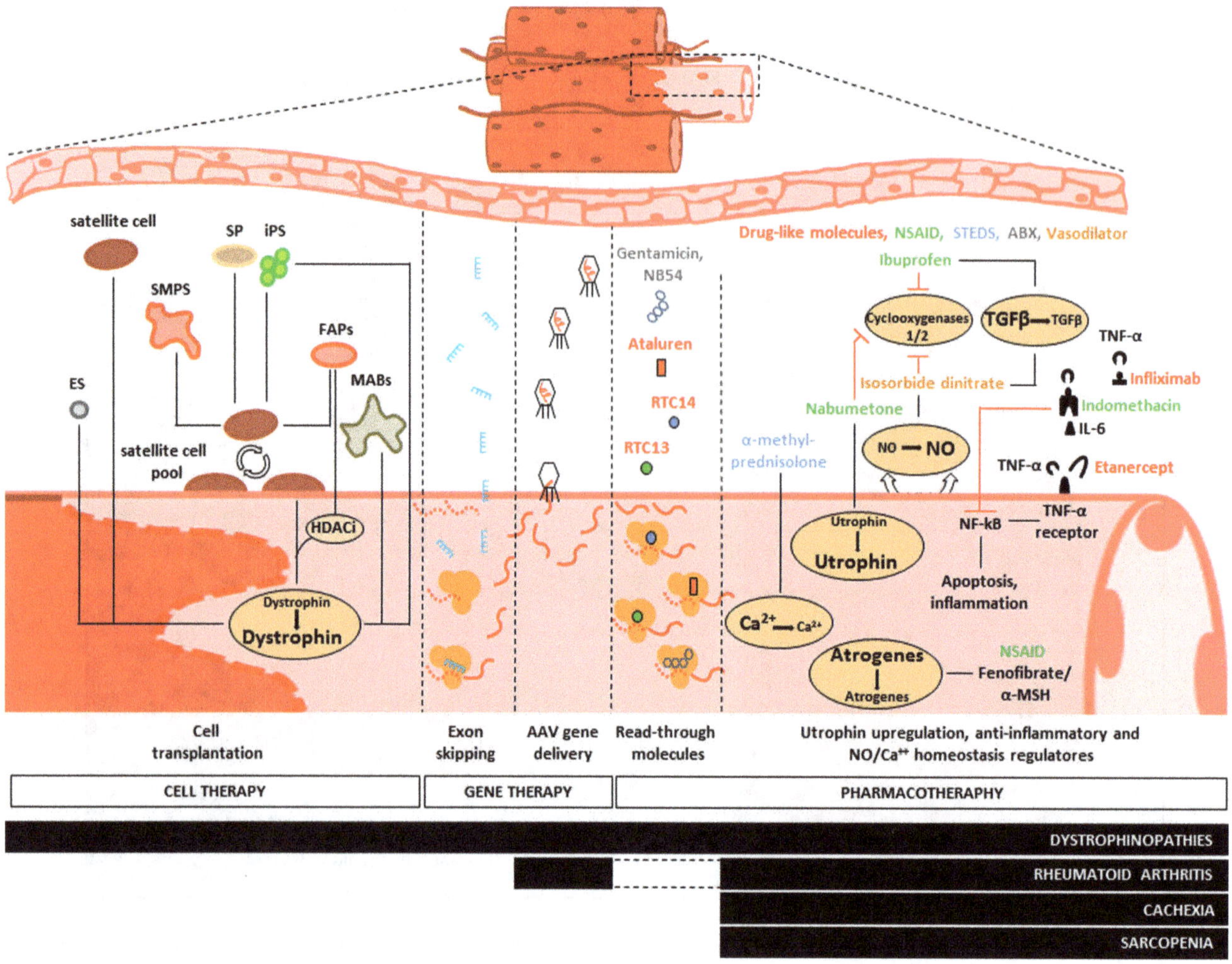

FIGURE 2 | Treatments of muscle diseases. Representative scheme of the main therapeutic approaches adopted to counteract muscle wasting. Pharmacotherapy aims to maintain muscle integrity by neutralization of ubiquitin-proteasome pathway (UPP), provoked by circulating pro-inflammatory stimuli (i.e., TNF-α and Il-6). Administration of non-steroidal anti-inflammatory drugs (NSAID, green), fenofibrates and steroids (STEDS, blue) reduces the overall expressions of atrogenes. It also stimulates utrophin expression and regulates the cytosolic homeostasis of NO and Ca^{++} elements, while drug-like molecules (red) and antibiotics (green) provide the "read-through" strategy to obtain semi-functional dystrophin protein. To date, NSAID and STEDS are the most diffused drugs to treat dystrophinopathies, cachexia syndrome, rheumatoid arthritis and sarcopenia. Gene therapy is experimentally adopted for dystrophinopathies treatments. Such method is based on the use of Adeno-associated viruses (AAV) and lentiviral vectors to mediate the delivery of micro-dystrophin or mini-utrophin and by use of exon skipping strategy to increase the endogenous expression of dystrophin (see text). Skeletal Myogenic Precursors (SMPS), Side Population (SP), Fibro-Adipogenic Progenitors (FAPs) and Mesoangioblasts (MABs) are potential candidates for cell therapeutic approaches of dystrophinopathies. MABs were recently enrolled in PhaseI/II clinical trial either for their ability to repopulate the endogenous pool of satellite cells and for their myogenic differentiation capability to produce dystrophin.

2002) or in combination with taurine (an aminoacid with antioxidant properties), as a candidate for pharmacological regulation of the cytosolic calcium flux in dystrophic muscles (Cozzoli et al., 2011).

The pharmacological efforts aiming to counteract muscle degeneration in dystrophinopathies mainly point to stabilize the muscular membrane integrity. This is the case of drugs designed to increase the expression level of native utrophin, as a mechanisms used to compensate for the dystrophin lack (Tinsley et al., 1998; Gilbert et al., 1999). Nabumetone is a novel promising small molecule with anti-inflammatory properties (COX1 and 2 inhibitor) that *in vitro* can activate the promoter of the A isoform of utrophin (Moorwood et al., 2011). The administration of aminoglycosides antibiotics (i.e., Gentamicin, NB54) (Barton-Davis et al., 1999; Politano et al., 2003; Nudelman et al., 2009) and read-through compounds such as RTC13, RTC14 (Kayali et al., 2012), or ataluren (PTC124) (Hamed, 2006; Finkel, 2010) has been proposed as a new strategy to induce ribosomal read-through of premature termination mutations, to obtain a full-length dystrophin protein in patients with DMD and Becker Muscular Dystrophy (BMD) (**Figure 2**). Various pro-inflammatory stimuli are involved in cancer mediated muscle wasting (Todorov et al., 1996; Suzuki et al., 2013), RA (Gomez-Sanmiguel et al., 2013) and sarcopenia (Malafarina et al., 2012).

In this case the pharmacological approaches used so far aim to counteract the biological activity of secreted pro-inflammatory mediators, such as interleukins (Il-1β, IL-6), interferon gamma (IFN-γ), tumor necrosis factor alpha (TNF-α) (Todorov et al., 1996) and proteolysis inducing factor (PIF) (Todorov et al., 1999). Unfortunately, anti-cytokine therapy aimed to block TNF-α by administration of Infliximab (monoclonal TNF antibody) or Etanercept (soluble TNF-α receptor) in cancer patients showed only poor ameliorative effects on cachexia pathophysiology (Gueta et al., 2010; Wu et al., 2013), whereas in patients with RA mediated cachexia, Etanercept was shown to reduced mortality (Morgan et al., 2014) and ameliorate the muscular function (Marcora et al., 2006). Indomethacin showed anti-cachectic effects in muscles from tumor bearing mice by inducing reduction in the levels of NF-kappaB, TNF-α and IL-6 (Zhou et al., 2003). Notably, dithiocarbamate inhibits IL-6 synthesis (Nai et al., 2007). Other treatments proposed in *in vivo* models in order to counteract oxidative and inflammatory burden in cancer-mediated muscle wasting are based on administration of glycine (Ham et al., 2013), simvastatin (Palus et al., 2013), eicosapentaenoic acid (Vaughan et al., 2012) and use of proteasome inhibitors to block the ubiquitin-proteasome pathway (Zhang et al., 2013). Such treatments efficiently counteract the expression of genes associated with the muscle protein breakdown observed in cancer cachexia (i.e., Atrogin-1 and MuRF-1) On the contrary, fenofibrate, a PPARα agonist (Castillero et al., 2011), and α-Melanocyte-stimulating hormone (α-MSH) (Gomez-Sanmiguel et al., 2013) ameliorate the pathophysiology of muscles in an adjuvant-induced arthritis rat model by preventing the overexpression of Atrogin-1, MuRF-1, and myostatin observed in RA (Castillero et al., 2011; Gomez-Sanmiguel et al., 2013). Pharmacological treatments used to counteract the progressive loss of skeletal muscle mass observed in sarcopenia are based on the administration of ghrelin, testosterone, Growth Hormone (GH), myostatin inhibitors and supplementation of vitamin D (Malafarina et al., 2012). Therapeutically, despite the efforts spent so far for sarcopenia treatment, only few results have been achieved in terms of increased muscle mass and strength, and decrease of muscle catabolism. Because vitamin D levels decrease with elderly, promising results were obtained in dietary supplementation of vitamin D in aged people, specially in muscle functional improvement (Malafarina et al., 2012).

GENE THERAPY

Gene replacement strategy was historically conceived to counteract the lack of dystrophin that affects DMD and BDM patients. Transgenic mice (mdx), dogs with X-linked muscular dystrophy (GRMD), and non-human primates (cynomolgus macaques) are examples of animal models extensively used to test novel methods for dystrophin gene delivery. Adeno-associated viruses (AAV) and lentivirus based vectors mediate efficient delivery of micro-dystrophin or mini-utrophin (Cerletti et al., 2003) and provide an alternative option for dystrophin-deficient mdx mouse (Gregorevic et al., 2004, 2006; Yoshimura et al., 2004; Liu et al., 2005; Rodino-Klapac et al., 2007), in non-human primate animal models (Rodino-Klapac et al., 2007) and Golden Retriever Muscular Dystrophy (GRMD) dogs (Cerletti et al., 2003; Sampaolesi et al., 2006; Koo et al., 2011). Nevertheless, all the dystrophin delivery methods proposed so far showed poor restoration of dystrophin within a small area of the skeletal muscle tissue targeted and only a partial improvement of the contractile properties (Rodino-Klapac et al., 2013) (**Figure 2**). Since deletions of single or multiple exons in the dystrophin gene are the most pathogenic mutations in DMD and BDM, antisense-mediated exon skipping (Douglas and Wood, 2013) represents a promising additional strategy adopted to increase dystrophin expression in DMD and BDM models, by restoring the genetic reading frame. Notably, this can be obtained either by single- (Van Deutekom et al., 2007; Jorgensen et al., 2009; Kinali et al., 2009) or multi-exon skipping approaches (Aartsma-Rus et al., 2006; McClorey et al., 2006; Goyenvalle et al., 2012). So far, many antisense oligonucleotide, such as morpholino oligomers (PMOs) and 2′O-methylphosphorothioate oligoribonucleotides (2′OMe), have been synthetized and successfully tested both *in vitro* and *in vivo* (Benedetti et al., 2013). They act by targeting of specific exons allowing their skipping during the splicing of dystrophin mRNA (**Figure 2**). In 2007 van Deutekom and colleagues tested the ability of PRO051oligonucleotide to restore dystrophin into the *tibialis anterior* of 4 DMD patients. In 2009 Kinali and colleagues treated the *extensor digitorum brevis* of 7 DMD patients with morpholino splice-switching oligonucleotide (AVI-4658) (Kinali et al., 2009). These trials provided evidences for local restoration of dystrophin in the treated muscles and for the safety of the protocols adopted (Van Deutekom et al., 2007).

However, because myoastin negatively affects skeletal muscle growth, AAV-mediated gene delivery of myostatin inhibitors (i.e., MRPO) has been proposed as a therapeutic strategy to maintain muscle mass (Morine et al., 2010) and improve the contraction force (Qiao et al., 2008) in both mdx mice (Qiao et al., 2008; Morine et al., 2010) and dogs (Qiao et al., 2009). Noteworthy, gene therapy AAV-mediated approaches were also used to restore structural, such as sarcoglycans (Sampaolesi et al., 2003), and non-structural proteins (Goonasekera et al., 2011). In fact, it is known that cytosolic alteration of Ca^{2+} flux observed in muscular dystrophies leads to sarcolemmal instability. This could be reduced by overexpressing the sarcoplasmic reticulum Ca^{2+} ATPase 1 (SERCA1) in both mdx and δ-sarcoglycan-null ($Sgcd^{-/-}$) mice (Goonasekera et al., 2011). Preclinical studies about the therapeutic applications of AAV-based gene delivery strategies were also performed to treat RA (Dai and Rabie, 2007). In particular, because the synovial lining is poorly transduced, subsynovial muscle tissues have been predominantly transfected in various RA models to investigate the effects of anti-inflammatory mediators such as IL-4 (Cottard et al., 2000) and IL-10 (Apparailly et al., 2002) either in mice (Cottard et al., 2000; Apparailly et al., 2002) as well as in human and murine synovial cell lines (Katakura et al., 2004).

CELL THERAPY

As already previously mentioned, satellite cells are quiescent unipotent stem cells, located underneath the basal lamina of adult skeletal muscle fibers (Mauro, 1961). They are formed during the second wave of embryonic myogenesis after which they exit the cell cycle, contributing significantly to the first post-natal muscle growth (Gros et al., 2005; Kassar-Duchossoy et al., 2005; Relaix et al., 2005). In case of muscle damages, satellite cells can re-enter the cell cycle resulting in an increasing number of myogenic progenitors able to fuse and form new muscle fibers (Huard et al., 2002; Jarvinen et al., 2005; Tedesco et al., 2010; Wang and Rudnicki, 2012). Given their natural commitment, it has been easy to consider satellite cells as the leading candidate for muscle regeneration in dystrophic mice (Partridge et al., 1989). In the case of transplantation of individual fibers into the *tibialis anterior* of irradiated mdx mice (specific treatment used to remove the existing population of satellite cells), satellite cells of the fiber donor expand, repopulating the endogenous pool, and differentiate into functional myofibers. $Pax7^+/CD34^+/GFP^+$ satellite cells, isolated from the diaphragm of Pax3::GFP mice, proved a good cellular model for the treatment of irradiated mdx muscles, resulting in restoration of the expression of dystrophin in many skeletal fibers and reconstitution of the pool of resident satellites cells (Montarras et al., 2005) (**Figure 2**). It has been shown by *in vivo* imaging that a single $CD34^+$/integrinα^+ satellite cell can replenish the resident satellite pool that, in the presence of further damage, can quickly re-enter a new wave of proliferation, generating new myofibers (Sacco et al., 2008). Fifty years of studies about the role of stem cells in skeletal muscle regeneration have identified a complex pattern of expression for surface markers within the endogenous pool of satellite cells (Rinaldi and Perlingeiro, 2013). Specific subpopulations of satellite cells positive for CD34 (Beauchamp et al., 2000), M-cadherin (Irintchev et al., 1994), $\alpha7\beta1$-integrin (Burkin and Kaufman, 1999; Gnocchi et al., 2009), syndecan-3/4 (Cornelison et al., 2004), the chemokine receptor CXCR4 (Ratajczak et al., 2003) barx2 (Meech et al., 2012) and caveolin-1 (Volonte et al., 2005) have been identified and investigated for their *in vitro*, as well as *in vivo*, therapeutic potential.

The intra-muscular injections, however, have revealed some significant problems. One of the major limitations on the use of satellite cells in therapy is the cell heterogeneity. The variable rate of satellite cell homing after transplantation of a single myofiber could be due to the cell heterogeneity and their functional niche of origin. Moreover, satellite cells show limited migratory ability, reduced myogenic capacity when expanded *in vitro*, while the host immune rejection still represents a major issue when satellite cells are used for transplantation (Mouly et al., 2005; Kuang and Rudnicki, 2008). Nevertheless, many others methodological issues concerning intramuscular cell transplantation of myogenic stem cells in the treatment of dystrophinopathies have been partially solved by a further basic knowledge of the skeletal muscle stem cell biology, achieved in the recent years by both clinical and pre-clinical data (Hill et al., 2006; Skuk and Tremblay, 2011; Brack and Rando, 2012).

Recently, interesting results have been obtained by the prospective isolation of skeletal myogenic precursors (SMPS) (**Figure 2**), a distinct population of the satellite cells pool, characterized by the expression of Cxcr4 and β1integrin and the absence of CD45, Sca1 and Mac1(Sherwood et al., 2004). Once injected into immunodeficient mdx muscles, SMPS contribute to the muscle regeneration (up to 94%) and to the satellite cell pool. SMPS need to be injected freshly isolated, in order to have beneficial effects. Although their migratory capacity remains limited to the areas surrounding the site of injection, the contractile force of limb muscles was significantly higher in the treated mice compared to controls (Cerletti et al., 2008).

A subpopulation of progenitors associated with skeletal muscles is a so-called SP. SP cells are defined as myogenic cells $SCA1^+/CD45^+$ (Polesskaya et al., 2003; Seale et al., 2004), unable to retain the intercalating Hoechst 33342 dyes (Gussoni et al., 1999; Polesskaya et al., 2003; Montanaro et al., 2004). When co-cultured with myoblasts, they can fuse to form myotubes *in vitro* and, if injected into the femoral artery in mice $mdx5^{cv}$ mice, can contribute up to 5–8% of the regenerated fibers (Perez et al., 2009). Remarkable results were obtained with the isolation of a rare subset (0.25%) of SP cells, identified as $SCA1^+/ABCG2^+/Syndecan4^+/Pax7^+$ cells (Tanaka et al., 2009). Once injected, those cells in muscle treated with 1.2% $BaCl_2$ regenerate up to 30% of the fibers and, surprisingly, reconstitute up to 75% of the endogenous satellite pool (Tanaka et al., 2009). However, the muscle damage induced by $BaCl_2$ is not a commonly accepted model of regeneration and this must be taken into account when interpreting these results. Another class of myogenic precursor was isolated from the population of endothelial cells in human muscles, through the prospective isolation of cells by FACS $CD56^+/CD34^+/CD144^+$ (Okada et al., 2008). These myoendothelial progenitors, after injection into injured muscle of SCID mice can be grafted into existing muscle fibers and form neofibres (Tamaki et al., 2002). A population of muscle-interstitial cells, referred to as FAPs, was recently identified. FAPs have been shown to mediate the beneficial effects of histone deacetylase inhibitors (HDACi) in mdx mice (Mozzetta et al., 2013). HDACi are known as promoters of endogenous regeneration and functional recovery of dystrophic muscles in the mdx mouse. They act by increasing the fiber size and reducing both the fibrosis and the fat deposition (Minetti et al., 2006). FAPs isolated from young dystrophic subjects show a minimal myogenic commitment that can be implemented by HDACi at the expense of their fibro-adipogenic potential. In addition, HDACi enhance FAPs ability to promote differentiation of adjacent satellite cells (**Figure 2**).

In recent years, a new class of stem cells associated with vasculatures and termed mesoangioblasts (MABs) have been studied as potential therapeutic protocols to threat dystrophic muscles (**Figure 2**). MABs were originally isolated from the dorsal aorta of the embryo (E9.5) (Minasi et al., 2002) and then from adult skeletal muscles in mice, dogs, and humans (Tonlorenzi et al., 2007; Quattrocelli et al., 2012). MABs are positive for several markers, including CD34, SMA, Pdgfrα, Pdgfrβ, Ng2, and AP, supporting the hypothesis that they belong to a subgroup of pericytes. MABs are multipotent as highlighted by their myogenic, osteogenic, chondrogenic, and adipogenic differentiation potential observed in quail-chick chimeras and *in vitro* and *in vivo* experiments in mouse model. After intra-arterial injection in dystrophic muscles of *Scga*-null mice or GRMD dogs, MABs are able to regenerate (up to 50%) muscle architecture, with functionality (Sampaolesi et al., 2006). Similarly, promised results were obtained with the transplantation of human MABs in immunodeficient mdx mice (Sampaolesi et al., 2003). Building up on those promising preclinical studies a Phase I/II clinical trial of donor mesoangioblasts transplantation from HLA-identical donors in 5 DMD patients is nearing completion (EudraCT Number: 2011-000176-33). However, due the ethical rules, several limitations are present in this first attempt of stem cell systemic delivery in DMD patients. First, the age of the patients and progression of the disease were advanced in the enrolled patients. Second, cell dose was quite low, from 1/5 to 1/10 of that administered to the GRMD dogs. Third, injections were limited into the femoral arteries, confining the cell treatment mainly to the muscles downstream the femoral artery. Taken into account those limitations, this trial will give important information about the safety of systemic delivery of adult stem cells in DMD patients. This trial will also hopefully answer some questions regarding the capability of donor stem cells to migrate towards regenerating muscles and undergo myogenic differentiation, by producing dystrophin.

In the last few years there is a growing interest about the therapeutic prospective offered by pluripotent stem cells. Embryonic Stem (ES) cells have been isolated from the inner cell mass of the blastocyst in mouse (Evans and Kaufman, 1981; Martin, 1981) and in human (Thomson et al., 1998), showing pluripotent features. Mouse and human ES cells can efficiently differentiate into the three germ layers, mesoderm, ectoderm and endoderm and a consistent number of studies showed their myogenic differentiation potential *in vitro* and *in vivo* (Bhagavati and Xu, 2005; Barberi et al., 2007; Filareto et al., 2012). The therapeutic use of ES cells has been strongly debated in the scientific community, mainly because of limitations linked to immune rejection and ethical concerns. However, part of these obstacles has been overcome by a pioneering study of Yamanaka in 2006 (Takahashi and Yamanaka, 2006) showing that induced pluripotent stem (iPS) cells can be generated from somatic cells. In addition, a very recent paper published in Nature showed that is possible to generate pluripotent stem cells by STAP, stimulus-triggered acquisition of pluripotency (Obokata et al., 2014). Basically, pluripotent conversion can be achieved by brief exposition of low-passage source cells to acidic conditions (pH 5.7). Since STAP reprogramming takes a very short period, only few days unlike transgene- or chemical-induced iPS cell conversion, it could be clinically relevant for tailoring cell therapy approaches.

To date, the use of iPS cells to potentially correct the dystrophic phenotype has been reported in several studies on murine (Mizuno et al., 2010; Darabi et al., 2011; Quattrocelli et al., 2011; Filareto et al., 2013) and human iPS cells (Darabi et al., 2012). Preclinical evidences show that myoblasts and mesenchymal cells derived from human ES and iPS can efficiently fuse with mature muscle fibers (Awaya et al., 2012; Goudenege et al., 2012) and improve the performances of engrafted muscles (Darabi et al., 2012) (**Figure 2**). After introduction of factor-based reprogramming, generation of iPS cells is feasible from any kind of cell population. However, iPS cells own an epigenetic memory, which results in a biased cell-differentiation towards the cell lineage of its source. This is probably due to the conservation of epigenetic marks, like CpG island (CGI) methylation and histone modifications, after reprogramming (Kim et al., 2010; Polo et al., 2010). Also iPS cells generated from murine skeletal MABs upon teratoma analysis differentiated with a significantly greater efficiency towards skeletal myocytes compared to fibroblast-reprogrammed iPS cells (Quattrocelli et al., 2011). If the myogenic memory will be confirmed in human iPS cells, this phenomenon could have an unpredicted impact for future translational studies.

Overall, these evidences suggest that, although all the efforts made so far on the use of pluripotent stem cells have been focalized on dystrophinopathies, the therapeutic use of iPS and ES cells could be an extraordinary potential clinical tool useful in the treatment of any skeletal muscle degenerations.

NEW CHALLENGE: MICRORNAS AND THEIR THERAPEUTIC POTENTIAL

In the early '90 a 22 nt non-coding transcript RNA, lin-4, was identified in *C. elegans*. It represses the expression of lin-14, a nuclear protein necessary for the larval development (Lee et al., 1993; Wightman et al., 1993). This discovery was the trigger for thousands of subsequent publications regarding the identification of micro inhibitory RNAs (miRNAs) in early embryogenesis (Berardi et al., 2012) and in cardiac and skeletal myogenesis (Ge and Chen, 2011; Crippa et al., 2012). miRNAs target sites in the 3′UTR of the mRNA leading to inhibition of mRNA translation and/or enhanced mRNA degradation, thus resulting in the decrease of protein expression levels (Djuranovic et al., 2011). miRNAs are generally transcribed by RNA polymerase II, as a primary miRNA (pri-miRNA)s then the RNase III enzyme Drosha removes hairpins from pri-miRNAs generating pre-miRNAs. In the cytoplasm, the pre-miRNA is further cleaved by the RNase III enzyme Dicer to generate mature miRNAs.

Highly expressed miRNAs in skeletal muscle tissue are termed myomiRs, which include miR-1, miR-133a, miR133-b, miR-206, miR-208, miR208b, miR486, and miR-499 (Van Rooij et al., 2008). They can be responsible for metabolic changes in skeletal muscle tissue (**Figure 3**). For example, muscular hypertrophy in Texel sheep is caused by a point mutation in the 3′UTR of myostatin RNA messengers, which creates a target site for miR-1 and miR-206 (Clop et al., 2006). Those miRNAs are abundant in the skeletal muscle tissue and can negatively affect myostatin expression, one of the most effective repressor of muscle growth. However, since another possible target for miR-206 is utrophin, a valuable substitute of dystrophin, several researchers believe that miR-206 can be responsible to sustain the dystrophic phenotype (Rosenberg et al., 2006). Transgenic mice for gain and loss of function studies are necessary to shed light in those controversies.

miRNA are also critic regulators for muscle wasting. In fact, possible targets for miR-486 are PTEN (phosphatase and tensin homolog) and FoxO1A, elements of the PI3/Akt pathway (Small et al., 2010) involved in muscle wasting and apoptosis. The activity of miR-486 results in muscle hypertrophy, since it leads to the activation of mTOR via PTEN inhibiton, and to the reduction of the ubiquitin ligase expression, which sustains atrophy in skeletal muscle tissue. The expression profiles of miR-486 strongly support its role in muscle homeostasis, since it is decreased in denervated muscles and almost absent in Duchenne patients (Eisenberg et al., 2007).

miR-1 and miR-133 modulate skeletal and cardiac muscle growth and differentiation. miR-1 promotes skeletal muscle

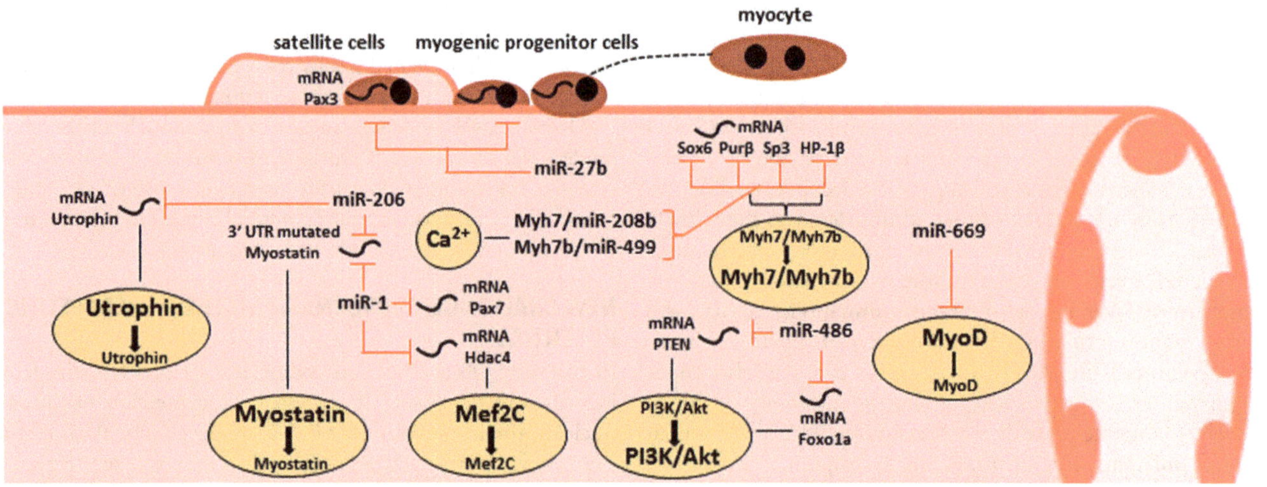

FIGURE 3 | The roles of miRNA in skeletal muscle homeostasis and dysfunction. Representative scheme of the main miRNAs involved in skeletal muscle functions. Specific miRNAs are critical for satellite cell activation (miR-27b) or for skeletal muscle differentiation (miR-1) and can be induced for therapeutic approaches. Other miRNAs are involved in muscle metabolism and they are able to modulate the AKT/PI3K pathway. Two miRNA families are peculiar for their opposite dual biological functions: miR-669 can inhibit MyoD causing a benefit in cardiac progenitors but in the same time reduced myogenic potential in skeletal muscle progenitors; miR-206 can induce hypertrophy by targeting mutated 3′UTR of myostatin messengers and can sustain dystrophic phenotype by inhibiting utrophin expression.

differentiation by targeting the histone deacetylase 4 (*HDAC4*), that in turn represses Mef2C, an essential muscle transcription factor. On the contrary, miR-133 stimulates myoblast proliferation by targeting *SRF* (Chen et al., 2006), while miR-206 promotes myoblast differentiation targeting the mRNA of *PolA1* (Kim et al., 2006), a DNA polymerase subunit. MyoD and myogenin can regulate miR-206 expression by binding specific elements in the enhancer region upstream miR-206 gene. Overexpression of miR-27b causes premature differentiation of muscle satellite cells: once myoblasts exit the cell cycle, miR-27 indeed targets the 3′UTR of *Pax3* (Crist et al., 2009).

The fine-tuned expression of miR-499 and miR-208b plays a role in the control of skeletal muscle performance. In response to calcium signaling, miR-208b and miR-499 indeed reinforce slow fiber conversion by inducing the expression of β -MHC and Myh7b (Van Rooij et al., 2009). They were considered initially as MyomiRs since they are encoded by introns of their host myosin genes Myh7 and Myh7b. These two intronic miRNAs target the transcriptional repressors of slow myofiber genes, including Sox6, Purβ, Sp3, and HP-1β, (Van Rooij et al., 2009). Recently, we have also identified a microRNA family, called miR-669, involved in the muscle lineage switch (Crippa et al., 2011) and used them as therapeutic molecules for long term treatments (Quattrocelli et al., 2013) in an animal model of limb girdle muscular dystrophy type 2E. Up to now, crucial information concerning the effects of miR669 in human setting for cardiac and skeletal muscle differentiation are still missing.

In summary, the possibility to increase the pool of myogenic stem cells, induce hypertrophy or reduce atrophic cell signaling by the perturbation of miRNA expression profiles offers a new opportunity to re-establish the skeletal muscle homeostasis lost in the wide range of muscolo-skeletal disorders (**Figure 3**).

CONCLUDING REMARKS

In conclusion, stem cell research will ride the third millennium as highlighted by the Nobel Prize in Physiology or Medicine 2012 jointly conferred to John Gurdon and Shinya Yamanaka for their discoveries on cell reprogramming which paved the way for new therapeutic horizons. We accumulated evidences that stem cell therapy with donor adult cells has produced dramatic amelioration in dystrophic mice and dogs. However, their finite lifespan and replication capacity, limit their therapeutic potential. Several types or subtypes of resident stem cells have been isolated and characterized from adult skeletal muscles. Further translational studies are still necessary to get molecular insights on how to improve the myogenic potential of each cell type. Moreover, it will be relevant to reveal the molecular and epigenetic signatures of myogenic progenitors to identify all molecules involved in the crosstalk among the different pools. In addition, several articles have documented a subset of miRNAs that regulate myogenic cell proliferation, differentiation, and contractility. The possibility to improve myogenic commitment of stem cells by targeting the expression of specific miRNAs is now implicated in several preclinical studies (Crippa et al., 2012). New insights into additional mechanism of post-transcriptional regulation mediated by lncRNAs are desirable since they have an impact on the distribution of miRNA molecules on their targets (Twayana et al., 2013). In the following years miRNA technologies combined to stem cell treatments will test novel therapeutic strategies for skeletal muscle disorders.

Muscle progenitors may be generated from patient iPS cells, genetically modified, systemically injected, then recruited to and integrated in the areas of damage. This would circumvent problems related to allogeneic transplantation and difficulty in obtaining autologous stem cells. The novel reprogramming methods

(Obokata et al., 2014) do not require nuclear transfer or genetic manipulation and thus they are more suitable for translational studies with clinical implications. It is interesting that such a great potential has not been explored yet in cachexia and sarcopenia, where it could be employed avoiding genetic manipulation. However, the enormous research impetus on regenerative medicine and stem cell-based therapy could strongly influence the future scientific directions. Emerging literature supports the hypothesis that downregulating myonuclear apoptosis might preserve muscle mass and function in the elderly. In principle, employing pharmacological or genetic interventions to target muscle protein turnover, autophagy and myogenic stem cell function may provide a more thorough protection against muscle aging and atrophy. These multi-therapeutic approaches will face several challenges, including the clear determination of feasible therapeutic windows for each specific intervention, especially if systemic delivery is employed. Nevertheless, pursuing this path is certainly worth in order to relieve the individual and societal burden associated with muscular degeneration.

ACKNOWLEDGMENTS

The Translational Cardiomyology laboratory is supported by CARE-MIFP7, Association française contre les myopathies (AFM), CARIPLO FOUNDATION, Fonds Wetenschappelijk Onderzoek (FWO), Geconcerteerde Onderzoeksacties (GOA), Interuniversity Attraction Poles (IUAP), and Onderzoekstoelagen (OT) grants. Emanuele Berardi is a postdoctoral fellow supported by FWO and Maurilio Sampaolesi is recipient of an Excellentiefinanciering KUL Project grant. The authors would like to thanks also Paolo Luban and Rondoufonds voor Duchenne Onderzoek for kind donations. We appreciated Jan Deprest, Paul Holvoet, Danny Huylebroeck, Arnold Luttun, Frank Luyten, Karin Sipido, Catherine Verfaillie, An Zwijsen for critical discussion. The authors would like to thank Christina Vochten and Vicky Raets for professional secretarial service.

REFERENCES

Aartsma-Rus, A., Kaman, W. E., Weij, R., Den Dunnen, J. T., Van Ommen, G. J., and Van Deutekom, J. C. (2006). Exploring the frontiers of therapeutic exon skipping for Duchenne muscular dystrophy by double targeting within one or multiple exons. *Mol. Ther.* 14, 401–407. doi: 10.1016/j.ymthe.2006.02.022

Abdel-Hamid, H., and Clemens, P. R. (2012). Pharmacological therapies for muscular dystrophies. *Curr. Opin. Neurol.* 25, 604–608. doi: 10.1097/Wco.0b013e328357f44c

Apparailly, F., Millet, V., Noel, D., Jacquet, C., Sany, J., and Jorgensen, C. (2002). Tetracycline-inducible interleukin-10 gene transfer mediated by an adeno-associated virus: application to experimental arthritis. *Hum. Gene Ther.* 13, 1179–1188. doi: 10.1089/104303402320138961

Awaya, T., Kato, T., Mizuno, Y., Chang, H., Niwa, A., Umeda, K., et al. (2012). Selective development of myogenic mesenchymal cells from human embryonic and induced pluripotent stem cells. *PLoS ONE* 7:e51638. doi: 10.1371/journal.pone.0051638

Barberi, T., Bradbury, M., Dincer, Z., Panagiotakos, G., Socci, N. D., and Studer, L. (2007). Derivation of engraftable skeletal myoblasts from human embryonic stem cells. *Nat. Med.* 13, 642–648. doi: 10.1038/nm1533

Barton-Davis, E. R., Cordier, L., Shoturma, D. I., Leland, S. E., and Sweeney, H. L. (1999). Aminoglycoside antibiotics restore dystrophin function to skeletal muscles of mdx mice. *J. Clin. Invest.* 104, 375–381. doi: 10.1172/JCI7866

Beauchamp, J. R., Heslop, L., Yu, D. S., Tajbakhsh, S., Kelly, R. G., Wernig, A., et al. (2000). Expression of CD34 and Myf5 defines the majority of quiescent adult skeletal muscle satellite cells. *J. Cell Biol.* 151, 1221–1234. doi: 10.1083/jcb.151.6.1221

Benedetti, S., Hoshiya, H., and Tedesco, F. S. (2013). Repair or replace? Exploiting novel gene and cell therapy strategies for muscular dystrophies. *FEBS J.* 280, 4263–4280. doi: 10.1111/febs.12178

Berardi, E., Pues, M., Thorrez, L., and Sampaolesi, M. (2012). miRNAs in ESC differentiation. *Am. J. Physiol. Heart Circ. Physiol.* 303, H931–H939. doi: 10.1152/ajpheart.00338.2012

Bhagavati, S., and Xu, W. (2005). Generation of skeletal muscle from transplanted embryonic stem cells in dystrophic mice. *Biochem. Biophys. Res. Commun.* 333, 644–649. doi: 10.1016/j.bbrc.2005.05.135

Blake, D. J., Weir, A., Newey, S. E., and Davies, K. E. (2002). Function and genetics of dystrophin and dystrophin-related proteins in muscle. *Physiol. Rev.* 82, 291–329. doi: 10.1152/physrev.00028.2001

Bodine, S. C., Latres, E., Baumhueter, S., Lai, V. K. M., Nunez, L., Clarke, B. A., et al. (2001). Identification of ubiquitin ligases required for skeletal muscle atrophy. *Science* 294, 1704–1708. doi: 10.1126/science.1065874

Bonifati, M. D., Ruzza, G., Bonometto, P., Berardinelli, A., Gorni, K., Orcesi, S., et al. (2000). A multicenter, double-blind, randomized trial of deflazacort versus prednisone in Duchenne muscular dystrophy. *Muscle Nerve* 23, 1344–1347. doi: 10.1002/1097-4598(200009)23:9<1344::AID-MUS4>3.0.CO;2-F

Brack, A. S., and Rando, T. A. (2012). Tissue-specific stem cells: lessons from the skeletal muscle satellite cell. *Cell Stem Cell* 10, 504–514. doi: 10.1016/j.stem.2012.04.001

Bruera, E. (1997). ABC of palliative care. Anorexia, cachexia, and nutrition. *BMJ* 315, 1219–1222. doi: 10.1136/bmj.315.7117.1219

Burkin, D. J., and Kaufman, S. J. (1999). The alpha7beta1 integrin in muscle development and disease. *Cell Tissue Res.* 296, 183–190. doi: 10.1007/s004410051279

Castillero, E., Nieto-Bona, M. P., Fernandez-Galaz, C., Martin, A. I., Lopez-Menduina, M., et al. (2011). Fenofibrate, a PPAR{alpha} agonist, decreases atrogenes and myostatin expression and improves arthritis-induced skeletal muscle atrophy. *Am. J. Physiol. Endocrinol. Metab.* 300, E790–E799. doi: 10.1152/ajpendo.00590.2010

Cerletti, M., Jurga, S., Witczak, C. A., Hirshman, M. F., Shadrach, J. L., Goodyear, L. J., et al. (2008). Highly efficient, functional engraftment of skeletal muscle stem cells in dystrophic muscles. *Cell* 134, 37–47. doi: 10.1016/j.cell.2008.05.049

Cerletti, M., Negri, T., Cozzi, F., Colpo, R., Andreetta, F., Croci, D., et al. (2003). Dystrophic phenotype of canine X-linked muscular dystrophy is mitigated by adenovirus-mediated utrophin gene transfer. *Gene Ther.* 10, 750–757. doi: 10.1038/sj.gt.3301941

Chen, J. F., Mandel, E. M., Thomson, J. M., Wu, Q. L., Callis, T. E., Hammond, S. M., et al. (2006). The role of microRNA-1 and microRNA-133 in skeletal muscle proliferation and differentiation. *Nat. Genet.* 38, 228–233. doi: 10.1038/Ng1725

Clop, A., Marcq, F., Takeda, H., Pirottin, D., Tordoir, X., Bibe, B., et al. (2006). A mutation creating a potential illegitimate microRNA target site in the myostatin gene affects muscularity in sheep. *Nat. Genet.* 38, 813–818. doi: 10.1038/ng1810

Cornelison, D. D., Wilcox-Adelman, S. A., Goetinck, P. F., Rauvala, H., Rapraeger, A. C., and Olwin, B. B. (2004). Essential and separable roles for Syndecan-3 and Syndecan-4 in skeletal muscle development and regeneration. *Genes Dev.* 18, 2231–2236. doi: 10.1101/gad.1214204

Cottard, V., Mulleman, D., Bouille, P., Mezzina, M., Boissier, M. C., and Bessis, N. (2000). Adeno-associated virus-mediated delivery of IL-4 prevents collagen-induced arthritis. *Gene Ther.* 7, 1930–1939. doi: 10.1038/sj.gt.3301324

Cozzoli, A., Rolland, J. F., Capogrosso, R. F., Sblendorio, V. T., Longo, V., Simonetti, S., et al. (2011). Evaluation of potential synergistic action of a combined treatment with alpha-methyl-prednisolone and taurine on the mdx mouse model of Duchenne muscular dystrophy. *Neuropathol. Appl. Neurobiol.* 37, 243–256. doi: 10.1111/j.1365-2990.2010.01106.x

Crippa, S., Cassano, M., Messina, G., Galli, D., Galvez, B. G., Curk, T., et al. (2011). miR669a and miR669q prevent skeletal muscle differentiation in postnatal cardiac progenitors. *J. Cell Biol.* 193, 1197–1212. doi: 10.1083/jcb.201011099

Crippa, S., Cassano, M., and Sampaolesi, M. (2012). Role of miRNAs in muscle stem cell biology: proliferation, differentiation and death. *Curr. Pharm. Des.* 18, 1718–1729. doi: 10.2174/138161212799859620

Crist, C. G., Montarras, D., Pallafacchina, G., Rocancourt, D., Cumano, A., Conway, S. J., et al. (2009). Muscle stem cell behavior is modified by microRNA-27 regulation of Pax3 expression. *Proc. Natl. Acad. Sci. U.S.A.* 106, 13383–13387. doi: 10.1073/pnas.0900210106

Dai, J., and Rabie, A. B. M. (2007). The use of recombinant adeno-associated virus for skeletal gene therapy. *Orthod. Craniofac. Res.* 10, 1–14. doi: 10.1111/j.1601-6343.2007.00381.x

D'Angelo, M. G., Gandossini, S., Martinelli Boneschi, F., Sciorati, C., Bonato, S., Brighina, E., et al. (2012). Nitric oxide donor and non steroidal anti inflammatory drugs as a therapy for muscular dystrophies: evidence from a safety study with pilot efficacy measures in adult dystrophic patients. *Pharmacol. Res* 65, 472–479. doi: 10.1016/j.phrs.2012.01.006

Darabi, R., Arpke, R. W., Irion, S., Dimos, J. T., Grskovic, M., Kyba, M., et al. (2012). Human ES- and iPS-derived myogenic progenitors restore DYSTROPHIN and improve contractility upon transplantation in dystrophic mice. *Cell Stem Cell* 10, 610–619. doi: 10.1016/j.stem.2012.02.015

Darabi, R., Pan, W., Bosnakovski, D., Baik, J., Kyba, M., and Perlingeiro, R. C. (2011). Functional myogenic engraftment from mouse iPS cells. *Stem Cell Rev.* 7, 948–957. doi: 10.1007/s12015-011-9258-2

Djuranovic, S., Nahvi, A., and Green, R. (2011). A parsimonious model for gene regulation by miRNAs. *Science* 331, 550–553. doi: 10.1126/science.1191138

Douglas, A. G., and Wood, M. J. (2013). Splicing therapy for neuromuscular disease. *Mol. Cell. Neurosci.* 56, 169–185. doi: 10.1016/j.mcn.2013.04.005

Eisenberg, I., Eran, A., Nishino, I., Moggio, M., Lamperti, C., Amato, A. A., et al. (2007). Distinctive patterns of microRNA expression in primary muscular disorders. *Proc. Natl. Acad. Sci. U.S.A.*104, 17016–17021. doi: 10.1073/pnas.0708115104

Emery, A. E. H. (2002). The muscular dystrophies. *Lancet* 359, 687–695. doi: 10.1016/S0140-6736(02)07815-7

Evans, M. J., and Kaufman, M. H. (1981). Establishment in culture of pluripotential cells from mouse embryos. *Nature* 292, 154–156. doi: 10.1038/292154a0

Fearon, K., Strasser, F., Anker, S. D., Bosaeus, I., Bruera, E., Fainsinger, R. L., et al. (2011). Definition and classification of cancer cachexia: an international consensus. *Lancet Oncol.* 12, 489–495. doi: 10.1016/S1470-2045(10)70218-7

Filareto, A., Darabi, R., and Perlingeiro, R. C. (2012). Engraftment of ES-derived myogenic progenitors in a severe mouse model of muscular dystrophy. *J. Stem Cell Res. Ther.* 10:S10-001. doi: 10.4172/2157-7633.S10-001

Filareto, A., Parker, S., Darabi, R., Borges, L., Iacovino, M., Schaaf, T., et al. (2013). An *ex vivo* gene therapy approach to treat muscular dystrophy using inducible pluripotent stem cells. *Nat. Commun.* 4, 1549. doi: 10.1038/ncomms2550

Finkel, R. S. (2010). Read-through strategies for suppression of nonsense mutations in Duchenne/Becker muscular dystrophy: aminoglycosides and ataluren (PTC124). *J. Child Neurol.* 25, 1158–1164. doi: 10.1177/0883073810371129

Ge, Y., and Chen, J. (2011). MicroRNAs in skeletal myogenesis. *Cell Cycle* 10, 441–448. doi: 10.4161/cc.10.3.14710

Gilbert, R., Nalbantoglu, J., Petrof, B. J., Ebihara, S., Guibinga, G. H., Tinsley, J. M., et al. (1999). Adenovirus-mediated utrophin gene transfer mitigates the dystrophic phenotype of mdx mouse muscles. *Hum. Gene Ther.* 10, 1299–1310. doi: 10.1089/10430349950017987

Gnocchi, V. F., White, R. B., Ono, Y., Ellis, J. A., and Zammit, P. S. (2009). Further characterisation of the molecular signature of quiescent and activated mouse muscle satellite cells. *PLoS ONE* 4:E5205. doi: 10.1371/Journal.Pone.0005205

Goldstein, J. A., and Mcnally, E. M. (2010). Mechanisms of muscle weakness in muscular dystrophy. *J. Gen. Physiol.* 136, 29–34. doi: 10.1085/jgp.201010436

Gomes, M. D., Lecker, S. H., Jagoe, R. T., Navon, A., and Goldberg, A. L. (2001). Atrogin-1, a muscle-specific F-box protein highly expressed during muscle atrophy. *Proc. Natl. Acad. Sci. U.S.A.* 98, 14440–14445. doi: 10.1073/pnas.251541198

Gomez-Sanmiguel, A. B., Martin, A. I., Nieto-Bona, M. P., Fernandez-Galaz, C., Lopez-Menduina, M., Villanua, M. A., et al. (2013). Systemic alpha-melanocyte-stimulating hormone administration decreases arthritis-induced anorexia and muscle wasting. *Am. J. Physiol. Regul. Integr. Comp. Physiol.* 304, R877–R886. doi: 10.1152/ajpregu.00447.2012

Goonasekera, S. A., Lam, C. K., Millay, D. P., Sargent, M. A., Hajjar, R. J., Kranias, E. G., et al. (2011). Mitigation of muscular dystrophy in mice by SERCA overexpression in skeletal muscle. *J. Clin. Invest.* 121, 1044–1052. doi: 10.1172/JCI43844

Goudenege, S., Lebel, C., Huot, N. B., Dufour, C., Fujii, I., Gekas, J., et al. (2012). Myoblasts derived from normal hESCs and dystrophic hiPSCs efficiently fuse with existing muscle fibers following transplantation. *Mol. Ther.* 20, 2153–2167. doi: 10.1038/mt.2012.188

Goyenvalle, A., Wright, J., Babbs, A., Wilkins, V., Garcia, L., and Davies, K. E. (2012). Engineering multiple U7snRNA constructs to induce single and multiexon-skipping for Duchenne muscular dystrophy. *Mol. Ther.* 20, 1212–1221. doi: 10.1038/mt.2012.26

Gregorevic, P., Allen, J. M., Minami, E., Blankinship, M. J., Haraguchi, M., Meuse, L., et al. (2006). rAAV6-microdystrophin preserves muscle function and extends lifespan in severely dystrophic mice. *Nat. Med.* 12, 787–789. doi: 10.1038/nm1439

Gregorevic, P., Blankinship, M. J., Allen, J. M., Crawford, R. W., Meuse, L., Miller, D. G., et al. (2004). Systemic delivery of genes to striated muscles using adeno-associated viral vectors. *Nat. Med.* 10, 828–834. doi: 10.1038/nm1085

Griggs, R. C., Moxley, R. T. 3rd., Mendell, J. R., Fenichel, G. M., Brooke, M. H., Pestronk, A., et al. (1991). Prednisone in Duchenne dystrophy. A randomized, controlled trial defining the time course and dose response. Clinical Investigation of Duchenne Dystrophy Group. *Arch. Neurol.* 48, 383–388. doi: 10.1001/archneur.1991.00530160047012

Griggs, R. C., Moxley, R. T. 3rd., Mendell, J. R., Fenichel, G. M., Brooke, M. H., Pestronk, A., et al. (1993). Duchenne dystrophy: randomized, controlled trial of prednisone (18 months) and azathioprine (12 months). *Neurology* 43, 520–527. doi: 10.1212/WNL.43.3_Part_1.520

Gros, J., Manceau, M., Thome, V., and Marcelle, C. (2005). A common somitic origin for embryonic muscle progenitors and satellite cells. *Nature* 435, 954–958. doi: 10.1038/Nature03572

Gueta, I., Altman, A., and Shoenfeld, Y. (2010). [The effect of blocking TNF-alpha in patients with cancer-related cachexia and anorexia]. *Harefuah* 149, 512–514, 550, 551.

Gumerson, J. D., and Michele, D. E. (2011). The dystrophin-glycoprotein complex in the prevention of muscle damage. *J. Biomed. Biotechnol.* 2011:210797. doi: 10.1155/2011/210797

Gussoni, E., Soneoka, Y., Strickland, C. D., Buzney, E. A., Khan, M. K., Flint, A. F., et al. (1999). Dystrophin expression in the mdx mouse restored by stem cell transplantation. *Nature* 401, 390–394. doi: 10.1038/43922

Ham, D. J., Murphy, K. T., Chee, A., Lynch, G. S., and Koopman, R. (2013). Glycine administration attenuates skeletal muscle wasting in a mouse model of cancer cachexia. *Clin. Nutr.* doi: 10.1016/j.clnu.2013.06.013. [Epub ahead of print].

Hamed, S. A. (2006). Drug evaluation: PTC-124–a potential treatment of cystic fibrosis and Duchenne muscular dystrophy. *IDrugs* 9, 783–789.

He, W. A., Berardi, E., Cardillo, V. M., Acharyya, S., Aulino, P., Thomas-Ahner, J., et al. (2013). NF-κB-mediated Pax7 dysregulation in the muscle microenvironment promotes cancer cachexia. *J. Clin. Invest.* 123, 4821–4835. doi: 10.1172/JCI68523

Hill, E., Boontheekul, T., and Mooney, D. J. (2006). Designing scaffolds to enhance transplanted myoblast survival and migration. *Tissue Eng.* 12, 1295–1304. doi: 10.1089/ten.2006.12.1295

Huard, J., Li, Y., and Fu, F. H. (2002). Current concepts review - Muscle injuries and repair: current trends in research. *J. Bone Joint Surg. Am.* 84A, 822–832.

Irintchev, A., Zeschnigk, M., Starzinski-Powitz, A., and Wernig, A. (1994). Expression pattern of M-cadherin in normal, denervated, and regenerating mouse muscles. *Dev. Dyn.* 199, 326–337. doi: 10.1002/aja.1001990407

Jarvinen, T. A. H. J., Jarvinen, T. L. N., Kaariainen, M., Kalimo, A., and Jarvinen, M. (2005). Muscle injuries - Biology and treatment. *Am. J. Sports Med.* 33, 745–764. doi: 10.1177/0363546505274714

Jensen, T. E., and Richter, E. A. (2012). Regulation of glucose and glycogen metabolism during and after exercise. *J. Physiol.* 590, 1069–1076. doi: 10.1113/jphysiol.2011.224972

Jorgensen, L. H., Larochelle, N., Orlopp, K., Dunant, P., Dudley, R. W., Stucka, R., et al. (2009). Efficient and fast functional screening of microdystrophin constructs *in vivo* and *in vitro* for therapy of duchenne muscular dystrophy. *Hum. Gene Ther.* 20, 641–650. doi: 10.1089/hum.2008.162

Kassar-Duchossoy, L., Giacone, E., Gayraud-Morel, B., Jory, A., Gomes, D., and Tajbakhsh, S. (2005). Pax3/Pax7 mark a novel population of primitive myogenic cells during development. *Genes Dev.* 19, 1426–1431. doi: 10.1101/Gad.345505

Katakura, S., Jennings, K., Watanabe, S., Adachi, E., Thornton, S., Gao, G. P., et al. (2004). Recombinant adeno-associated virus preferentially transduces human, compared to mouse, synovium: implications for arthritis therapy. *Mod. Rheumatol.* 14, 18–24. doi: 10.1007/s10165-003-0260-7

Kayali, R., Ku, J. M., Khitrov, G., Jung, M. E., Prikhodko, O., and Bertoni, C. (2012). Read-through compound 13 restores dystrophin expression and improves muscle function in the mdx mouse model for Duchenne muscular dystrophy. *Hum. Mol. Genet.* 21, 4007–4020. doi: 10.1093/hmg/dds223

Kim, H. K., Lee, Y. S., Sivaprasad, U., Malhotra, A., and Dutta, A. (2006). Muscle-specific microRNA miR-206 promotes muscle differentiation. *J. Cell Biol.* 174, 677–687. doi: 10.1083/jcb.200603008

Kim, K., Doi, A., Wen, B., Ng, K., Zhao, R., Cahan, P., et al. (2010). Epigenetic memory in induced pluripotent stem cells. *Nature* 467, 285–290. doi: 10.1038/nature09342

Kinali, M., Arechavala-Gomeza, V., Feng, L., Cirak, S., Hunt, D., Adkin, C., et al. (2009). Local restoration of dystrophin expression with the morpholino oligomer AVI-4658 in Duchenne muscular dystrophy: a single-blind, placebo-controlled, dose-escalation, proof-of-concept study. *Lancet Neurol.* 8, 918–928. doi: 10.1016/S1474-4422(09)70211-X

Koo, T., Okada, T., Athanasopoulos, T., Foster, H., Takeda, S., and Dickson, G. (2011). Long-term functional adeno-associated virus-microdystrophin expression in the dystrophic CXMDj dog. *J. gene Med.* 13, 497–506. doi: 10.1002/jgm.1602

Kuang, S., and Rudnicki, M. A. (2008). The emerging biology of satellite cells and their therapeutic potential. *Trends Mol. Med.* 14, 82–91. doi: 10.1016/j.molmed.2007.12.004

Laviano, A., Meguid, M. M., and Rossi-Fanelli, F. (2003). Cancer anorexia: clinical implications, pathogenesis, and therapeutic strategies. *Lancet Oncol.* 4, 686–694. doi: 10.1016/S1470-2045(03)01247-6

Lee, R. C., Feinbaum, R. L., and Ambros, V. (1993). The c-elegans heterochronic gene lin-4 encodes small rnas with antisense complementarity to lin-14. *Cell* 75, 843–854. doi: 10.1016/0092-8674(93)90529-Y

Leung, D. G., and Wagner, K. R. (2013). Therapeutic advances in muscular dystrophy. *Ann. Neurol.* 74, 404–411. doi: 10.1002/Ana.23989

Lim, S. S., Vos, T., Flaxman, A. D., Danaei, G., Shibuya, K., Adair-Rohani, H., et al. (2012). A comparative risk assessment of burden of disease and injury attributable to 67 risk factors and risk factor clusters in 21 regions, 1990–2010: a systematic analysis for the Global Burden of Disease Study 2010. *Lancet* 380, 2224–2260. doi: 10.1016/S0140-6736(12)61766-8

Liu, M., Yue, Y., Harper, S. Q., Grange, R. W., Chamberlain, J. S., and Duan, D. (2005). Adeno-associated virus-mediated microdystrophin expression protects young mdx muscle from contraction-induced injury. *Mol. Ther.* 11, 245–256. doi: 10.1016/j.ymthe.2004.09.013

Malafarina, V., Uriz-Otano, F., Iniesta, R., and Gil-Guerrero, L. (2012). Sarcopenia in the elderly: diagnosis, physiopathology and treatment. *Maturitas* 71, 109–114. doi: 10.1016/j.maturitas.2011.11.012

Marcora, S. M., Chester, K. R., Mittal, G., Lemmey, A. B., and Maddison, P. J. (2006). Randomized phase 2 trial of anti-tumor necrosis factor therapy for cachexia in patients with early rheumatoid arthritis. *Am. J. Clin. Nutr.* 84, 1463–1472.

Martin, G. R. (1981). Isolation of a pluripotent cell line from early mouse embryos cultured in medium conditioned by teratocarcinoma stem cells. *Proc. Natl. Acad. Sci. U.S.A.* 78, 7634–7638. doi: 10.1073/pnas.78.12.7634

Mauro, A. (1961). Satellite cell of skeletal muscle fibers. *J. Biophys. Biochem. Cytol.* 9, 493–495. doi: 10.1083/jcb.9.2.493

McClorey, G., Moulton, H. M., Iversen, P. L., Fletcher, S., and Wilton, S. D. (2006). Antisense oligonucleotide-induced exon skipping restores dystrophin expression *in vitro* in a canine model of DMD. *Gene Ther.* 13, 1373–1381. doi: 10.1038/sj.gt.3302800

Meech, R., Gonzalez, K. N., Barro, M., Gromova, A., Zhuang, L., Hulin, J. A., et al. (2012). Barx2 is expressed in satellite cells and is required for normal muscle growth and regeneration. *Stem Cells* 30, 253–265. doi: 10.1002/stem.777

Minasi, M. G., Riminucci, M., De Angelis, L., Borello, U., Berarducci, B., Innocenzi, A., et al. (2002). The meso-angioblast: a multipotent, self-renewing cell that originates from the dorsal aorta and differentiates into most mesodermal tissues. *Development* 129, 2773–2784.

Minetti, G. C., Colussi, C., Adami, R., Serra, C., Mozzetta, C., Parente, V., et al. (2006). Functional and morphological recovery of dystrophic muscles in mice treated with deacetylase inhibitors. *Nat. Med.* 12, 1147–1150. doi: 10.1038/Nm1479

Mizuno, Y., Chang, H., Umeda, K., Niwa, A., Iwasa, T., Awaya, T., et al. (2010). Generation of skeletal muscle stem/progenitor cells from murine induced pluripotent stem cells. *FASEB J.* 24, 2245–2253. doi: 10.1096/fj.09-137174

Montanaro, F., Liadaki, K., Schienda, J., Flint, A., Gussoni, E., and Kunkel, L. M. (2004). Demystifying SP cell purification: viability, yield, and phenotype are defined by isolation parameters. *Exp. Cell Res.* 298, 144–154. doi: 10.1016/j.yexcr.2004.04.010

Montarras, D., Morgan, J., Collins, C., Relaix, F., Zaffran, S., Cumano, A., et al. (2005). Direct isolation of satellite cells for skeletal muscle regeneration. *Science* 309, 2064–2067. doi: 10.1126/science.1114758

Moorwood, C., Lozynska, O., Suri, N., Napper, A. D., Diamond, S. L., and Khurana, T. S. (2011). Drug discovery for Duchenne muscular dystrophy via utrophin promoter activation screening. *PLoS ONE* 6:e26169. doi: 10.1371/journal.pone.0026169

Morgan, C. L., Emery, P., Porter, D., Reynolds, A., Young, A., Boyd, H., et al. (2014). Treatment of rheumatoid arthritis with etanercept with reference to disease-modifying anti-rheumatic drugs: long-term safety and survival using prospective, observational data. *Rheumatology* 53, 186–194. doi: 10.1093/rheumatology/ket333

Morine, K. J., Bish, L. T., Pendrak, K., Sleeper, M. M., Barton, E. R., and Sweeney, H. L. (2010). Systemic myostatin inhibition via liver-targeted gene transfer in normal and dystrophic mice. *PLoS ONE* 5:e9176. doi: 10.1371/journal.pone.0009176

Mouly, V., Aamiri, A., Perie, S., Mamchaoui, K., Barani, A., Bigot, A., et al. (2005). Myoblast transfer therapy: is there any light at the end of the tunnel? *Acta Myol.* 24, 128–133.

Moxley, R. T. 3rd., Ashwal, S., Pandya, S., Connolly, A., Florence, J., Mathews, K., et al. (2005). Practice parameter: corticosteroid treatment of Duchenne dystrophy: report of the Quality Standards Subcommittee of the American Academy of Neurology and the Practice Committee of the Child Neurology Society. *Neurology* 64, 13–20. doi: 10.1212/01.WNL.0000148485.00049.B7

Mozzetta, C., Consalvi, S., Saccone, V., Tierney, M., Diamantini, A., Mitchell, K. J., et al. (2013). Fibroadipogenic progenitors mediate the ability of HDAC inhibitors to promote regeneration in dystrophic muscles of young, but not old Mdx mice. *EMBO Mol. Med.* 5, 626–639. doi: 10.1002/emmm.201202096

Nai, Y. J., Jiang, Z. W., Wang, Z. M., Li, N., and Li, J. S. (2007). Prevention of cancer cachexia by pyrrolidine dithiocarbamate (PDTC) in colon 26 tumor-bearing mice. *JPEN* 31, 18–25. doi: 10.1177/014860710703100118

Nielsen, S., and Pedersen, B. K. (2008). Skeletal muscle as an immunogenic organ. *Curr. Opin. Pharmacol.* 8, 346–351. doi: 10.1016/j.coph.2008.02.005

Nudelman, I., Rebibo-Sabbah, A., Cherniavsky, M., Belakhov, V., Hainrichson, M., Chen, F., et al. (2009). Development of novel aminoglycoside (NB54) with reduced toxicity and enhanced suppression of disease-causing premature stop mutations. *J. Med. Chem.* 52, 2836–2845. doi: 10.1021/jm801640k

Obokata, H., Wakayama, T., Sasai, Y., Kojima, K., Vacanti, M. P., Niwa, H., et al. (2014). Stimulus-triggered fate conversion of somatic cells into pluripotency. *Nature* 505, 641–647. doi: 10.1038/nature12968

Okada, M., Payne, T. R., Zheng, B., Oshima, H., Momoi, N., Tobita, K., et al. (2008). Myogenic endothelial cells purified from human skeletal muscle improve cardiac function after transplantation into infarcted myocardium. *J. Am. Coll. Cardiol.* 52, 1869–1880. doi: 10.1016/j.jacc.2008.07.064

Palus, S., Von Haehling, S., Flach, V. C., Tschirner, A., Doehner, W., Anker, S. D., et al. (2013). Simvastatin reduces wasting and improves cardiac function as well as outcome in experimental cancer cachexia. *Int. J. Cardiol.* 168, 3412–3418. doi: 10.1016/j.ijcard.2013.04.150

Partridge, T. A., Morgan, J. E., Coulton, G. R., Hoffman, E. P., and Kunkel, L. M. (1989). Conversion of mdx myofibres from dystrophin-negative to -positive by injection of normal myoblasts. *Nature* 337, 176–179. doi: 10.1038/337176a0

Pedersen, B. K., and Febbraio, M. A. (2008). Muscle as an endocrine organ: focus on muscle-derived interleukin-6. *Physiol. Rev.* 88, 1379–1406. doi: 10.1152/physrev.90100.2007

Perez, A. L., Bachrach, E., Illigens, B. M. W., Jun, S. J., Bagden, E., Steffen, L., et al. (2009). Cxcr4 enhances engraftment of muscle progenitor cells. *Muscle Nerve* 40, 562–572. doi: 10.1002/Mus.21317

Polesskaya, A., Seale, P., and Rudnicki, M. A. (2003). Wnt signaling induces the myogenic specification of resident CD45(+) adult stem cells during muscle regeneration. *Cell* 113, 841–852. doi: 10.1016/S0092-8674(03)00437-9

Politano, L., Nigro, G., Nigro, V., Piluso, G., Papparella, S., Paciello, O., et al. (2003). Gentamicin administration in Duchenne patients with premature stop codon. Preliminary results. *Acta Myol.* 22, 15–21.

Polo, J. M., Liu, S., Figueroa, M. E., Kulalert, W., Eminli, S., Tan, K. Y., et al. (2010). Cell type of origin influences the molecular and functional properties of mouse induced pluripotent stem cells. *Nat. Biotechnol.* 28, 848–855. doi: 10.1038/nbt.1667

Qiao, C., Li, J., Jiang, J., Zhu, X., Wang, B., and Xiao, X. (2008). Myostatin propeptide gene delivery by adeno-associated virus serotype 8 vectors enhances muscle growth and ameliorates dystrophic phenotypes in mdx mice. *Hum. Gene Ther.* 19, 241–254. doi: 10.1089/hum.2007.159

Qiao, C., Li, J., Zheng, H., Bogan, J., Yuan, Z., Zhang, C., et al. (2009). Hydrodynamic limb vein injection of adeno-associated virus serotype 8 vector carrying canine myostatin propeptide gene into normal dogs enhances muscle growth. *Hum. Gene Ther.* 20, 1–10. doi: 10.1089/hum.2008.135

Quattrocelli, M., Crippa, S., Montecchiani, C., Camps, J., Cornaglia, A. I., Boldrin, L., et al. (2013). Long-term miR-669a therapy alleviates chronic dilated cardiomyopathy in dystrophic mice. *J. Am. Heart Assoc.* 2:e000284. doi: 10.1161/JAHA.113.000284

Quattrocelli, M., Palazzolo, G., Floris, G., Schöffski, P., Anastasia, L., Orlacchio, A., et al. (2011). Intrinsic cell memory reinforces myogenic commitment of pericyte-derived iPSCs. *J. Pathol.* 223, 593–603. doi: 10.1002/path.2845

Quattrocelli, M., Palazzolo, G., Perini, I., Crippa, S., Cassano, M., and Sampaolesi, M. (2012). Mouse and human mesoangioblasts: isolation and characterization from adult skeletal muscles. *Methods Mol. Biol.* 798, 65–76. doi: 10.1007/978-1-61779-343-1_4

Ratajczak, M. Z., Majka, M., Kucia, M., Drukala, J., Pietrzkowski, Z., Peiper, S., et al. (2003). Expression of functional CXCR4 by muscle satellite cells and secretion of SDF-1 by muscle-derived fibroblasts is associated with the presence of both muscle progenitors in bone marrow and hematopoietic stem/progenitor cells in muscles. *Stem Cells* 21, 363–371. doi: 10.1634/stemcells.21-3-363

Relaix, F., Rocancourt, D., Mansouri, A., and Buckingham, M. (2005). A Pax3/Pax7-dependent population of skeletal muscle progenitor cells. *Nature* 435, 948–953. doi: 10.1038/Nature03594

Rinaldi, F., and Perlingeiro, R. C. (2013). Stem cells for skeletal muscle regeneration: therapeutic potential and roadblocks. *Transl. Res.* doi: 10.1016/j.trsl.2013.11.006. [Epub ahead of print].

Rodino-Klapac, L. R., Janssen, P. M., Montgomery, C. L., Coley, B. D., Chicoine, L. G., Clark, K. R., et al. (2007). A translational approach for limb vascular delivery of the micro-dystrophin gene without high volume or high pressure for treatment of Duchenne muscular dystrophy. *J. Trans. Med.* 5:45. doi: 10.1186/1479-5876-5-45

Rodino-Klapac, L. R., Janssen, P. M., Shontz, K. M., Canan, B., Montgomery, C. L., Griffin, D., et al. (2013). Micro-dystrophin and follistatin co-delivery restores muscle function in aged DMD model. *Hum. Mol. Genet.* 22, 4929–4937. doi: 10.1093/hmg/ddt342

Rosenberg, M. I., Georges, S. A., Asawachaicharn, A., Analau, E., and Tapscott, S. J. (2006). MyoD inhibits Fstl1 and Utrn expression by inducing transcription of miR-206. *J. Cell Biol.* 175, 77–85. doi: 10.1083/jcb.200603039

Ruegg, U. T., Nicolas-Metral, V., Challet, C., Bernard-Helary, K., Dorchies, O. M., Wagner, S., et al. (2002). Pharmacological control of cellular calcium handling in dystrophic skeletal muscle. *Neuromuscul. Disord.* 12(Suppl. 1), S155–S161. doi: 10.1016/S0960-8966(02)00095-0

Sacco, A., Doyonnas, R., Kraft, P., Vitorovic, S., and Blau, H. M. (2008). Self-renewal and expansion of single transplanted muscle stem cells. *Nature* 456, 502–506. doi: 10.1038/Nature07384

Sampaolesi, M., Blot, S., D'Antona, G., Granger, N., Tonlorenzi, R., Innocenzi, A., et al. (2006). Mesoangioblast stem cells ameliorate muscle function in dystrophic dogs. *Nature* 444, 574–579. doi: 10.1038/nature05282

Sampaolesi, M., Torrente, Y., Innocenzi, A., Tonlorenzi, R., D'Antona, G., Pellegrino, M. A., et al. (2003). Cell therapy of alpha-sarcoglycan null dystrophic mice through intra-arterial delivery of mesoangioblasts. *Science* 301, 487–492. doi: 10.1126/science.1082254

Scott, D., Blizzard, L., Fell, J., and Jones, G. (2011). The epidemiology of sarcopenia in community living older adults: what role does lifestyle play? *J. Cachexia Sarcopenia Muscle* 2, 125–134. doi: 10.1007/s13539-011-0036-4

Seale, P., Ishibashi, J., Scime, A., and Rudnicki, M. A. (2004). Pax7 is necessary and sufficient for the myogenic specification of CD45(+): Sca1(+) stem cells from injured muscle. *PLoS Biol.* 2:e130. doi: 10.1371/journal.pbio.0020130

Sherwood, R. I., Christensen, J. L., Conboy, I. M., Conboy, M. J., Rando, T. A., Weissman, I. L., et al. (2004). Isolation of adult mouse myogenic progenitors: Functional heterogeneity of cells within and engrafting skeletal muscle. *Cell* 119, 543–554. doi: 10.1016/j.cell.2004.10.021

Skuk, D., and Tremblay, J. P. (2011). Intramuscular cell transplantation as a potential treatment of myopathies: clinical and preclinical relevant data. *Exp. Opin. Biol. Ther.* 11, 359–374. doi: 10.1517/14712598.2011.548800

Small, E. M., O'Rourke, J. R., Moresi, V., Sutherland, L. B., McAnally, J., Gerard, R. D., et al. (2010). Regulation of PI3-kinase/Akt signaling by muscle-enriched microRNA-486. *Proc. Natl. Acad. Sci. U.S.A.* 107, 4218–4223. doi: 10.1073/pnas.1000300107

Suzuki, H., Asakawa, A., Amitani, H., Nakamura, N., and Inui, A. (2013). Cancer cachexia–pathophysiology and management. *J. Gastroenterol.* 48, 574–594. doi: 10.1007/s00535-013-0787-0

Takahashi, K., and Yamanaka, S. (2006). Induction of pluripotent stem cells from mouse embryonic and adult fibroblast cultures by defined factors. *Cell* 126, 663–676. doi: 10.1016/j.cell.2006.07.024

Tamaki, T., Akatsuka, A., Ando, K., Nakamura, Y., Matsuzawa, H., Hotta, T., et al. (2002). Identification of myogenic-endothelial progenitor cells in the interstitial spaces of skeletal muscle. *J. Cell Biol.* 157, 571–577. doi: 10.1083/jcb.200112106

Tanaka, K. K., Hall, J. K., Troy, A. A., Cornelison, D. D. W., Majka, S. M., and Olwin, B. B. (2009). Syndecan-4-expressing muscle progenitor cells in the SP engraft as satellite cells during muscle regeneration. *Cell Stem Cell* 4, 217–225. doi: 10.1016/j.stem.2009.01.016

Tedesco, F. S., Dellavalle, A., Diaz-Manera, J., Messina, G., and Cossu, G. (2010). Repairing skeletal muscle: regenerative potential of skeletal muscle stem cells. *J. Clin. Invest.* 120, 11–19. doi: 10.1172/JCI40373

Thomson, J. A., Itskovitz-Eldor, J., Shapiro, S. S., Waknitz, M. A., Swiergiel, J. J., Marshall, V. S., et al. (1998). Embryonic stem cell lines derived from human blastocysts. *Science* 282, 1145–1147. doi: 10.1126/science.282.5391.1145

Tinsley, J., Deconinck, N., Fisher, R., Kahn, D., Phelps, S., Gillis, J. M., et al. (1998). Expression of full-length utrophin prevents muscular dystrophy in mdx mice. *Nat. Med.* 4, 1441–1444. doi: 10.1038/4033

Tisdale, M. J. (2002). Cachexia in cancer patients. *Nat. Rev. Cancer* 2, 862–871. doi: 10.1038/nrc927

Todorov, P., Cariuk, P., McDevitt, T., Coles, B., Fearon, K., and Tisdale, M. (1996). Characterization of a cancer cachectic factor. *Nature* 379, 739–742. doi: 10.1038/379739a0

Todorov, P. T., Field, W. N., and Tisdale, M. J. (1999). Role of a proteolysis-inducing factor (PIF) in cachexia induced by a human melanoma (G361). *Br. J. Cancer* 80, 1734–1737. doi: 10.1038/sj.bjc.6690590

Tonlorenzi, R., Dellavalle, A., Schnapp, E., Cossu, G., and Sampaolesi, M. (2007). Isolation and characterization of mesoangioblasts from mouse, dog, and human tissues. *Curr. Protoc. Stem Cell Biol.* Chapter 2: Unit 2B.1. doi: 10.1002/9780470151808.sc02b01s3

Twayana, S., Legnini, I., Cesana, M., Cacchiarelli, D., Morlando, M., and Bozzoni, I. (2013). Biogenesis and function of non-coding RNAs in muscle differentiation and in Duchenne muscular dystrophy. *Biochem. Soc. Trans.* 41, 844–849. doi: 10.1042/BST20120353

Van Deutekom, J. C., Janson, A. A., Ginjaar, I. B., Frankhuizen, W. S., Aartsma-Rus, A., Bremmer-Bout, M., et al. (2007). Local dystrophin restoration with antisense oligonucleotide PRO051. *N. Engl. J. Med.* 357, 2677–2686. doi: 10.1056/NEJMoa073108

Van Rooij, E., Liu, N., and Olson, E. N. (2008). MicroRNAs flex their muscles. *Trends Genet.* 24, 159–166. doi: 10.1016/j.tig.2008.01.007

Van Rooij, E., Quiat, D., Johnson, B. A., Sutherland, L. B., Qi, X. X., Richardson, J. A., et al. (2009). A Family of microRNAs encoded by myosin genes governs myosin expression and muscle performance. *Dev. Cell* 17, 662–673. doi: 10.1016/j.devcel.2009.10.013

Vaughan, V. C., Sullivan-Gunn, M., Hinch, E., Martin, P., and Lewandowski, P. A. (2012). Eicosapentaenoic acid and oxypurinol in the treatment of muscle wasting in a mouse model of cancer cachexia. *PLoS ONE* 7:e45900. doi: 10.1371/journal.pone.0045900

Volonte, D., Liu, Y., and Galbiati, F. (2005). The modulation of caveolin-1 expression controls satellite cell activation during muscle repair. *FASEB J.* 19, 237–239. doi: 10.1096/fj.04-2215fje

Wang, Y. X., and Rudnicki, M. A. (2012). Satellite cells, the engines of muscle repair. *Nature Rev. Mol. Cell Biol.* 13, 127–133. doi: 10.1038/nrm3265

Wightman, B., Ha, I., and Ruvkun, G. (1993). Posttranscriptional regulation of the heterochronic gene lin-14 by lin-4 mediates temporal pattern formation in *C. elegans*. *Cell* 75, 855–862. doi: 10.1016/0092-8674(93)90530-4

Wu, C., Fernandez, S. A., Criswell, T., Chidiac, T. A., Guttridge, D., Villalona-Calero, M., et al. (2013). Disrupting cytokine signaling in pancreatic cancer: a phase I/II study of etanercept in combination with gemcitabine in patients with advanced disease. *Pancreas* 42, 813–818. doi: 10.1097/MPA.0b013e318279b87f

Yoshimura, M., Sakamoto, M., Ikemoto, M., Mochizuki, Y., Yuasa, K., Miyagoe-Suzuki, Y., et al. (2004). AAV vector-mediated microdystrophin expression in a relatively small percentage of mdx myofibers improved the mdx phenotype. *Mol. Ther.* 10, 821–828. doi: 10.1016/j.ymthe.2004.07.025

Zhang, L., Tang, H., Kou, Y., Li, R., Zheng, Y., Wang, Q., et al. (2013). MG132-mediated inhibition of the ubiquitin-proteasome pathway ameliorates cancer cachexia. *J. Cancer Res. Clin. Oncol.* 139, 1105–1115. doi: 10.1007/s00432-013-1412-6

Zhou, W., Jiang, Z. W., Tian, J., Jiang, J., Li, N., and Li, J. S. (2003). Role of NF-kappaB and cytokine in experimental cancer cachexia. *World J. Gastroenterol.* 9, 1567–1570.

18

CD13 promotes mesenchymal stem cell-mediated regeneration of ischemic muscle

M. Mamunur Rahman[1], Jaganathan Subramani[1,2], Mallika Ghosh[1], Jiyeon K. Denninger[1], Kotaro Takeda[1], Guo-Hua Fong[1], Morgan E. Carlson[3,4]* and Linda H. Shapiro[1]*

[1] Center for Vascular Biology, University of Connecticut Health Center, Farmington, CT, USA
[2] Department of Anesthesiology, Texas Tech University Health Sciences Center, Lubbock, TX, USA
[3] Center on Aging, University of Connecticut Health Center, Farmington, CT, USA
[4] Drug Discovery, Genomics Institute of the Novartis Research Foundation, San Diego, CA, USA

***Correspondence:**
Morgan E. Carlson, Center on Aging, University of Connecticut Health Center, 263 Farmington Ave., Farmington, CT 06030, USA
e-mail: mcarlson@gnf.org;
Linda H. Shapiro, Center for Vascular Biology, University of Connecticut Health Center, 263 Farmington Ave., Farmington, CT 06030, USA
e-mail: lshapiro@neuron.uchc.edu

Mesenchymal stem cells (MSCs) are multipotent, tissue-resident cells that can facilitate tissue regeneration and thus, show great promise as potential therapeutic agents. Functional MSCs have been isolated and characterized from a wide array of adult tissues and are universally identified by the shared expression of a core panel of MSCs markers. One of these markers is the multifunctional cell surface peptidase CD13 that has been shown to be expressed on human and murine MSCs from many tissues. To investigate whether this universal expression indicates a functional role for CD13 in MSC biology we isolated, expanded and characterized MSCs from bone marrow of wild type (WT) and CD13^{KO} mice. Characterization of these cells demonstrated that both WT and CD13^{KO} MSCs expressed the full complement of MSC markers (CD29, CD44, CD49e, CD105, Sca1), showed comparable proliferation rates and were capable of differentiating toward the adipogenic and osteogenic lineages. However, MSCs lacking CD13 were unable to differentiate into vascular cells, consistent with our previous characterization of CD13 as an angiogenic regulator. Compared to WT MSCs, adhesion and migration on various extracellular matrices of CD13^{KO} MSCs were significantly impaired, which correlated with decreased phospho-FAK levels and cytoskeletal alterations. Crosslinking human MSCs with activating CD13 antibodies increased cell adhesion to endothelial monolayers and induced FAK activation in a time dependent manner. In agreement with these *in vitro* data, intramuscular injection of CD13^{KO} MSCs in a model of severe ischemic limb injury resulted in significantly poorer perfusion, decreased ambulation, increased necrosis and impaired vascularization compared to those receiving WT MSCs. This study suggests that CD13 regulates FAK activation to promote MSC adhesion and migration, thus, contributing to MSC-mediated tissue repair. CD13 may present a viable target to enhance the efficacy of mesenchymal stem cell therapies.

Keywords: CD13, mesenchymal stem cells, adhesion, cell transplantation, hindlimb ischemia

INTRODUCTION

Stem cells have the amazing capacity to contribute to the growth and healing of many different types of tissues and hold tremendous promise as therapeutic tools in many diseases. However, the realization of optimal stem cell therapy is critically dependent on the successful retention of implanted cells at the site of injury and their effective incorporation into the damaged tissue. Mesenchymal stem cells (MSC) are a potential source of stem cells that have been shown to be effective in a range of cellular therapies in tissue engineering and regenerative medicine, but the biologic mechanisms underlying their function are just being elucidated. This knowledge is clearly essential to improving and optimizing stem cell therapies going forward.

While no single cell surface marker unequivocally identifies MSCs from all tissues, consensus in the field has proposed three minimal criteria to distinguish MSCs from other hematopoietic stem cells (Dominici et al., 2006). Characteristic MSCs (1) adhere to plastic, (2) express a characteristic pattern of cell surface molecules, and (3) can be differentiated into chondroblasts, adipocytes and osteoblasts *in vitro*. Additional cell surface markers have been identified as being expressed on MSCs, but as they are also expressed on other cells are not always included in the profile. CD13 is a member of this latter group and has been shown to be expressed on embryonic and adult stem cells isolated from numerous sources (Aust et al., 2004; Covas et al., 2005; Fan et al., 2005; Musina et al., 2005; Trubiani et al., 2005; Seeberger et al., 2006). However, potential functional roles for CD13 in these cells have not been investigated.

CD13 is a type II zinc-dependent metallopeptidase (also known as aminopeptidase N) that is found on the surface of all myeloid cells in addition to pericytes, activated endothelial cells, and subsets of organ-specific epithelial cells (Funk et al., 1994;

Jamur et al., 2005; Mina-Osorio, 2008; Armulik et al., 2011). It is a multifunctional protein with both enzyme-dependent and independent functions that contribute to adhesion, cell migration, angiogenesis, inflammatory trafficking, adhesion, antigen presentation, and endocytosis (Shipp and Look, 1993; Bhagwat et al., 2003; Luan and Xu, 2007; Petrovic et al., 2007; Winnicka et al., 2010; Ghosh et al., 2012; Pereira et al., 2013; Rahman et al., 2013; Subramani et al., 2013).

In this study, we phenotypically and functionally characterized bone marrow-derived MSC from wild type and $CD13^{KO}$ mice. Isolated cells of both genotypes expressed normal profiles of characteristic stem cell markers and were capable of differentiation into the adipogenic and osteogenic lineages. However, functional analysis showed that CD13 is important for optimal MSC adhesion, migration and vascular network formation. In addition, FAK phosphorylation is diminished and cytoskeletal architecture is disrupted in $CD13^{KO}$ MSCs. Finally, $CD13^{KO}$ MSC were impaired in their ability to mediate the recovery of perfusion in a murine model of hind limb ischemia *in vivo*.

MATERIALS AND METHODS

ANIMALS

Global $CD13^{KO}$ mice were generated at the Gene Targeting and Transgenic Facility at the University of Connecticut Health Center (Winnicka et al., 2010) and back-crossed for 10 generations to the FVB strain (The Jackson Laboratory, Bar Harbor, ME). All animals were housed under specific pathogen-free conditions with 12 h light/dark cycle and controlled temperature at the University of Connecticut Health Center animal facilities in accordance with Institutional and Office of Laboratory Animal Welfare guidelines. 7–8 weeks old mice were used for all experiments.

BONE MARROW DERIVED MESENCHYMAL STEM CELLS ISOLATION AND CULTURE

MSC were isolated and cultured as previously described (Peister et al., 2004). Briefly, the femurs and tibiae were removed, cleaned, and flushed the marrow cells from 6 to 8 weeks old WT and $CD13^{KO}$ mice. Total mononuclear cells were cultured in DMEM, with 15% FBS on plastic dishes at 37°C in 5% humidified CO_2. After 24 h., non-adherent cells were washed off and adherent cells were expanded. When adherent cells were confluent (defined as passage 0), they were continuously cultured as MSCs until passage 3. All primary cell experiments used cells at passage 4–7 to avoid both hematopoietic cells contamination and long-term culture effects.

HUMAN BONE MARROW MESENCHYMAL STEM CELL CULTURE

Human MSCs were purchased from Thermo Scientific (#SV30110.02) and cultured with mesenchymal stem cell medium (MSCM) from ScienCell (#7501) that is a complete medium designed for optimal growth of normal human MSCs *in vitro*.

REVERSE TRANSCRIPTION PCR ANALYSIS

The total cellular RNA was isolated from the wild type MSCs (WT-MSCs) and $CD13^{KO}$ MSCs (KO-MSCs). PCR amplification was performed using Invitrogen Superscript III Reverse Transcriptase and other reagents according to manufacturer's instructions (Invitrogen Corporation, Carlsbad, CA). For PCR, we used primers for Sca1, CD29, CD44, CD49e, and CD105. All of the primer sequences were determined using established GenBank sequences. Duplicate PCR reactions were amplified using primers designed GAPDH as a control for analysis by agarose gel electrophoresis.

FLOW CYTOMETRIC ASSESSMENT OF CELLULAR INFILTRATION

Flow cytometric analysis was used to characterize the phenotypes of the MSCs. Cells were lifted with trypsin/EDTA and counted. About 1×10^5 cells (in 100 µl PBS/0.5% bovine serum albumin/2 mmol/l EDTA) were incubated with fluorescence-labeled monoclonal antibodies against mouse CD29, CD49e, CD34, CD45, CD11b at 4°C for 30 min. All antibodies were purchased from Biolegend. Flow cytometry was performed on LSRII (Becton Dickinson) and the data analyzed with FlowJo software (Tree Star).

ADIPOGENIC AND OSTEOGENIC DIFFERENTIATION

Passage 4 MSCs were incubated to differentiate into adipocytes and osteoblasts in corresponding induction medium for 3 weeks (Peister et al., 2004). For adipogenesis, the cultures were incubated in DMEM that was supplemented with 15%FBS, 100 U/mL penicillin, 100 µg/ml streptomycin, 12 mM L-glutamine, 5 µg/ml insulin (Sigma), 50 µM indomethacin (Sigma), 1×10^{-6} M dexamethasone, and 0.5 µM 3-isobutyl-1-methylxanthine (IBMX; Sigma). The medium was changed 2 times per week for 3 weeks. The cells were fixed with 10% formalin for 20 min at RT and stained with 0.5% Oil Red O (Sigma) in methanol (Sigma) for 20 min at RT. For osteogenesis, the cultures were then incubated in DMEM that was supplemented with 15% FBS, 100 U/mL penicillin, 100 µg/ml streptomycin, 12 mM L-glutamine, 20 mM β-glycerol phosphate (Sigma, St Louis, MO), 50 ng/ml thyroxine (Sigma), 1 nM dexamethasone (Sigma), and 0.5 µM ascorbate 2-phosphate (Sigma). The media was changed 2 times per week for 3 weeks. The cells were fixed with 10% formalin for 20 min at RT and stained with Alizarin Red, pH 4.1 (Sigma) for 20 min at RT.

ADHESION ASSAYS

Wells of a 96-well plate (Reacti-bind™, Pierce Biotechnology) were coated with fibronectin (10 µg/ml), Matrigel (1:100 dilution), or 1% gelatin overnight at 4°C, washed, blocked with 100 µl 1% boiled BSA for 1 h at room temperature. Cells (1×10^4 /well/150 µl) were plated for 60 min at 37°C, washed three times, and stained with 0.5% crystal violet for 30 min. Plates were washed six times with PBS, solubilized with 100 µl 1% SDS solution and adhesion was quantified with a spectrophotometer at 595 nm (Mina-Osorio et al., 2008; Kim et al., 2012).

MTT PROLIFERATION ASSAY OF MSCs

Cells were plated at a density of 6000 cells/ well/ 200 µl in a 96 well plate (None and Fibronectin coated) and were incubated with complete medium. MTT (20 µl, 5 mg/ml) was added to each well at indicated time points and incubated for 3.5 h. MTT converted in living cells was solubilized with 4 mM HCl, 0.1% Nonidet P-40 (NP40) in isopropanol and absorbance measured at 595/655 nm.

CELL MIGRATION AND INVASION ASSAYS

Cell migration and invasion assays were performed using a BD FluoroBlok 24-multiwell insert system (BD Biosciences). The inserts contain a fluorescence-blocking, 8-μm pore size membrane. The FluoroBlok allow quantification of the number of cells that have migrated through the pores by microscope. To study cell migration, MSCs were suspended in serum-free DMEM medium, and seeded on a BD Falcon FluoroBlok 24-multiwell insert (0.25 ml of cells suspension, 1×10^4 cells per top chamber). To study cell invasion, the FluoroBlok were coated with Matrigel (1:5 dilutions) for 2 h at 37°C. MSCs were suspended in serum-free DMEM medium, and seeded on coated FluoroBlok (0.25 ml of cells suspension, 1×10^5 cells per top chamber). The bottom chambers contained 0.75 ml of 10% FBS contained DMEM medium. Cells were incubated in the FluoroBlok multiwell insert system for 4 h. (migration) and for 6 h (invasion) at 37°C in a humidified atmosphere of 5% CO_2. Carefully cut the FluoroBlok and coverslipped on slides using Dapi Vectashield mounting medium (Vector Laboratories, Burlingame, CA). Photographs and of migrated cells were taken with Axiocam MRC camera (0.63X magnification) attached to Zeiss Axioplan 2 microscope using a 10x objectives and counted them.

ENDOTHELIAL CELL NETWORK FORMATION ASSAY

WT and CD13^{KO} MSCs (1×10^5) were seeded on Matrigel (BD Biosciences, Bedford, MA) coated 24 well plates with DMEM (10% FBS). After 12 h, images were acquired at 20X magnification (2X objective) using a Nikon T-BPA camera attached to the Nikon Eclipse TE2000-U. The software used was SPOT version 4.1. Three individual experiments were performed. Total numbers of branch points per well were enumerated.

WESTERN BLOTTING

Isolated primary MSCs were lysed in ice-cold buffer (1% NP40 lysis buffer with protease and phosphatase inhibitors). Equal amount of protein from each group were separated by SDS-PAGE and transferred on to PVDF membrane and incubated with respective primary antibodies; CD13 monoclonal antibody for mouse CD13 (SL-13, custom made by ProMab Biotechnologies, Inc. Richmond, CA); 452 for human CD13 (Dr. Meenhard Herlyn, Philadelphia, PA); pFAK 397, pFAK925, and tFAK (cell signaling); β-Actin (Sigma); followed by incubation with horseradish peroxidase-conjugated secondary antibodies. The antigen-antibody complexes were detected with the use of a chemiluminescence reagent kit (Thermoscientific).

HISTOLOGY AND IMMUNOHISTOCHEMISTRY

Mouse or human MSCs were cultured on slides and fixed in 4% paraformaldehyde solution, permeabilized with 0.2% Triton X-100 for 10 min, and blocked with 5% BSA for 1 h. Cells were incubated with SL-13 (dilution 1/500) for mouse CD13 staining; 452 mAb (dilution 1/250) for human CD13 staining; pFAK397 and pFAK925 (cell signaling) for pFAK staining overnight followed by fluorescence secondary antibody (dilution 1/1000) for 1 h at room temperature. For F-actin staining cells were incubated with TRITC-phalloidin (Sigma-Aldrich, 1/100 dilution) for 1 h. overnight followed by fluorescence secondary antibody (dilution 1/1000) for 1 h at room temperature.

After completing blood flow assessments over 21 days, gastrocnemius muscles were dissected, fixed in 4% paraformaldehyde for 24 h, dehydrated, embedded in paraffin, and sectioned at 7 μm thickness. After deparaffinization and rehydration, antigen retrieval was done with citrate buffer pH 6 and sections blocked and incubated overnight at 4°C with primary antibodies followed by fluorescent secondary antibody for 1 h at room temperature. The capillaries were visualized by immunofluorescent staining with anti-CD31 (Santa Cruz Biotechnology) (dilution 1/200). Respective fluorophore-conjugated secondary antibodies (Molecular Probes, Carlsbad, CA) (dilution 1/1000) were used. The slides were coverslipped using Dapi Vectashield mounting medium (Vector Laboratories, Burlingame, CA). The capillary density is assessed relative to the number of muscle fibers. Muscle regeneration (fibers with centrally located nuclei/total fiber #) in the crural muscle was analyzed by haematoxylin and eosin staining.

Tissue sections were photographed with Optronics camera attached to Ziess Axioskop 2 plus microscope using the Zeiss Achroplan 20X objective and images were captured using MagnaFire SP 2.1B software. Fluorescence images were photographed with Axiocam MRC camera (0.63X magnification) attached to Zeiss Axioplan 2 microscope using a 10x, 20X, 40X or 63X objectives. For fluorescence quantification all of the images were acquired at the same exposure.

QUANTITATIVE CELL ADHESION ASSAY AND CD13 CROSS-LINKING

Monolayer adhesion assays were performed as described previously (Mina-Osorio et al., 2008). In brief, human MSCs (1×10^5) were labeled with calcein for 30 min at 37°C followed by treating with activating anti-CD13 452 mAb for 30 min with or without, washed and allowed to adhere to HUVEC monolayer cells for 45 min, lysed and fluorescence read at 485/530 nm and expressed as relative fluorescence unit (RFU).

For cross-linking of CD13 on human MSCs, cells were incubated with control anti-CD13 452 mAb in culture medium for 0, 5, 15, and 30 min at 37°C in a humidified 5% CO2 incubator. Immediately after cross-linking, the reaction was stopped by adding 5 mL of cold PBS and washed once. Cells were lysed in 1.0% NP-40 lysis buffer (20.0 mM HEPES pH 7.4, 150 mM NaCl, and 1.0% NP-40) with protease inhibitor cocktail (Roche) and phosphatase inhibitors. Lysates were cleared by centrifugation at 7000 rpm for 15 min. Proteins or immunoprecipitates were diluted with 4X sample buffer and resolved by 10% SDS-PAGE and electrotransfered onto a polyvinylidene difluoride membrane (Millipore, Bedford, MA) followed by probing with pFAK397 (1:1000), followed by HRP-conjugated secondary Abs (1:5000) and detected using the ECL- kit (Thermoscientific, USA). The blot also stripped for tFAK and β-Actin detection.

HINDLIMB ISCHEMIA MODEL AND CELL TRANSPLANTATION

All animal procedures were performed in accordance with the guidelines approved by the Animal Care Committee of the University of Connecticut. Surgical grade anesthesia was induced by intraperitoneal injection of Ketamine (100 mg/kg) and Xylazine (10 mg/kg). The right femoral artery was ligated proximal to the deep femoral artery and distal to saphenous artery. The deep femoral artery, superficial branches and bifurcation of the popliteal artery were cauterized, and the femoral artery was completely removed between the two ligatures avoiding injury of the femoral vein and nerve to preclude influence of inflammation and edema on arteriogenesis and angiogenesis. Postoperative analgesia was provided with buprenorphine (0.05 mg/kg). After 4 h., the injection of PBS, wild type MSC (WT-MSC), and CD13^{KO} MSC (KO-MSC) were performed intramuscularly by injecting cells (2×10^6) resuspended in PBS at three different points (20 μl in each point) into the gastrocnemius muscles of wild type mice with a 27 g needle (Kim et al., 2012).

LASER-DOPPLER PERFUSION IMAGING

Non-invasive measurements of superficial hindlimb perfusion were obtained before and 0, 3, 7, 14, and 21 days after ligation using a Laser Doppler perfusion imager (model LDI2-IR, Moor Instruments, Wilmington, DE) that was modified for high resolution and depth of penetration (2 mm) with and 830 nm wavelength infrared 2.5 mW laser diode, 100 μm beam diameter,

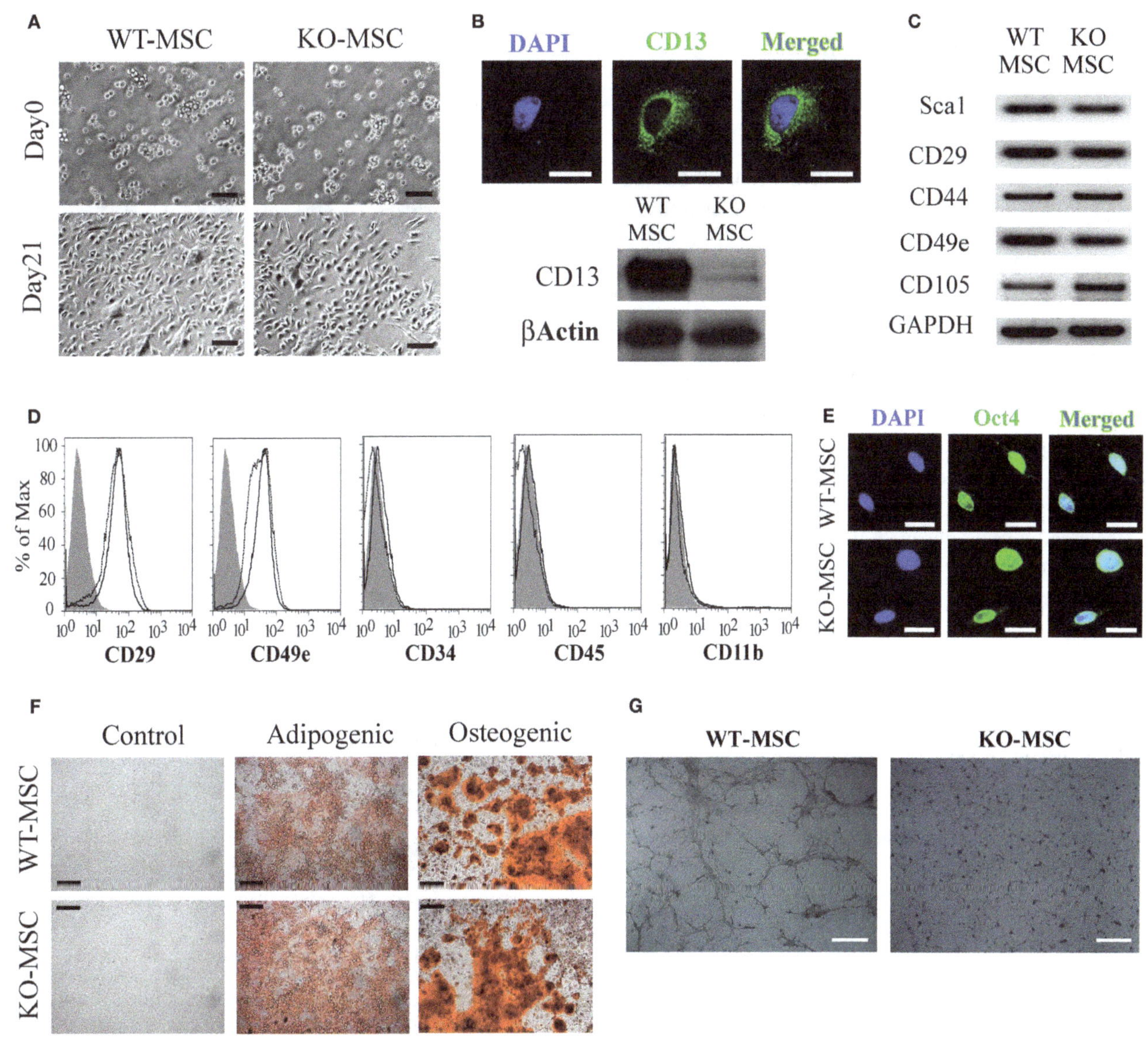

FIGURE 1 | Mesenchymal stem cell culture and characterization. (A) Phase contrast image of BM derived MSCs at Day 0 and Day 21(Bar = 100 μm). **(B)** CD13 expression in WT-MSCs by fluorescence immunostaining (Bar = 20 μm) and protein expression of CD13 in WT-MSC. **(C)** RT PCR analysis of stem cell expression profiles. **(D)** Flow cytometric analysis of MSCs. Cells were characteristically positive for CD29, CD49e and negative for CD19, CD31, and CD34. Unstained;WT-MSC; KO-MSC–. **(E)** Both WT-MSC and KO-MSC expressed transcription factor OCT3/4 (Bar = 20 μm). **(F)** Confluent MSCs were transferred to adipogenic and osteogenic medium for 3 weeks. Adipocytes were detected by oil red O staining and osteoblasts by alizarin red staining (Bar = 200 μm). **(G)** 1×10^5 cells were seeded on Matrigel coated 6-well plates and incubated for 12 h. cells isolated from CD13^{KO} mice are unable to form capillary networks and form fewer branches (Bar = 200 μm).

and 15 kHz bandwidth. At each time point, an average of 4 measurements per animal was made on anesthetized (1.5% isoflurane on an isothermal heating pad). To avoid the influence of light and temperature, the results were expressed as a ratio of perfusion in the right (ischemic) vs. left [non-ischemic (NI)] limb (Limbourg et al., 2009).

IN VIVO ASSESSMENT OF LIMB FUNCTION AND ISCHEMIC DAMAGE

Semi quantitative assessment of impaired use of the ischemic limb (ambulation score) was performed using the following criterion: 3 = most severe, unable to use the foot, dragging foot; 2 = no dragging, but no plantar flexion (ability to flex the ankle); 1 = positive plantar flexion; and 0 = able to flex toes to grasp cage in response to gentle traction on the tail (Stabile et al., 2003). Semi quantitative measurement of the ischemic damage (necrosis score) was also assessed (1 to 5 = one to five fingernails damaged, 6 to 10 = one to five fingers fully damaged, 11 = total paw damage).

QUANTIFICATION OF CELL ENGRAFTMENT IN ISCHEMIC HINDLIMBS

Cell engraftment in the ischemic hindlimb was quantified by histological analysis. Briefly, red fluorescent dye PKH26 labeled WT-MSC (2×10^6) and green fluorescent dye PKH67 labeled KO-MSC (2×10^6) were injected into ischemic hindlimbs of wild type mice. After 7 days, the ischemic hindlimbs were harvested, and tissue sections were embedded and sectioned. Five fields from four tissue sections were randomly selected, and the number of labeled cells was counted in each field (Kim et al., 2012).

STATISTICAL ANALYSIS

The data were represented as mean ± s.e.m. of the indicated number of measurements. Statistical differences between groups were analyzed by using unpaired, two-tailed t-test or One-Way ANOVA. Differences were considered significant at $p < 0.05$.

RESULTS

MESENCHYMAL STEM CELL CULTURE AND CHARACTERIZATION

To determine if CD13 contributes to the biologic function of stem cells we isolated MSCs from the bone marrow of wild type and $CD13^{KO}$ mice. Cells of both genotypes were grossly visually similar upon isolation and throughout the experimental culture period (**Figure 1A**) and as expected, the CD13 protein was abundantly expressed on wild type but not $CD13^{KO}$ MSCs (**Figure 1B**). RT-PCR and flow cytometric analyses illustrated that cultured cells of both genotypes expressed equivalent levels of the characteristic cell surface MSC markers (**Figures 1C,D**). Similarly, immunofluorescent staining for the pluripotency marker Oct4 verified the multipotent potential of both wild type and $CD13^{KO}$ MSCs (**Figure 1E**). Furthermore, characterization of cultured wild type and $CD13^{KO}$ MSCs showed comparable capacities to form adipocytes and osteoclasts under conditions reported to induce adipogenic and osteogenic differentiation (**Figure 1F**). Interestingly, and consistent with our previous data implicating CD13 as a functional regulator of angiogenesis (Pasqualini et al., 2000; Bhagwat et al., 2001, 2003; Petrovic et al., 2007) $CD13^{KO}$ MSCs were incapable of forming endothelial networks (**Figure 1G**). These results confirmed CD13 as a MSC marker and suggest that CD13 is not necessary for the formation of MSC in the bone marrow or their short-term survival *in vitro* after isolation. However, CD13 is required for MSC to differentiate toward some but not all cell lineages.

$CD13^{KO}$ MESENCHYMAL STEM CELLS ARE FUNCTIONALLY IMPAIRED

We have previously demonstrated that CD13 functions as an adhesion molecule regulating monocyte-endothelial interactions (Mina-Osorio et al., 2008; Subramani et al., 2013) and is required for endothelial cell invasion (Bhagwat et al., 2003; Petrovic et al., 2007). To determine if CD13 functioned similarly in MSCs we

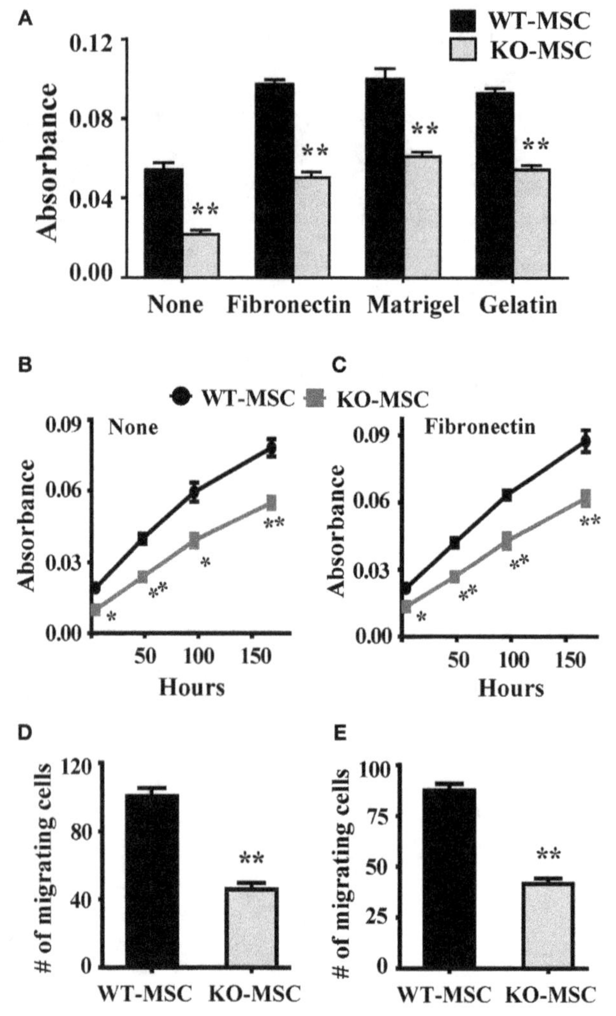

FIGURE 2 | Lack of CD13 impairs MSC adhesion, proliferation, migration, and invasion. **(A)** Adhesion assay: Cells (1×10^4) were seeded in 96 well plates coated separately with fibronectin, Matrigel, or gelatin and allowed to adhere for 1 h at 37°C. After PBS wash, adherent cells were detected by MTT assay. $n = 6$, $^{**}P < 0.01$. **(B,C)** Proliferation assay: Cells (0.5×10^4) were seeded in 96 well plate and cell proliferation detected by MTT assay at the indicated time points. $n = 6$, $^{*}P < 0.05$, $^{**}P < 0.01$. **(D)** Migration assay: 1×10^4 cells were seeded in FluoroBlok chambers. After 4 h. incubation the cells were stained with DAPI and counted. $n = 4$, $^{**}P < 0.01$. **(E)** Invasion assay: 1×10^5 cells were seeded on Matrigel (1:5 dilution) coated FluoroBlok chambers. After 6 h. incubation the cells were counted. $n = 4$, $^{**}P < 0.01$.

tested wild type and CD13^{KO} MSCs in *in vitro* in adhesion, migration and invasion assays; functions that are dependent on adhesion. Assessment of MSC adhesion to matrix proteins contained in preparations of human fibronectin, Matrigel or gelatin (**Figure 2A**) indicated that CD13^{KO} MSCs are significantly less adherent than wild type cells to all ECM proteins tested, suggesting that this effect is not strictly matrix or ligand dependent and that CD13 plays a more universal role in cell attachment. In contrast, proliferation rates as measured by the MTT assay are similar over time (**Figures 2B,C**), although lower initial absorbance readings for CD13^{KO} cells in this assay likely reflect their overall reduced adherence. Similar to our results in endothelial cells, both migration and invasion of MSC toward chemotactic stimuli were impaired (**Figures 2D,E**). Therefore, lack of CD13 hinders MSC functions *in vitro*, consistent with a loss in adhesive properties.

ADHESION-REGULATING SIGNAL TRANSDUCTION PATHWAYS ARE ALTERED IN CD13^{KO} MSCs

Adhesion to the extracellular matrix via adhesion molecules activates well-characterized signal transduction cascades that induce intracellular alterations in the cytoskeleton. Staining for intracellular F-actin in wild type and CD13^{KO} MSCs with phalloidin shows an obvious disruption of cytoskeletal integrity in the absence of CD13 (**Figure 3A**). Accordingly, dramatic reductions in phosphorylation of FAK at residues 397 and 925 and a nearly

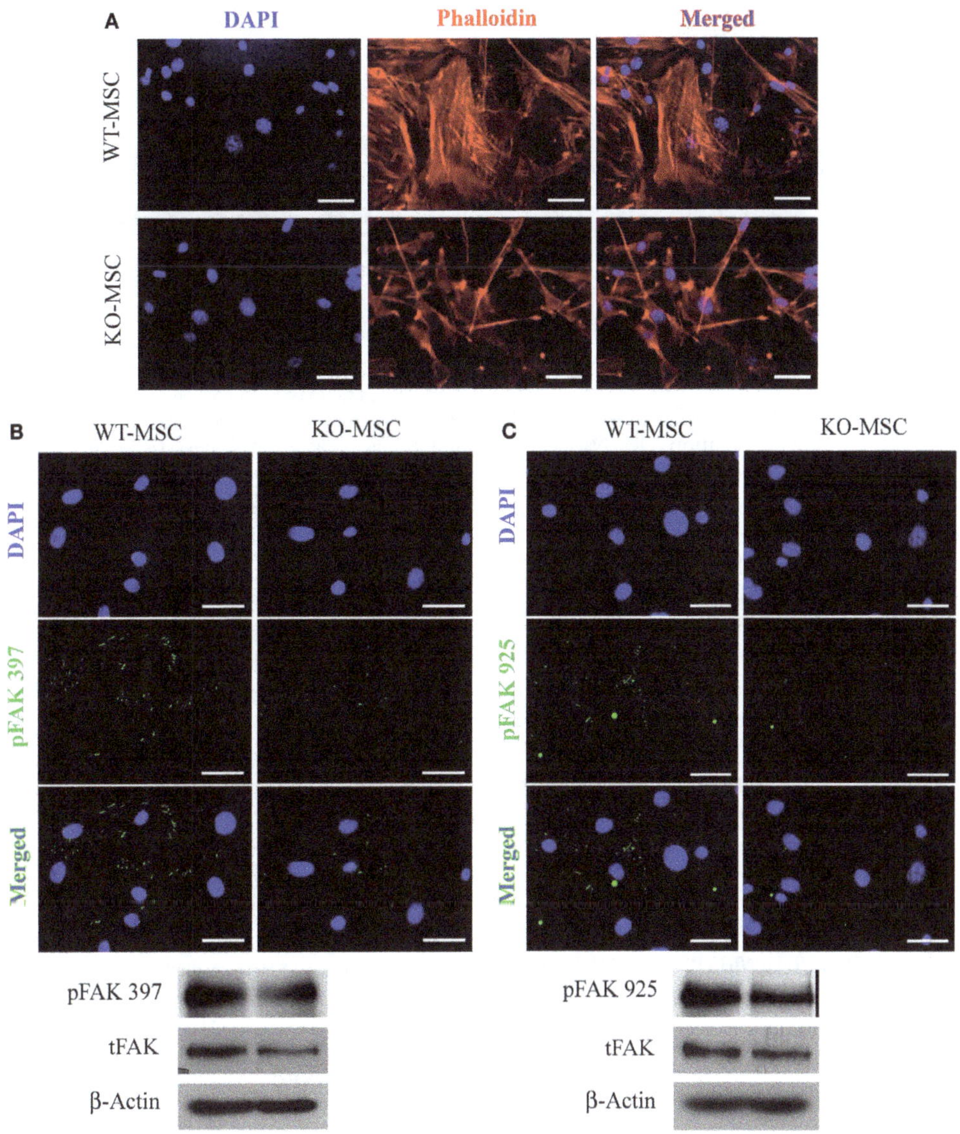

FIGURE 3 | Mesenchymal stem cell defects in CD13^{KO} mice are cell intrinsic. (A) phalloidin-stained MSC cells isolated from injured muscles of CD13^{KO} mice showed remarkable cytoskeletal disruption compared to cells from WT mice; Objective 40X (Bar = 100 μm). **(B,C)** Immunofluorescent detection of FAK phosphorylation at tyrosine residues 397 **(B)** and 925 **(C)**. Protein lysates of MSC were probed for phospho-FAK (Y397) and phospho-FAK (Y925) with β-actin as the loading control. CD13^{KO} MSCs expressed lower levels of phospho-FAK protein (Bar = 20 μm).

complete absence of focal adhesions clearly indicate severely disordered adhesion processes, although total FAK protein levels are unchanged (**Figures 3B,C**) suggesting CD13 regulates MSC adhesion via FAK activation as we have previously shown in monocytes (Subramani et al., 2013).

CD13 ACTIVATION INDUCES ADHESION AND FAK ACTIVATION IN HUMAN MSCs

We have demonstrated that activation of CD13 with a ligand mimicking monoclonal antibody increases monocyte adhesion to endothelial cells (Mina-Osorio et al., 2008; Subramani et al., 2013). CD13 is also prominently expressed in human MSCs (hMSC, **Figure 4A**) and may similarly mediate MSC-endothelial adhesion. Crosslinking of hMSC CD13 with the activating mAb 452 induces cell-cell adhesion (**Figure 4B**) and FAK phosphorylation (**Figure 4C**), suggesting that CD13 can function as a signal transducing adhesion molecule to mediate MSC adhesion, migration and invasion.

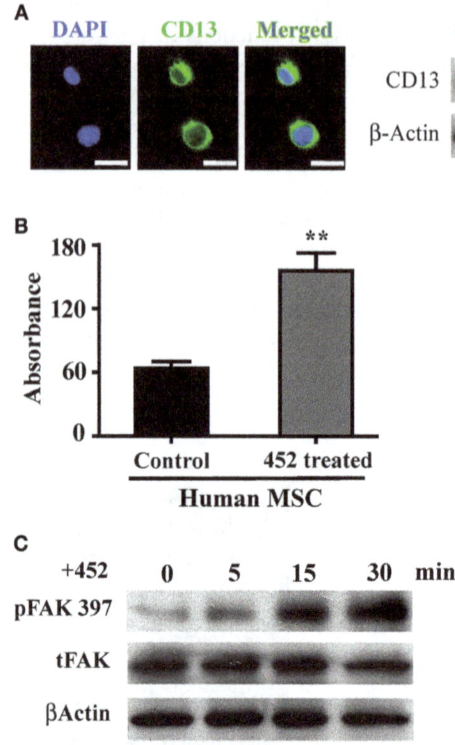

FIGURE 4 | CD13 activation increases monolayer adhesion and FAK phosphorylation in human MSCs. (A) Human mesenchymal stem cells also express CD13 by immunofluorescence (green); Objective 63X (Bar = 20 μm) and immunoblot of human cell lysates. **(B)** Colorimetric quantification of adhesion of human MSCs treated with the CD13 activating mAb 452 to HUVEC monolayers. Data represents the mean ± s.e.m. $n = 3$ from two independent experiments (** $P < 0.01$). **(C)** CD13 crosslinking with activating mAb 452 temporally induces FAK tyrosine phosphorylation in human MSCs.

CD13^{KO} MESENCHYMAL STEM CELLS ARE IMPAIRED IN ENHANCING WOUND HEALING *IN VIVO*

It is well established that administration of exogenous MSCs substantially contributes to wound repair in the hind-limb ischemia model of angiogenesis. To assess the effect of the lack of CD13 in MSC function *in vivo*, we removed the femoral artery and collateral vessels from single flanks of WT mice and injected randomized animals either with purified WT or CD13^{KO} MSCs or PBS control into the surgery site. Laser Doppler imaging of blood flow immediately following ligation clearly showed that the ligated leg is poorly perfused (blue color) relative to the contralateral leg (**Figure 5A**, day 0), but that circulation is progressively re-established over a period of 3 weeks (**Figure 5A**). In agreement with published studies, this revascularization is significantly improved in the animals injected with wild type MSCs compared to animals injected with vehicle control (**Figure 5B**). In contrast, injection of CD13^{KO} MSCs showed a significant and prolonged delay in recovery of blood flow over 21 days post-injury, suggesting that impaired MSC adhesion *in vitro* predicts reduced MSC function *in vivo* in the absence of CD13. In agreement with this result, we found reduced ambulatory capacity (impaired limb function, **Figure 5C**) and a higher degree of paw necrosis in the CD13^{KO} animals (**Figures 5D,E**).

MUSCLE GENERATION AND CAPILLARY FORMATION ARE IMPAIRED IN MICE INJECTED WITH CD13^{KO} MSC FOLLOWING ISCHEMIC INJURY

In vivo

Histologic analysis of muscles from animals receiving WT MSCs at 21 days post-surgery/injection showed clear evidence of regenerating muscle as illustrated by numerous myofibers with centrally located nuclei (WT- **Figure 6A**) where vehicle controls showed marked metaplasia with loss of myofibers and decreased muscle regeneration characteristic of impaired muscle recovery **Figure 6A**, PBS (Limbourg et al., 2009). While CD13^{KO} MSCs contribute to healing, muscle recovery is noticeably reduced (**Figure 6A**, KO and **Figure 6C**). Similarly, femoral artery removal results in hypoxia that triggers a robust angiogenic response and exogenously administered MSCs can enhance this revascularization of injured tissue (Limbourg et al., 2009). Immunofluorescent analysis of the vascular response to injury indicate that the density of CD31+ endothelial cell-lined luminal capillaries is significantly decreased in muscles of mice receiving CD13^{KO} MSCs (**Figures 6B,D**). In addition, these structures appeared more immature with fewer characteristic branches in recipients of CD13^{KO} MSCs, confirming our *in vitro* observations that CD13 is required for angiogenesis and suggesting that CD13 promotes MSC-mediated wound healing and revascularization in this model of ischemic injury.

CD13 PROLONGS THE SURVIVAL AND ENGRAFTMENT OF MESENCHYMAL STEM CELLS

The impaired muscle regeneration in recipients of CD13^{KO} MSCs suggests that CD13-dependent adhesion is important for the engraftment of MSC. To estimate the relative engraftment potential of WT and CD13^{KO} MSCs in ischemic hindlimbs, we directly transplanted a total of 2×10^6 differentially PKH dye-labeled cells of each genotype into the ischemic region

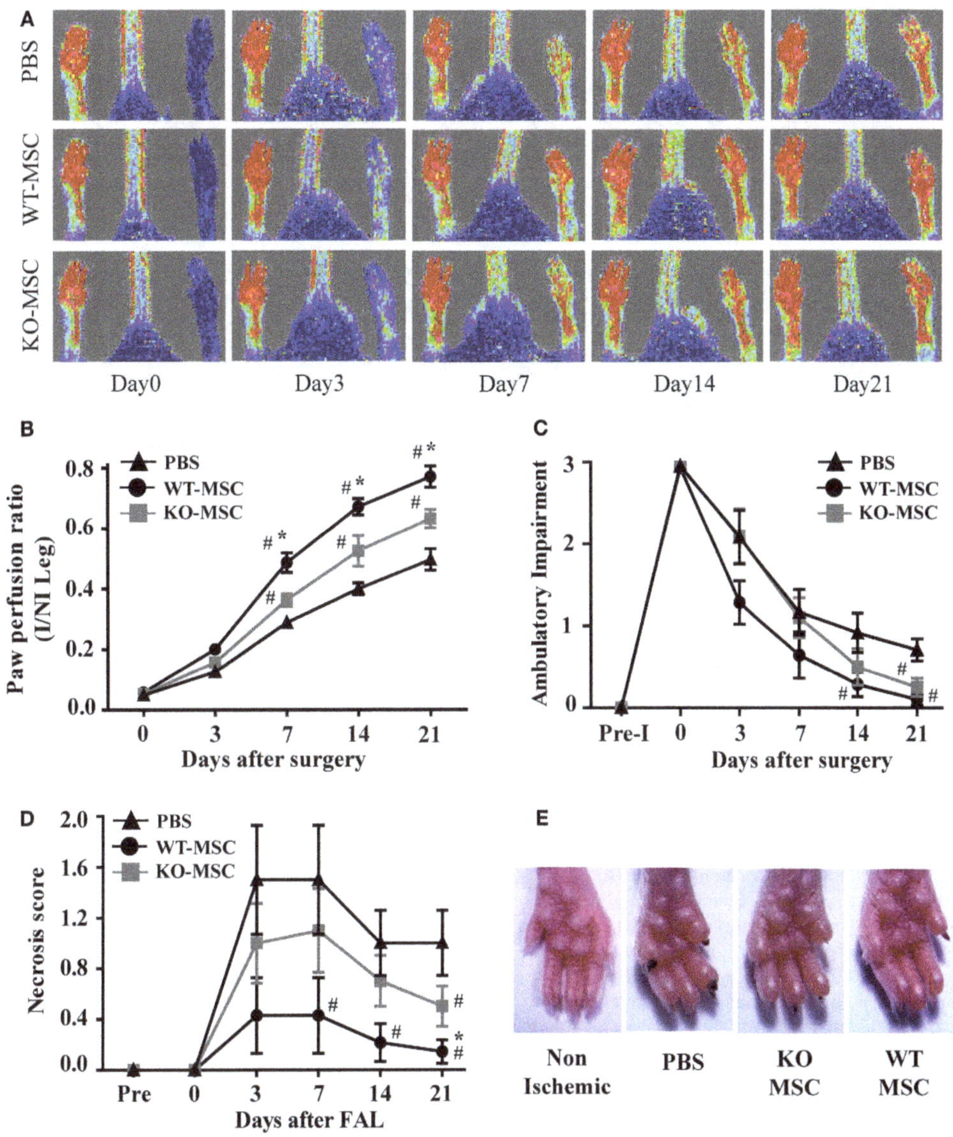

FIGURE 5 | Lack of CD13 on exogenously administered MSCs impairs perfusion recovery in an *in vivo* hindlimb ischemia model. (A) Laser Doppler flow imaging of perfusion in mice at the indicated time points. Representative color-coded images of three groups (PBS, WT-MSC, and KO-MSC) of mice on day 0, 3, 7, 14, and 21 after surgery and cell transplantation assessed by laser Doppler imaging. Red indicates highest perfusion velocity, green intermediate, and blue, lowest velocity. **(B)** Cumulative results for PBS ($n = 7$), WT-MSC ($n = 6$), and KO-MSC ($n = 8$) injected mice are shown graphically as ratios of blood flow in ischemic limb (I) to that in the non-ischemic limb (NI) at each time point. Functional assessment of ischemic muscles. Cumulative results are shown graphically as **(C)** the ambulatory impairment score; **(D)** ischemic tissue damage score as described in Methods. **(E)** Images of Non-ischemic and PBS, WT-MSC, and KO-MSC injected ischemic paw. Black nail indicates necrosis. $^{\#}P < 0.05$ compare to PBS and $^{*}P < 0.05$ compare to KO-MSC; (score assessment criteria in Methods).

of the hindlimb injury. 7 days post-injury/transplantation, hindlimb tissues were collected and analyzed for the number of dye labeled cells remaining in the wound by fluorescence microscopy (**Figures 7A,B**). Significantly higher numbers of transplanted WT MSCs were detected in tissues (PKH+/nuclear-DAPI+) than CD13^{KO} MSCs (**Figure 7C**), suggesting that CD13 regulates the function of transplanted MSCs in the wound; potentially at the level of retention, survival, or engraftment potential, thus, significantly contributing to the ability of exogenous MSCs to facilitate wound healing in ischemic injury.

DISCUSSION

CD13 was originally identified as a marker of myeloid leukemia and normal hematopoietic cells of the myeloid lineage (Subcomittee, 1984) and was subsequently discovered to be identical to the cell surface peptidase Aminopeptidase N (Look et al., 1989). Further studies by our group and others have

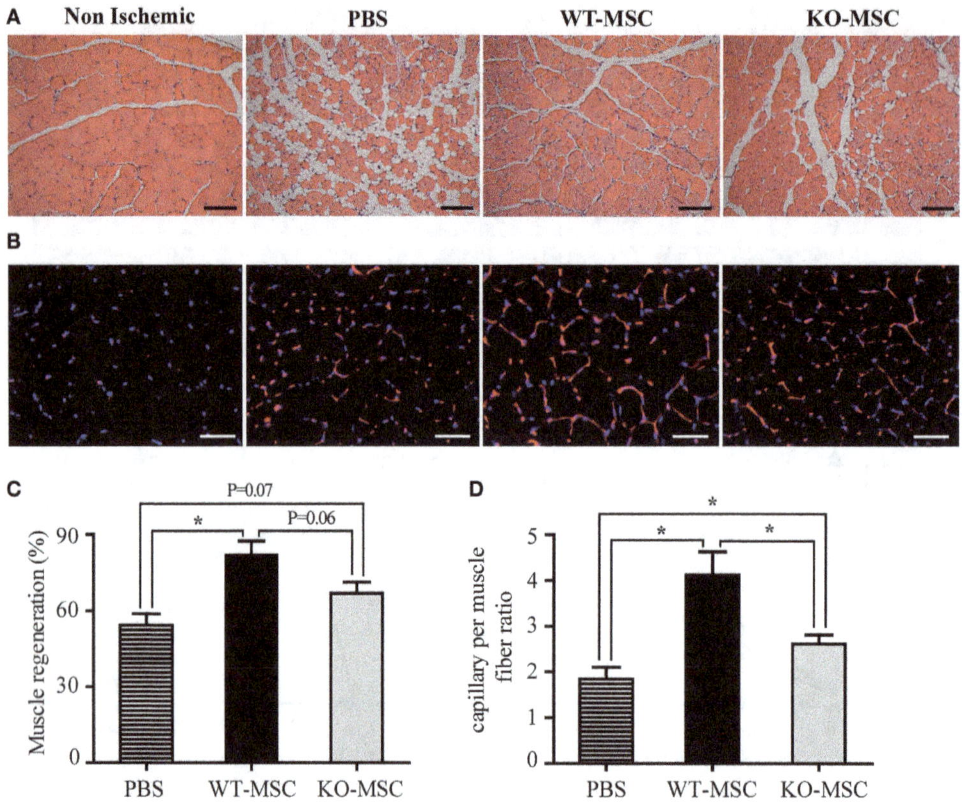

FIGURE 6 | Muscle regeneration and capillary formation are impaired in mice injected with CD13^{KO} MSC following ischemic injury. (A) Hematoxylin and eosin (H&E) staining of gastrocnemius muscle regeneration was confirmed by the presence of multiple, centrally located myocyte nuclei, 20X objective; Bar = 100 μm. **(B)** Capillaries were visualized by immunofluorescent staining with CD31 (red) and nuclei with DAPI (blue); Objective, 40X objective; Bar = 50 μm. **(C)** The area of the injured tissue was compared among PBS, WT-MSC, and KO-MSC groups. A significant increase in muscle regeneration (average) was observed in WT-MSC group compared with PBS group at day 21. **(D)** The ratio of capillary density per fiber was measured in ischemic gastrocnemius muscles. Capillary density was significantly increased in WT-MSC compared with other groups, PBS and KO-MSC. All data were quantified by ImagePro Plus. Values are shown as mean ± s.e.m. (*$P < 0.05$) (PBS $n = 7$; WT-MSC $n = 6$; KO-MSC $n = 6$).

identified numerous functional roles for this molecule in various tissues in addition to hematopoietic cells, some of which are enzyme-dependent [cleavage of bioactive peptides (Gros et al., 1985), reabsorption of amino acids (McClellan and Garner, 1980)] and others that are independent of its enzymatic activity [viral receptor (Yeager et al., 1992), adhesion molecule (Mina-Osorio et al., 2008), endocytic mediator (Ghosh et al., 2012) and angiogenic regulator (Bhagwat et al., 2001)]. The prominent and pervasive expression of CD13 on embryonic and adult stem cells of numerous origins (Aust et al., 2004; Covas et al., 2005; Fan et al., 2005; Musina et al., 2005; Trubiani et al., 2005; Seeberger et al., 2006) prompted the current investigation into possible roles for this multifunctional molecule on MSC biology. Comparison of the *in vitro* and *in vivo* properties of bone marrow-derived mesenchymal stem cell populations isolated from wild type and CD13^{KO} mice showed that MSC-expressed CD13 serves many of the functions that have been demonstrated on other cells and that lack of CD13 on MSCs has profound effects on the ability of exogenously administered cells to contribute to healing of skeletal muscle following severe ischemic injury.

Initial characterization of our global CD13^{KO} animals showed that unchallenged mice are healthy and fertile with essentially normal hematopoietic profiles and physiologic myeloid functions (Winnicka et al., 2010), similar to the normal expression profiles of stem cell markers and proliferation rates we observed in freshly isolated bone marrow derived MSCs. Interestingly, although both wild type and CD13^{KO} MSCs express the pluripotency marker Oct4 and can differentiate into cells characteristic of the osteogenic and adipogenic lineages, MSCs lacking CD13 are unable to form vascular networks *in vitro*. This finding is in agreement our previous work demonstrating that CD13 regulates angiogenesis by transducing signals important to the formation of endothelial filopodia (Petrovic et al., 2007), but also raises the intriguing possibility that CD13 may specify or determine endothelial cell fate. Consistent with this notion, we have shown that transcription factors that mediate CD13 expression in myeloid cells also direct the differentiation of myeloid progenitor cells to macrophages (Hegde et al., 1998, 1999), suggesting that CD13 may also be involved in mechanisms that program the differentiation of specific cell lineages. Studies investigating this interesting possibility are ongoing in our laboratory.

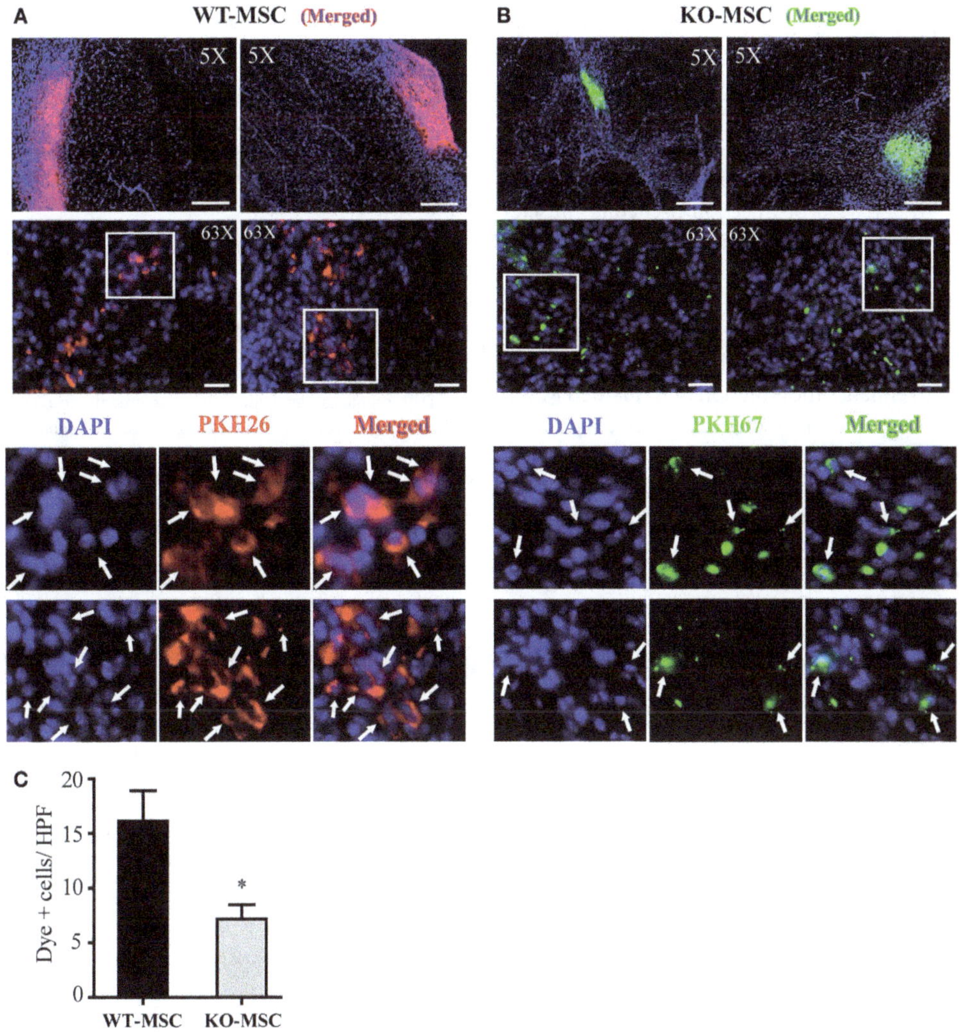

FIGURE 7 | Engraftment of MSCs *in vivo*. Representative images of localized PKH26 (red) labeled WT-MSCs **(A)** and PKH67 (green) labeled KO-MSCs **(B)** at 7 days after cell injection. **(C)** Quantification of engrafted MSCs. Dye positive cells was quantified. $*P < 0.05$ WT-MSC vs. KO-MSC. 5X objective, Bar = 500 μm; 63X objective, Bar = 50 μm.

We have also shown that CD13 is a homotypic adhesion molecule that mediates inflammatory interactions between monocytes and endothelial cells and activation of CD13 induces signal transduction, cytoskeletal reorganization and increased adhesion to regulate inflammatory monocyte trafficking (Mina-Osorio et al., 2008; Subramani et al., 2013). In the current study, we demonstrate that phosphorylation of the critical focal adhesion kinase FAK and subsequent adhesion of CD13^{KO} MSCs to the extracellular matrix is also significantly reduced. FAK phosphorylation/activation regulates adhesion, which is fundamental to the processes of MSC survival, migration and invasion that control the ability of MSCs to integrate, survive and contribute to healing at the site of injury (Song et al., 2007; Hu et al., 2011; Liao et al., 2012; Meng et al., 2013). Therefore, the reduced adhesive capacity of MSCs resulting from the loss of CD13 profoundly affects essential, cell intrinsic functions and likely forms the basis of the diminished muscle regeneration seen upon CD13^{KO} MSC treatment.

In keeping with the defective CD13^{KO} MSC morphogenesis and capillary network formation, we also find that capillary density is decreased and the capillaries that are formed are immature and poorly branched in the injuries of recipients of the CD13^{KO} MSCs, clearly contributing to reduced functional recovery. In support of this notion, we have found that angiogenesis is universally impaired in CD13^{KO} animals subjected to ischemic injury models (Pereira et al., 2013; Rahman et al., 2013) or tumors (Pasqualini et al., 2000; Bhagwat et al., 2003). Alternatively, the implanted MSCs have been described as a minor source of healthy precursor cells and wild type tissue-resident endothelial precursors are critical for neovessel formation in the wound. This data would argue that the decrease in angiogenesis and lessened regeneration in the CD13^{KO} may be due to reduced survival or retention of the MSCs in the wound, as these are a rich source of paracrine factors that serve to enhance repair by endogenous cells (Williams and Hare, 2011). Indeed, studies in cardiac cell therapy suggest that only a fraction of the donor cells actually integrate long-term, but rather function more short-term by secreting cytokines that stimulate differentiation of tissue-resident precursors, inhibit fibrosis, increase survival, suppress inflammation, and promote angiogenesis (Schulman and Hare, 2012). We find that by 7 days post-injection, ischemic muscles receiving $CD13^{KO}$ MSCs contained significantly fewer labeled cells than recipients of wild type MSCs, which is consistent with reduced survival or retention of cells lacking CD13 at the site of injection. Interestingly, our observation that activation of CD13 on MSCs induces their adhesion suggests that activation of CD13 may be a mechanism to enhance the adhesion of implanted MSCs to improve integration, paracrine secretion, revascularization, muscle regeneration, and perfusion recovery.

Collectively, our results clearly indicate that CD13 plays a protective role in MSC-mediated skeletal muscle repair, which we believe is primarily due to defects in MSC adhesion and angiogenesis. The multifunctional nature of this molecule is consistent with CD13's regulation of multiple aspects of healing following ischemic injury in the muscle and may be a potentially viable target to improve MSC therapy.

AUTHOR CONTRIBUTIONS

Developed study concept: M. Mamunur Rahman, Linda H. Shapiro, Jiyeon K. Denninger, Kotaro Takeda, Guo-Hua Fong, Morgan E. Carlson. Designed experiments: M. Mamunur Rahman, Jiyeon K. Denninger, Linda H. Shapiro, Morgan E. Carlson. Performed experiments: M. Mamunur Rahman, Mallika Ghosh, Jaganathan Subramani. Interpreted data: M. Mamunur Rahman, Linda H. Shapiro, Morgan E. Carlson, Mallika Ghosh, Jaganathan Subramani. Wrote manuscript: M. Mamunur Rahman, Linda H. Shapiro, Morgan E. Carlson.

ACKNOWLEDGMENTS

We would like to thank Dr. Kevin Claffey for use of his microscope. In addition we thank the staff of the UCHC Gene Targeting and Transgenic Facility (GTTF) and the Histology Core Facility. This work was supported by Public Health Service grant HL-70694 from the National Heart, Lung and Blood Institute and the State of Connecticut Stem Cell Research Program grant #09-SCA-UCHC-009.

REFERENCES

Armulik, A., Genove, G., and Betsholtz, C. (2011). Pericytes: developmental, physiological, and pathological perspectives, problems, and promises. *Dev. Cell* 21, 193–215. doi: 10.1016/j.devcel.2011.07.001

Aust, L., Devlin, B., Foster, S. J., Halvorsen, Y. D., Hicok, K., du Laney, T., et al. (2004). Yield of human adipose-derived adult stem cells from liposuction aspirates. *Cytotherapy* 6, 7–14. doi: 10.1080/14653240310004539

Bhagwat, S. V., Lahdenranta, J., Giordano, R., Arap, W., Pasqualini, R., and Shapiro, L. H. (2001). CD13/APN is activated by angiogenic signals and is essential for capillary tube formation. *Blood* 97, 652–659. doi: 10.1182/blood.V97.3.652

Bhagwat, S. V., Petrovic, N., Okamoto, Y., and Shapiro, L. H. (2003). The angiogenic regulator CD13/APN is a transcriptional target of ras signaling pathways in endothelial morphogenesis. *Blood* 101, 1818–1826. doi: 10.1182/blood-2002-05-1422

Covas, D. T., Piccinato, C. E., Orellana, M. D., Siufi, J. L., Silva, W. A. Jr., Proto-Siqueira, R., et al. (2005). Mesenchymal stem cells can be obtained from the human saphena vein. *Exp. Cell Res.* 309, 340–344. doi: 10.1016/j.yexcr.2005.06.005

Dominici, M., Le Blanc, K., Mueller, I., Slaper-Cortenbach, I., Marini, F., Krause, D., et al. (2006). Minimal criteria for defining multipotent mesenchymal stromal cells. the international society for cellular therapy position statement. *Cytotherapy* 8, 315–317. doi: 10.1080/14653240600855905

Fan, C. G., Tang, F. W., Zhang, Q. J., Lu, S. H., Liu, H. Y., Zhao, Z. M., et al. (2005). Characterization and neural differentiation of fetal lung mesenchymal stem cells. *Cell Transplant.* 14, 311–321. doi: 10.3727/000000005783983070

Funk, P. E., Kincade, P. W., and Witte, P. L. (1994). Native associations of early hematopoietic stem cells and stromal cells isolated in bone marrow cell aggregates. *Blood* 83, 361–369.

Ghosh, M., Mcauliffe, B., Subramani, J., Basu, S., and Shapiro, L. H. (2012). CD13 regulates dendritic cell cross-presentation and T cell responses by inhibiting receptor-mediated antigen uptake. *J. Immunol.* 188, 5489–5499. doi: 10.4049/jimmunol.1103490

Gros, C., Giros, B., and Schwartz, J. C. (1985). Identification of aminopeptidase M as an enkephalin-inactivating enzyme in rat cerebral membranes. *Biochemistry* 24, 2179–2185. doi: 10.1021/bi00330a011

Hegde, S. P., Kumar, A., Kurschner, C., and Shapiro, L. H. (1998). c-Maf interacts with c-Myb to regulate transcription of an early myeloid gene during differentiation. *Mol. Cell. Biol.* 18, 2729–2737.

Hegde, S. P., Zhao, J., Ashmun, R. A., and Shapiro, L. H. (1999). c-Maf induces monocytic differentiation and apoptosis in bipotent myeloid progenitors. *Blood* 94, 1578–1589.

Hu, X., Wei, L., Taylor, T. M., Wei, J., Zhou, X., Wang, J. A., et al. (2011). Hypoxic preconditioning enhances bone marrow mesenchymal stem cell migration via Kv2.1 channel and FAK activation. *Am. J. Physiol. Cell Physiol.* 301, C362–C372. doi: 10.1152/ajpcell.00013.2010

Jamur, M. C., Grodzki, A. C., Berenstein, E. H., Hamawy, M. M., Siraganian, R. P., and Oliver, C. (2005). Identification and characterization of undifferentiated mast cells in mouse bone marrow. *Blood* 105, 4282–4289. doi: 10.1182/blood-2004-02-0756

Kim, S. W., Zhang, H. Z., Kim, C. E., An, H. S., Kim, J. M., and Kim, M. H. (2012). Amniotic mesenchymal stem cells have robust angiogenic properties and are effective in treating hindlimb ischaemia. *Cardiovasc. Res.* 93, 525–534. doi: 10.1093/cvr/cvr328

Liao, X., Lu, S., Zhuo, Y., Winter, C., Xu, W., and Wang, Y. (2012). Visualization of Src and FAK activity during the differentiation process from HMSCs to osteoblasts. *PLoS ONE* 7:e42709. doi: 10.1371/journal.pone.0042709

Limbourg, A., Korff, T., Napp, L. C., Schaper, W., Drexler, H., and Limbourg, F. P. (2009). Evaluation of postnatal arteriogenesis and angiogenesis in a mouse model of hind-limb ischemia. *Nat. Protoc.* 4, 1737–1746. doi: 10.1038/nprot.2009.185

Look, A. T., Ashmun, R. A., Shapiro, L. H., and Peiper, S. C. (1989). Human myeloid plasma membrane glycoprotein CD13 (gp150) is identical to aminopeptidase N. *J. Clin. Invest.* 83, 1299–1307. doi: 10.1172/JCI114015

Luan, Y., and Xu, W. (2007). The structure and main functions of aminopeptidase N. *Curr. Med. Chem.* 14, 639–647. doi: 10.2174/092986707780059571

McClellan, J. B. Jr., and Garner, C. W. (1980). Purification and properties of human intestine alanine aminopeptidase. *Biochim. Biophys. Acta* 613, 160–167. doi: 10.1016/0005-2744(80)90202-8

Meng, F., Rui, Y., Xu, L., Wan, C., Jiang, X., and Li, G. (2013). Aqp1 enhances migration of bone marrow mesenchymal stem cells through regulation of FAK and beta-catenin. *Stem Cells Dev.* 23, 66–75. doi: 10.1089/scd.2013.0185

Mina-Osorio, P. (2008). The moonlighting enzyme CD13: old and new functions to target. *Trends Mol. Med.* 14, 361–371. doi: 10.1016/j.molmed.2008.06.003

Mina-Osorio, P., Winnicka, B., O'Conor, C., Grant, C. L., Vogel, L. K., Rodriguez-Pinto, D., et al. (2008). CD13 is a novel mediator of monocytic/endothelial cell adhesion. *J. Leukoc. Biol.* 84, 448–459. doi: 10.1189/jlb.1107802

Musina, R. A., Bekchanova, E. S., and Sukhikh, G. T. (2005). Comparison of mesenchymal stem cells obtained from different human tissues. *Bull. Exp. Biol. Med.* 139, 504–509. doi: 10.1007/s10517-005-0331-1

Pasqualini, R., Koivunen, E., Kain, R., Lahdenranta, J., Sakamoto, M., Stryhn, A., et al. (2000). Aminopeptidase N is a receptor for tumor-homing peptides and a target for inhibiting angiogenesis. *Cancer Res.* 60, 722–727.

Peister, A., Mellad, J. A., Larson, B. L., Hall, B. M., Gibson, L. F., and Prockop, D. J. (2004). Adult stem cells from bone marrow (MSCs) isolated from different strains of inbred mice vary in surface epitopes, rates of proliferation, and differentiation potential. *Blood* 103, 1662–1668. doi: 10.1182/blood-2003-09-3070

Pereira, F. E., Cronin, C., Ghosh, M., Zhou, S. Y., Agosto, M., Subramani, J., et al. (2013). CD13 is essential for inflammatory trafficking and infarct healing following permanent coronary artery occlusion in mice. *Cardiovasc. Res.* 100, 74–83. doi: 10.1093/cvr/cvt155

Petrovic, N., Schacke, W., Gahagan, J. R., O'Conor, C. A., Winnicka, B., Conway, R. E., et al. (2007). CD13/APN regulates endothelial invasion and filopodia formation. *Blood* 110, 142–150. doi: 10.1182/blood-2006-02-002931

Rahman, M. M., Ghosh, M., Subramani, J., Fong, G. H., Carlson, M., and Shapiro, L. H. (2013). CD13 regulates anchorage and differentiation of the skeletal muscle satellite stem cell population in ischemic injury. *Stem Cells* doi: 10.1002/stem.1610. [Epub ahead of print].

Schulman, I. H., and Hare, J. M. (2012). Key developments in stem cell therapy in cardiology. *Regen. Med.* 7, 17–24. doi: 10.2217/rme.12.80

Seeberger, K. L., Dufour, J. M., Shapiro, A. M., Lakey, J. R., Rajotte, R. V., and Korbutt, G. S. (2006). Expansion of mesenchymal stem cells from human pancreatic ductal epithelium. *Lab. Invest.* 86, 141–153. doi: 10.1038/labinvest.3700377

Shipp, M. A., and Look, A. T. (1993). Hematopoietic differentiation antigens that are membrane-associated enzymes: cutting is the key! *Blood* 82, 1052–1070.

Song, H., Chang, W., Lim, S., Seo, H. S., Shim, C. Y., Park, S., et al. (2007). Tissue transglutaminase is essential for integrin-mediated survival of bone marrow-derived mesenchymal stem cells. *Stem Cells* 25, 1431–1438. doi: 10.1634/stemcells.2006-0467

Stabile, E., Burnett, M. S., Watkins, C., Kinnaird, T., Bachis, A., la Sala, A., et al. (2003). Impaired arteriogenic response to acute hindlimb ischemia in CD4-knockout mice. *Circulation* 108, 205–210. doi: 10.1161/01.CIR.0000079225.50817.71

Subcomittee, I.-W. N. (1984). Nomenclature for clusters of differentiation (CD) of antigens defined on human leukocyte populations. IUIS-WHO nomenclature subcommittee. *Bull. World Health Organ.* 62, 809–815.

Subramani, J., Ghosh, M., Rahman, M. M., Caromile, L. A., Gerber, C., Rezaul, M., et al. (2013). Tyrosine phosphorylation of CD13 regulates inflammatory cell-cell adhesion and monocyte trafficking. *J. Immunol.* 191, 3905–3912. doi: 10.4049/jimmunol.1301348

Trubiani, O., di Primio, R., Traini, T., Pizzicannella, J., Scarano, A., Piattelli, A., et al. (2005). Morphological and cytofluorimetric analysis of adult mesenchymal stem cells expanded *ex vivo* from periodontal ligament. *Int. J. Immunopathol. Pharmacol.* 18, 213–221.

Williams, A. R., and Hare, J. M. (2011). Mesenchymal stem cells: biology, pathophysiology, translational findings, and therapeutic implications for cardiac disease. *Circ. Res.* 109, 923–940. doi: 10.1161/CIRCRESAHA.111.243147

Winnicka, B., O'Conor, C., Schacke, W., Vernier, K., Grant, C. L., Fenteany, F. H., et al. (2010). CD13 is dispensable for normal hematopoiesis and myeloid cell functions in the mouse. *J. Leukoc. Biol.* 88, 347–359. doi: 10.1189/jlb.0210065

Yeager, C. L., Ashmun, R. A., Williams, R. K., Cardellichio, C. B., Shapiro, L. H., Look, A. T., et al. (1992). Human aminopeptidase N is a receptor for human coronavirus 229E. *Nature* 357, 420–422. doi: 10.1038/357420a0

19

Sphingosine 1-phosphate axis: A new leader actor in skeletal muscle biology

Chiara Donati*[1,2], *Francesca Cencetti*[1,2] *and Paola Bruni*[1,2]

[1] *Dipartimento di Scienze Biomediche, Sperimentali e Cliniche, University of Florence, Florence, Italy*
[2] *Istituto Interuniversitario di Miologia, Italy*

Correspondence:
Paola Bruni, Dipartimento di Scienze Biomediche, Sperimentali e Cliniche, Viale GB Morgagni 50, 50134 Florence, Italy
e-mail: paola.bruni@unifi.it

Sphingosine 1-phosphate (S1P) is a bioactive lipid involved in the regulation of biological processes such as proliferation, differentiation, motility, and survival. Here we review the role of S1P in the biology and homeostasis of skeletal muscle. S1P derives from the catabolism of sphingomyelin and is produced by sphingosine phosphorylation catalyzed by sphingosine kinase (SK). S1P can act either intracellularly or extracellularly through specific ligation to its five G protein-coupled receptors (GPCR) named S1P receptors (S1PR). Many experimental findings obtained in the last 20 years demonstrate that S1P and its metabolism play a multifaceted role in the regulation of skeletal muscle regeneration. Indeed, this lipid is known to activate muscle-resident satellite cells, regulating their proliferation and differentiation, as well as mesenchymal progenitors such as mesoangioblasts that originate outside skeletal muscle, both involved in tissue repair following an injury or disease. The molecular mechanism of action of S1P in skeletal muscle cell precursors is highly complex, especially because S1P axis is under the control of a number of growth factors and cytokines, canonical regulators of skeletal muscle biology. Moreover, this lipid is crucially involved in the regulation of skeletal muscle contractile properties, responsiveness to insulin, fatigue resistance and tropism. Overall, on the basis of these findings S1P signaling appears to be an appealing pharmacological target for improving skeletal muscle repair. Nevertheless, further understanding is required on the regulation of S1P downstream signaling pathways and the expression of S1PR. This article will resume our current knowledge on S1P signaling in skeletal muscle, hopefully stimulating further investigation in the field, aimed at individuating novel molecular targets for ameliorating skeletal muscle regeneration and reducing fibrosis of the tissue after a trauma or due to skeletal muscle diseases.

Keywords: sphingosine 1-phosphate, skeletal muscle, skeletal muscle progenitors, satellite cells, muscle regeneration, insulin responsiveness, myoblasts, skeletal muscle metabolism

INTRODUCTION ON SKELETAL MUSCLE

Skeletal muscle represents about 40% of the entire body weight. The functional and structural constituent of skeletal muscle is the myofiber, multinucleated cell that derives from the fusion of mesodermal precursors named myoblasts. Each myofiber is delimited by the basal lamina and is composed of myofibrils of actin and myosin, organized as a sarcomere, the functional unit of skeletal muscle. On the basis of their physiological features, muscle fibers can be distinguished into slow contracting, fatigue resistant fibers and fast contracting, fatigue sensitive fibers.

Skeletal muscle exerts physiological roles relevant for the control of body metabolism since it accounts for bloodstream aminoacid disposal in fasting condition and for removing excess glucose by favoring glycogen accumulation in response to insulin after a meal. Moreover, by releasing heat during force generation it contributes to body temperature maintenance.

During development, the number of myofibers following myoblast fusion increase, while in adulthood skeletal muscle is stable beyond infrequent fusion of satellite cells to compensate physiologic turnover. Following a trauma, injury, or disease skeletal muscle has indeed the potential to regenerate thanks to an highly orchestrated process driven by satellite cells and their niche (Yin et al., 2013).

Satellite cells are the resident stem cells of the skeletal muscle, located between the basal lamina of muscle fibers and the plasma membrane. Even if it is known that satellite cells derive from somites, their exact progenitor cell is still elusive. Satellite cells are quiescent in adult skeletal muscle and represent 3–6% of the total nuclei in the fiber (Tedesco et al., 2010). When activated, they start proliferating and can generate in few days a large number of myofibers: it has been demonstrated that few as seven satellite cells transplanted into irradiated muscle of dystrophic immune-deficient mice led to an increase of 100 new muscle fibers with thousands of myonuclei (Collins et al., 2005). Activated satellite cells cultured on plastic collagen-coated dishes are named "satellite cell-derived myoblasts" or myogenic precursor cells distinct from a functional and molecular point of view from freshly isolated satellite cells, possibly due to the absence of their niche (Dhawan and Rando, 2005; Pallafacchina et al., 2010). Stem cells can self-renew in asymmetric and symmetric division. In asymmetric division the parental stem cell divides into two different daughter cells, one remains stem cell, the other fated to differentiate. In symmetric division the parental stem cell gives rise to two daughter stem cells of equal stemness. Satellite cells can undergo asymmetric and symmetric division and non-canonical Wnt signaling plays a role in the regulation of self-renewal (Chargé and Rudnicki, 2004; Troy et al., 2012). A number of satellite cell markers have been identified such as Pax3, Pax7, Myf5, M-cadherin, cMet, CD34, CXCR4, although they are not unique and there is not complete correspondence between mouse and human (Yin et al., 2013).

In addition to satellite cells, other skeletal muscle progenitors including pericytes (Dellavalle et al., 2011), mesoangioblasts (Minasi et al., 2002), bone marrow stem cells (LaBarge and Blau, 2002), and interstitial cells (Mitchell et al., 2010) located outside the myofiber, have been demonstrated to have the ability to regenerate skeletal muscle, although to a negligible extent compared with satellite cells (Judson et al., 2013). Nowadays there is a great interest in understanding the molecular mechanisms of skeletal muscle regeneration since it will permit the development of cell therapies for skeletal muscle diseases such as muscular dystrophies (Tedesco et al., 2010), a group of inherited disorders characterized by progressive muscle wasting and depletion of the satellite cell pool after extensive cycle of regeneration (Carlson and Conboy, 2007; Chakkalakal et al., 2012; Pannérec et al., 2012; García-Prat et al., 2013). Muscular dystrophies are indeed very difficult to treat because skeletal muscle is composed of hundreds of millions of post-mitotic nuclei.

SPHINGOLIPID METABOLISM AND SPHINGOSINE 1-PHOSPHATE FORMATION

During the last 20 years, sphingolipids, initially considered structural component of eukaryotic membranes, have been highlighted as a crucial molecules involved in the regulation of fundamental biological processes such as cell migration, survival, proliferation, differentiation, adhesion, and implicated in inflammation, tumorigenesis, immunity and vascular development (Hannun and Obeid, 2008; Maceyka et al., 2012). In this review we will focus on the role of the bioactive sphingolipid sphingosine 1-phosphate (S1P), its metabolism, its receptors and its cross-talk with growth factors and cytokines in skeletal muscle biology and physiology.

Ceramide, a largely known effector of stress responses (Zeidan and Hannun, 2010) plays a central role in sphingolipid metabolism. The first step in the *de novo* pathway of ceramide production is the condensation reaction catalyzed by the enzyme serine palmitoyl transferase to form dihydrosphingosine from palmitoyl-CoA and the aminoacid serine. Dihydrosphingosine is then acylated by the action of ceramide synthase to dihydroceramide which is then desaturated to ceramide by the enzyme ceramide desaturase. Ceramide can be also generated by the breakdown of membrane sphingomyelins, catalyzed by the action of various sphingomyelinases or by the degradation of complex glycosphingolipids by the action of glucosylceramidases. The acyl chain of ceramide is then removed by the action of ceramidases and the amino alcohol sphingosine is produced. Sphingosine can be reconverted to ceramide by the action of ceramide synthase via the so-called salvage pathway mechanism. Sphingosine can be phosphorylated in an ATP-dependent manner to S1P by the enzymes sphingosine kinase (SK) 1 and SK2. S1P can be dephosphorylated back to sphingosine by the action of two specific S1P phosphatases and by three lipid phosphate phosphatases. Alternatively, S1P is irreversibly degraded by the action of S1P lyase (SPL) into hexadecenal and phosphoethanolamine.

SK1 is a cytosolic enzyme which contains residues that bind acidic phospholipids that contribute to its intracellular localization (Stahelin et al., 2005). Numerous agonists have been reported to be able to activate SK1, including growth factors, hormones, cytokines, and G protein-coupled receptors (GPCR) ligands. Following ERK phosphorylation at serine 225, SK1 translocates to plasma membrane where its substrate sphingosine is localized (Pitson et al., 2003). The regulation of SK localization within the cell is the major mechanism by which the enzyme affects sphingolipid metabolism since only minute increases in the activity are reported following stimulation with different agonists. Once produced, S1P, precisely partitioned into plasma membrane microdomains, is then locally released to activate S1P receptors (S1PR) acting in autocrine and/or paracrine manner. This process is called "inside-out" signaling. Different transporters have been implicated in S1P export such as the ATP binding cassette transporters, ABCC1 (Mitra et al., 2006), ABCA1 (Sato et al., 2007), ABCG2 (Takabe et al., 2010), and more recently the specific spinster 2 (Spns2) (Kawahara et al., 2009); however, no information on their role in skeletal muscle is presently available. Additionally, since the chloride ion channel CFTR has a role in mediating S1P transport and signaling in heart (Meissner et al., 2012) and lack of CFTR causes functional alteration in skeletal muscle (Divangahi et al., 2009), it will be of interest to further investigate this issue.

In contrast to SK1, SK2 is localized in several intracellular compartments such as endoplasmic reticulum, nucleus, and mitochondria. Even if it is known that ERK-mediated phosphorylation is required for SK2 activation, the exact mechanism of SK2 regulation is still elusive. While SK1-formed S1P is rapidly exported outside the cell through the transporters localized at the plasma membrane, SK2-produced S1P at the level of mitochondria and endoplasmic reticulum is likely rapidly degraded or dephosphorylated by SPL and phosphatases present in close proximity. Therefore, SK2 has, in respect to SK1, an enhanced ability to recycle sphingoid bases for ceramide synthesis (Le Stunff et al., 2007). Compared to SK1, less is known about the mechanism of SK2 regulation. It has been reported that EGF and phorbol ester (Hait et al., 2007) activates the enzyme. Moreover, under hypoxia an increase in SK2 protein level and enzymatic activity has been demonstrated (Schnitzer et al., 2009).

Bioactive S1P can either function as ligand of a family of GPCR named S1PR and through intracellular targets, some of them recently identified. There are five specific S1PR, $S1PR_{1-5}$, all with low nM Kd values. Since these receptors couple to multiple α subunits of heterotrimeric G proteins and are differentially expressed in diverse cell types and tissues, they induce the activation of different downstream targets such as ERK, Rac, Rho, JNK, adenylyl cyclase, phospholipase C, thus evoking distinct, sometimes overlapping or opposite, biological responses. While $S1P_{1-3}$ are ubiquitously expressed, $S1P_4$ and $S1P_5$ are tissue specific, being mostly expressed in the lymphoid and central nervous system, respectively (Spiegel and Milstien, 2003). $S1P_1$ plays a crucial role in angiogenesis, indeed its deletion in mice is embryonic lethal due to hemorrhage for incomplete vascular maturation since pericytes do not migrate to the nascent endothelial tubes (Liu et al., 2000). $S1P_2$ null mice are deaf indicating that $S1P_2$ is required for proper development of the auditory and vestibular systems (Kono et al., 2007). Unlike $S1P_1$ null mice, $S1P_3$ deletion in mice do not generate any obvious phenotype.

A number of cytokines and growth factors have been reported to regulate the expression of the enzymes of S1P metabolism (Lebman and Spiegel, 2008). In addition to S1PR transactivation following stimulation with growth factors and cytokines, S1P ligation to its receptors also transactivates growth factor tyrosine kinase receptors. This mutual functional cross-talk regulates fundamental biological processes such as growth, differentiation, and motility in various cell types.

Many data reported in literature support that the intracellular role of S1P is that of counteracting the biological actions of ceramide in the so-called "rheostat model" where the S1P-forming enzyme SK plays a crucial role. Although S1P was discovered as intracellular messenger (Olivera and Spiegel, 1993), only recently, some of the intracellular targets of S1P have begun to be identified. SK2 present in the nucleus has been demonstrated to form a complex with histone H3 and histone deacetylases (HDACs). SK2-produced S1P binds to and inhibits HDAC1/2, thus contributing to the regulation of the epigenetic control of specific genes (Hait et al., 2009). Instead, tumor necrosis factor receptor associated factor 2 (TRAF2), a crucial component in NFkB signaling triggered by TNFα, has been reported as intracellular target for S1P produced by SK1. Indeed, S1P formed by SK1, which is known to co-localize with TRAF2 (Xia et al., 2002) has been found to bind to TRAF2 and stimulate its dormant ubiquitin ligase activity upstream of NFkB activation (Alvarez et al., 2010). Moreover, SK2-produced S1P in the mitochondrion binds *in vitro* and *in vivo* to prohibitin 2, a conserved protein that regulates mitochondrial assembly and function. SK2 null mice display reduced mitochondria respiration, suggesting that S1P/prohibitin 2 interaction is physiologically relevant for mitochondrial function (Strub et al., 2011).

BIOLOGICAL ROLE OF S1P IN SATELLITE CELLS

A number of recently published papers support the role of S1P axis in the regulation of muscle resident satellite cell biology. Indeed, S1P was identified as one of the few extracellular cues capable of stimulating quiescent satellite cells to enter the cell cycle (Nagata et al., 2006). Inhibition of S1P formation by incubation with the SK inhibitor dimethylsphingosine (DMS) significantly reduced satellite cell activation in response to mitogen and impaired satellite cell-driven muscle regeneration in response to *in vivo* damage induced by cardiotoxin. Moreover, the authors showed that the degradation of the sphingomyelin inner leaflet pool accounts for the generation of S1P, then regulating satellite cell activation. In line with these findings, Calise et al. have characterized the S1PR involved in the mitogenic effect of S1P and the underlying mechanism of action (Calise et al., 2012). Satellite cells express 4 out of 5 S1PR, $S1PR_{1-4}$, being $S1P_3$ the most expressed one in growing conditions. Indeed, by utilizing specific receptor antagonist and siRNA silencing, S1P was demonstrated to stimulate labeled thymidine incorporation by engagement of $S1P_2$ and $S1P_3$ in a PI3K-dependent manner. Moreover, the authors demonstrated also that S1P positively stimulates satellite cell migration via specific ligation to $S1P_1$ and $S1P_4$. This latter finding, for the first time, highlights the role of $S1P_4$ in skeletal muscle beyond its already established relevance in lymphoid tissue. Very recently it has been shown that $S1P_3$ suppresses cell cycle progression in murine satellite cells (Fortier et al., 2013). Indeed, satellite cells isolated from $S1P_3$ null mice showed enhanced *ex-vivo* proliferation, while retrovirally-mediated constitutive expression of $S1P_3$ inhibited cell proliferation of satellite cells.

BIOLOGICAL ROLE OF S1P IN OTHER SKELETAL MUSCLE PROGENITORS

Skeletal muscle regeneration, besides being due to the presence of resident satellite cells in skeletal muscle, is carried on, *in vivo* or after transplantation, by progenitors that originates outside the basal lamina such as pericytes, interstitial cells, mesoangioblasts, and adipose tissue-derived mesenchymal stem cells (ASC). The characterization of the molecular mechanism of the myogenic potential of these progenitors is nowadays of great interest since such kind of knowledge could be applied in the development of cell therapies for diseases characterized by skeletal muscle degeneration. S1P axis has been shown to play a role in the regulation of fundamental biological parameters such as proliferation, migration and differentiation of multipotent adult stem cells such as mesoangioblasts (Donati et al., 2007a, 2009, 2011), and ASC (Nincheri et al., 2009).

Mesoangioblasts (Minasi et al., 2002) are vascular progenitors associated with dorsal aorta in avian and mammalian species, that when transplanted *in vivo* give rise to multiple mesodermal cell types such as osteoblasts, chondrocytes, and muscle cells. They show an extensive ability of *in vitro* self-renewing and upon injection, are able to cross the endothelial barrier and can fuse with muscle fibers, contributing to their regeneration. Indeed, mesoangioblasts have been demonstrated to contribute to muscle regeneration in animal models of muscular dystrophy such as α-sarcoglycan null mice (Sampaolesi et al., 2003) and golden retriever dystrophic dogs (Sampaolesi et al., 2006). $S1P_{1-3}$ were detected at mRNA level in mesoangioblasts with $S1P_3$ the predominantly expressed receptor. S1P has been demonstrated to potently stimulate mesoangioblast proliferation in $S1P_2$-dependent manner (Donati et al., 2007a). Moreover, the bioactive sphingolipid successfully contrasted the apoptosis induced by different apoptogenic stimuli, without engagement of S1PR. It is important to note that pre-treatment of mesoangioblasts with S1P enhanced their survival when injected in the tibialis anterior muscle of α-sarcoglycan null dystrophic mice, further supporting a role for the sphingolipid in preventing programmed cell death. Moreover, the SK/S1P axis was found to be involved in the anti-apoptotic action exerted by TGFβ in these cells (Donati et al., 2009). RNA silencing or overexpression of dominant negative mutant form of SK1 highlighted a key role of SK1 but not SK2 in mediating TGFβ pro-survival action. The cytokine increased SK activity and up-regulated SK1 expression which was down-regulated by the apoptotic challenge. A successive study demonstrated the crucial role of the cross-talk between S1P and TGFβ in the biology of mesoangioblasts. Data obtained by a cDNA microarray study, validated by real time PCR and immunofluorescence microscopy approaches, highlighted that S1P exerts a strong differentiating action of mesoangioblasts toward smooth muscle cells. Interestingly it was shown that S1P axis was required by TGFβ to exert its differentiating activity toward smooth muscle on mesoangioblasts. The study individuated also the transcription factor GATA6 as a novel player in the complex transcriptional regulation of mesoangioblast differentiation to smooth muscle. S1P up-regulated the expression of GATA6 which was responsible for the enhanced expression of smooth muscle contractile proteins. By specific silencing of GATA6 it was demonstrated that the transcription factor was critical also in the pro-differentiating activity of TGFβ (Donati et al., 2011).

ASC are mesenchymal stem cells able to differentiate into different mesodermal lineages (Chamberlain et al., 2007). Being relatively easy to isolate and able to rapidly proliferate *in vitro*, these cells are promising in the development of cell therapy tools. S1P administration to ASC up-regulated the expression of smooth muscle protein markers, induced the appearance of calcium currents and of actin cytoskeleton reorganization typical of smooth muscle cells. S1P differentiating action was found to rely on $S1P_2$ engagement while $S1P_3$ role was less critical (Nincheri et al., 2009).

BIOLOGICAL ROLE OF S1P SIGNALING AXIS IN MYOBLASTS

C2C12 cell line is a subclone of the parental C2 cells which differentiate into myotubes in appropriate culture condition, after serum deprivation (Yaffe and Saxel, 1977; Blau et al., 1985). This model is therefore widely used as a tool to study the myogenic differentiation process and the involved molecular mechanisms.

C2C12 cells express 4 out of 5 S1PR, $S1P_{1-4}$, being $S1P_1$ the most expressed receptor (Meacci et al., 2003; Bruni and Donati, 2013; Donati et al., 2013). Earlier reports showed that in C2C12 cells exogenous S1P activates a number of signaling pathways: indeed it induced a rapid stimulation of phospholipase D activity (Meacci et al., 1999) and a transient and rapid membrane association of RhoA (Meacci et al., 2000) in a PKC-dependent manner. Moreover, the bioactive lipid was demonstrated to induce Ca^{2+} mobilization in a $S1P_{2/3}$-dependent manner (Meacci et al., 2002). Interestingly, differentiation of C2C12 myoblasts into myotubes was accompanied by deep changes in expression of S1PR. Indeed, $S1P_2$ was down-regulated while $S1P_3$ was up-regulated in differentiated cells (Meacci et al., 2003), suggesting that $S1P_2$ plays a role in myoblasts but is dispensable in myotubes. The crucial role of $S1P_2$ in myogenic differentiation of C2C12 myoblasts was demonstrated in a later study, where S1P was shown to exert via this receptor subtype a negative action on serum-induced proliferation and to act as a potent inducer of differentiation (Donati et al., 2005). The role of $S1P_2$ was demonstrated by pharmacological and genetic approaches. The involvement of $S1P_2$ in myogenic differentiation was further confirmed by a subsequent report where the compound K6PC5, a synthetic derivative of ceramide, previously shown to induce SK1 activation in keratinocytes (Kwon et al., 2007), stimulated myoblast differentiation in a $S1P_2$-dependent manner (Bernacchioni et al., 2011).

$S1P_2$ was also identified as the responsible for the inhibitory effect on myoblast directional motility and insulin like growth factor-1 (IGF-1)-induced chemotaxis exerted by S1P in C2C12 myoblasts (Becciolini et al., 2006), in line with the anti-migratory action of this receptor demonstrated in other cell systems (Arikawa et al., 2003; Lepley et al., 2005). In this study was also established the involvement of RhoA activation in the negative regulation of cell motility.

During muscle regeneration, following satellite cell activation and migration to the site of lesion, inhibition of myoblast motility and differentiation into myotubes takes place in a highly orchestrated manner. In view of its role as muscle pleiotropic regulatory molecule, S1P exerts a dual role on cell migration, stimulating at first migration of activated satellite cells (Calise et al., 2012) and then inhibiting that of C2C12 myoblasts (Becciolini et al., 2006), subsequently to a timely remodeling of S1PR expression pattern, thus favoring skeletal muscle repair (**Table 1**).

During *in vitro* differentiation of C2C12 myoblasts, a small population of cells, named reserve cells remains undifferentiated, thus resembling quiescent satellite cells (Yoshida et al., 1998). The analysis of the role of S1PR in regulating cell proliferation highlighted that in reserve cells, S1P, via specific coupling to $S1P_1$, stimulates cell proliferation similarly to what demonstrated in satellite cells but differently from what shown in myoblasts (Rapizzi et al., 2008). In view of the finely regulated expression of S1PR during commitment and differentiation of myogenic precursors which drive different biological outcomes of the bioactive lipid, future studies are required to characterize the specific molecular mechanisms regulating the differential expression of S1PR and their coupling.

Successive studies have elucidated some downstream events implicated in the promyogenic effect of the sphingolipid. Indeed, exogenous addition of S1P to C2C12 myoblasts up-regulated the expression of the gap junctional protein connexin-43 (Squecco et al., 2006), and the transient receptor potential cation channel, a component of the stretch activated channel (Formigli et al., 2007; Meacci et al., 2010).

The role of S1P metabolism, with special attention to SK, the enzyme responsible for S1P production, in the regulation of C2C12 cell growth and differentiation has been highlighted. Indeed, the expression of SK1 was found to be enhanced in differentiating myoblasts (Meacci et al., 2008). Additionally, when overexpressed, SK1 was responsible for a significative reduction of

Table 1 | Role of sphingosine 1-phosphate on cell proliferation and migration in myoblasts and activated satellite cells.

	Cell Proliferation	Cell Migration
C2C12 Myoblasts	↓	↓
Activated Satellite Cells	↑	↑

myoblast proliferation rate, while it enhanced the appearance of a differentiated phenotype and the expression of myogenic marker proteins. On the contrary, when SK1 was silenced or a dominant negative mutant form of the enzyme was overexpressed, myoblast proliferation was increased and myogenic differentiation rate was reduced. The role of $S1P_2$ in myogenic differentiation was also confirmed in this study, since when the receptor was silenced, the pro-myogenic action of SK1 overexpression was abolished. Therefore, although in the literature SK1 has been reported to have a mitogenic role (Maceyka et al., 2012), in myoblasts this enzyme displays an opposite biological effect.

As outlined above, SK activity is under the control of a variety of growth factors, cytokines, neurotransmitters, and hormones (Maceyka et al., 2012), which leads to the existence of functional cross-talks further complicating S1P signaling. Following the demonstration of the role of SK1 in myogenesis, several reports have shown that a number of growth factors and cytokine, known as crucial regulator of skeletal muscle biology, co-opt S1P signaling (**Figures 1**, **2**). The pro-inflammatory cytokine TNFα, which is critically implicated in the remodeling of skeletal muscle (Li and Schwartz, 2001), at low doses has been shown to translocate SK1 to membrane and, via $S1P_2$ engagement, to stimulate C2C12 myoblast differentiation (Donati et al., 2007b). Notably, IGF-1, one of the most important physiological regulator of skeletal muscle regeneration (Pedersen and Febbraio, 2012), activates both SK isoforms, SK1 and SK2, and via specific transactivation of $S1P_2$, exerts its myogenic action (Bernacchioni et al., 2012). Moreover, IGF-1 is also responsible for SK-dependent transactivation of $S1P_1$ and $S1P_3$ that in turn reduce the mitogenic effect of the growth factor.

Interestingly, also platelet derived growth factor (PDGF), another growth factor relevant for the biology and the repair of skeletal muscle (Husmann et al., 1996), exerts a negative role on myoblast proliferation via selective SK1 activation and $S1P_1$ transactivation. Moreover, S1P inside-out signaling and $S1P_1$ engagement appear to be necessary for conveying of PDGF-induced chemotactic action. It is important to note that despite the importance of $S1P_1$ engagement in the biological action of IGF-1 and PDGF in myoblasts, $S1P_1$ down-regulation or pharmacological inhibition did not affect the biological responses evoked by exogenously added S1P (Donati et al., 2005; Becciolini et al., 2006). This observation suggests that spatial regulation of S1P generation inside the cell is critical for determining the subset of engaged receptors, its final biological outcomes and that $S1P_1$ is not freely accessible to its ligand from outside the cell. Indeed, structural evidence indicated that ligand binding to $S1P_1$ occurs by initial delivery of S1P to the exterior portion of membrane followed by a lateral diffusion into the receptor binding pocket (O'Sullivan and Dev, 2013).

SK/S1P axis is also exploited by TGFβ to transmit its pro-fibrotic, anti-differentiating action in C2C12 myoblasts (Cencetti et al., 2010). Unfortunately, during muscle regeneration, the transdifferentiation of myoblasts and muscle resident fibroblasts into myofibroblasts give rise to muscle fibrosis that reduces muscle contractile properties and impairs full muscular recovery. The cytokine TGFβ plays a crucial role in the promotion of the fibrosis onset and in the inhibition of myogenesis (McLennan and Koishi, 2002); importantly, the inhibition of TGFβ signaling pathway has been shown to ameliorate the chronic degenerative fibrosis of dystrophic muscles (Cohn et al., 2007). Indeed, TGFβ induced a Smad-dependent up-regulation of SK1 expression and activation, which, in contrast to what expected on the basis of the previously demonstrated SK1 role in myogenesis (Donati et al., 2005; Meacci et al., 2008), redirected the final S1P biological outcome from being promyogenic to profibrotic since the cytokine induced also a profound remodeling of S1PR expression pattern, at least at mRNA levels. This was responsible for readdressing the pro-myogenic role mediated through $S1P_2$ to a pro-fibrotic role mediated by $S1P_3$, which following TGFβ administration, became the most expressed receptor. These data support the concept that interfering with $S1P_3$ signaling might favor therapeutic intervention to reduce skeletal muscle fibrosis.

Very recently a new signaling pathway related to TGFβ-induced apoptosis has been identified in C2C12 myoblasts which relies on Rho kinase-2 stimulation, subsequent to SMAD-dependent TGFβ-induced $S1P_4$ up-regulation and transactivation via SK2 (Cencetti et al., 2013). This finding supports the notion that $S1P_4$ is up-regulated by TGFβ and is relevant for the apoptotic action of the cytokine in skeletal muscle.

BIOLOGICAL ROLE OF S1P IN SKELETAL MUSCLE

Skeletal muscle has the ability to adapt to different physiological and pathological conditions since it displays a high degree of

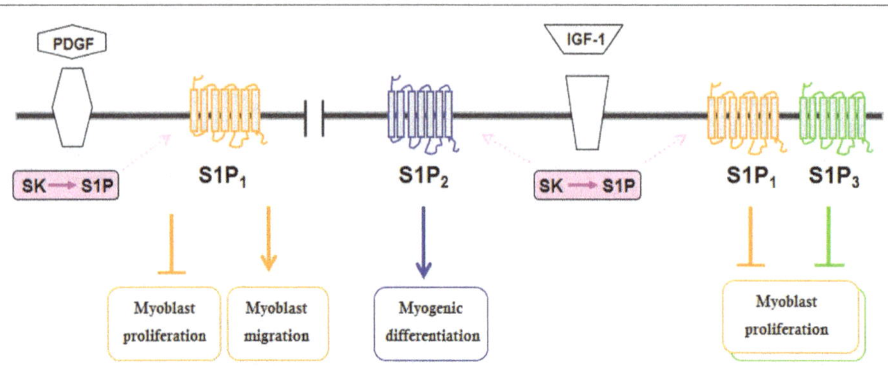

FIGURE 1 | Schematic diagram of the biological actions evoked by S1PR transactivation by some growth factors in C2C12 myoblasts.

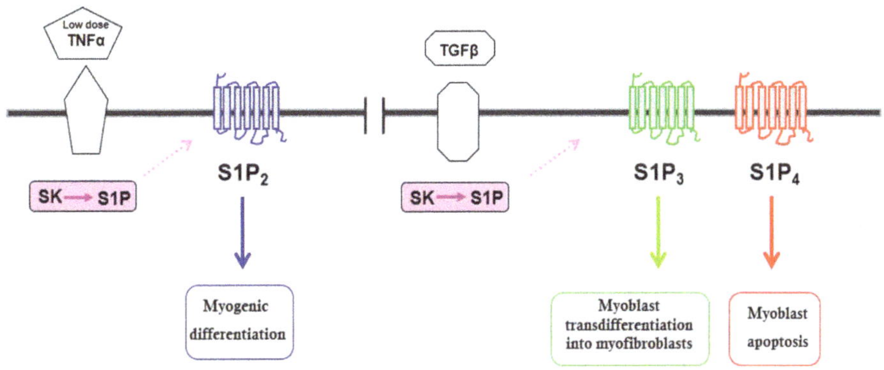

FIGURE 2 | Schematic diagram of the biological actions evoked by S1PR transactivation by some cytokines in C2C12 myoblasts.

plasticity. The size of skeletal muscle fibers results from a balance between protein synthesis and degradation, and varies as a consequence of physiological and pathological circumstances. The increase of individual muscle fibers, i.e., hypertrophy, occurs when protein synthesis exceeds protein degradation in response to hormonal stimulation or mechanical overload. A reduction in skeletal muscle mass and fiber size, i.e., atrophy, occurs in response to catabolic hormonal stimulation, denervation, aging, cancer, bed rest, and starvation (Schiaffino et al., 2013). S1P has been reported to be involved in the regulation of some physiological properties of skeletal muscle such as muscle contractility, fatigue, and adaptation.

Indeed, S1P has been shown to affect the excitation-contraction coupling in fibers isolated from murine extensor digitorum longus (EDL). The bioactive lipid modulated the voltage threshold and the inward calcium current through the dihydropyridine receptor in a $S1P_3$-dependent manner although the experiments were carried out in the presence of the unspecific receptor antagonist suramin (Bencini et al., 2003).

Zanin et al. (2008) has demonstrated a trophic role for S1P in a rat model of denervation atrophy. S1P, delivered to the muscle through a mini osmotic pump, significantly reduced the negative effects of denervation on muscle mass and cross sectional area (CSA) after 7 and 14 days of regeneration. Moreover, despite its established anti-proliferative and pro-apoptotic role (Bruni and Donati, 2008), also sphingosine exerted a trophic effect, likely due to its conversion to S1P catalyzed by SK, as suggested by the abolishment of the positive action of the sphingolipid in the presence of DMS. Moreover, by real time PCR, $S1P_1$, and $S1P_3$ were found to be selectively expressed, and subjected to down-regulation upon denervation.

The decline in the ability of skeletal muscle to generate force after a strenuous exercise is named muscle fatigue. The process is reversible and depends on multiple factors such as the intensity and the duration of the contraction and the type of fibers of the muscles. Exogenous S1P has been found able of reducing muscle fatigue of EDL muscles (Danieli-Betto et al., 2005). Interestingly, administration of sphingosine significantly diminished the tension decline. Since sphingosine effect was reduced in the presence of the unselective SK inhibitor DMS, it was deduced that the mechanism of action implicates S1P production through SK activation. Indeed the effect of sphingosine, but not that of S1P, was abolished in the absence of Ca^{2+}, suggesting a Ca^{2+}-dependent mechanism of activation of SK.

The role of S1P signaling in skeletal muscle regeneration has been firstly demonstrated in mouse and rat models after myotoxic injury induced by bupivacaine (Danieli-Betto et al., 2010). The administration of S1P after muscle damage induced a significant increase of CSA while the neutralization of circulating S1P by administration of an anti-S1P antibody abolished fiber growth. Western blotting analysis of S1PR expression in muscle lysates during rat soleus regeneration showed dynamic changes of S1PR at protein level suggesting their putative role during regeneration. The S1P-induced increase of regenerating fiber growth was inhibited by a selective $S1P_1$ agonist and augmented by a selective $S1P_{1/3}$ antagonist, supporting a negative role of $S1P_1$ and a positive role of $S1P_3$ in the early phases of regeneration. In contrast, a very recent study demonstrated that in $S1P_3$ null mice acute muscle regeneration was enhanced and that genetic ablation of $S1P_3$ in mdx mice produced a less severe dystrophic phenotype (Fortier et al., 2013). Further studies are therefore required to clarify the exact role of $S1P_3$ in skeletal muscle regeneration.

Herr et al. (2003) have demonstrated that mutation in the gene that encodes for the homolog of SPL generates Sply mutants in fruit fly that do not catalyze S1P degradation and accumulate S1P. In these mutants the thoracic flight muscles degenerate due to the absence of fibers in the dorsal longitudinal muscles. These findings highlight the importance of sphingolipid metabolism in muscle homeostasis, crucial for adult muscle development and integrity.

Presently, beside mammalian models to study muscular dystrophy including mouse, dog and cat, genetically tractable models have been established in *Danio rerio* and *Drosophila melanogaster* (Shcherbata et al., 2007). Very recently, a paper published by Pantoja et al. (2013), demonstrated that suppression of *wunen*, an homolog of lipid phosphate phosphatase 3, suppresses dystrophic muscle phenotype measured by evaluation of correct localization of the titin-homolog, projectin, in sarcomeres and functional movements. The authors demonstrated that wunen suppression acts through the elevation of S1P levels, since analogous findings were obtained altering S1P levels genetically via down-regulation of SPL or up-regulation of serine palmitoyl-CoA transferase, or pharmacologically by oral administration of SPL inhibitors. The same authors have very recently demonstrated that an increase of S1P levels via administration of an SPL inhibitor positively affected acute muscle regeneration of dystrophic mdx mice. The beneficial effects of S1P on increased muscle fiber size, force, diminished fibrosis, and fat accumulation were linked to the ability of S1P of increasing the number of myogenic cells (Ieronimakis et al., 2013).

The role of $S1P_2$ *in vivo* in the early phases of regeneration has been demonstrated recently by Germinario et al. (2012) after injection of notexin in two mouse model of $S1P_2$ deficiency: the $S1P_2$ null mice and wild-type mice systemically administered with the $S1P_2$ antagonist JTE-013. Indeed, the absence of $S1P_2$ or its blockade delayed the regeneration of skeletal muscle measured as soleus CSA. Interestingly, the systemic administration of an anti-S1P antibody, which induced a reduction of soleus fiber growth in wild-type mice was ineffective in the absence of $S1P_2$.

Microarray study revealed that during mouse skeletal muscle regeneration following notexin injury, while *sphk1* gene is upregulated at early time points, *sgpl1* gene is induced several days post injury (Loh et al., 2012). SPL is expressed at very low level in skeletal muscle at rest, while is up-regulated in response to ischemia (Kumar and Saba, 2009) and radiation (Bandhuvula et al., 2011). The specific requirement for SK1 to support muscle regeneration and satellite cell recruitment has been demonstrated in SK1 null mice. Interestingly the plasma of dystrophic mdx mice display reduced S1P levels, comparable to that of SK1 null mice, probably due to a significant up-regulation of *sgpl1* rather than down-regulation of *sphK1* or *sphK2* genes. Tetrahydroxybutylimidazole, unspecific inhibitor of SPL, improved the number of regenerating fibers in dystrophic muscles and satellite cell activation. The combination of pharmacological inhibitors, S1PR antagonists and plasmid constructs *in vitro* showed that S1P recruits satellite cells through activation on $S1PR_2$/Rho GTPase/STAT3 signaling axis (Loh et al., 2012).

BIOLOGICAL ROLE OF S1P IN INSULIN RESPONSIVENESS OF SKELETAL MUSCLE

Skeletal muscle plays a crucial role in the regulation of whole body metabolism. In response to insulin, in fed condition, skeletal muscle is responsible for glucose removal from the bloodstream thus contributing to the majority of glucose disposal for the building-up of glycogen. Since skeletal muscle utilizes the majority of body glucose, reduced insulin responsiveness in skeletal muscle leads to the development of metabolic syndrome (McGarry, 2002). SK1/S1P axis has recently been implicated in the regulation of glucose metabolism. In C2C12 myoblasts pharmacological inhibition of SK1 reduced insulin-stimulated glucose uptake while its overexpression mimicked *in vivo* insulin action. Moreover, overexpression of SK1 gene reduced blood glucose level in diabetic mice (Ma et al., 2007). In keeping with the role of S1P as insulin-mimetic cue, a study has reported that in C2C12 myoblasts S1P, through engagement of $S1P_2$, produces a transient burst of reactive oxygen species which is sensed by protein tyrosine phosphatase-1B, the main negative regulator of insulin receptor phosphorylation, which undergoes inhibition. This blockade provokes a ligand-independent trans-phosphorylation of insulin receptor and a strong increase in glucose uptake (Rapizzi et al., 2009). This study appears to provide the possible mechanistic explanation of the insulin-mimetic action of SK1 overexpression, highlighting a feedback responsible for the sustained activation of insulin receptor. Since in this study possible implications of S1P-directed insulin signaling in diabetes were not established, future studies are required aimed at clarifying whether impaired S1P signaling contributes to the development of insulin resistance and whether improvement of S1P/$S1P_2$ signaling would be beneficial for glucose disposal by skeletal muscle.

In addition to the role of elevated triacylglycerol levels in skeletal muscle for the development of insulin sensitivity (McGarry, 2002), a number of reports support the role of ceramide for diminished insulin responsiveness. Taking into account that SK plays a crucial role in the regulation of the relative levels of ceramide/sphingosine and S1P, it will be of crucial interest in the future to understand whether the biological effects observed as consequence of SK overexpression are due to specific S1P-induced signaling or rather to diminution of ceramide cellular levels.

In this line, transgenic mice overexpressing SK1 display improved insulin sensitivity compared to wild-type animal after a 6 week high fat diet, due to increased SK activity in skeletal muscle and decreased intracellular ceramide content (Bruce et al., 2012). The same authors have demonstrated that daily treatment with FTY720, that acts as functional antagonist of S1PR and has been reported to inhibit the activity of ceramide synthase *in vitro* (Berdyshev et al., 2009; Lahiri et al., 2009), for 6 weeks after an high fat diet improved mice glucose tolerance, insulin uptake and Akt phosphorylation through ceramide, diacylglycerol, and triacylglycerol reduction in muscle (Bruce et al., 2013). Interestingly, the expression levels of the enzymes involved in sphingolipid metabolism were not altered.

It has been demonstrated that treatment with palmitate in C2C12 myotubes increased S1P as consequence of increased expression and activity of SK1 (Hu et al., 2009). Very recently, in the context of free fatty acid oversupply it has been shown that SK1 is regulated at transcriptional level by the transcription factor PPARα in C2C12 cells (Ross et al., 2013). Moreover, specifically in skeletal muscle palmitate treatment induced the expression of IL-6 and its downstream signaling in a SK1- and $S1P_3$-dependent manner. IL-6 expression, which is up-regulated in diet-induced obese mice, was attenuated in SK1 null mice. IL-6 produced by skeletal muscle is the prototype of an emerging class of cytokines named myokines which mediate the cross-talk between muscle and other tissues. The role of IL-6 and its signaling in skeletal muscle of obese mice remain unaddressed in this study. Since several studies have reported that muscular IL-6 has a role in metabolism rather than in inflammation, working as an energy sensor and as a lipolytic factor (Pedersen and Febbraio, 2012), the role of SK in the regulation of IL-6 expression and release by skeletal muscle should also be therefore further investigated in other experimental settings.

CONCLUSION

Overall, the here reported experimental findings highlight the fundamental role of S1P signaling axis in skeletal muscle biology.

Future studies will confidently dissect in detail the molecular mechanisms that regulate S1P metabolism and S1PR expression in the various aspects of skeletal muscle biology and hopefully they will bring to characterize the therapeutic potential of S1P signaling pathway in skeletal muscle diseases.

ACKNOWLEDGMENTS

This work was supported in part by funds from the University of Florence, Fondazione Cassa di Risparmio di Lucca e PRIN 2009 to Paola Bruni.

REFERENCES

Alvarez, S. E., Harikumar, K. B., Hait, N. C., Allegood, J., Strub, G. M., Kim, E. Y., et al. (2010). Sphingosine-1-phosphate is a missing cofactor for the E3 ubiquitin ligase TRAF2. *Nature* 465, 1084–1088. doi: 10.1038/nature09128

Arikawa, K., Takuwa, N., Yamaguchi, H., Sugimoto, N., Kitayama, J., Nagawa, H., et al. (2003). Ligand-dependent inhibition of B16 melanoma cell migration and invasion via endogenous S1P2 G protein-coupled receptor. Requirement of inhibition of cellular RAC activity. *J. Biol. Chem.* 278, 32841–32851. doi: 10.1074/jbc.M305024200

Bandhuvula, P., Honbo, N., Wang, G. Y., Jin, Z. Q., Fyrst, H., Zhang, M., et al. (2011). S1P lyase: a novel therapeutic target for ischemia-reperfusion injury of the heart. *Am. J. Physiol. Heart Circ. Physiol.* 300, H1753–H1761. doi: 10.1152/ajpheart.00946.2010

Becciolini, L., Meacci, E., Donati, C., Cencetti, F., Rapizzi, E., and Bruni, P. (2006). Sphingosine 1-phosphate inhibits cell migration in C2C12 myoblasts. *Biochim. Biophys. Acta* 1761, 43–51. doi: 10.1016/j.bbalip.2006.01.006

Bencini, C., Squecco, R., Piperio, C., Formigli, L., Meacci, E., Nosi, D., et al. (2003). Effects of sphingosine 1-phosphate on excitation-contraction coupling in mammalian skeletal muscle. *J. Muscle Res. Cell. Motil.* 24, 539–554. doi: 10.1023/B:JURE.0000009898.02325.58

Berdyshev, E. V., Gorshkova, I., Skobeleva, A., Bittman, R., Lu, X., Dudek, S. M., et al. (2009). FTY720 inhibits ceramide synthases and up-regulates dihydrosphingosine 1-phosphate formation in human lung endothelial cells. *J. Biol. Chem.* 284, 5467–5477. doi: 10.1074/jbc.M805186200

Bernacchioni, C., Cencetti, F., Blescia, S., Donati, C., and Bruni, P. (2012). Sphingosine kinase/sphingosine 1-phosphate axis: a new player for insulin-like growth factor-1-induced myoblast differentiation. *Skelet. Muscle* 2, 15. doi: 10.1186/2044-5040-2-15

Bernacchioni, C., Cencetti, F., Kwon, M. J., Gwak, H. S., Jeong, S. K., Bruni, P., et al. (2011). The sphingosine kinase activator K6PC-5 stimulates C2C12 myoblast differentiation. *Int. J. Immunopathol. Pharmacol.* 24, 55–62.

Blau, H. M., Pavlath, G. K., Hardeman, E. C., Chiu, C. P., Silberstein, L., Webster, S. G., et al. (1985). Plasticity of the differentiated state. *Science* 230, 758–766. doi: 10.1126/science.2414846

Bruce, C. R., Risis, S., Babb, J. R., Yang, C., Kowalski, G. M., Selathurai, A., et al. (2012). Overexpression of sphingosine kinase 1 prevents ceramide accumulation and ameliorates muscle insulin resistance in high-fat diet-fed mice. *Diabetes* 61, 3148–3155. doi: 10.2337/db12-0029

Bruce, C. R., Risis, S., Babb, J. R., Yang, C., Lee-Young, R. S., Henstridge, D. C., et al. (2013). The sphingosine-1-phosphate analog FTY720 reduces muscle ceramide content and improves glucose tolerance in high fat-fed male mice. *Endocrinology* 154, 65–76. doi: 10.1210/en.2012-1847

Bruni, P., and Donati, C. (2008). Pleiotropic effects of sphingolipids in skeletal muscle. *Cell. Mol. Life Sci.* 65, 3725–3736. doi: 10.1007/s00018-008-8236-6

Bruni, P., and Donati, C. (2013). Role of sphingosine 1-phosphate in skeletal muscle cell biology. *Handb. Exp. Pharmacol.* 216, 457–467. doi: 10.1007/978-3-7091-1511-4_23

Calise, S., Blescia, S., Cencetti, F., Bernacchioni, C., Donati, C., and Bruni, P. (2012). Sphingosine 1-phosphate stimulates proliferation and migration of satellite cells: role of S1P receptors. *Biochim. Biophys. Acta* 1823, 439–450. doi: 10.1016/j.bbamcr.2011.11.016

Carlson, M. E., and Conboy, I. M. (2007). Loss of stem cell regenerative capacity within aged niches. *Aging Cell* 6, 371–382. doi: 10.1111/j.1474-9726.2007.00286.x

Cencetti, F., Bernacchioni, C., Nincheri, P., Donati, C., and Bruni, P. (2010). Transforming growth factor-beta1 induces transdifferentiation of myoblasts into myofibroblasts via up-regulation of sphingosine kinase-1/S1P3 axis. *Mol. Biol. Cell* 21, 1111–1124. doi: 10.1091/mbc.E09-09-0812

Cencetti, F., Bernacchioni, C., Tonelli, F., Roberts, E., Donati, C., and Bruni, P. (2013). TGFβ1 evokes myoblast apoptotic response via a novel signaling pathway involving S1P4 transactivation upstream of Rho-kinase-2 activation. *FASEB J.* 27, 4532–4546. doi: 10.1096/fj.13-228528

Chakkalakal, J. V., Jones, K. M., Basson, M. A., and Brack, A. S. (2012). The aged niche disrupts muscle stem cell quiescence. *Nature* 490, 355–360. doi: 10.1038/nature11438

Chamberlain, G., Fox, J., Ashton, B., and Middleton, J. (2007). Concise review: mesenchymal stem cells: their phenotype, differentiation capacity, immunological features, and potential for homing. *Stem Cells* 25, 2739–2749. doi: 10.1634/stemcells.2007-0197

Chargé, S. B., and Rudnicki, M. A. (2004). Cellular and molecular regulation of muscle regeneration. *Physiol. Rev.* 84, 209–238. doi: 10.1152/physrev.00019.2003

Cohn, R. D., van Erp, C., Habashi, J. P., Soleimani, A. A., Klein, E. C., Lisi, M. T., et al. (2007). Angiotensin II type 1 receptor blockade attenuates TGF-beta-induced failure of muscle regeneration in multiple myopathic states. *Nat. Med.* 13, 204–210. doi: 10.1038/nm1536

Collins, C. A., Olsen, I., Zammit, P. S., Heslop, L., Petrie, A., Partridge, T. A., et al. (2005). Stem cell function, self-renewal, and behavioral heterogeneity of cells from the adult muscle satellite cell niche. *Cell* 122, 289–301. doi: 10.1016/j.cell.2005.05.010

Danieli-Betto, D., Germinario, E., Esposito, A., Megighian, A., Midrio, M., Ravara, B., et al. (2005). Sphingosine 1-phosphate protects mouse extensor digitorum longus skeletal muscle during fatigue. *Am. J. Physiol. Cell Physiol.* 288, C1367–C1373. doi: 10.1152/ajpcell.00246.2004

Danieli-Betto, D., Peron, S., Germinario, E., Zanin, M., Sorci, G., Franzoso, S., et al. (2010). Sphingosine 1-phosphate signaling is involved in skeletal muscle regeneration. *Am. J. Physiol. Cell Physiol.* 298, C550–C558. doi: 10.1152/ajpcell.00072.2009

Dellavalle, A., Maroli, G., Covarello, D., Azzoni, E., Innocenzi, A., Perani, L., et al. (2011). Pericytes resident in postnatal skeletal muscle differentiate into muscle fibres and generate satellite cells. *Nat. Commun.* 2, 499. doi: 10.1038/ncomms1508

Dhawan, J., and Rando, T. A. (2005). Stem cells in postnatal myogenesis: molecular mechanisms of satellite cell quiescence, activation and replenishment. *Trends Cell Biol.* 15, 666–673. doi: 10.1016/j.tcb.2005.10.007

Divangahi, M., Balghi, H., Danialou, G., Comtois, A. S., Demoule, A., Ernest, S., et al. (2009). Lack of CFTR in skeletal muscle predisposes to muscle wasting and diaphragm muscle pump failure in cystic fibrosis mice. *PLoS Genet.* 5:e1000586. doi: 10.1371/journal.pgen.1000586

Donati, C., Cencetti, F., and Bruni, P. (2013). New insights into the role of sphingosine 1-phosphate and lysophosphatidic acid in the regulation of skeletal muscle cell biology. *Biochim. Biophys. Acta* 1831, 176–184. doi: 10.1016/j.bbalip.2012.06.013

Donati, C., Cencetti, F., De Palma, C., Rapizzi, E., Brunelli, S., Cossu, G., et al. (2009). TGFbeta protects mesoangioblasts from apoptosis via sphingosine kinase-1 regulation. *Cell. Signal.* 21, 228–236. doi: 10.1016/j.cellsig.2008.10.007

Donati, C., Cencetti, F., Nincheri, P., Bernacchioni, C., Brunelli, S., Clementi, E., et al. (2007a). Sphingosine 1-phosphate mediates proliferation and survival of mesoangioblasts. *Stem Cells* 25, 1713–1719. doi: 10.1634/stemcells.2006-0725

Donati, C., Nincheri, P., Cencetti, F., Rapizzi, E., Farnararo, M., and Bruni, P. (2007b). Tumor necrosis factor-alpha exerts pro-myogenic action in C2C12 myoblasts via sphingosine kinase/S1P2 signaling. *FEBS Lett.* 581, 4384–4388. doi: 10.1016/j.febslet.2007.08.007

Donati, C., Marseglia, G., Magi, A., Serrati, S., Cencetti, F., Bernacchioni, C., et al. (2011). Sphingosine 1-phosphate induces differentiation of mesoangioblasts towards smooth muscle. A role for GATA6. *PLoS ONE* 6:e20389. doi: 10.1371/journal.pone.0020389

Donati, C., Meacci, E., Nuti, F., Becciolini, L., Farnararo, M., and Bruni, P. (2005). Sphingosine 1-phosphate regulates myogenic differentiation: a major role for S1P2 receptor. *FASEB J.* 19, 449–451. doi: 10.1096/fj.04-1780fje

Formigli, L., Meacci, E., Sassoli, C., Squecco, R., Nosi, D., Chellini, F., et al. (2007). Cytoskeleton/stretch-activated ion channel interaction regulates myogenic differentiation of skeletal myoblasts. *J. Cell. Physiol.* 211, 296–306. doi: 10.1002/jcp.20936

Fortier, M., Figeac, N., White, R. B., Knopp, P., and Zammit, P. S. (2013). Sphingosine-1-phosphate receptor 3 influences cell cycle progression in muscle satellite cells. *Dev. Biol.* 382, 504–516. doi: 10.1016/j.ydbio.2013.07.006

García-Prat, L., Sousa-Victor, P., and Muñoz-Cánoves, P. (2013). Functional dysregulation of stem cells during aging: a focus on skeletal muscle stem cells. *FEBS J.* 280, 4051–4062. doi: 10.1111/febs.12221

Germinario, E., Peron, S., Toniolo, L., Betto, R., Cencetti, F., Donati, C., et al. (2012). S1P2 receptor promotes mouse skeletal muscle regeneration. *J. Appl. Physiol.* 113, 707–713. doi: 10.1152/japplphysiol.00300.2012

Hait, N. C., Allegood, J., Maceyka, M., Strub, G. M., Harikumar, K. B., Singh, S. K., et al. (2009). Regulation of histone acetylation in the nucleus by sphingosine-1-phosphate. *Science* 325, 1254–1257. doi: 10.1126/science.1176709

Hait, N. C., Bellamy, A., Milstien, S., Kordula, T., and Spiegel, S. (2007). Sphingosine kinase type 2 activation by ERK-mediated phosphorylation. *J. Biol. Chem.* 282, 12058–12065. doi: 10.1074/jbc.M609559200

Hannun, Y. A., and Obeid, L. M. (2008). Principles of bioactive lipid signalling: lessons from sphingolipids. *Nat. Rev. Mol. Cell Biol.* 9, 139–150. doi: 10.1038/nrm2329

Herr, D. R., Fyrst, H., Phan, V., Heinecke, K., Georges, R., Harris, G. L., et al. (2003). Sply regulation of sphingolipid signaling molecules is essential for Drosophila development. *Development* 130, 2443–2453. doi: 10.1242/dev.00456

Hu, W., Bielawski, J., Samad, F., Merrill, A. H. Jr., and Cowart, L. A. (2009). Palmitate increases sphingosine-1-phosphate in C2C12 myotubes via upregulation of sphingosine kinase message and activity. *J. Lipid Res.* 50, 1852–1862. doi: 10.1194/jlr.M800635-JLR200

Husmann, I., Soulet, L., Gautron, J., Martelly, I., and Barritault, D. (1996). Growth factors in skeletal muscle regeneration. *Cytokine Growth Factor Rev.* 7, 249–258. doi: 10.1016/S1359-6101(96)00029-9

Ieronimakis, N., Pantoja, M., Hays, A. L., Dosey, T. L., Qi, J., Fischer, K. A., et al. (2013). Increased sphingosine-1-phosphate improves muscle regeneration in acutely injured mdx mice. *Skelet. Muscle* 3, 20. doi: 10.1186/2044-5040-3-20

Judson, R. N., Zhang, R. H., and Rossi, F. M. (2013). Tissue-resident mesenchymal stem/progenitor cells in skeletal muscle: collaborators or saboteurs. *FEBS J.* 280, 4100–4108. doi: 10.1111/febs.12370

Kawahara, A., Nishi, T., Hisano, Y., Fukui, H., Yamaguchi, A., and Mochizuki, N. (2009). The sphingolipid transporter spns2 functions in migration of zebrafish myocardial precursors. *Science* 323, 524–527. doi: 10.1126/science.1167449

Kono, M., Belyantseva, I. A., Skoura, A., Frolenkov, G. I., Starost, M. F., Dreier, J. L., et al. (2007). Deafness and stria vascularis defects in S1P2 receptor-null mice. *J. Biol. Chem.* 282, 10690–10696. doi: 10.1074/jbc.M700370200

Kumar, A., and Saba, J. D. (2009). Lyase to live by: sphingosine phosphate lyase as a therapeutic target. *Expert Opin. Ther. Targets* 13, 1013–1025. doi: 10.1517/14728220903039722

Kwon, Y. B., Kim, C. D., Youm, J. K., Gwak, H. S., Park, B. D., Lee, S. H., et al. (2007). Novel synthetic ceramide derivatives increase intracellular calcium levels and promote epidermal keratinocyte differentiation. *J. Lipid Res.* 48, 1936–1943. doi: 10.1194/jlr.M700185-JLR200

LaBarge, M. A., and Blau, H. M. (2002). Biological progression from adult bone marrow to mononucleate muscle stem cell to multinucleate muscle fiber in response to injury. *Cell* 111, 589–601. doi: 10.1016/S0092-8674(02) 01078-4

Lahiri, S., Park, H., Laviad, E. L., Lu, X., Bittman, R., and Futerman, A. H. (2009). Ceramide synthesis is modulated by the sphingosine analog FTY720 via a mixture of uncompetitive and noncompetitive inhibition in an Acyl-CoA chain length-dependent manner. *J. Biol. Chem.* 284, 16090–16098. doi: 10.1074/jbc.M807438200

Lebman, D. A., and Spiegel, S. (2008). Cross-talk at the crossroads of sphingosine-1-phosphate, growth factors, and cytokine signaling. *J. Lipid Res.* 49, 1388–1394. doi: 10.1194/jlr.R800008-JLR200

Lepley, D., Paik, J. H., Hla, T., and Ferrer, F. (2005). The G protein-coupled receptor S1P2 regulates Rho/Rho kinase pathway to inhibit tumor cell migration. *Cancer Res.* 65, 3788–3795. doi: 10.1158/0008-5472.CAN-04-2311

Le Stunff, H., Giussani, P., Maceyka, M., Lepine, S., Milstien, S., and Spiegel, S. (2007). Recycling of sphingosine is regulated by the concerted actions of sphingosine-1-phosphate phosphohydrolase 1 and sphingosine kinase 2. *J. Biol. Chem.* 282, 34372–34380. doi: 10.1074/jbc.M703329200

Li, Y. P., and Schwartz, R. J. (2001). TNF-alpha regulates early differentiation of C2C12 myoblasts in an autocrine fashion. *FASEB J.* 15, 1413–1415. doi: 10.1096/fj.00-0632fje

Liu, Y., Wada, R., Yamashita, T., Mi, Y., Deng, C. X., Hobson, J. P., et al. (2000). Edg-1, the G protein-coupled receptor for sphingosine-1-phosphate, is essential for vascular maturation. *J. Clin. Invest.* 106, 951–961. doi: 10.1172/JCI10905

Loh, K. C., Leong, W. I., Carlson, M. E., Oskouian, B., Kumar, A., Fyrst, H., et al. (2012). Sphingosine-1-phosphate enhances satellite cell activation in dystrophic muscles through a S1PR2/STAT3 signaling pathway. *PLoS ONE* 7:e37218. doi: 10.1371/journal.pone.0037218

Ma, M. M., Chen, J. L., Wang, G. G., Wang, H., Lu, Y., Li, J. F., et al. (2007). Sphingosine kinase 1 participates in insulin signalling and regulates glucose metabolism and homeostasis in KK/Ay diabetic mice. *Diabetologia* 50, 891–900. doi: 10.1007/s00125-006-0589-5

Maceyka, M., Harikumar, K. B., Milstien, S., and Spiegel, S. (2012). Sphingosine-1-phosphate signaling and its role in disease. *Trends Cell Biol.* 22, 50–60. doi: 10.1016/j.tcb.2011.09.003

McGarry, J. D. (2002). Banting lecture 2001: dysregulation of fatty acid metabolism in the etiology of type 2 diabetes. *Diabetes* 51, 7–18. doi: 10.2337/diabetes.51.1.7

McLennan, I. S., and Koishi, K. (2002). The transforming growth factor-betas: multifaceted regulators of the development and maintenance of skeletal muscles, motoneurons and Schwann cells. *Int. J. Dev. Biol.* 46, 559–567.

Meacci, E., Bini, F., Sassoli, C., Martinesi, M., Squecco, R., Chellini, F., et al. (2010). Functional interaction between TRPC1 channel and connexin-43 protein: a novel pathway underlying S1P action on skeletal myogenesis. *Cell. Mol. Life Sci.* 67, 4269–4285. doi: 10.1007/s00018-010-0442-3

Meacci, E., Cencetti, F., Donati, C., Nuti, F., Farnararo, M., Kohno, T., et al. (2003). Down-regulation of EDG5/S1P2 during myogenic differentiation results in the specific uncoupling of sphingosine 1-phosphate signalling to phospholipase D. *Biochim. Biophys. Acta* 1633, 133–142. doi: 10.1016/S1388-1981(03)00106-9

Meacci, E., Cencetti, F., Formigli, L., Squecco, R., Donati, C., Tiribilli, B., et al. (2002). Sphingosine 1-phosphate evokes calcium signals in C2C12 myoblasts via Edg3 and Edg5 receptors. *Biochem. J.* 362(Pt 2), 349–357. doi: 10.1042/0264-6021:3620349

Meacci, E., Donati, C., Cencetti, F., Romiti, E., and Bruni, P. (2000). Permissive role of protein kinase C alpha but not protein kinase C delta in sphingosine 1-phosphate-induced Rho A activation in C2C12 myoblasts. *FEBS Lett.* 482, 97–101. doi: 10.1016/S0014-5793(00)02039-1

Meacci, E., Nuti, F., Donati, C., Cencetti, F., Farnararo, M., and Bruni, P. (2008). Sphingosine kinase activity is required for myogenic differentiation of C2C12 myoblasts. *J. Cell. Physiol.* 214, 210–220. doi: 10.1002/jcp.21187

Meacci, E., Vasta, V., Donati, C., Farnararo, M., and Bruni, P. (1999). Receptor-mediated activation of phospholipase D by sphingosine 1-phosphate in skeletal muscle C2C12 cells. A role for protein kinase C. *FEBS Lett.* 457, 184–188. doi: 10.1016/S0014-5793(99)01033-9

Meissner, A., Yang, J., Kroetsch, J. T., Sauvé, M., Dax, H., Momen, A., et al. (2012). Tumor necrosis factor-α-mediated downregulation of the cystic fibrosis transmembrane conductance regulator drives pathological sphingosine-1-phosphate signaling in a mouse model of heart failure. *Circulation* 125, 2739–2750. doi: 10.1161/CIRCULATIONAHA.111.047316

Minasi, M. G., Riminucci, M., De Angelis, L., Borello, U., Berarducci, B., Innocenzi, A., et al. (2002). The meso-angioblast: a multipotent, self-renewing cell that originates from the dorsal aorta and differentiates into most mesodermal tissues. *Development* 129, 2773–2783.

Mitchell, K. J., Pannerec, A., Cadot, B., Parlakian, A., Besson, V., Gomes, E. R., et al. (2010). Identification and characterization of a non-satellite cell muscle resident progenitor during postnatal development. *Nat. Cell Biol.* 12, 257–266. doi: 10.1038/ncb2025

Mitra, P., Oskeritzian, C. A., Payne, S. G., Beaven, M. A., Milstien, S., and Spiegel, S. (2006). Role of ABCC1 in export of sphingosine-1-phosphate from mast cells. *Proc. Natl. Acad. Sci. U.S.A.* 103, 16394–16399. doi: 10.1073/pnas.0603734103

Nagata, Y., Partridge, T. A., Matsuda, R., and Zammit, P. S. (2006). Entry of muscle satellite cells into the cell cycle requires sphingolipid signaling. *J. Cell Biol.* 174, 245–253. doi: 10.1083/jcb.200605028

Nincheri, P., Luciani, P., Squecco, R., Donati, C., Bernacchioni, C., Borgognoni, L., et al. (2009). Sphingosine 1-phosphate induces differentiation of adipose tissue-derived mesenchymal stem cells towards smooth muscle cells. *Cell. Mol. Life Sci.* 66, 1741–1754. doi: 10.1007/s00018-009-9181-8

Olivera, A., and Spiegel, S. (1993). Sphingosine 1-phosphate as second messenger in cell proliferation induced by PDGF and FCS mitogens. *Nature* 365, 557–560. doi: 10.1038/365557a0

O'Sullivan, C., and Dev, K. K. (2013). The structure and function of the S1P1 receptor. *Trends Pharmacol. Sci.* 34, 401–412. doi: 10.1016/j.tips.2013.05.002

Pallafacchina, G., Francois, S., Regnault, B., Czarny, B., Dive, V., Cumano, A., et al. (2010). An adult tissue-specific stem cell in its niche: a gene profiling analysis of *in vivo* quiescent and activated muscle satellite cells. *Stem Cell Res.* 4, 77–91. doi: 10.1016/j.scr.2009.10.003

Pannérec, A., Marazzi, G., and Sassoon, D. (2012). Stem cells in the hood: the skeletal muscle niche. *Trends Mol. Med.* 18, 599–606. doi: 10.1016/j.molmed.2012.07.004

Pantoja, M., Fischer, K. A., Ieronimakis, N., Reyes, M., and Ruohola-Baker, H. (2013). Genetic elevation of sphingosine 1-phosphate suppresses dystrophic muscle phenotypes in Drosophila. *Development* 140, 136–146. doi: 10.1242/dev.087791

Pedersen, B. K., and Febbraio, M. A. (2012). Muscles, exercise and obesity: skeletal muscle as a secretory organ. *Nat. Rev. Endocrinol.* 8, 457–465. doi: 10.1038/nrendo.2012.49

Pitson, S. M., Moretti, P. A., Zebol, J. R., Lynn, H. E., Xia, P., Vadas, M. A., et al. (2003). Activation of sphingosine kinase 1 by ERK1/2-mediated phosphorylation. *EMBO J.* 22, 5491–5500. doi: 10.1093/emboj/cdg540

Rapizzi, E., Donati, C., Cencetti, F., Nincheri, P., and Bruni, P. (2008). Sphingosine 1-phosphate differentially regulates proliferation of C2C12 reserve cells and myoblasts. *Mol. Cell. Biochem.* 314, 193–199. doi: 10.1007/s11010-008-9780-y

Rapizzi, E., Taddei, M. L., Fiaschi, T., Donati, C., Bruni, P., and Chiarugi, P. (2009). Sphingosine 1-phosphate increases glucose uptake through trans-activation of insulin receptor. *Cell. Mol. Life Sci.* 66, 3207–3218. doi: 10.1007/s00018-009-0106-3

Ross, J. S., Hu, W., Rosen, B., Snider, A. J., Obeid, L. M., and Cowart, L. A. (2013). Sphingosine kinase 1 is regulated by PPARalpha in response to free fatty acids and is essential for skeletal muscle IL-6 production and signaling in diet-induced obesity. *J. Biol. Chem.* 288, 22193–22206. doi: 10.1074/jbc.M113.477786

Sampaolesi, M., Blot, S., D'Antona, G., Granger, N., Tonlorenzi, R., Innocenzi, A., et al. (2006). Mesoangioblast stem cells ameliorate muscle function in dystrophic dogs. *Nature* 444, 574–579. doi: 10.1038/nature05282

Sampaolesi, M., Torrente, Y., Innocenzi, A., Tonlorenzi, R., D'Antona, G., Pellegrino, M. A., et al. (2003). Cell therapy of alpha-sarcoglycan null dystrophic mice through intra-arterial delivery of mesoangioblasts. *Science* 301, 487–492. doi: 10.1126/science.1082254

Sato, K., Malchinkhuu, E., Horiuchi, Y., Mogi, C., Tomura, H., Tosaka, M., et al. (2007). Critical role of ABCA1 transporter in sphingosine 1-phosphate release from astrocytes. *J. Neurochem.* 103, 2610–2619. doi: 10.1111/j.1471-4159.2007.04958.x

Schiaffino, S., Dyar, K. A., Ciciliot, S., Blaauw, B., and Sandri, M. (2013). Mechanisms regulating skeletal muscle growth and atrophy. *FEBS J.* 280, 4294–4314. doi: 10.1111/febs.12253

Schnitzer, S. E., Weigert, A., Zhou, J., and Brune, B. (2009). Hypoxia enhances sphingosine kinase 2 activity and provokes sphingosine-1-phosphate-mediated chemoresistance in A549 lung cancer cells. *Mol. Cancer Res.* 7, 393–401. doi: 10.1158/1541-7786.MCR-08-0156

Shcherbata, H. R., Yatsenko, A. S., Patterson, L., Sood, V. D., Nudel, U., Yaffe, D., et al. (2007). Dissecting muscle and neuronal disorders in a Drosophila model of muscular dystrophy. *EMBO J.* 26, 481–493. doi: 10.1038/sj.emboj.7601503

Spiegel, S., and Milstien, S. (2003). Sphingosine 1 phosphate: an enigmatic signalling lipid. *Nat. Rev. Mol. Cell Biol.* 4, 397–407. doi: 10.1038/nrm1103

Squecco, R., Sassoli, C., Nuti, F., Martinesi, M., Chellini, F., Nosi, D., et al. (2006). Sphingosine 1-phosphateinduces myoblast differentiation through Cx43 protein expression: a role for a gap junction-dependent and -independent function. *Mol. Biol. Cell* 17, 4896–4910. doi: 10.1091/mbc.E06-03-0243

Stahelin, R. V., Hwang, J. H., Kim, J. H., Park, Z. Y., Johnson, K. R., Obeid, L. M., et al. (2005). The mechanism of membrane targeting of human sphingosine kinase 1. *J. Biol. Chem.* 280, 43030–43038. doi: 10.1074/jbc.M507574200

Strub, G. M., Paillard, M., Liang, J., Gomez, L., Allegood, J. C., Hait, N. C., et al. (2011). Sphingosine-1-phosphate produced by sphingosine kinase 2 in mitochondria interacts with prohibitin 2 to regulate complex IV assembly and respiration. *FASEB J.* 25, 600–612. doi: 10.1096/fj.10-167502

Takabe, K., Kim, R. H., Allegood, J. C., Mitra, P., Ramachandran, S., Nagahashi, M., et al. (2010). Estradiol induces export of sphingosine 1-phosphate from breast cancer cells via ABCC1 and ABCG2. *J. Biol. Chem.* 285, 10477–10486. doi: 10.1074/jbc.M109.064162

Tedesco, F. S., Dellavalle, A., Diaz-Manera, J., Messina, G., and Cossu, G. (2010). Repairing skeletal muscle: regenerative potential of skeletal muscle stem cells. *J. Clin. Invest.* 120, 11–19. doi: 10.1172/JCI40373

Troy, A., Cadwallader, A. B., Fedorov, Y., Tyner, K., Tanaka, K. K., and Olwin, B. B. (2012). Coordination of satellite cell activation and self-renewal by Par-complex-dependent asymmetric activation of p38α/β MAPK. *Cell Stem Cell* 11, 541–553. doi: 10.1016/j.stem.2012.05.025

Xia, P., Wang, L., Moretti, P. A., Albanese, N., Chai, F., Pitson, S. M., et al. (2002). Sphingosine kinase interacts with TRAF2 and dissects tumor necrosis factor-alpha signaling. *J. Biol. Chem.* 277, 7996–8003. doi: 10.1074/jbc.M111423200

Yaffe, D., and Saxel, O. (1977). Serial passaging and differentiation of myogenic cells isolated from dystrophic mouse muscle. *Nature* 270, 725–727. doi: 10.1038/270725a0

Yin, H., Price, F., and Rudnicki, M. A. (2013). Satellite cells and the muscle stem cell niche. *Physiol. Rev.* 93, 23–67. doi: 10.1152/physrev.00043.2011

Yoshida, N., Yoshida, S., Koishi, K., Masuda, K., and Nabeshima, Y. (1998). Cell heterogeneity upon myogenic differentiation: down-regulation of MyoD and Myf-5 generates 'reserve cells.' *J. Cell Sci.* 111(Pt 6), 769–779.

Zanin, M., Germinario, E., Dalla Libera, L., Sandona, D., Sabbadini, R. A., Betto, R., et al. (2008). Trophic action of sphingosine 1-phosphate in denervated rat soleus muscle. *Am. J. Physiol. Cell Physiol.* 294, C36–C46. doi: 10.1152/ajpcell.00164.2007

Zeidan, Y. H., and Hannun, Y. A. (2010). The acid sphingomyelinase/ceramide pathway: biomedical significance and mechanisms of regulation. *Curr. Mol. Med.* 10, 454–466. doi: 10.2174/156652410791608225

20

A metabolic link to skeletal muscle wasting and regeneration

René Koopman[1], C. Hai Ly[2] and James G. Ryall[2]*

[1] Clinical Nutrition and Muscle and Exercise Metabolism Group, The University of Melbourne, Melbourne, VIC, Australia
[2] Stem Cell Metabolism and Regenerative Medicine Group, Basic and Clinical Myology Laboratory, Department of Physiology, The University of Melbourne, Melbourne, VIC, Australia

***Correspondence:**
James G. Ryall, Stem Cell Metabolism and Regenerative Medicine Group, Basic and Clinical Myology Laboratory, Department of Physiology, The University of Melbourne, Melbourne, VIC 3010, Australia
e-mail: jgryall@gmail.com

Due to its essential role in movement, insulating the internal organs, generating heat to maintain core body temperature, and acting as a major energy storage depot, any impairment to skeletal muscle structure and function may lead to an increase in both morbidity and mortality. In the context of skeletal muscle, altered metabolism is directly associated with numerous pathologies and disorders, including diabetes, and obesity, while many skeletal muscle pathologies have secondary changes in metabolism, including cancer cachexia, sarcopenia and the muscular dystrophies. Furthermore, the importance of cellular metabolism in the regulation of skeletal muscle stem cells is beginning to receive significant attention. Thus, it is clear that skeletal muscle metabolism is intricately linked to the regulation of skeletal muscle mass and regeneration. The aim of this review is to discuss some of the recent findings linking a change in metabolism to changes in skeletal muscle mass, as well as describing some of the recent studies in developmental, cancer and stem-cell biology that have identified a role for cellular metabolism in the regulation of stem cell function, a process termed "metabolic reprogramming."

Keywords: metabolism, satellite cells, stem cells, cell fate, glycolysis

INTRODUCTION

Metabolism is loosely defined as the collection of enzymatic reactions essential for life, and can be catabolic/anabolic and exothermic/endothermic in nature. While in a constant state of flux, these reactions reach equilibrium (homeostasis) and are maintained in the absence of altered energy supply or demand. However, a sustained change in metabolism can have serious implications for an individual and can lead to an increase in both morbidity and mortality. In the context of skeletal muscle, altered metabolism is associated with numerous pathologies and disorders, including diabetes, obesity, Pompe's disease, McArdle disease and numerous mitochondrial disorders (Angelini and Semplicini, 2010; Raben et al., 2012; Russell et al., 2013), while many skeletal muscle pathologies have secondary changes in metabolism, including cancer cachexia, age-related muscle wasting and weakness (termed sarcopenia) and the muscular dystrophies (Ryall et al., 2008; Russell et al., 2013). Furthermore, the importance of cellular metabolism in the regulation of skeletal muscle stem cells is beginning to receive significant attention (Ryall, 2013). Thus, it is clear that skeletal muscle metabolism is intricately linked to the regulation of skeletal muscle mass and regeneration. The aim of this review is to discuss some of the recent findings regarding the role of metabolic dysfunction in skeletal muscle wasting and weakness, as well as to highlight potential novel therapeutic targets for future drug discovery and development. Finally, as cellular metabolism is beginning to receive increased attention in the regulation of stem cell identity, we discuss some of the implications for the regulation of skeletal muscle stem cell activity and regeneration following injury. However, before addressing these topics in detail, a brief overview of the major metabolic pathways will be discussed.

CELLULAR METABOLISM IN SKELETAL MUSCLE

Energy in the form of adenosine triphosphate (ATP) is essential for cells to conduct the processes necessary for life, and depletion of ATP can lead to necrosis or apoptosis (Tsujimoto, 1997). The conversion of ATP to adenosine diphosphate (ADP) or adenosine monophosphate (AMP) and inorganic phosphate (P_i) is exothermic and liberates energy that can be harnessed to fuel enzymatic reactions. Cellular ATP is derived from the breakdown of fats (via fatty acid oxidation, FAO), carbohydrates (via glycolysis) and proteins (via proteolysis) to pyruvate and/or acetyl CoA which, in the presence of oxygen, can be converted to ATP in the mitochondria via oxidative phosphorylation (OXPHOS). The majority of ATP is generated via glycolysis in the cytoplasm and OXPHOS in the mitochondria, with the relative contribution of each process dependent on a range of factors, including substrate and oxygen availability, and cellular energy demand (Salway, 2012).

Briefly, FAO involves an energy consuming reaction which converts FA and Co-enzyme A (Co-A) to fatty acyl-CoA (FA-CoA) and is catalyzed by the enzyme fatty acyl-CoA synthetase. FA-CoA cannot be directly transported across the mitochondrial inner membrane and must first be converted to an acyl carnitine derivative and then reconverted to FA-CoA inside the mitochondria. FAO involves a stepwise process of dehydrogenation of acyl-CoA to acetyl-CoA which can then be metabolized by the tricarboxylic acid cycle (TCA) and the mitochondrial electron transport chain (ETC, Salway, 2012, **Figure 1**).

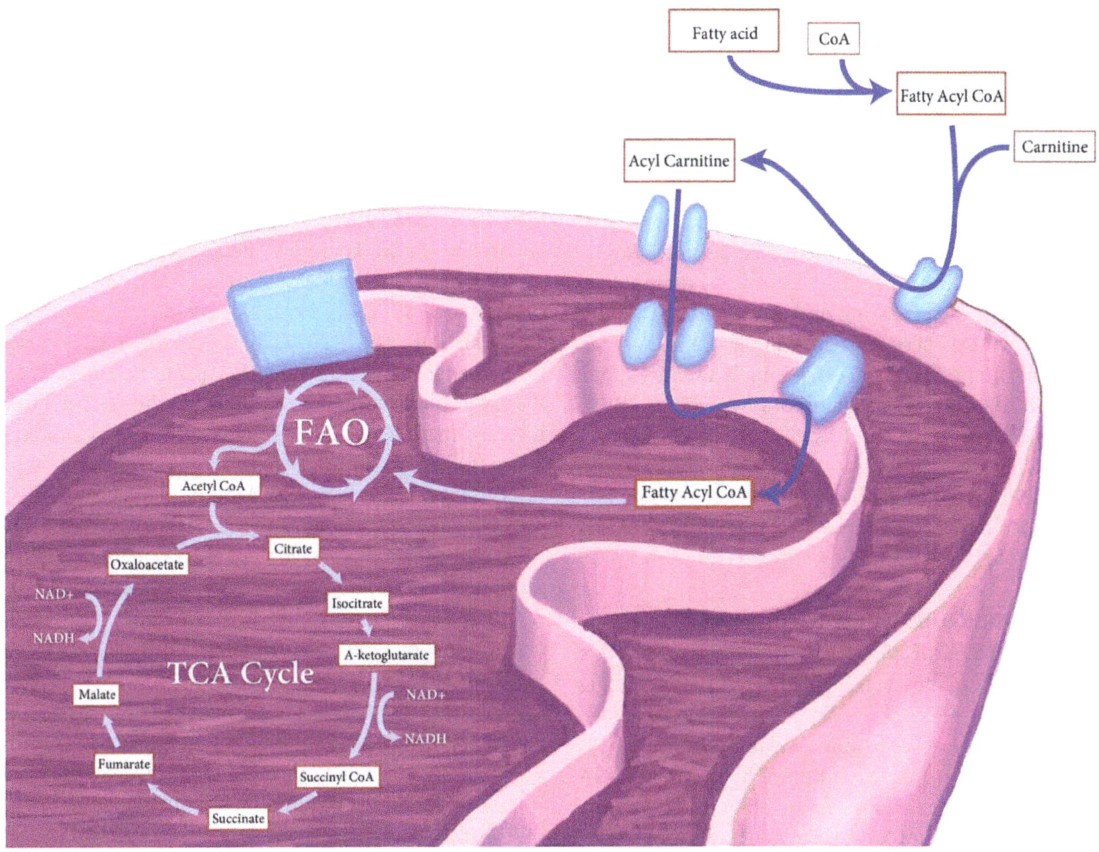

FIGURE 1 | Schematic of the process of fatty-acid oxidation (FAO) in cells. Fatty-acid-CoA (FA-CoA) is converted to an acyl carnitine derivative in the mitochondrial membrane, acylcarnitine is then converted back to FA-CoA within the mitochondria where it undergoes a series of dehydrogenation reactions to form acetyl-CoA. Acetyl-CoA, in turn enters the tricarboxylic acid (TCA) cycle to generate NADH to drive complex I, and succinate to drive complex II of the mitochondrial electron transport chain.

Glucose is metabolized by almost all organisms in a cytosolic process termed glycolysis which yields two molecules of ATP per molecule of glucose. Circulating glucose enters a cell predominantly via a family of transmembrane glucose transporters (GLUT1-11), with several isoforms each being specific to certain tissues. Once inside the cell, glucose is converted to glucose-6-phosphate (G6P) by hexokinase in an ATP consuming reaction, following which G6P is converted first to fructose-6-phosphate (F6P) and then to fructose-1-6-bisphosphate (F1,6BP). The conversion to F1,6BP is irreversible and is considered the step at which glucose is committed to glycolysis (Lunt and Vander Heiden, 2011). This reaction is catalyzed by phosphofructokinase 1 (PFK1); an enzyme allosterically controlled by levels of ATP, such that abundant levels of ATP inhibits PFK1. Cleavage of F1,6BP generates two molecules of glyceraldehyde-3-phosphate (G3P), which are then converted to phosphoenolpyruvate (PEP). The final step of glycolysis involves the conversion of PEP to pyruvate to release ATP; a reaction catalyzed by the enzyme pyruvate kinase (PK) (Lunt and Vander Heiden, 2011). Under aerobic conditions pyruvate is transported into the mitochondria and converted to acetyl-CoA for OXPHOS. Under anaerobic conditions, lactate dehydrogenase (LDH) reduces pyruvate to lactate, which is then shunted into the extracellular space via the monocarboxylate transporter and then transported to the liver for gluconeogenesis (Salway, 2012).

In the presence of oxygen, mitochondrial acetyl-CoA generated via FAO or glycolysis enters the tricarboxylic acid (TCA) cycle where the acetyl group is transferred to oxaloacetate to form citrate. Through a series of well described reactions (**Figure 1**), citrate is converted first into its structural isomer, isocitrate and then α-ketoglutarate; reactions that lead to the production of NADH, H^+ and CO_2. Further decarboxylation of α-ketoglutarate liberates additional NADH and H^+ and a high energy thioester, succinyl-CoA. Succinyl-CoA undergoes phosphorylation to form succinate and then further oxidation and hydration steps to reform oxaloacetate and additional NADH and H^+. The NADH and H^+ produced via the TCA cycle are then used to drive the mitochondrial electron transport chain (ETC) for the generation of ATP (Lunt and Vander Heiden, 2011). Clearly skeletal muscle metabolism is strictly regulated by substrate availability, presence of oxygen and energy demand, which in turn also regulate muscle protein metabolism and cell size.

METABOLIC DISTURBANCES LEADING TO ALTERATIONS IN SKELETAL MUSCLE MASS

The preservation of skeletal muscle function is crucial for maintaining an independent lifestyle and the capacity to perform the activities of daily living. Generally considered to be the result of a balance between protein synthesis and degradation, skeletal muscle mass is carefully regulated through the actions of numerous complementary and (sometimes) interacting pathways. Any disruption to this careful balance of protein synthesis and degradation can have serious consequences. The role of metabolism in the progression of muscle wasting and weakness in individual disorders has previously been described in detail for diabetes, obesity (Akhmedov and Berdeaux, 2013), Pompe's disease (Raben et al., 2012), McArdles disease (Angelini and Semplicini, 2010) and several mitochondrial disorders (Russell et al., 2013). As such, our aim is to describe some of the more recent discoveries linking specific metabolic signaling pathways to muscle wasting and weakness, with a specific focus on the central role of mechanistic target of rapamycin (mTOR).

THE mTOR COMPLEX 1 SIGNALING PATHWAY REGULATES DIURNAL VARIATIONS IN PROTEIN SYNTHESIS

Protein turnover in skeletal muscle is highly responsive to changes in substrate availability (Rennie et al., 1982). It is generally accepted that acute changes in substrate availability, amino acids (AAs) in particular, modulate protein synthesis by altering mRNA translation. Many laboratories have shown that the signaling pathway involving mTOR complex I (mTORC1) plays a crucial role in the control of initiation and elongation of mRNA translation (Bodine et al., 2001; Bolster et al., 2003; Dreyer et al., 2006). The mTORC1 signaling pathway integrates a wide variety of extra- and intracellular signals, including insulin (and its related growth factors), nutrient (glucose and amino acids) availability, and cellular energy status to regulate protein synthesis, autophagy, cell growth and metabolism (Laplante and Sabatini, 2012). The activity of mTORC1 determines the activity of downstream effectors such as the 70-kDa S6 protein kinase (S6K1) and the eukaryotic initiation factor 4E-binding protein (4E-BP1) (Kimball et al., 2002). Both play key regulatory roles in modulating translation initiation, and control the binding of mRNA to the 40S ribosomal subunit (Kimball et al., 2002).

mTORC1 activity is controlled amongst others, by its upstream regulator, the tuberous sclerosis complex (TSC1-TSC2, Dodd and Tee, 2012). Activation of this complex stimulates the GTPase function of Rheb, a small GTPase that acts as a proximal key activator of mTORC1, which leads to a reduction in Rheb-induced mTORC1 activation. In contrast, inactivation of the TSC1-TSC2 complex results in the accumulation of GTP-bound Rheb and thus activation of mTORC1 (Dodd and Tee, 2012). Clearly, the activity of the TSC1-TSC2 complex and Rheb-mTORC1 interaction are critical for the correct operation of the mTORC1 pathway in response to changes in homeostasis.

Given that protein synthesis requires a plentiful supply of amino acids and energy (ATP), it is not surprising that mTORC1 signaling is under strict regulation. Increased availability of AAs strongly stimulates muscle protein synthesis (Rennie et al., 1982; Volpi et al., 1998, 1999; Paddon-Jones et al., 2004, 2006). Besides serving as a substrate for polypeptide biosynthesis, the essential AAs (EAAs), but not the non-essential AAs (NEAAs), have been shown to directly activate regulatory proteins in mRNA translation, thereby increasing muscle protein synthesis. Noteworthy, the latter event does not require increased NEAA availability (Volpi et al., 2003). The branched-chain AA, leucine, is of particular interest since it has the unique ability to directly increase signaling through mTORC1 and its downstream targets 4E-BP1 and S6K1 and ribosomal S6. Therefore, leucine represents the main anabolic signal responsible for the post-prandial increase in muscle protein synthesis (Smith et al., 1992; Norton and Layman, 2006).

Dickinson et al. (2011) have provided clear evidence that, in humans, rapamycin injection prior to EAA intake prevents the expected increase in protein synthesis and attenuates the increase in mTORC1-signaling, supporting a fundamental role for mTORC1 activation as a key-regulator of protein synthesis in response to increased AA availability. A detailed discussion about how cells sense AAs and how these signals are communicated to mTORC1 is beyond the scope of this review as we aim to focus in more detail how changes in glucose metabolism alter the activity of this particular pathway, instead the reader is directed to a number of recent excellent reviews (Dodd and Tee, 2012; Laplante and Sabatini, 2012).

One important example of the importance of mTOR in the metabolic regulation of muscle mass can be observed during the process of age-related muscle wasting and weakness (sarcopenia). While the effect of ageing and sarcopenia on mTOR associated signaling in skeletal muscle in the fasted state has been investigated in detail its role remains unclear. Some reports in humans suggest that mTOR and S6K1 protein expression (Cuthbertson et al., 2005) or phosphorylation status (Li et al., 2012) are reduced in muscles from elderly individuals, whereas others report no difference in the fasted state (Guillet et al., 2004; Drummond et al., 2008a). Importantly however, following the administration of EAA (with or without carbohydrates), elderly humans have a blunted increase in mTOR (Cuthbertson et al., 2005), and S6K1 (Guillet et al., 2004; Cuthbertson et al., 2005) phosphorylation compared with young controls, resulting in an attenuated (Cuthbertson et al., 2005) or delayed (Drummond et al., 2008a) anabolic response. These studies indicate that the skeletal muscle response to alterations in glucose and AA availability is compromised in the elderly, and could be a result of a defect in either the ability of the muscle to respond, or detect, a change in energy availability.

AMP ACTIVATED PROTEIN KINASE AS A NEGATIVE REGULATOR OF SKELETAL MUSCLE MASS

The most well-studied energy sensor in skeletal muscle is the 5′-AMP-activated protein kinase (AMPK) (Steinberg and Kemp, 2009). AMPK is activated by an elevation in the AMP/ATP ratio leading to inhibition of energy consuming anabolic processes such as protein synthesis and stimulation of catabolic energy producing processes such as glycolysis, FAO and protein degradation (Steinberg et al., 2010). AMPK is thought to regulate mTORC1 signaling either via 1) phosphorylation of TSC2, leading to increased GTPase activity of Rheb; 2) direct phosphorylation of mTOR at Thr2446 preventing stimulatory phosphorylation on

Ser2448; or 3) the phosphorylation and dissociation of the critical mTORC1 protein, Raptor (Steinberg and Kemp, 2009, **Figure 2**).

Pharmacological activation of AMPK using 5-Aminoimidazole-4-carboxamide ribonucleotide (AICAR) suppresses phosphorylation of mTOR and 4E-BP1 and induces atrophy in C2C12 myotubes *in vitro* (Zhao et al., 2010). On the other hand, knock-down of AMPKα1/2 subunits has been shown to increase myotube diameter, associated with a marked increase in S6K1 and protein synthesis rate (Lantier et al., 2010), an effect that was found to be ablated following treatment with rapamycin. In addition, skeletalmuscle-specific deficient AMPKα1/2 KO mice have increased muscle mass with bigger myofibers and S6K1 signaling (Lantier et al., 2010). AMPK activity is rapidly suppressed when muscles are exposed to increasing concentrations of either leucine or glucose that stimulate increases in muscle protein synthesis and signaling through mTORC1 (Saha et al., 2010). Conversely, activation of AMPK by AICAR reduced leucine- and glucose-stimulated increases in protein synthesis and mTOR phosphorylation (Saha et al., 2010). Clearly, AMPK can modulate mTORC1 signaling which is one of the mechanisms by which protein synthesis can be reduced during cellular stress.

Based on the described relationship between AMPK activity and signaling through mTOR, one would expect that reduced protein synthesis in metabolic diseases are associated with increased levels of AMPK activity. However, the role of AMPK in altered protein metabolism in sarcopenia, obesity and diabetes is unclear. Some reports demonstrate reductions in AMPK signaling in skeletal muscle samples collected from elderly humans (Li et al., 2012), whereas others report no change in the fasted state and increased AMPK phosphorylation following amino acid ingestion (Drummond et al., 2008b). In muscle samples from obese and type 2 diabetes patients, AMPK expression and activation are not significantly different from controls (Hojlund et al., 2004; Steinberg et al., 2004), suggesting that changes in AMPK signaling may not be the primary defect preceding metabolic changes associated with these conditions (Steinberg and Kemp, 2009).

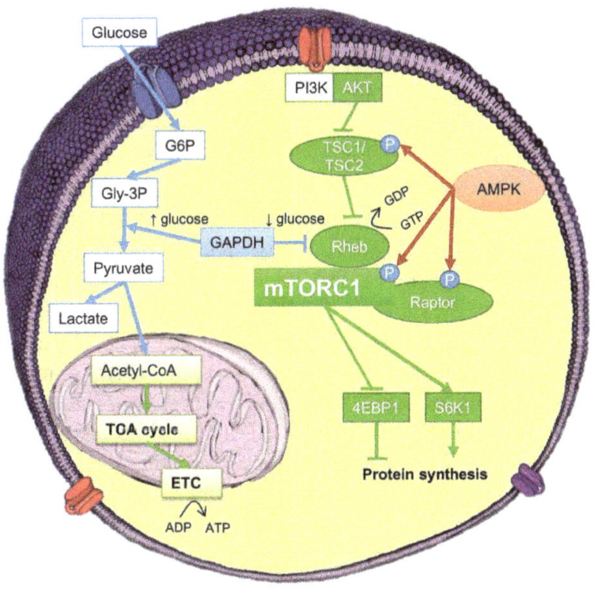

FIGURE 2 | Considered one of the master regulators of protein synthesis, mammalian target of rapamycin (mTOR) is perfectly positioned to receive feedback regarding the cellular energy status. During levels of high glycolytic flux, the ADP/ATP ratio is low, and so AMPK activity is reduced, furthermore, GAPDH is prevented from interacting with the small GTPaseRheb. Together, these pathways lead to elevated mTOR complex I (mTORCI) signaling, and protein synthesis.

GLYCOLYTIC FLUXIN SKELETAL MUSCLE CAN DIRECTLY REGULATE mTORC1 ACTIVITY

AMPK mediated signaling is not the only way cellular stress or a change in homeostasis signals to mTORC1 to regulate protein synthesis. Recently, it has been demonstrated that glycolysis is linked to the mTORC1 pathway via the direct binding of glyceraldehyde-3-phosphate dehydrogenase (GAPDH) to Rheb in HEK293 and mouse embryo fibroblasts (Lee et al., 2009). The GAPDH-mediated reaction in glycolysis is substrate limited, therefore, GAPDH is well suited to monitor the glycolytic flux. The glycolytic flux regulates the interaction between GAPDH and Rheb, and this interaction inhibits mTORC1 signaling by preventing Rheb from binding to mTOR (Dodson et al., 2013). GAPDH regulates the binding of Rheb to mTOR in a manner that is dependent upon glycolytic intermediates and is independent of the nucleotide-charged status of Rheb. High glycolytic flux suppresses the interaction between GAPDH and Rheb and thus allows Rheb to activate mTORC1, whereas low glycolytic flux enhances the binding of GAPDH and Rheb, ultimately suppressing mTORC1 signaling (Lee et al., 2009, **Figure 2**). Thus, the GAPDH-Rheb axis may be responsible for more close cross talk between the glycolytic and the mTORC1 pathways, whereas the AMPK-dependent pathways may be responsive to other conditions that alter the AMP/ATP ratio (**Figure 2**).

The idea that the rate of glycolysis controls more than just carbohydrate metabolism in muscle *in vivo* is supported by a recent study by Luo et al. (2013). These authors demonstrated that during the development and progression of colorectal cancer, expression of the secreted autophagy-inducing stress protein HMGB1 increased in the muscle of tumor bearing mice. HMGB1administration resulted in a reduction in the protein expression of pyruvate kinase muscle (PKM) isoform 1 leading to a reduction in PKM activity, which was associated with a reduced phosphorylation status of mTOR, increased autophagy, and increased utilization of AAs, glutamine in particular, to produce intermediates for the TCA cycle (Luo et al., 2013). These results are in line with previous observations from Saha et al. (2010) showing that increased glucose availability (25 vs. 5.5 mM) increased mTOR related signaling, independent of changes in ATP/AMP/ADP and creatine phosphate (Saha et al., 2010), but associated with increased lactate-to-pyruvate ratio. These data suggest 1) a higher flux through glycolysis; and 2) decreased NAD^+-to-NADH ratio. These changes may suppress the interaction between GAPDH and Rheb and thus allow Rheb to activate mTORC1, and/or reduce the abundance of the NAD^+-dependent histone/protein deacetylase SIRT1, ultimately reducing the activity of AMPK

(Ruderman et al., 2010). The potential role of PKM and SIRT1in skeletal muscle regeneration will be discussed in more detail below.

A NOVEL ROLE FOR NON-ESSENTIAL AMINO ACIDS IN THE REGULATION OF PROTEIN METABOLISM AND OXIDATIVE STRESS IN SKELETAL MUSCLE

Although NEAAs are generally believed not to be important for the regulation of protein synthesis under normal conditions, studies have indicated that some of these AAs can manipulate muscle protein metabolism during conditions of (chronic low-grade) inflammation or oxidative stress; e.g., during ageing (Wheeler et al., 1999; Roth et al., 2003). AAs such as glutamine and glycine are thought to modulate the production of inflammatory cytokines; thereby reducing the negative impact of these cytokines on protein metabolism.

Originally proposed to serve solely as a metabolic fuel or protein precursor for rapidly dividing cells, glutamine has been found to directly (or indirectly) regulate the expression of many genes related to metabolism, signal transduction, cell defense and repair, and to inhibit the activation of intracellular signaling pathways associated with cellular stress, such as the p38 MAP kinase and ERK pathways (for review see Curi et al., 2005). Examples of specific glutamine target molecules that help protect cells from inflammation and oxidative stress, include the increased expression of heat shock protein 72 and glutathione (Wischmeyer, 2006). Although the mechanism of action of glutamine has been studied in detail, the signaling mechanisms by which glycine can prevent or reduce cellular oxidative stress, and regulate protein synthesis/breakdown, metabolism, and the development of skeletal muscle, are not well understood.

Glycine is a simple NEAA consisting of a single carbon molecule attached to an amino and a carboxyl group. Glycine is often considered biologically neutral and sometimes used as an is onitrogenous control. However, evidence is emerging that glycine administration activates glycine-gated chloride channels in inflammatory cells, thereby effectively reducing $[Ca^{2+}]_i$, cytokine production, and whole-body (systemic) inflammation in several models (Zhong et al., 2003; Roth, 2007). Since increased inflammation plays a key role in the loss of skeletal muscle and adipose tissue with cancer cachexia, we recently tested the hypothesis that increasing glycine availability could represent a simple, safe and promising treatment to reduce wasting (Ham et al., 2013). We found that glycine treatment prevented ~50% of the cancer-induced loss in muscle mass and helped maintain muscle strength in tumor bearing mice. In addition, glycine reduced skeletal muscle IL-6 and F4/80 mRNA (a marker of macrophages) expression, and tended to reduce the oxidized glutathione/total glutathione ratio indicative of a reduction in oxidative stress. Finally, glycine treatment partially prevented the tumor-induced reduction in eIF-3f protein, a key protein in the regulation of mTORC1 binding to S6K1 (Lagirand-Cantaloube et al., 2008), normally seen in cachetic mice. These data suggest that during wasting conditions, the NEAA glycine can modulate anabolic signaling through mTORC1 (Ham et al., 2013). Clearly, glycine affects metabolism in multiple ways, but the exact cellular mechanisms of its action are not completely understood.

LINKING SKELETAL MUSCLE METABOLISM TO SATELLITE CELL BIOLOGY AND REGENERATION

In addition to the important role of metabolism in the regulation of protein balance and skeletal muscle mass, a developing body of literature has identified metabolism as playing an important role in the regulation of cell-fate during the specification and subsequent differentiation of stem-cells, a process that has been termed "metabolic reprogramming" (Lunt and Vander Heiden, 2011; Ryall, 2013).

SKELETAL MUSCLE STEM CELLS—THE SATELLITE CELL

Skeletal muscle is capable of remarkable regeneration in response to injury or trauma, a property conferred on skeletal muscle by the presence of a resident population of stem cells, the satellite cell (SC, Brack and Rando, 2012; Relaix and Zammit, 2012; Yin et al., 2013). First identified by Alexander Mauro in 1961, the SC sits in a unique anatomical location between the sarcolemma of the muscle fiber and the basement membrane that envelops the fiber (Mauro, 1961). The physical space surrounding the SC is termed the "SC niche" (Bentzinger et al., 2013). Interestingly, SCs have been found to co-localize with blood vessels (Christov et al., 2007; Ryall, 2013), placing them in an optimal position to respond to intrinsic signals from both the skeletal muscle fiber itself and changes in the systemic environment.

In healthy adult skeletal muscle, the majority of SCs exist in a quiescent state, outside of the cell cycle, in a state termed G_0. In response to injury or trauma, the SC leaves the quiescent state and enters the cell cycle at G_1 (activation). The SC then becomes specified to the myogenic lineage (specification/commitment) and progresses through the cell-cycle (proliferation). After several rounds of proliferation, SCs exit the cell cycle and undergo differentiation and fusion to form an immature myotube. Finally, these myotubes mature and grow to form mature myofibers. In this manner, SCs can efficiently repair damaged muscle fibers. Importantly, a small population of SCs exit the cell cycle early and return to the G_0 quiescent state, thus ensuring that the SC pool is replenished. Each of these steps is regulated through the coordinated expression of a family of transcription factors—the myogenic regulatory factors (MRFs); MyoD, Myf5, Myogenin, and MRF4 (MRFs, Brack and Rando, 2012; Bentzinger et al., 2013; Yin et al., 2013).

Although many other cell types such as $PW1^+$ (Paternally expressed 3 protein)/$Pax7^-$ interstitial cells (PIC), mesoangioblasts and mesenchymal stem cells have been proposed to contribute to myofiber regeneration (Dellavalle et al., 2007; Pannerec et al., 2013), work by Sambasivan and colleagues demonstrated that ablation of SCs led to failure of skeletal muscle regeneration (Sambasivan et al., 2011). These results suggest that while these "secondary" cell types contribute to regeneration they cannot replace the role of SCs. Thus, the remainder of this discussion will focus on SCs, as defined by the presence of the Pax7 transcription factor.

Advances in cell isolation techniques combined with the use of large scale gene arrays has provided a global view of quiescent SCs and insight into the regulation of SC quiescence and subsequent activation. Fukada et al. (2007) studied gene expression of quiescent and proliferating SCs, by combining fluorescence activated cell sorting (FACS) to isolate a pure subpopulation of SCs, followed by microarray analyses on either freshly isolated SCs (quiescent) or *ex vivo* activated and proliferating SCs. SCs were FACS isolated from a mononuclear suspension using fluorescently labeled antibodies for SM/C-2.6 (target antigen currently unknown) and CD45, with SM/C-2.6^+ and $CD45^-$ cells defined as the SC population. Utilizing microarray technology, 507 genes were identified with greater than five-fold differential expression in the quiescent vs. the proliferating SC populations. As expected, genes involved in the negative regulation of cell cycle progression were enriched in quiescent SCs. Interestingly, genes encoding regulators of cell-cell adhesion molecules, resistance to oxidative stress, and lipid transporter activity were also enriched in quiescent SCs (Fukada et al., 2007). It has been proposed that signaling through cell-cell adhesion molecules maintains SCs in an undifferentiated quiescent state, while resistance to oxidative stress is essential for all stem cell populations, so as to prevent free radical induced damage to the DNA. However, the importance of lipid transport and FAO in quiescent SCs has yet to be investigated.

In support for a role of FAO in the regulation of a stem-cell population, Ito and colleagues have shown that FAO may play a role in regulating hematopoietic stem-cell (HPSC) fate decisions (Ito et al., 2012). In this study the authors focussed on the role of peroxisome proliferator-activated receptor δ (PPARδ), which has been implicated in nutrient sensing and transcriptional regulation of genes involved in FA transport and FAO during stem-cell self-renewal (Takahashi et al., 2007). The inhibition of PPARδ or FAO in the context of HPSCs led to a decrease in self-renewal, and a decrease in the ratio of asymmetric to symmetric division in these cells. In contrast, treatment of HPSCs with a PPARδ agonist improved the maintenance of the HPSC population and increased the proportion of asymmetric divisions (Ito et al., 2012). This exciting study provided evidence that the PPARδ-FAO pathway may play an important role in the control of stem cell fate and, in particular, the control of asymmetric division of HPSCs.

METABOLIC REPROGRAMMING—LINKING METABOLISM TO TRANSCRIPTION AND THE REGULATION OF STEM CELL FATE

The first evidence linking a change in cellular metabolism to a change in cell state was provided by Otto Warburg in 1956, who found that tumor cells preferentially utilized the glycolytic pathway even in the presence of oxygen (Warburg, 1956). This process was referred to as aerobic glycolysis, and later the "Warburg effect." Since this seminal finding a significant body of work has focussed on the altered metabolism that occurs in tumor cells, and it has recently been proposed as a core hallmark of cancer (Ward and Thompson, 2012). Interestingly, a process of metabolic transformation has been identified in stem-cell populations during changes in cell-fate, with an explosion of interest in this area over the last 2–3 years. Through advances in developmental, cancer and stem-cell biology, it has become apparent that changes in cellular metabolism play a large role in the regulation of stem cell function—a process termed "metabolic reprogramming." Studies in embryonic stem cells (ESCs), and induced pluripotent stem cells (iPSCs) revealed that in these highly proliferative populations there is an increased reliance upon glycolysis and a reduced level of OXPHOS, compared with cells undergoing differentiation (Folmes et al., 2011; Zhang et al., 2011, 2012). The increased reliance on glycolysis has been attributed to the requirement of these cells to have access to a large supply of carbon and nitrogen for the generation of new biomass in these proliferating cells (Lunt and Vander Heiden, 2011, **Figure 3**). In contrast, studies in adult stem cell populations (that exist in a quiescent state, such as human T cells and resting B cells) have indicated that these cell populations rely upon FAO and OXPHOS, and upregulate markers of glycolysis upon a shift toward active proliferation (Wang et al., 2011; Le et al., 2012).

Clearly, the energetic demands and need for new biomass will differ for SCs during periods of quiescence, proliferation and differentiation. Thus, SCs must reprogram their metabolic profile to match these altered conditions. Evidence of a link between metabolism, SC identity and transplant efficiency has been provided by a recent study focussed on caloric restriction (CR, Cerletti et al., 2012). Mice were given a diet consisting of 60% of the caloric intake of standard *ad lib* fed mice for 12 weeks. At the completion of this dietary intervention there was an increase in total SC number, increased SC mitochondrial abundance and OXPHOS activity, and an increased proliferative capacity of SCs. Furthermore, the increase in OXPHOS activity observed in SCs isolated from CR mice was associated with a two-fold increase in the transplant efficiency of these cells (Cerletti et al., 2012). Interestingly, when control SCs were transplanted into a CR host

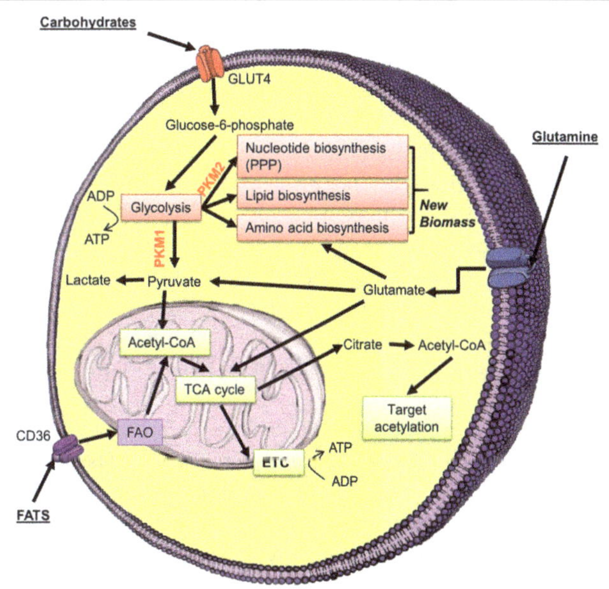

FIGURE 3 | Highly proliferative cell populations, such as some tumors, ESCs, iPSCs, and SCs require a ready supply of carbon and nitrogen for the generation of new biomass (nucleotides, proteins, phospholipids). To achieve this, many highly proliferative cell populations switch to a predominantly glycolytic based metabolism, but upregulate the PKM2 splice isoform of pyruvate kinase. In this manner, proliferating cells can build up sufficient glycolytic intermediates for the biomass necessary for cell division.

animal there was a similar improvement in transplant efficiency; indicating that both intrinsic SC factors and the host environment may influence the overall efficacy of SC transplant therapies (Cerletti et al., 2012).

The "golden age of biochemistry" in the first half of the 20th century helped define the majority of the metabolic pathways responsible for nutrient breakdown, however, it is only recently that a potential link between metabolism and cellular identity has been proposed (Deberardinis et al., 2008; Daley, 2012; Deberardinis and Thompson, 2012). As the metabolic state of a cell reflects the integrated response to both intracellular energy demands and the extracellular environment, alterations to either can lead to changes in metabolite balances (NAD^+/NADH, ADP/ATP, GDP/GTP), cellular pH, oxygen availability, small molecules (acetyl-CoA, methionine), voltage gradients and many more. All of these metabolically regulated changes can lead to differential regulation of transcription, and changes in cell identity (Lu and Thompson, 2012).

Acetyl-CoA and histone acetylation

Chromatin structure and organization is carefully regulated through a series of dynamic post-translational modifications, including (but not limited to) acetylation, methylation, phosphorylation, and ubiquitination. These modifications can alter the accessibility of the DNA to transcription initiating factors. One common histone modification, acetylation, has been found to be regulated in a metabolic dependant manner (Wellen et al., 2009; Lu and Thompson, 2012). Histone acetylation occurs via the actions of a histone acetyltransferase (HAT) in a reaction that transfers the acetyl group from acetyl-CoA to a specific residue (typically lysine) on the histone tail. In a study by Wellen et al. (2009) glucose was found to be the primary source of acetyl-CoA used in histone acetylation via conversion of mitochondrial derived acetate, induced by the enzyme ATP-citrate lyase (ACL). In this study, the authors used siRNA to demonstrate that ACL is essential for histone, but not protein acetylation. These results suggest that the acetyl pool used for protein acetylation may not be the same as that used for histone acetylation (Rathmell and Newgard, 2009). Importantly, a switch in substrate availability/utilization could lead to a rapid alteration in acetyl-CoA availability and histone acetylation status. Whether such a switch exists in SCs, and what role it may have, remains an intriguing possibility.

NAD^+ and the sirtuin family of histone/protein deacetylases

The class III family of histone/protein deacetylases, the sirtuin family, consists of seven members, all of which contain a conserved core catalytic domain and differ in their C- and N-terminal domains (Ryall, 2012). Unlike class I and II histone deacetylases (HDACs), sirtuins require NAD^+ for their deacetylase activity. One of the best described sirtuins, SIRT1 acts as a catalyst to transfer the acetyl group of the protein target to NAD^+ to produce nicotinamide (NAM), 2′-O-acetyl-ADP ribose, and the deacetylated target protein. Due to the reliance upon NAD^+, SIRT1 can be considered as an "energy sensor" that is activated in response to an increase in NAD^+ availability. At the level of whole skeletal muscle SIRT1 has been found to target a range of histone and protein targets, including histones H3K9 and H4K16, and the transcription factors PGC1α, MyoD, and FoxO1/3a (Fulco et al., 2003, 2008; Vaquero et al., 2006).

In 2003 Fulco and colleagues identified SIRT1 as an important regulator of skeletal muscle gene expression (Fulco et al., 2003). In this study the authors demonstrated that increased SIRT1 activity lead to inhibition of C2C12 differentiation, and reduced the expression of Myogenin (*Myog*) a master regulator of differentiation. In a follow up study, these authors went on to demonstrate that during periods of reduced nutrient availability, C2C12 differentiation was inhibited in both a SIRT1 and NAD^+ dependent manner. Interestingly, the NAD^+ salvage enzyme nicotinamide phosphoribosyltransferase (Nampt, responsible for the conversion of nicotinamide back to NAD^+) was found to mediate the effects of nutrient deprivation on myogenic differentiation (Fulco et al., 2008). However, the role of SIRT1 (and indeed NAD^+) has yet to be investigated in SCs, particularly during important cell fate decisions such as myogenic commitment and the process of differentiation.

While SIRT1 is the best described of the sirtuin family (in the context of skeletal muscle), there exists six other mammalian sirtuins all of which have been found to regulate metabolism in many tissues (Chang and Guarente, 2013). Currently, very little is known about the role (if any) of SIRT2-6 in SCs, however a number of recent studies have begun to identify a role for some of these deacetylases in skeletal muscle. SIRT3 is localized to the mitochondria and has been found to promote the activity of a number of important mitochondrial enzymes, including pyruvate dehydrogenase, in a deacetylation dependent manner (Fernandez-Marcos et al., 2012; Jing et al., 2013). The SIRT4 isoform (also localized to the mitochondria) can regulate lipid metabolism via deacetylation of the malonyl CoA decarboxylase (MCD) enzyme leading to its inhibition and subsequent lipogenesis (Laurent et al., 2013). Finally, SIRT6 has been found to (indirectly) negatively regulate AKT phosphorylation, and subsequent hypoglycaemia via increased transport of glucose into skeletal muscle (Xiao et al., 2010).

Serine/glycine metabolism and histone methylation

Similarly to the requirement for acetyl-CoA for histone acetylation, histone methylation requires S-adenosyl (SAM) methionine as a methyl-donor. Shyh-Chang and colleagues have recently demonstrated a requirement for the amino acid threonine in histone H3K4 trimethylation (H3K4me3) in pluripotent mouse embryonic stem cells (mESC, Shyh-Chang et al., 2013). Interestingly, these authors determined that threonine was a requirement for H3K4me3 and H3K4me2, but not H3K4me1, H3K9me3, H3K27me3 or H3K26me3, suggesting that threonine levels regulate the methylation status of specific lysine residues. However, similarly to acetyl-CoA metabolism, the role of threonine metabolism in SC quiescence, proliferation and differentiation has not been investigated.

Utilizing chromatin immunoprecipitation, followed by whole genome sequencing (ChIPseq), it is possible to obtain a global enrichmentprofile of specific histone modifications. Liu and colleagues used ChIPseq to analyse the global expression profile of histone H3K4me3 and H3K27me3 in FACS isolated quiescent and proliferating SCs (Liu et al., 2013), and found that while both quiescent and proliferating SCs exhibited similar H3K4me3 profiles, the global level of H3K27me3 was significantly enriched. As expected (due to its link to gene silencing) many genes that were down regulated in proliferating SCs exhibited a dramatic enrichment of H3K27me3 throughout the gene body. In a previous study by Juan and colleagues, the histone methyltransferase Ezh2 was found to be an essential regulator of SC identity and self-renewal. While not present in quiescent SCs, Ezh2 was rapidly upregulated in activated and proliferating SCs, leading to H3K27me3 and inhibiting the expression of transcription factors known to regulate non-myogenic lineages (Juan et al., 2011).

Differential splicing of pyruvate kinase, and histone phosphorylation

Differential splicing of PKM at exons 9 and 10 has been found to be an important regulator of the decision to shunt glycolytic intermediates for breakdown to acetyl-CoA (which will enter the mitochondria and the TCA cycle), or to instead enter the PPP to produce nucleotides, proteins and phospholipids for cell growth (Gupta et al., 2011; Macintyre and Rathmell, 2011). Inclusion of exon 9 produces PKM1, which catalyzes the dephosphorylation of phosphoenolpyruvate (PEP), and promotes the entry of pyruvate into the mitochondria for conversion to acetyl-CoA. In contrast, exon 10 inclusion produces the PKM2 splice isoform which has a reduced affinity for PEP, and leads to the build-up of glycolytic intermediates available for entry into the PPP (Gupta et al., 2011). Interestingly, highly proliferative stem-cells such as ESCs and tumor cells exhibit preferential transcription of PKM2—indicating that PKM may play an important role in the process of stem-cell metabolic reprogramming (Lv et al., 2011; Ye et al., 2012). Similarly, proliferating C2C12 cells exhibit preferential transcription of the PKM2 splice isoform, which has been proposed to be essential to allow the cells to generate sufficient intermediates for the generation of new macromolecules (Harada et al., 1995; David et al., 2010).

A LINK BETWEEN SKELETAL MUSCLE FIBER METABOLISM AND SATELLITE CELL DENSITY

The space that surrounds the SC between the basal lamina and sarcolemma has been termed the "SC niche" (Lander et al., 2012). The majority of adult stem-cells have been found to localize to a specialized niche, and a number of exciting studies have proposed that SC function can be regulated via changes to the niche environment (Gilbert et al., 2010; Chakkalakal et al., 2012). It is interesting to postulate that the metabolic milieu of the SC niche may be different from that of the muscle fiber and/or the extracellular space. Thus muscle damage would be expected to destroy the niche and expose the SC to an altered metabolic environment, leading to rapid changes in both nutrient uptake and intracellular metabolism.

In addition to the local niche milieu (open to influence via changes in the systemic environment), SC numbers can be influenced by the fiber they are attached to, with an increased number of SCs associated with fibers that are predominantly oxidative (slow, type I fibers), compared with fibers that rely primarily on glycolysis (fast, type II fibers) (Putman et al., 2001; Christov et al., 2007). However, whether this is due to direct signaling from the fiber to the SC population and what role the metabolic status of the fiber may play in SC biology, has yet to be investigated.

Both physiological and pathological changes in metabolism can influence stem-cell number and function. Interestingly, interventions that promote a shift in skeletal muscle metabolism from glycolysis to OXPHOS, such as chronic low-frequency stimulation (LFS) of the peroneal nerve (a model of endurance exercise training), have been observed to lead to an increase in SC number (Putman et al., 1999, 2001). While LFS is a well characterized model in regards to effects on whole muscle and single fiber metabolism, very little is known regarding the effects on SC metabolism.

CONCLUSIONS

While a wealth of information exists on the role of metabolism in health and disease, it is only more recently that we are beginning to appreciate the close link between metabolism and skeletal muscle wasting and regeneration. The studies presented in the current discussion have identified numerous ways in which metabolism can directly influence protein synthesis and transcription. It is in this manner that metabolic remodeling can play a large role in both physiologic and pathologic adaptations during a disruption in homeostasis. However, it is also clear that significant questions remain regarding the role of metabolism in skeletal muscle, particularly with reference to its role in regulating SC biology and skeletal muscle regeneration.

ACKNOWLEDGMENTS

James G. Ryall is supported by an Overseas Biomedical Research Fellowship from the National Health and Medical Research Council of Australia.

REFERENCES

Akhmedov, D., and Berdeaux, R. (2013). The effects of obesity on skeletal muscle regeneration. *Front. Physiol.* 4:371. doi: 10.3389/fphys.2013.00371

Angelini, C., and Semplicini, C. (2010). Metabolic myopathies: the challenge of new treatments. *Curr. Opin. Pharmacol.* 10, 338–345. doi: 10.1016/j.coph.2010.02.006

Bentzinger, C. F., Wang, Y. X., Dumont, N. A., and Rudnicki, M. A. (2013). Cellular dynamics in the muscle satellite cell niche. *EMBO Rep.* 14, 1062–1072. doi: 10.1038/embor.2013.182

Bodine, S. C., Stitt, T. N., Gonzalez, M., Kline, W. O., Stover, G. L., Bauerlein, R., et al. (2001). Akt/mTOR pathway is a crucial regulator of skeletal muscle hypertrophy and can prevent muscle atrophy *in vivo*. *Nat. Cell Biol.* 3, 1014–1019. doi: 10.1038/ncb1101-1014

Bolster, D. R., Kubica, N., Crozier, S. J., Williamson, D. L., Farrell, P. A., Kimball, S. R., et al. (2003). Immediate response of mammalian target of rapamycin (mTOR)-mediated signalling following acute resistance exercise in rat skeletal muscle. *J. Physiol.* 553, 213–220. doi: 10.1113/jphysiol.2003.047019

Brack, A. S., and Rando, T. A. (2012). Tissue-specific stem cells: lessons from the skeletal muscle satellite cell. *Cell Stem Cell* 10, 504–514. doi: 10.1016/j.stem.2012.04.001

Cerletti, M., Jang, Y. C., Finley, L. W., Haigis, M. C., and Wagers, A. J. (2012). Short-term calorie restriction enhances skeletal muscle stem cell function. *Cell Stem Cell* 10, 515–519. doi: 10.1016/j.stem.2012.04.002

Chakkalakal, J. V., Jones, K. M., Basson, M. A., and Brack, A. S. (2012). The aged niche disrupts muscle stem cell quiescence. *Nature* 490, 355–360. doi: 10.1038/nature11438

Chang, H. C., and Guarente, L. (2013). SIRT1 and other sirtuins in metabolism. *Trends Endocrinol. Metab.* doi: 10.1016/j.tem.2013.12.001. [Epub ahead of Print].

Christov, C., Chretien, F., Abou-Khalil, R., Bassez, G., Vallet, G., Authier, F. J., et al. (2007). Muscle satellite cells and endothelial cells: close neighbors and privileged partners. *Mol. Biol. Cell* 18, 1397–1409. doi: 10.1091/mbc.E06-08-0693

Curi, R., Lagranha, C. J., Doi, S. Q., Sellitti, D. F., Procopio, J., Pithon-Curi, T. C., et al. (2005). Molecular mechanisms of glutamine action. *J. Cell. Physiol.* 204, 392–401. doi: 10.1002/jcp.20339

Cuthbertson, D., Smith, K., Babraj, J., Leese, G., Waddell, T., Atherton, P., et al. (2005). Anabolic signaling deficits underlie amino acid resistance of wasting, aging muscle. *FASEB J.* 19, 422–424. doi: 10.1096/fj.04-2640fje

Daley, G. Q. (2012). Cellular alchemy and the golden age of reprogramming. *Cell* 151, 1151–1154. doi: 10.1016/j.cell.2012.11.016

David, C. J., Chen, M., Assanah, M., Canoll, P., and Manley, J. L. (2010). HnRNP proteins controlled by c-Myc deregulate pyruvate kinase mRNA splicing in cancer. *Nature* 463, 364–368. doi: 10.1038/nature08697

Deberardinis, R. J., Lum, J. J., Hatzivassiliou, G., and Thompson, C. B. (2008). The biology of cancer: metabolic reprogramming fuels cell growth and proliferation. *Cell Metab.* 7, 11–20. doi: 10.1016/j.cmet.2007.10.002

Deberardinis, R. J., and Thompson, C. B. (2012). Cellular metabolism and disease: what do metabolic outliers teach us? *Cell* 148, 1132–1144. doi: 10.1016/j.cell.2012.02.032

Dellavalle, A., Sampaolesi, M., Tonlorenzi, R., Tagliafico, E., Sacchetti, B., Perani, L., et al. (2007). Pericytes of human skeletal muscle are myogenic precursors distinct from satellite cells. *Nat. Cell Biol.* 9, 255–267. doi: 10.1038/ncb1542

Dickinson, J. M., Fry, C. S., Drummond, M. J., Gundermann, D. M., Walker, D. K., Glynn, E. L., et al. (2011). Mammalian target of rapamycin complex 1 activation is required for the stimulation of human skeletal muscle protein synthesis by essential amino acids. *J. Nutr.* 141, 856–862. doi: 10.3945/jn.111.139485

Dodd, K. M., and Tee, A. R. (2012). Leucine and mTORC1: a complex relationship. *Am. J. Physiol. Endocrinol. Metab.* 302, E1329–E1342. doi: 10.1152/ajpendo.00525.2011

Dodson, M., Darley-Usmar, V., and Zhang, J. (2013). Cellular metabolic and autophagic pathways: traffic control by redox signaling. *Free Radic Biol. Med.* 63, 207–221. doi: 10.1016/j.freeradbiomed.2013.05.014

Dreyer, H. C., Fujita, S., Cadenas, J. G., Chinkes, D. L., Volpi, E., and Rasmussen, B. B. (2006). Resistance exercise increases AMPK activity and reduces 4E-BP1 phosphorylation and protein synthesis in human skeletal muscle. *J. Physiol.* 576, 613–624. doi: 10.1113/jphysiol.2006.113175

Drummond, M. J., Bell, J. A., Fujita, S., Dreyer, H. C., Glynn, E. L., Volpi, E., et al. (2008a). Amino acids are necessary for the insulin-induced activation of mTOR/S6K1 signaling and protein synthesis in healthy and insulin resistant human skeletal muscle. *Clin. Nutr.* 27, 447–456. doi: 10.1016/j.clnu.2008.01.012

Drummond, M. J., Dreyer, H. C., Pennings, B., Fry, C. S., Dhanani, S., Dillon, E. L., et al. (2008b). Skeletal muscle protein anabolic response to resistance exercise and essential amino acids is delayed with aging. *J. Appl. Physiol.* 104, 1452–1461. doi: 10.1152/japplphysiol.00021.2008

Fernandez-Marcos, P. J., Jeninga, E. H., Canto, C., Harach, T., De Boer, V. C., Andreux, P., et al. (2012). Muscle or liver-specific Sirt3 deficiency induces hyperacetylation of mitochondrial proteins without affecting global metabolic homeostasis. *Sci. Rep.* 2, 425. doi: 10.1038/srep00425

Folmes, C. D., Nelson, T. J., Martinez-Fernandez, A., Arrell, D. K., Lindor, J. Z., Dzeja, P. P., et al. (2011). Somatic oxidative bioenergetics transitions into pluripotency-dependent glycolysis to facilitate nuclear reprogramming. *Cell Metab.* 14, 264–271. doi: 10.1016/j.cmet.2011.06.011

Fukada, S., Uezumi, A., Ikemoto, M., Masuda, S., Segawa, M., Tanimura, N., et al. (2007). Molecular signature of quiescent satellite cells in adult skeletal muscle. *Stem Cells* 25, 2448–2459. doi: 10.1634/stemcells.2007-0019

Fulco, M., Cen, Y., Zhao, P., Hoffman, E. P., McBurney, M. W., Sauve, A. A., et al. (2008). Glucose restriction inhibits skeletal myoblast differentiation by activating SIRT1 through AMPK-mediated regulation of Nampt. *Dev. Cell* 14, 661–673. doi: 10.1016/j.devcel.2008.02.004

Fulco, M., Schiltz, R. L., Iezzi, S., King, M. T., Zhao, P., Kashiwaya, Y., et al. (2003). Sir2 regulates skeletal muscle differentiation as a potential sensor of the redox state. *Mol. Cell* 12, 51–62. doi: 10.1016/S1097-2765(03)00226-0

Gilbert, P. M., Havenstrite, K. L., Magnusson, K. E., Sacco, A., Leonardi, N. A., Kraft, P., et al. (2010). Substrate elasticity regulates skeletal muscle stem cell self-renewal in culture. *Science* 329, 1078–1081. doi: 10.1126/science.1191035

Guillet, C., Prod'homme, M., Balage, M., Gachon, P., Giraudet, C., Morin, L., et al. (2004). Impaired anabolic response of muscle protein synthesis is associated with S6K1 dysregulation in elderly humans. *FASEB J.* 18, 1586–1587. doi: 10.1096/fj.03-1341fje

Gupta, R. K., Rosen, E. D., and Spiegelman, B. M. (2011). Identifying novel transcriptional components controlling energy metabolism. *Cell. Metab.* 14, 739–745. doi: 10.1016/j.cmet.2011.11.007

Ham, D. J., Murphy, K. T., Chee, A., Lynch, G. S., and Koopman, R. (2013). Glycine administration attenuates skeletal muscle wasting in a mouse model of cancer cachexia. *Clin. Nutr.* doi: 10.1016/j.clnu.2013.06.013. [Epub ahead of print].

Harada, Y., Nakamura, M., and Asano, A. (1995). Temporally distinctive changes of alternative splicing patterns during myogenic differentiation of C2C12 cells. *J. Biochem.* 118, 780–790.

Hojlund, K., Mustard, K. J., Staehr, P., Hardie, D. G., Beck-Nielsen, H., Richter, E. A., et al. (2004). AMPK activity and isoform protein expression are similar in muscle of obese subjects with and without type 2 diabetes. *Am. J. Physiol. Endocrinol. Metab.* 286, E239–E244. doi: 10.1152/ajpendo.00326.2003

Ito, K., Carracedo, A., Weiss, D., Arai, F., Ala, U., Avigan, D. E., et al. (2012). A PML-PPAR-delta pathway for fatty acid oxidation regulates hematopoietic stem cell maintenance. *Nat. Med.* 18, 1350–1358. doi: 10.1038/nm.2882

Jing, E., O'Neill, B. T., Rardin, M. J., Kleinridders, A., Ilkeyeva, O. R., Ussar, S., et al. (2013). Sirt3 regulates metabolic flexibility of skeletal muscle through reversible enzymatic deacetylation. *Diabetes* 62, 3404–3417. doi: 10.2337/db12-1650

Juan, A. H., Derfoul, A., Feng, X., Ryall, J. G., Dell'Orso, S., Pasut, A., et al. (2011). Polycomb EZH2 controls self-renewal and safeguards the transcriptional identity of skeletal muscle stem cells. *Genes Dev.* 25, 789–794. doi: 10.1101/gad.2027911

Kimball, S. R., Farrell, P. A., and Jefferson, L. S. (2002). Invited review: role of insulin in translational control of protein synthesis in skeletal muscle by amino acids or exercise. *J. Appl. Physiol.* 93, 1168–1180. doi: 10.1152/japplphysiol.00221.2002

Lagirand-Cantaloube, J., Offner, N., Csibi, A., Leibovitch, M. P., Batonnet-Pichon, S., Tintignac, L. A., et al. (2008). The initiation factor eIF3-f is a major target for atrogin1/MAFbx function in skeletal muscle atrophy. *EMBO J.* 27, 1266–1276. doi: 10.1038/emboj.2008.52

Lander, A. D., Kimble, J., Clevers, H., Fuchs, E., Montarras, D., Buckingham, M., et al. (2012). What does the concept of the stem cell niche really mean today? *BMC Biol.* 10:19. doi: 10.1186/1741-7007-10-19

Lantier, L., Mounier, R., Leclerc, J., Pende, M., Foretz, M., and Viollet, B. (2010). Coordinated maintenance of muscle cell size control by AMP-activated protein kinase. *FASEB J.* 24, 3555–3561. doi: 10.1096/fj.10-155994

Laplante, M., and Sabatini, D. M. (2012). mTOR signaling in growth control and disease. *Cell* 149, 274–293. doi: 10.1016/j.cell.2012.03.017

Laurent, G., German, N. J., Saha, A. K., De Boer, V. C., Davies, M., Koves, T. R., et al. (2013). SIRT4 coordinates the balance between lipid synthesis and catabolism by repressing malonyl CoA decarboxylase. *Mol. Cell* 50, 686–698. doi: 10.1016/j.molcel.2013.05.012

Le, A., Lane, A. N., Hamaker, M., Bose, S., Gouw, A., Barbi, J., et al. (2012). Glucose-independent glutamine metabolism via TCA cycling for proliferation and survival in B cells. *Cell Metab.* 15, 110–121. doi: 10.1016/j.cmet.2011.12.009

Lee, M. N., Ha, S. H., Kim, J., Koh, A., Lee, C. S., Kim, J. H., et al. (2009). Glycolytic flux signals to mTOR through glyceraldehyde-3-phosphate dehydrogenase-mediated regulation of Rheb. *Mol. Cell. Biol.* 29, 3991–4001. doi: 10.1128/mcb.00165-09

Li, M., Verdijk, L. B., Sakamoto, K., Ely, B., Van Loon, L. J., and Musi, N. (2012). Reduced AMPK-ACC and mTOR signaling in muscle from older men, and effect of resistance exercise. *Mech. Ageing Dev.* 133, 655–664. doi: 10.1016/j.mad.2012.09.001

Liu, L., Cheung, T. H., Charville, G. W., Hurgo, B. M., Leavitt, T., Shih, J., et al. (2013). Chromatin modifications as determinants of muscle stem cell quiescence and chronological aging. *Cell Rep.* 4, 189–204. doi: 10.1016/j.celrep.2013.05.043

Lu, C., and Thompson, C. B. (2012). Metabolic regulation of epigenetics. *Cell Metab.* 16, 9–17. doi: 10.1016/j.cmet.2012.06.001

Lunt, S. Y., and Vander Heiden, M. G. (2011). Aerobic glycolysis: meeting the metabolic requirements of cell proliferation. *Annu. Rev. Cell Dev. Biol.* 27, 441–464. doi: 10.1146/annurev-cellbio-092910-154237

Luo, Y., Yoneda, J., Ohmori, H., Sasaki, T., Shimbo, K., Eto, S., et al. (2013). Cancer usurps skeletal muscle as an energy repository. *Cancer Res.* 74, 330–340. doi: 10.1158/0008-5472.CAN-13-1052

Lv, L., Li, D., Zhao, D., Lin, R., Chu, Y., Zhang, H., et al. (2011). Acetylation targets the M2 isoform of pyruvate kinase for degradation through chaperone-mediated autophagy and promotes tumor growth. *Mol. Cell* 42, 719–730. doi: 10.1016/j.molcel.2011.04.025

Macintyre, A. N., and Rathmell, J. C. (2011). PKM2 and the tricky balance of growth and energy in cancer. *Mol. Cell.* 42, 713–714. doi: 10.1016/j.molcel.2011.06.003

Mauro, A. (1961). Satellite cell of skeletal muscle fibers. *J. Biophys. Biochem. Cytol.* 9, 493–495. doi: 10.1083/jcb.9.2.493

Norton, L. E., and Layman, D. K. (2006). Leucine regulates translation initiation of protein synthesis in skeletal muscle after exercise. *J. Nutr.* 136, 533S–537S.

Paddon-Jones, D., Sheffield-Moore, M., Katsanos, C. S., Zhang, X. J., and Wolfe, R. R. (2006). Differential stimulation of muscle protein synthesis in elderly humans following isocaloric ingestion of amino acids or whey protein. *Exp. Gerontol.* 41, 215–219. doi: 10.1016/j.exger.2005.10.006

Paddon-Jones, D., Sheffield-Moore, M., Zhang, X. J., Volpi, E., Wolf, S. E., Aarsland, A., et al. (2004). Amino acid ingestion improves muscle protein synthesis in the young and elderly. *Am. J. Physiol. Endocrinol. Metab.* 286, E321–E328. doi: 10.1152/ajpendo.00368.2003

Pannerec, A., Formicola, L., Besson, V., Marazzi, G., and Sassoon, D. A. (2013). Defining skeletal muscle resident progenitors and their cell fate potentials. *Development* 140, 2879–2891. doi: 10.1242/dev.089326

Putman, C. T., Dusterhoft, S., and Pette, D. (1999). Changes in satellite cell content and myosin isoforms in low-frequency-stimulated fast muscle of hypothyroid rat. *J. Appl. Physiol.* 86, 40–51.

Putman, C. T., Sultan, K. R., Wassmer, T., Bamford, J. A., Skorjanc, D., and Pette, D. (2001). Fiber-type transitions and satellite cell activation in low-frequency-stimulated muscles of young and aging rats. *J. Gerontol. A Biol. Sci. Med. Sci.* 56, B510–B519. doi: 10.1093/gerona/56.12.B510

Raben, N., Wong, A., Ralston, E., and Myerowitz, R. (2012). Autophagy and mitochondria in Pompe disease: nothing is so new as what has long been forgotten. *Am. J. Med. Genet. C Semin. Med. Genet.* 160C, 13–21. doi: 10.1002/ajmg.c.31317

Rathmell, J. C., and Newgard, C. B. (2009). Biochemistry. A glucose-to-gene link. *Science* 324, 1021–1022. doi: 10.1126/science.1174665

Relaix, F., and Zammit, P. S. (2012). Satellite cells are essential for skeletal muscle regeneration: the cell on the edge returns centre stage. *Development* 139, 2845–2856. doi: 10.1242/dev.069088

Rennie, M. J., Edwards, R. H., Halliday, D., Matthews, D. E., Wolman, S. L., and Millward, D. J. (1982). Muscle protein synthesis measured by stable isotope techniques in man: the effects of feeding and fasting. *Clin. Sci. (Lond.)* 63, 519–523.

Roth, E. (2007). Immune and cell modulation by amino acids. *Clin. Nutr.* 26, 535–544. doi: 10.1016/j.clnu.2007.05.007

Roth, E., Zellner, M., Wessner, B., Strasser, E., Manhart, N., Oehler, R., et al. (2003). Glycine–an inert amino acid comes alive. *Nutrition* 19, 817–818. doi: 10.1016/S0899-9007(03)00100-X

Ruderman, N. B., Xu, X. J., Nelson, L., Cacicedo, J. M., Saha, A. K., Lan, F., et al. (2010). AMPK and SIRT1: a long-standing partnership? *Am. J. Physiol. Endocrinol. Metab.* 298, E751–E760. doi: 10.1152/ajpendo.00745.2009

Russell, A. P., Foletta, V. C., Snow, R. J., and Wadley, G. D. (2013). Skeletal muscle mitochondria: a major player in exercise, health and disease. *Biochim. Biophys. Acta.* doi: 10.1016/j.bbagen.2013.11.016. [Epub ahead of print].

Ryall, J. G. (2012). The role of sirtuins in the regulation of metabolic homeostasis in skeletal muscle. *Curr. Opin. Clin. Nutr. Metab. Care* 15, 561–566. doi: 10.1097/MCO.0b013e3283590914

Ryall, J. G. (2013). Metabolic reprogramming as a novel regulator of skeletal muscle development and regeneration. *FEBS J.* 280, 4004–4013. doi: 10.1111/febs.12189

Ryall, J. G., Schertzer, J. D., and Lynch, G. S. (2008). Cellular and molecular mechanisms underlying age-related skeletal muscle wasting and weakness. *Biogerontology* 9, 213–228. doi: 10.1007/s10522-008-9131-0

Saha, A. K., Xu, X. J., Lawson, E., Deoliveira, R., Brandon, A. E., Kraegen, E. W., et al. (2010). Downregulation of AMPK accompanies leucine- and glucose-induced increases in protein synthesis and insulin resistance in rat skeletal muscle. *Diabetes* 59, 2426–2434. doi: 10.2337/db09-1870

Salway, J. (2012). *Medical Biochemistry at a Glance.* West Sussex: John Wiley and Sons, Ltd.

Sambasivan, R., Yao, R., Kissenpfennig, A., Van Wittenberghe, L., Paldi, A., Gayraud-Morel, B., et al. (2011). Pax7-expressing satellite cells are indispensable for adult skeletal muscle regeneration. *Development* 138, 3647–3656. doi: 10.1242/dev.067587

Shyh-Chang, N., Daley, G. Q., and Cantley, L. C. (2013). Stem cell metabolism in tissue development and aging. *Development* 140, 2535–2547. doi: 10.1242/dev.091777

Smith, K., Barua, J. M., Watt, P. W., Scrimgeour, C. M., and Rennie, M. J. (1992). Flooding with L-[1-13C] leucine stimulates human muscle protein incorporation of continuously infused L-[1-13C] valine. *Am. J. Physiol.* 262, E372–E376.

Steinberg, G. R., and Kemp, B. E. (2009). AMPK in Health and Disease. *Physiol. Rev.* 89, 1025–1078. doi: 10.1152/physrev.00011.2008

Steinberg, G. R., O'Neill, H. M., Dzamko, N. L., Galic, S., Naim, T., Koopman, R., et al. (2010). Whole body deletion of AMP-activated protein kinase {beta}2 reduces muscle AMPK activity and exercise capacity. *J. Biol. Chem.* 285, 37198–37209. doi: 10.1074/jbc.M110.102434

Steinberg, G. R., Smith, A. C., Van Denderen, B. J., Chen, Z., Murthy, S., Campbell, D. J., et al. (2004). AMP-activated protein kinase is not down-regulated in human skeletal muscle of obese females. *J. Clin. Endocrinol. Metab.* 89, 4575–4580. doi: 10.1210/jc.2004-0308

Takahashi, S., Tanaka, T., and Sakai, J. (2007). New therapeutic target for metabolic syndrome: PPARdelta. *Endocr. J.* 54, 347–357. doi: 10.1507/endocrj.KR-99

Tsujimoto, Y. (1997). Apoptosis and necrosis: intracellular ATP level as a determinant for cell death modes. *Cell Death Differ.* 4, 429–434. doi: 10.1038/sj.cdd.4400262

Vaquero, A., Scher, M. B., Lee, D. H., Sutton, A., Cheng, H. L., Alt, F. W., et al. (2006). SirT2 is a histone deacetylase with preference for histone H4 Lys 16 during mitosis. *Genes Dev.* 20, 1256–1261. doi: 10.1101/gad.1412706

Volpi, E., Ferrando, A. A., Yeckel, C. W., Tipton, K. D., and Wolfe, R. R. (1998). Exogenous amino acids stimulate net muscle protein synthesis in the elderly. *J. Clin. Invest.* 101, 2000–2007. doi: 10.1172/JCI939

Volpi, E., Kobayashi, H., Sheffield-Moore, M., Mittendorfer, B., and Wolfe, R. R. (2003). Essential amino acids are primarily responsible for the amino acid stimulation of muscle protein anabolism in healthy elderly adults. *Am. J. Clin. Nutr.* 78, 250–258.

Volpi, E., Mittendorfer, B., Wolf, S. E., and Wolfe, R. R. (1999). Oral amino acids stimulate muscle protein anabolism in the elderly despite higher first-pass splanchnic extraction. *Am. J. Physiol.* 277, E513–E520.

Wang, R., Dillon, C. P., Shi, L. Z., Milasta, S., Carter, R., Finkelstein, D., et al. (2011). The transcription factor Myc controls metabolic reprogramming upon T lymphocyte activation. *Immunity* 35, 871–882. doi: 10.1016/j.immuni.2011.09.021

Warburg, O. (1956). On the origin of cancer cells. *Science* 123, 309–314. doi: 10.1126/science.123.3191.309

Ward, P. S., and Thompson, C. B. (2012). Metabolic reprogramming: a cancer hallmark even warburg did not anticipate. *Cancer Cell* 21, 297–308. doi: 10.1016/j.ccr.2012.02.014

Wellen, K. E., Hatzivassiliou, G., Sachdeva, U. M., Bui, T. V., Cross, J. R., and Thompson, C. B. (2009). ATP-citrate lyase links cellular metabolism to histone acetylation. *Science* 324, 1076–1080. doi: 10.1126/science.1164097

Wheeler, M. D., Ikejema, K., Enomoto, N., Stacklewitz, R. F., Seabra, V., Zhong, Z., et al. (1999). Glycine: a new anti-inflammatory immunonutrient. *Cell. Mol. Life Sci.* 56, 843–856. doi: 10.1007/s000180050030

Wischmeyer, P. E. (2006). The glutamine story: where are we now? *Curr. Opin. Crit. Care* 12, 142–148. doi: 10.1097/01.ccx.0000216582.87674.a4

Xiao, C., Kim, H. S., Lahusen, T., Wang, R. H., Xu, X., Gavrilova, O., et al. (2010). SIRT6 deficiency results in severe hypoglycemia by enhancing both basal and insulin-stimulated glucose uptake in mice. *J. Biol. Chem.* 285, 36776–36784. doi: 10.1074/jbc.M110.168039

Ye, J., Mancuso, A., Tong, X., Ward, P. S., Fan, J., Rabinowitz, J. D., et al. (2012). Pyruvate kinase M2 promotes de novo serine synthesis to sustain mTORC1 activity and cell proliferation. *Proc. Natl. Acad. Sci. U.S.A.* 109, 6904–6909. doi: 10.1073/pnas.1204176109.

Yin, H., Price, F., and Rudnicki, M. A. (2013). Satellite cells and the muscle stem cell niche. *Physiol. Rev.* 93, 23–67. doi: 10.1152/physrev.00043.2011

Zhang, J., Khvorostov, I., Hong, J. S., Oktay, Y., Vergnes, L., Nuebel, E., et al. (2011). UCP2 regulates energy metabolism and differentiation potential of human pluripotent stem cells. *EMBO J.* 30, 4860–4873. doi: 10.1038/emboj.2011.401

Zhang, J., Nuebel, E., Daley, G. Q., Koehler, C. M., and Teitell, M. A. (2012). Metabolic regulation in pluripotent stem cells during reprogramming and self-renewal. *Cell Stem Cell* 11, 589–595. doi: 10.1016/j.stem.2012.10.005

Zhao, J. X., Yan, X., Tong, J. F., Means, W. J., McCormick, R. J., Zhu, M. J., et al. (2010). Mouse AMP-activated protein kinase gamma3 subunit R225Q mutation affecting mouse growth performance when fed a high-energy diet. *J. Anim. Sci.* 88, 1332–1340. doi: 10.2527/jas.2009-2376

Zhong, Z., Wheeler, M. D., Li, X., Froh, M., Schemmer, P., Yin, M., et al. (2003). L-Glycine: a novel antiinflammatory, immunomodulatory, and cytoprotective agent. *Curr. Opin. Clin. Nutr. Metab. Care* 6, 229–240. doi: 10.1097/01.mco.0000058609.19236.a4

Permissions

All chapters in this book were first published by Frontiers; hereby published with permission under the Creative Commons Attribution License or equivalent. Every chapter published in this book has been scrutinized by our experts. Their significance has been extensively debated. The topics covered herein carry significant findings which will fuel the growth of the discipline. They may even be implemented as practical applications or may be referred to as a beginning point for another development.

The contributors of this book come from diverse backgrounds, making this book a truly international effort. This book will bring forth new frontiers with its revolutionizing research information and detailed analysis of the nascent developments around the world.

We would like to thank all the contributing authors for lending their expertise to make the book truly unique. They have played a crucial role in the development of this book. Without their invaluable contributions this book wouldn't have been possible. They have made vital efforts to compile up to date information on the varied aspects of this subject to make this book a valuable addition to the collection of many professionals and students.

This book was conceptualized with the vision of imparting up-to-date information and advanced data in this field. To ensure the same, a matchless editorial board was set up. Every individual on the board went through rigorous rounds of assessment to prove their worth. After which they invested a large part of their time researching and compiling the most relevant data for our readers.

The editorial board has been involved in producing this book since its inception. They have spent rigorous hours researching and exploring the diverse topics which have resulted in the successful publishing of this book. They have passed on their knowledge of decades through this book. To expedite this challenging task, the publisher supported the team at every step. A small team of assistant editors was also appointed to further simplify the editing procedure and attain best results for the readers.

Apart from the editorial board, the designing team has also invested a significant amount of their time in understanding the subject and creating the most relevant covers. They scrutinized every image to scout for the most suitable representation of the subject and create an appropriate cover for the book.

The publishing team has been an ardent support to the editorial, designing and production team. Their endless efforts to recruit the best for this project, has resulted in the accomplishment of this book. They are a veteran in the field of academics and their pool of knowledge is as vast as their experience in printing. Their expertise and guidance has proved useful at every step. Their uncompromising quality standards have made this book an exceptional effort. Their encouragement from time to time has been an inspiration for everyone.

The publisher and the editorial board hope that this book will prove to be a valuable piece of knowledge for researchers, students, practitioners and scholars across the globe.

List of Contributors

Dmitry Akhmedov and Rebecca Berdeaux
Department of Integrative Biology and Pharmacology and Graduate School of Biomedical Sciences, University of Texas Health Science Center at Houston, Houston, TX, USA

Patrick F. Connolly and Howard O. Fearnhead
Pharmacology and Therapeutics, National University of Ireland Galway, Galway, Ireland

Richard Jäger
Department of Natural Sciences, Bonn-Rhein-Sieg University of Applied Sciences, Rheinbach, Germany

Heather Manring and Noah Weisleder
Department of Physiology and Cell Biology, Davis Heart and Lung Research Institute, The Ohio State University Wexner Medical Center, Columbus, OH, USA

Eduardo Abreu and Leticia Brotto
Muscle Biology Research Group, School of Nursing and Health Studies, University of Missouri-Kansas City, Kansas City, MO, USA

Marco Brotto
Muscle Biology Research Group, School of Nursing and Health Studies, University of Missouri-Kansas City, Kansas City, MO, USA
Basic Medical Sciences Pharmacology, School of Medicine, University of Missouri-Kansas City, Kansas City, MO, USA
Basic Medical Sciences Pharmacology, School of Pharmacy, University of Missouri-Kansas City, Kansas City, MO, USA

Eric S. Folker
Department of Biology, Boston College, Chestnut Hill, MA, USA

Keith G. Avin
Department of Physical Medicine and Rehabilitation, University of Pittsburgh, Pittsburgh, PA, USA
Division of Geriatric Medicine, Department of Medicine, University of Pittsburgh, PA, USA

Paul M. Coen
Division of Endocrinology and Metabolism, Department of Medicine, University of Pittsburgh, Pittsburgh, PA, USA
Department of Health and Physical Education, University of Pittsburgh, Pittsburgh, PA, USA

Mary K. Baylies
Department of Development al Biology, Sloan-Kettering Institute, New York, NY, USA

Wan Huang and Gwendolyn A. Sowa
Department of Physical Medicine and Rehabilitation, University of Pittsburgh, Pittsburgh, PA, USA

Donna B. Stolz
Department of Cell Biology and Physiology, University of Pittsburgh, Pittsburgh, PA, USA

John J. Dubé, Bret H. Goodpaster and Robert M. O'Doherty
Division of Endocrinology and Metabolism, Department of Medicine, University of Pittsburgh, Pittsburgh, PA, USA

Fabrisia Ambrosio
Department of Physical Medicine and Rehabilitation, University of Pittsburgh, Pittsburgh, PA, USA
McGowan Institute for Regenerative Medicine, University of Pittsburgh, Pittsburgh, PA, USA

Sarah M. Senf
Department of Physical Therapy, University of Florida, Gainesville, FL, USA

Carmen Bertoni
Department of Neurology, David Geffen School of Medicine, University of California Los Angeles, CA, USA

Sunita Mathur and Dina Brooks
Department of Physical Therapy, University of Toronto, Toronto, ON, Canada

Celso R. F. Carvalho
Department of Physical Therapy, University of São Paulo, São Paulo, Brazil

Mirella Meregalli, Andrea Farini, Clementina Sitzia and Yvan Torrente
Stem Cell Laboratory, Dipartimento di Fisiopatologia Medico-Chirurgica e dei Trapianti, Centro Dino Ferrari, Fondazione IRCCS Ca' Granda Ospedale Maggiore Policlinico, Università degli Studi di Milano, Milano, Italy

Kathryn H. Myburgh
Muscle Research Group, Department of Physiological Sciences, Stellenbosch University, Stellenbosch, South Africa

Naomi E. Brooks
Health and Exercise Science Research Group, School of Sport, University of Stirling, Stirling, UK

Donna M. D'Souza, Dhuha Al-Sajee and Thomas J. Hawke
Department of Pathology and Molecular Medicine, McMaster University, Hamilton, ON, Canada

So-ichiro Fukada, Yuran Ma, Takuji Ohtani, Yoko Watanabe, Satoshi Murakami and Masahiko Yamaguchi
Laboratory of Molecular and Cellular Physiology, Graduate School of Pharmaceutical Sciences, Osaka University, Osaka, Japan

Leslie M. Baehr
Department of Physiology and Membrane Biology, University of California, Davis, Davis, CA, USA

Matthew Tunzi
Department of Neurobiology, Physiology, and Behavior, University of California, Davis, Davis, CA, USA

Sue C. Bodine
Department of Physiology and Membrane Biology, University of California, Davis, Davis, CA, USA
Department of Neurobiology, Physiology, and Behavior, University of California, Davis, Davis, CA, USA

Justin G. Boyer and Andrew Ferrier
Ottawa Hospital Research Institute, Regenerative Medicine Program, Ottawa, ON, Canada
Department of Cellular and Molecular Medicine, University of Ottawa, Ottawa, ON, Canada

Rashmi Kothary
Ottawa Hospital Research Institute, Regenerative Medicine Program, Ottawa, ON, Canada
Department of Cellular and Molecular Medicine, University of Ottawa, Ottawa, ON, Canada
Department of Medicine, University of Ottawa, Ottawa, ON, Canada

Jeffrey Kim , Morgan E. Carlson and Bruce A. Watkins
Center on Aging, University of Connecticut Health Center, Farmington, CT, USA

Akiyoshi Uezumi and Kunihiro Tsuchida
Division for Therapies against Intractable Diseases, Institute for Comprehensive Medical Science, Fujita Health University, Aichi, Japan

Madoka Ikemoto-Uezumi
Department of Regenerative Medicine, National Center for Geriatrics and Gerontology, National Institute for Longevity Sciences, Aichi, Japan

Emanuele Berardi
Translational Cardiomyology Laboratory, Department of Development and Reproduction, KUL University of Leuven, Leuven, Belgium
Interuniversity Institute of Myology, Italy

Daniela Annibali
Laboratory of Cell Metabolism and Proliferation, Vesalius Research Center, Vlaamse Institute voor Biotechnologie, Leuven, Belgium

Marco Cassano
Interuniversity Institute of Myology, Italy
School of Life Sciences, Ecole Polytechnique Fédérale de Lausanne, Lausanne, Switzerland

Stefania Crippa
Interuniversity Institute of Myology, Italy
Department of Medicine, University of Lausanne Medical School, Lausanne, Switzerland

Maurilio Sampaolesi
Translational Cardiomyology Laboratory, Department of Development and Reproduction, KUL University of Leuven, Leuven, Belgium
Interuniversity Institute of Myology, Italy
Division of Human Anatomy, Department of Public Health, Experimental and Forensic Medicine, University of Pavia, Pavia, Italy

M. Mamunur Rahman, Mallika Ghosh, Jiyeon K. Denninger, Kotaro Takeda, Guo-Hua Fong and Linda H. Shapiro
Center for Vascular Biology, University of Connecticut Health Center, Farmington, CT, USA

Jaganathan Subramani
Center for Vascular Biology, University of Connecticut Health Center, Farmington, CT, USA
Department of Anesthesiology, Texas Tech University Health Sciences Center, Lubbock, TX, USA

Morgan E. Carlson
Center on Aging, University of Connecticut Health Center, Farmington, CT, USA
Drug Discovery, Genomics Institute of the Novartis Research Foundation, San Diego, CA, USA

Chiara Donati, Francesca Cencetti and Paola Bruni
Dipartimento di Scienze Biomediche, Sperimentali e Cliniche, University of Florence, Florence, Italy
Istituto Interuniversitario di Miologia, Italy

René Koopman
Clinical Nutrition and Muscle and Exercise Metabolism Group, The University of Melbourne, Melbourne, VIC, Australia

C. Hai Ly and James G. Ryall
Stem Cell Metabolism and Regenerative Medicine Group, Basic and Clinical Myology Laboratory, Department of Physiology, The University of Melbourne, Melbourne, VIC, Australia

Index

A
Anabolism, 180, 223
Anti-inflammatory Drugs, 94, 181-182
Apoptotic Cells, 13-16, 18-21, 144

B
Basal Level, 14
Bone Morphogenetic Protein, 85, 133

C
Calcium Handling, 28, 32, 34, 190
Canonical Notch Signaling, 123, 130
Cardiovascular Diseases, 23, 45
Caspase Activation, 13-14, 18-22
Catabolism, 30-31, 180, 183, 204, 222
Cell Migration, 14-15, 18, 20-21, 41, 194, 202, 205, 207, 211-212
Cell-autonomous, 13-17, 19, 147, 149-150, 152
Cellular Mechanism, 25
Central Nervous System, 124, 145, 206
Centronuclear Myopathies, 25-26, 33
Chronic Inflammation, 5, 7, 81, 90, 181
Cytoskeleton, 18, 25, 35, 37-42, 44, 125, 129, 131, 197, 207, 211

D
Deconditioning, 76-77, 83
Diabetes Mellitus, 1, 9, 110-116
Distinct Mechanisms, 7, 40-41
Disuse Atrophy, 58, 77, 96-102, 104-108
Dystrophy, 4, 6, 10-11, 17, 20, 25, 28-33, 35-36, 42-44, 54, 57-59, 69-74, 84, 86, 91-95, 117, 124-132, 142, 147-148, 150, 152, 169, 173-174, 176, 178, 182-183, 187-190, 206, 213

F
Functional Overload, 89, 133-138, 140

G
Gastrocnemius Muscle, 3-4, 7, 108, 116, 200
Gene Correction, 59-61, 67, 71, 74
Gene Editing, 59-70, 72-73
Gene Regulation, 36-37, 39, 41-42, 107, 123
Gene Repair, 59, 61-64, 66, 68-73
Glioblastoma Cells, 14, 20

H
Heat Shock Proteins, 54, 58
Hematopoietic Stem Cells, 16, 92, 118, 123, 125, 130, 174, 202

I
Immobilization, 57, 88, 96-97, 99-108, 140
Immunofluorescent, 194, 196-198, 200
Insulin Sensitivity, 1, 8, 10, 154, 163, 167, 210
Intramuscular Injection, 2, 61, 192

L
Leptin Signaling, 2, 4, 6, 112
Lipids, 1-2, 8, 10-12, 30-31, 115, 156, 158-159, 161, 165-166
Lipotoxicity, 1-4, 9-11, 111
Lysophosphatidylcholine, 15, 21

M
Macrophages, 4-5, 8, 10, 16, 20, 22, 56, 78, 84, 87, 90-92, 94, 175, 178, 200, 218
Mesenchymal Stem Cells, 50, 71, 86, 88, 91-94, 174-177, 192-193, 196, 198, 202-203, 206-207, 211-212, 218
Metabolic Diseases, 110, 217
Metabolic Dysfunction, 2, 214
Metastasis, 14, 18, 20-21, 52
Microtubules, 37, 39-44, 105
Molecular Mechanisms, 31, 33, 42, 53, 101, 117, 124, 127, 149, 179-180, 205, 207, 222
Mouse Culture Systems, 40-41
Muscle Disorders, 24, 35-36, 59-61, 65, 68-69, 117-118, 124-127, 172
Muscle Dysfunction, 33, 54, 58, 76-77, 79-81
Muscle Fatigue, 23-24, 26, 28-32, 114, 209
Muscle Progenitor Cells, 2, 59-61, 67, 90, 95, 110, 131, 180, 189-190
Muscle Regeneration, 1-10, 12, 17-18, 23, 39, 43, 46, 49, 54, 56, 58, 70-72, 84, 87, 89-90, 92-93, 95, 101-102, 104-105, 107, 110-112, 114-118, 123-124, 128-132, 140, 152, 168-169, 172-173, 176-180, 184, 189-190, 198, 200-202, 204-212, 218, 221, 223
Muscle Satellite Cells, 6, 9, 11, 22, 73, 105, 107-110, 116, 118-119, 123, 125-132, 150, 175-178, 186-188, 190, 213, 222
Muscle Stem Cell, 8, 12, 51, 59, 94, 107, 109, 114-115, 117, 128-132, 152, 176, 187, 211-212, 214, 221
Muscular Disorders, 117, 125, 188
Muscular Dystrophies, 24-25, 44, 53, 57, 59, 61, 84, 119, 124, 127, 179, 181, 183, 187-188, 205, 214
Muscular Dystrophy, 6, 10-11, 17, 25, 28-29, 31-33, 35-36, 42-44, 54, 57-59, 69-74, 84, 91-95, 124-125, 127-132, 142, 147, 150, 152, 169, 174, 176, 178, 182-183, 187-190, 213
Musculoskeletal Disorders, 23, 26, 59, 180
Myoblasts, 3-8, 10-13, 16, 18, 36-37, 40, 61, 63-64, 67, 69, 72, 89-94, 99, 102, 106, 111, 113, 118-129, 131, 142, 146-147, 152, 154-156, 158-161, 163-166, 170, 177, 179, 184-189, 204, 207-213

Myodomains, 36, 40

Myofibers, 1-6, 10, 25, 35-37, 50-51, 55-57, 59, 63, 68, 86-87, 89-91, 100, 106, 108, 116-118, 120-121, 123-127, 130, 138, 142-145, 147-149, 156, 168-169, 171-174, 180-181, 184, 191, 198, 204, 217-218

Myogenic Memory, 126, 128, 185

Myostatin, 2, 5, 8-11, 79, 81-82, 87, 89-96, 100-109, 115, 126, 139-140, 144-145, 151-152, 174, 177-179, 183, 185-187, 189-190

Myostatin Gene Expression, 102-103, 140

Myotube Formation, 3-4, 7, 43, 125

N

Neutralization, 182, 209

Nuclear Movement, 35-43

O

Obesity, 1-3, 5-12, 58, 111, 114, 116, 155, 164-166, 169, 176, 213-214, 216-217, 221

Oligodeoxynucleotides, 59-60, 71

P

Pathological Conditions, 84, 168, 208

Pharmacological Inhibition, 16, 18, 208

Protein Balance, 76, 79, 218

Protein Degradation, 4, 32, 53, 79, 111, 115, 133, 136, 138, 209, 216

Protein Synthesis, 6-9, 11, 25, 30-32, 79, 84, 98, 102-103, 105-107, 133-140, 146, 209, 216-218, 221-223

Proteolysis, 24, 80, 101-102, 115, 136, 138-140, 180, 183, 190, 214

R

Regeneration, 1-12, 15-18, 20-23, 39, 43, 45-46, 49-51, 54-58, 68, 70-72, 79, 84, 87-90, 92-95, 100-102, 104-105, 107, 110-112, 114-118, 120, 123-125, 127-132, 140, 151-152, 168-169, 172-173, 176-180, 184, 187, 189-190, 192, 194, 198, 200-202, 204-212, 214, 218, 221, 223

Renal Fibrosis, 50, 52

S

Sarcopenia, 17, 23-24, 26-27, 29, 31-33, 45, 47, 49, 54, 113, 125-129, 131, 179-180, 182-183, 189, 214, 216-217

Satellite Cell Activation, 2, 4, 10, 56, 92-93, 105, 107-108, 128, 146, 190, 206-207, 210, 212-213, 223

Satellite Cells, 1-12, 17-18, 20, 22, 24, 36, 44, 59, 70, 73-74, 82, 84, 86-87, 89-90, 93, 95-97, 99-100, 105-111, 113-132, 143-144, 150-152, 164, 168-173, 175-184, 186-190, 204-207, 210-214, 222-223

Signal Transduction, 8-9, 13, 16, 25, 163, 166, 197, 201, 218

Skeletal Muscle, 1-13, 15, 21, 23-24, 26-35, 43-58, 69-74, 76-78, 80-87, 89-122, 124-133, 138-144, 146-152, 154-156, 162-174, 176-180, 183-190, 200, 202-218, 220-223

Skeletal Muscle Health, 29, 51, 97, 103, 110-113

Skeletal Muscle Regeneration, 1-4, 6-7, 10, 12, 49, 92-93, 102, 107, 115-118, 124, 128, 130-132, 152, 177, 179, 184, 189, 204-206, 209, 212, 218, 221, 223

Synaptophysin, 28-29, 33

T

Transgenic Mice, 3-4, 10, 22, 57, 102, 107, 129, 145, 148, 150, 152, 174, 185, 210

Translocation, 7, 40, 68, 102, 105, 132, 148, 152, 165

www.ingramcontent.com/pod-product-compliance
Lightning Source LLC
LaVergne TN
LVHW082212200926
848484LV00008B/2243
* 9 7 9 8 8 8 7 4 0 4 2 2 6 *